全国高等中医药院校中药学类专业双语规划教材
Bilingual Planned Textbooks for Chinese Materia Medica Majors in TCM Colleges and Universities

中药化学

Chemistry of Chinese Materia Medica

（供中药学类及相关专业使用）

(For Chinese Materia Medica and other related majors)

主　编　高增平　吴锦忠

主　审　魏　鑫（Sarepta Therapeutics Inc. USA）

　　　　彭江南（Morgan State University, USA）

副主编　曲　扬　马　涛　何细新　李　斌

编　者　（以姓氏笔画为序）

马　涛（北京中医药大学）　　　王　薇（陕西中医药大学）

王继彦（长春中医药大学）　　　曲　扬（辽宁中医药大学）

刘艾娟（北京中医药大学）　　　李　斌（江西中医药大学）

吴　霞（首都医科大学）　　　　吴锦忠（福建中医药大学）

何永志（天津中医药大学）　　　何细新（广州中医药大学）

辛　萍（哈尔滨医科大学）　　　张　薇（北京中医药大学）

邵　晶（甘肃中医药大学）　　　柴慧芳（贵州中医药大学）

高增平（北京中医药大学）　　　潘晓丽（成都中医药大学）

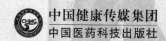

中国健康传媒集团

中国医药科技出版社

内 容 提 要

　　本教材是"全国高等中医药院校中药学类专业双语规划教材"之一，根据教育部相关文件精神和中药学类专业教学大纲基本要求，结合现行版《中国药典》和国家执业药师资格考试大纲要求编写而成，内容涵盖中药所含主要类型化学成分的结构特点、理化性质、提取分离、检识和结构鉴定等基本知识，同时还介绍了 30 味常用中药主要有效成分的结构特点、提取分离检识方法及质量控制标准等。

　　本教材正文部分采用以英文为主、专业词汇括号内中文标注的方式，具有便于通读、易于读懂的特点。在每章开头有"学习目标"中文版块，利于读者了解本章将要学习内容的重点；在每章结尾有"词汇表""重点小结"和"目标检测"中文版块，利于读者更好地掌握本章的重要知识点，并对学习效果进行自行检测，因此本教材具有方便学习、易于掌握重点知识、可自行检测学习效果等实用性强的特点。本教材为书网融合教材，即纸质教材有机融合电子教材、教学配套资源和数字化教学服务（在线教学、在线作业、在线考试）。

　　本教材可作为全国中医药院校中药学、中药资源学、中药制剂学、临床中药学、中药制药工程等相关专业的本科双语教学、留学生和研究生教学用书，也可作为中医药行业考试与培训及广大中医药工作者参考用书。

图书在版编目（CIP）数据

中药化学：汉英对照 / 高增平，吴锦忠主编 . —北京：中国医药科技出版社，2020.8

全国高等中医药院校中药学类专业双语规划教材

ISBN 978-7-5214-1869-9

Ⅰ.①中… Ⅱ.①高… ②吴… Ⅲ.①中药化学 – 双语教学 – 中医学院 – 教材 – 汉、英 Ⅳ.①R284

中国版本图书馆 CIP 数据核字（2020）第 097406 号

美术编辑 陈君杞

版式设计 辰轩文化

出版 **中国健康传媒集团** | 中国医药科技出版社

地址 北京市海淀区文慧园北路甲 22 号

邮编 100082

电话 发行：010-62227427 邮购：010-62236938

网址 www.cmstp.com

规格 889 × 1194 mm $\frac{1}{16}$

印张 29

字数 743 千字

版次 2020 年 8 月第 1 版

印次 2020 年 8 月第 1 次印刷

印刷 三河市万龙印装有限公司

经销 全国各地新华书店

书号 ISBN 978-7-5214-1869-9

定价 **89.00** 元

获取新书信息、投稿、为图书纠错，请扫码联系我们。

近些年随着世界范围的中医药热潮的涌动，来中国学习中医药学的留学生逐年增多，走出国门的中医药学人才也在增加。为了适应中医药国际交流与合作的需要，加快中医药国际化进程，提高来中国留学生和国际班学生的教学质量，满足双语教学的需要和中医药对外交流需求，培养优秀的国际化中医药人才，进一步推动中医药国际化进程，根据教育部、国家中医药管理局、国家药品监督管理局等部门的有关精神，在本套教材建设指导委员会主任委员成都中医药大学彭成教授等专家的指导和顶层设计下，中国医药科技出版社组织全国50余所高等中医药院校及附属医疗机构约420名专家、教师精心编撰了全国高等中医药院校中药学类专业双语规划教材，该套教材即将付梓出版。

本套教材共计23门，主要供全国高等中医药院校中药学类专业教学使用。本套教材定位清晰、特色鲜明，主要体现在以下方面。

一、立足双语教学实际，培养复合应用型人才

本套教材以高校双语教学课程建设要求为依据，以满足国内医药院校开展留学生教学和双语教学的需求为目标，突出中医药文化特色鲜明、中医药专业术语规范的特点，注重培养中医药技能、反映中医药传承和现代研究成果，旨在优化教育质量，培养优秀的国际化中医药人才，推进中医药对外交流。

本套教材建设围绕目前中医药院校本科教育教学改革方向对教材体系进行科学规划、合理设计，坚持以培养创新型和复合型人才为宗旨，以社会需求为导向，以培养适应中药开发、利用、管理、服务等各个领域需求的高素质应用型人才为目标的教材建设思路与原则。

二、遵循教材编写规律，整体优化，紧跟学科发展步伐

本套教材的编写遵循"三基、五性、三特定"的教材编写规律；以"必需、够用"为度；坚持与时俱进，注意吸收新技术和新方法，适当拓展知识面，为学生后续发展奠定必要的基础。实验教材密切结合主干教材内容，体现理实一体，注重培养学生实践技能训练的同时，按照教育部相关精神，增加设计性实验部分，以现实问题作为驱动力来培养学生自主获取和应用新知识的能力，从而培养学生独立思考能力、实验设计能力、实践操作能力和可持续发展能力，满足培养应用型和复合型人才的要求。强调全套教材内容的整体优化，并注重不同教材内容的联系与衔接，避免遗漏和不必要的交叉重复。

三、对接职业资格考试，"教考""理实"密切融合

本套教材的内容和结构设计紧密对接国家执业中药师职业资格考试大纲要求，实现教学与考试、理论与实践的密切融合，并且在教材编写过程中，吸收具有丰富实践经验的企业人员参与教材的编写，确保教材的内容密切结合应用，更加体现高等教育的实践性和开放性，为学生参加考试和实践工作打下坚实基础。

四、创新教材呈现形式，书网融合，使教与学更便捷更轻松

全套教材为书网融合教材，即纸质教材与数字教材、配套教学资源、题库系统、数字化教学服务有机融合。通过"一书一码"的强关联，为读者提供全免费增值服务。按教材封底的提示激活教材后，读者可通过 PC、手机阅读电子教材和配套课程资源（PPT、微课、视频等），并可在线进行同步练习，实时收到答案反馈和解析。同时，读者也可以直接扫描书中二维码，阅读与教材内容关联的课程资源，从而丰富学习体验，使学习更便捷。教师可通过 PC 在线创建课程，与学生互动，开展在线课程内容定制、布置和批改作业、在线组织考试、讨论与答疑等教学活动，学生通过 PC、手机均可实现在线作业、在线考试，提升学习效率，使教与学更轻松。此外，平台尚有数据分析、教学诊断等功能，可为教学研究与管理提供技术和数据支撑。需要特殊说明的是，有些专业基础课程，例如《药理学》等9种教材，起源于西方医学，因篇幅所限，在本次双语教材建设中纸质教材以英语为主，仅将专业词汇对照了中文翻译，同时在中国医药科技出版社数字平台"医药大学堂"上配套了中文电子教材供学生学习参考。

编写出版本套高质量教材，得到了全国知名专家的精心指导和各有关院校领导与编者的大力支持，在此一并表示衷心感谢。希望广大师生在教学中积极使用本套教材和提出宝贵意见，以便修订完善，共同打造精品教材，为促进我国高等中医药院校中药学类专业教育教学改革和人才培养做出积极贡献。

全国高等中医药院校中药学类专业双语规划教材
建设指导委员会

数字化教材编委会

主　编　高增平　吴锦忠

主　审　魏　鑫（Sarepta Therapeutics Inc. USA）

　　　　彭江南（Morgan State University, USA）

副主编　曲　扬　马　涛　何细新　李　斌

编　者　（以姓氏笔画为序）

马　涛（北京中医药大学）　　　王　薇（陕西中医药大学）

王继彦（长春中医药大学）　　　曲　扬（辽宁中医药大学）

刘艾娟（北京中医药大学）　　　李　斌（江西中医药大学）

吴　霞（首都医科大学）　　　　吴锦忠（福建中医药大学）

何永志（天津中医药大学）　　　何细新（广州中医药大学）

辛　萍（哈尔滨医科大学）　　　张　薇（北京中医药大学）

邵　晶（甘肃中医药大学）　　　柴慧芳（贵州中医药大学）

高增平（北京中医药大学）　　　潘晓丽（成都中医药大学）

前　言

　　中药化学是在中医药基本理论和临床用药经验指导下，运用现代科学理论和技术研究中药化学成分的一门学科。中医临床预防和治疗疾病的物质基础是中药化学成分，中药化学成分贯穿中药质量形成全过程，因此中药化学既是中药学相关专业的专业基础课程，又是专业课程，对指导中药材生产过程、中药资源开发利用、中药品质评价、中药新药研发、中药质量控制、中药临床应用等具有重要意义。

　　本教材是根据中药学类专业本科中药化学教学大纲的基本要求，结合现行版《中国药典》和国家执业药师职业资格考试大纲要求编写而成，全书共十二章。第一章绪论，介绍中药化学的基本概念、内容、应用及研究进展；第二章介绍中药化学成分的生物合成途径、分类及提取分离和结构鉴定方法；第三章至第十二章分别介绍中药所含主要类型化学成分的结构特征、理化性质、提取分离方法、检识方法、结构鉴定及30味中药实例，每一味中药实例包括来源、性味归经、功能主治、药理活性，主要有效成分，以及该药味的主要质量控制指标。既包含主要类型化学成分的基本理论知识，又以常用中药作为实际应用的例子，且融入了本学科研究的最新成果，使教材内容更加丰富。

　　本教材正文部分采用以英文为主、专业词汇括号内中文标注的方式编写，具有便于通读、易于读懂的特点。在英文部分，坚持语句语法简单化、专业词汇规范化的编写原则，逐句逐词斟酌，以利于教师准确施教，便于学生易学易懂，为本学科的英文科技论文阅读和写作能力的培养奠定基础。在每一章的开头都设计有"学习目标"中文版块，利于读者了解本章将要学习内容的重点；在每一章的结尾都设计有"词汇表""重点小结"和"目标检测"中文版块，在全书最后为读者提供了目标检测题目的答案。引导读者掌握重点，融会贯通，并对学习效果进行自我检测。另外在全书最后还特别设计了"岗位对接"中文版块，根据国家对中药执业药师考试大纲的要求，详细介绍执业中药师岗位需要重点掌握的中药化学相关知识。因此本教材具有方便学习、易于掌握重点知识、可自行检测学习效果等实用性强的特点。本教材为书网融合教材，即纸质教材有机融合电子教材、教学配套资源和数字化教学服务（在线教学、在线作业、在线考试）。

　　本教材编写分工如下：高增平（第一章，修稿、统稿）；李斌（第二章）；吴锦忠（第三章）；曲扬和何永志（第四章）；邵晶（第五章）；何细新（第六章）；王薇（第七章）；吴霞和张薇（第八章）；曲扬（第九章）；潘晓丽和辛萍（第十章）；马涛和王继彦（第十一章）；柴慧芳（第十二章）；张薇和刘艾娟（词汇表、英文语法）。美国 Sarepta Therapeutics Inc. 药事总监魏鑫女士和美国 Morgan State University 彭江南教授对本教材稿件进行了全面审阅。

1

本教材可作为全国中医药院校中药学、中药资源学、中药制剂学、临床中药学、中药制药工程及相关专业的本科双语教学、留学生和研究生教学用书，也可作为中医药行业考试与培训及广大中医药工作者参考用书。

　　在教材编写过程中，参考、引用了大量文献资料，因篇幅有限仅将主要参考书籍列在全书末尾，参加编写院校的领导和众多专家及同行都给予了热情的鼓励与支持，提出了很多宝贵意见和建议，在此一并表示衷心感谢！

　　教材编写立足"精品"，层层严格把关，但受编者水平所限，难免有不妥之处，希望广大师生和读者提出宝贵意见，以便日后再版时予以完善，使教材质量进一步提升。

编　者

2020 年 3 月

Chemistry of Chinese Materia Medica (CCMM) is a science that studies the chemical constituents of Chinese materia medica, by using physical, chemical and other modern scientific technologies, under the guidance of the basic theories and clinical experiences of Chinese medicine. CCMM offers professional training of principles and procedures of crude drug processing, developing new drugs or new applications of Chinese materia medica, quality assessment and control of Chinese materia medica, and clinical usage of Chinese materia medica. CCMM can also be taken as a basic class by students of other professions that relate to Chinese Materia Medica.

This textbook is compiled according to the basic requirements of the teaching syllabus of CCMM for undergraduate students majoring in Chinese Materia Medica, Chinese Pharmacopeia (current edition) and the syllabus of national licensed pharmacist qualification examination. There are 12 chapters in this textbook. Chapter 1 is the general introduction to CCMM, including the conceptions, contents, application and progress. Chapter 2 is general methods for chemical investigation of Chinese herbs, which mainly introduces the biosynthetic pathways, classification, extraction, isolation and structure determination of chemical constituents in Chinese herbs. Chapter 3–12 provide the structure characteristics, physicochemical properties, methods for extraction, isolation, identification, structure determination of main types of chemical constituents from Chinese herbs and 30 Chinese herbs are given as examples. The contents of each Chinese herb are introduced, including Biological Source, Property, Flavor, Channels Entered, Actions & Indications, Pharmacological Activities, Main Effective Chemical Constituents and Quality Control Standards. This textbook not only introduces the fundamental knowledge of main types of chemical constituents, also gives generally used Chinese herb as application example. Moreover, the contents of this textbook are enriched by some new progress in CCMM.

The body part of this textbook is mainly written in English, professional vocabulary being marked with Chinese translation in brackets. It is easy to read and understand. In the English part, the principles of sentence grammar simplification and professional vocabulary standardization are preferred. And it is carefully reviewed sentence by sentence and word by word, so as to help teachers teach accurately and students understand easily and establish foundation for training in English paper reading and writing skills. Each chapter starts with the module of "Learning Objective" in Chinese, which is helpful for readers to understand the key points of the chapter, and ends with the modules of both "Key Summary" and "Target Detection" in Chinese, and the answers are given in the end of this textbook, which can lead readers to grasp the key contents, understand thoroughly and carry out self-test for the relevant knowledge of this chapter. The module of "Post Docking" in Chinese is designed to introduce the required key knowledge of CCMM in the syllabus of national licensed Chinese pharmacist qualification examination. Therefore, this textbook with features of strong practicability is convenient to learn and easy to master key knowledge, and learning effect can be evaluated by self-test. In addition, this textbook is also equipped with digital teaching resources such as courseware and exercise test bank. Students can read the corresponding resources by scanning the two-dimensional code on the paper version of the textbook through their mobile phones, which makes the teaching resources more diversified and multi-dimensional, and realizes the interactive mode of "Book-Mobile terminal-Internet".

The comprehensive work of this textbook has called for collaborative effort of specialists from 13 universities of Chinese medicine in China and oversea experts. Gao Zengping (chapter 1, revise and draft text), Li Bin (chapter 2), Wu Jinzhong (chapter 3), Qu Yang and He Yongzhi (chapter 4), Shao Jing (chapter 5), He Xixin (chapter 6), Wang Wei (chapter 7), Wu Xia and Zhang Wei (chapter 8), Qu Yang (chapter 9), Pan Xiaoli and Xin Ping (chapter 10), Ma Tao and Wang Jiyan (chapter 11), Chai Huifang (chapter 12), Zhang Wei and Liu Aijuan (glossary, English grammar). Wei Xin (Director of Regulatory Affairs at Sarepta Therapeutics Inc. USA) and Peng Jiangnan (Assistant Professor at Morgan State University, USA) as reviewer.

This textbook can be used as the bilingual teaching textbook for undergraduate students, international students and graduate students majoring in Chinese Materia Medica, resource sciences of Chinese materia medica, pharmaceutics of Chinese materia medica, clinical Chinese materia medica, pharmaceutical engineering of Chinese materia medica and other related fields. It can also be a reference book for the examination and training of Chinese materia medica industry and researchers in Chinese materia medica.

In the process of compiling the textbook, a large number of literature materials are referenced. Due to the limited space, only the main reference materials are listed at the end of textbook. All the leaders, experts and peers participating in the compilation of this textbook provide warm encouragement and support and put forward valuable opinions and suggestions, which are highly appreciated by all editors.

The compilation of the textbook is based on the standard of "High-quality Textbook". It is strictly controlled from the aspects of compilation, review, editing and publishing. We hope that the teachers, students and readers would give criticism and correction so as to improve the quality of this textbook when it is republished in the future.

Editors

March, 2020

2

Contents

Chapter 1 General Introduction to Chemistry of Chinese Materia Medica

 学习目标

知识要求：
1. **掌握** 中药化学的含义及主要研究内容。
2. **熟悉** 中药化学的应用。
3. **了解** 中药化学的研究进展。

能力要求：

学会从理论基础、研究对象、研究内容、研究方法等方面分析中药化学与相近学科的异同，从而更好地理解中药化学的含义；理解中药化学知识在表征中药药性理论内涵、阐明中药有效物质基础及研发中药新药等方面的应用。

1 Conception of Chemistry of Chinese Materia Medica

Chemistry of Chinese Materia Medica (中药化学) may be defined as a science that studies the chemical constituents (化学成分) of Chinese materia medica (中药), by using physical, chemical and other modern scientific technologies, under the guidance of the basic theories and clinical experiences of Chinese medicine. It encompasses the knowledge of structural characteristics, physical and chemical properties, the methods of extraction (提取), isolation (分离), identification (检识) and structure (结构) determination of chemical constituents in Chinese materia medica. It also explores the biosynthesis (生合成), structure modification and structure-activity relationship (构效关系) of chemical constituents in Chinese materia medica.

The sources of Chinese materia medica include plants, animals and minerals but most of them are of plant origin. Therefore, Chinese materia medica is generally called Chinese herbal medicine or Chinese herb.

In general, every Chinese herb is a complex system that contains numerous natural compounds in a not well characterized matrix. The focus of Chemistry of Chinese Materia Medica is the effective constituents (有效成分), which are supposed to be responsible for the efficacy of the Chinese herb. In contrast, those compounds that are not responsible for the efficacy of the Chinese herb are called ineffective constituents

(无效成分). Actually, some known ineffective constituents [e.g. proteins (蛋白质), polysaccharides (多糖)] in the past have nowadays been proven to be effective. Therefore, effective or ineffective is not absolute. The effectiveness of a constituent depends on the herb in which the constituent presented and the development of sciences and technologies. With the remarkable development in the areas of separation (分离) science, spectroscopic (光谱的) technology and various available hyphenated (联用的) techniques, e.g. GC-MS, LC-MS, LC-NMR, LC-NMR-MS, CE-MS, more and more effective compounds have been isolated from or detected in Chinese herbs.

In general, each Chinese herb contains many effective constituents. These effective constituents may have similar structures, but sometimes their structures may be completely different. Maybe this is a plausible explanation of the multi-target therapy of Chinese herbs. The fraction containing a major effective constituent or a group of effective constituents with similar structures is called effective fraction (有效部位). For example, Notoginseng Total Saponins (三七总皂苷) from Notoginseng Radix et Rhizoma (三七) are a group of effective constituents with similar structures, Scutellaria Extract (黄芩提取物) from Scutellariae Radix (黄芩) is an effective fraction containing a major effective constituent, baicalin (黄芩苷).

All the phytochemical investigation and pharmacological screening of chemical constituents of Chinese herbs should be guided by the basic theories of Chinese medicine and centered on the clinical effects of this Chinese herb. For this reason, the Chemistry of Chinese Materia Medica is different from Phytochemistry (植物化学), Natural Products Chemistry (天然产物化学) or Natural Medicinal Chemistry (天然药物化学). Systematic TCM theories and rich clinical experiences provide directions in bioassay of Chinese herbs. Chinese medicine views the human body as an integrated organism, all organs and tissues working together. The same theory applies to Chinese herbs.

In general, an isolated single compound from a Chinese herb cannot represent the entire effect of the herb, many compounds in the herb working together to cure disease. All the effective constituents presented in a Chinese herb are called effective composition (有效物质基础) of this herb. Therefore, the purpose of the Chemistry of Chinese Materia Medica is to clarify the effective composition of the Chinese herb and reveal the relationship between the composition and the efficacy or nature of the herb.

Every Chinese herb has its own property (including cold, hot, warm and cool), flavor (including sour, bitter, sweet, pungent, salty, etc.) and channels entered (including Heart, Liver, Spleen, Lung, Kidney, Stomach, Gallbladder, Large intestine, Small intestine, etc.). All these correspond to the herb's effective composition and lay the foundation for its use in Chinese medicine. This is distinctly different from Phytochemistry, Natural Products Chemistry and Natural Medicinal Chemistry where no property, flavor, or channels are applied, and all the compounds from plants, natural sources, or natural drugs are studied as independent single compound. In the meantime, the Chemistry of Chinese Materia Medica and Phytochemistry, Natural Products Chemistry, Natural Medicinal Chemistry also have many similarities as they all use the same modern sciences and technologies (e.g. separation and spectroscopic technologies, etc.) for isolation, structure determination and modification, etc.

2　Application of Chemistry of Chinese Materia Medica

2.1　To Clarify the Effective Composition of Chinese Herbs

The core research objective of Chemistry of Chinese Materia Medica is phytochemical investigation of Chinese herbs. Many Chinese herbs have been studied of their chemical constituents and pharmacological activities. For example, many alkaloids including ephedrine (麻黄碱), pseudoephedrine (伪麻黄碱) and norephedrine (去甲基麻黄碱), etc. have been identified in Ephedrae Herba (麻黄) as effective constituents. However, the effective composition is not clear in many Chinese herbs and it seems to be impossible to know all the effective constituents in a Chinese herb. Therefore, exploration of the effective composition of Chinese herbs is still a central focus for Chemistry of Chinese Materia Medica.

The property and flavor of a Chinese herb is rooted in its effective composition. Different property (i.e. Hot, Cold, Warm, Cool, or Neutral) and flavor (i.e. Sour, Bitter, Sweet, Pungent, or Salty) are expected to correspond to different effective compositions. Each Chinese herb has its own effective composition responsible for its effectiveness and nature. Therefore, the study of Chemistry of Chinese Materia Medica will be helpful in clarifying the essence of basic theory in Chinese medicine.

We can understand the processing (炮制) mechanisms through effective constituent investigation. For example, vinegar-frying (醋炙) can increase the effect of Corydalis Rhizoma (延胡索) in relieving pain. After effective constituent investigation of Corydalis Rhizoma, we know that the alkaloids (生物碱) in Corydalis Rhizoma are major effective constituents and can form salts with vinegar in processing to improve the solubility of alkaloids in water. Some active compounds of Chinese herbs are both effective and toxic. The key factor is the quantity of the herb in a formula, therefore, proper dosage is very important. If the active/toxic compound is known, controlling the dosage (剂量) should be easy. For example, the raw Aconiti Radix (川乌) is too toxic to use, but the processed slices, Aconiti Radix Cocta (制川乌), can be used in clinic. Because the aconitine (乌头碱), hypaconitine (海帕乌头碱) and mesaconitine (美沙乌头碱) are major active/toxic compounds of Aconiti Radix, their structures contain ester bonds (酯键), which can be hydrolyzed (水解) in processing, so the content of these constituents can be controlled by standardizing the processing procedure. Therefore, the study of Chemistry of Chinese Materia Medica not only can make us understand the processing mechanism better, but also can guide us to make a reasonable processing procedure to ensure the efficacy and prevent toxication (中毒) of Chinese herbs.

Most of Chinese herbs are combined with others to form a multi-herb formula (复方) used in clinic to increase therapeutic effectiveness, to minimize the toxicity or side effects, to fit for the complex clinical situations, etc. When several herbs are combined together, their effective constituents are mixed and various reactions may occur. If the effective constituents of Chinese herbs are clearly identified, we may be able to intentionally enhance the beneficial reactions and reduce or prevent the harmful reactions. For example, baicalin, the effective constituent of Scutellariae Radix can be precipitated (沉淀) by berberine (小檗碱), the effective constituent of Coptidis Rhizoma (黄连) in water. So when they appear in a multi-herb formula together, they should be extracted with ethanol instead of water to avoid the combination of baicalin and berberine to form precipitate. Therefore, the study of Chemistry of Chinese Materia Medica can guide us in choosing suitable procedures for the preparation of multi-herb formulas.

It is interesting that a new publication reveals: the precipitate of baicalin (BA) and berberine (BBR), named natural self-assembled (自组装) BA-BBR nanoparticles (NPs), showed significant improvement of antibacterial and biofilm removal ability. This research strategy offers a reference for discovery of the principles of multi-herb formulas.

To sum up, although many researches reveal new discoveries of phytochemical investigations of Chinese herbs every year, the exact effective compositions of many Chinese herbs are yet to be explored.

2.2　To Facilitate the Development of New Chinese Patent Medicine

The study of Chemistry of Chinese Materia Medica can help enlarge the source of Chinese herbs or explore new source. For example, Ginseng Radix et Rhizoma (人参) is the dried root and rhizome of *Panax ginseng* C. A. Mey. Nowadays, the leaves of *Panax ginseng* C. A. Mey. also have become a Chinese herb, Ginseng Folium (人参叶), after comprehensive research on chemical constituents, pharmacological activities, toxicity and so on. Another example is Bovis Calculus (牛黄). It is the dried natural gallstone (胆结石) of *Bos taurus domesticus* Gmelin and its source is very rare and expensive. Bovis Calculus Artifactus (人工牛黄) is developed based on the understanding of Bovis Calculus's chemistry, pharmacology and biology through the application of Chemistry of Chinese Materia Medica and other disciplines.

The study of Chemistry of Chinese Herbs can provide high quality products (e.g. effective constituent, effective fraction) by using advanced isolation and purification techniques to produce modern preparations (制剂) such as injection (注射剂), tablet (片剂), aerosol (喷雾剂), granule (颗粒剂), capsule (胶囊剂), etc. More and more innovative medicines have been developed by using the knowledge of Chemistry of Chinese Materia Medica and other related subjects.

Quality is critical for the efficacy of Chinese herbs. Understanding of the chemical constituents in Chinese herbs is essential to control the quality of Chinese herbs. Chemistry of Chinese Materia Medica can provide the knowledge for investigating the chemical constituents of Chinese herbs and preparing reference substances for qualitative (定性的) and quantitative (定量的) analysis (分析) during setting up a quality control standard. The advancement of quality standards [including quantitative analysis standards and fingerprinting (指纹图谱) chromatography (色谱) standards, etc.] establishment in Chinese Pharmacopoeia (药典) [including crude drugs (药材), extracts (提取物), and preparations] is attributable to the Chemistry of Chinese Materia Medica.

All in all, the knowledge of Chemistry of Chinese Materia Medica applied in the whole process of Chinese medicinal industry from the source of Chinese herbs to the final products—new Chinese patent medicines (中成药).

2.3　To Benefit Other Related Subjects of Chinese Medicine

Chemistry of Chinese Materia Medica is not isolated. It has a close relationship with other subjects such as the Identification of Chinese Materia Medica (中药鉴定学), Processing of Chinese Materia Medica (中药炮制学), Pharmaceutics of Chinese Materia Medica (中药药剂学), Pharmacology of Chinese Materia Medica (中药药理学), etc. Chemistry of Chinese Materia Medica offers knowledge or tools for the following:

- Physical and chemical identification of Chinese herbs.
- Supporting the development of optimal processing conditions in order to have a better understanding in the mechanisms of processing.
- Supporting determination of suitable dosage forms.
- Developing suitable conditions for sample storage and manipulation.

In summary, Chemistry of Chinese Materia Medica is an important bridge between pharmaceutical and basic sciences. It plays a vital role in the field of Chinese medicine.

3   Progress of Chemistry of Chinese Materia Medica

3.1   Development in Effective Composition of Chinese Herbs

Although the complex multi-constituents of Chinese herbs make the study on effective composition of an herb or a multi-herb formula a challenge, some progress had been made in identifying chemical constituents responsible for the property and flavor of Chinese herbs. For example, most herbs with hot property contain volatile oils and alkaloids. The contents of amino acids, saccharides, Mn, Cu, Na and K in these herbs tend to be higher than that in herbs with cold property. In contrast, most cold property herbs contain saponins, and the quantity of Fe and Ca in these herbs tend to be higher than that in hot property herbs. Herbs with pungent flavor usually contain volatile oils, saponins and alkaloids. Sour flavored herbs mostly contain tannins and organic acids. Sweet flavored herbs mostly contain glycosides, proteins and saccharides. Bitter flavored herbs mostly contain alkaloids and glycosides. Therefore, the chemical structure and quantity of various constituents in Chinese herbs are closely related to their property and flavor. For better understanding the basic theory of Chinese Medicine, the relationship between the effective composition and the nature of the herb should be explored further.

In recent years, new theories and research methods have emerged and some valuable results have yielded.

A new theory regarding the nature of Chinese herb is that the flavors and properties of an herb can be split and combined. For example, the effective constituents and pharmacological activities of Evodiae Fructus (吴茱萸) have been investigated according to this new theory. The results have shown that the bitter constituents of Evodiae Fructus can stop vomiting and diarrhea, including alkaloids fraction 2, lactones, flavonoids, and so on; while the pungent constituents have anti-inflammatory activity and analgesic abilities, including alkaloids fraction 1, volatile oil, and so on. These results are consistent with the well-accepted effects of bitter and pungent flavors in theory of Chinese Medicine. Therefore, this demonstrates that the properties and flavors of Chinese herbs have corresponding effective chemical constituents. It is possible to split or combine these constituents to produce different effects that may be never recorded in Classics of Traditional Chinese Medicine.

It is noteworthy that a new strategy has been explored for paired-medicinein Chinese medicine. Scutellariae Radix-Coptidis Rhizoma is a paired-medicine which has been used for thousands of years

5

to effectively regulate intestinal flora and treat intestinal infection in clinics of China. Authors of this research choose the effective constituents, baicalin (BA) and berberin (BBR), from the two herbs to prepare natural self-assembled nanostructures and obtained BA-BBR nanoparticles (NPs). The research result showed that BA-BBR NPs has significant improvement of antibacterial and biofilm removal ability. This self-assembly strategy provides a new way of discovering the optimal unmodified combination of known effective constituents from Chinese herbs.

A three-element mathematical analysis model has been proposed to study the cold and hot property of Chinese herbs to elucidate the biological differences these properties may exert. The three elements are effective constituents, body-condition and biological response. This research model has the potential to explain the differences between hot and cold propertied herbs, and may stimulate new ideas for the study of the theory of Chinese Medicine.

Based on Chinese Medicine, every herb enters human body via its specific channel(s) to exert effect. The relationship between the distribution of effective constituents and the channels entered of a herb has been investigated by examining the metabolites of experimental animals. Metabonomics (代谢组学) and pharmacokinetics (药代动力学) play an important role in this setting.

Online analysis methods including bio-chromatography, liposome equilibrium dialysis (脂质体平衡透析), cell solid phase extraction, micro-dialysis (微透析) sampling coupled with HPLC or LC-MS, etc., are powerful tools for screening of the effective constituents of Chinese herbs.

3.2　Development in New Drug Research and Pharmaceutical Industry

Chemistry of Chinese Materia Medica supports new drug development from initial identification and isolation of effective constitutes or fractions to final scale-up production in pharmaceutical industry. Recently several new preparations produced from effective fractions of Chinese herbs were approved by China Food and Drug Administration (CFDA) for manufacturing.

Chemistry of Chinese Materia Medica plays an important role in developing resources of Chinese herbs. Some non-medicinal portions (非药用部位) of Chinese herbs in the past have been developed into medicinal portions by studying the effective constituents of the new portions. For example, the leaves, non-medicinal portion, of *Eucommia ulmoides* Oliv. and *Ginkgo biloba* L. in the past have become the resources of new Chinese herbs Eucommiae Folium (杜仲叶) and Ginkgo Folium (银杏叶) after a comprehensive research on chemical constituents, pharmacological activity and safty, etc. With technologies advance, more and more effective constituents have been isolated from Chinese herbs and structurally characterized. Some of them have been synthesized in laboratories. Further structure modifications or synthesis of analogues of the effective constituents may yield more safe and effective drugs. For example, artesunate (青蒿琥酯) and artemether (蒿甲醚) are semi-synthesized from artemisinin (青蒿素), which is isolated from Chinese herb Artemisiae Annuae Herba (青蒿).

3.3　Development of Quality Control for Chinese Herbs

The implementation of quality control for Chinese herbs is one of the key challenges in modernization of Chinese medicine. Chinese herbs are complex mixtures of numerous natural compounds. The complexity of the mixture needs highly selective and sensitive analytical methods to establish quality control for Chinese herbs. This is in contrast to most of chemical drugs that primarily contain a single compound to be analyzed. Chemistry of Chinese Materia Medica is at the forefront of developing methodologies to produce reference standards in support of quality control.

　　Chromatography is a powerful method in Chemistry of Chinese Materia Medica and is very useful for the quality control of Chinese herbs. TLC is widely used in the identification of Chinese herbs. HPLC is the most popular method for quantitative analysis and fingerprint. Fingerprint has included in the quality control standards for extracts, preparations and volatile oils from Chinese herbs in Chinese Pharmacopoeia.

　　There is an increased need for reliable methods of analysis and subsequent interpretation of the results or data. More and more new methods and techniques have been developed. For example, LC-MS, GC-MS, chemoinformatics (化学信息学) and chromatography fingerprint (色谱指纹图谱) are applied to evaluate the quality of Chinese herbs. In recent years, a new method, Integrated Spectrum-Effect Fingerprint (整合谱-效指纹图谱), has been proposed in some researches on herbs possessing antioxidant activity. This method provides information not only on the chemical constituents but also on the corresponding antioxidant activity by using online activity detection (HPLC-DAD-CL).

词　汇　表
An Alphabetical List of Words and Phrases

A		
Aconiti Radix	[əˈkɔnɪti][ˈreɪdɪks]	川乌
Aconiti Radix Cocta	[əˈkɔnɪti][ˈreɪdɪks][ˈkɔktə]	制川乌
aconitine	[əˈkɔnɪtiːn]	乌头碱
aerosol	[ˈeərəsɔːl]	喷雾剂
alkaloid	[ˈælkəlɔɪd]	生物碱
analysis	[əˈnæləsɪs]	分析
artemether	[ɑːtiˈmeðə]	蒿甲醚
Artemisiae Annuae Herba		青蒿
artemisinin	[ˌɑːtimiˈsaɪnɪn]	青蒿素
artesunate	[ˈɑːtiˌsuːnɪt]	青蒿琥酯
B		
baicalin	[ˈbeɪɪkəlɪn]	黄芩苷
berberine	[ˈbəːbəriːn]	小檗碱
biosynthesis	[ˌbaɪəuˈsɪnθɪsɪs]	生物合成
Bovis Calculus	[ˈbɔvɪs][ˈkælkjələs]	牛黄
Bovis Calculus Artifactus	[ˈbɔvɪs][ˈkælkjələs][ɑːtiˈfæktəs]	人工牛黄
C		
capsule	[ˈkæpsjuːl]	胶囊剂

(continued)

chemical constituent	['kemɪkl][kən'stɪtjuənt]	化学成分
Chemistry of Chinese Materia Medica	['kemɪstrɪ][əv][ˌtʃaɪ'ni:z][mə'tɪərɪə 'medɪkə]	中药化学
chemoinformatics	[keməˌɪnfə'metɪks]	化学信息学
Chinese materia medica	[ˌtʃaɪ'ni:z][mə'tɪərɪə 'medɪkə]	中药
Chinese patent medicine	[ˌtʃaɪ'ni:z]['peɪtənt]['medsn]	中成药
chromatography	[ˌkrəumə'tɔgrəfi]	色谱
chromatography fingerprint	[ˌkrəumə'tɔgrəfi]['fɪŋgəprɪnt]	色谱指纹图谱
Coptidis Rhizoma	['kɔptɪdɪs][raɪ'zəumə]	黄连
Corydalis Rhizoma	[kə'rɪdəlɪs] [raɪ'zəumə]	延胡索
crude drug	[kru:d][drʌg]	药材
D		
dosage	['dəusɪdʒ]	剂量
E		
effective composition	[ɪ'fektɪv][ˌkɔmpə'zɪʃn]	有效物质基础
effective constituent	[ɪ'fektɪv][kən'stɪtjuənt]	有效成分
effective fraction	[ɪ'fektɪv] ['frækʃn]	有效部位
Ephedrae Herba	[ɪ'fedrə] [hə:b]	麻黄
ephedrine	['efədri:n]	麻黄碱
ester bond	['estə][bɔnd]	酯键
Eucommiae Folium	['ju:kəmɪə]['fəulɪəm]	杜仲叶
Evodiae Fructus	[i:'vəudɪi:]['frʌktəs]	吴茱萸
extraction	[ɪk'strækʃn]	提取
extract	['ekstrækt]	提取物
F		
fingerprinting	['fɪŋgəprɪntɪŋ]	指纹图谱
G		
gallstone	['gɔ:lstəun]	胆结石
Ginkgo Folium	['gɪŋkgəu]['fəulɪəm]	银杏叶
Ginseng Folium	['dʒɪnseŋ]['fəulɪəm]	人参叶
Ginseng Radix et Rhizoma	['dʒɪnseŋ]['reɪdɪks][et][raɪ'zəumə]	人参
granule	['grænju:l]	颗粒剂
H		
hydrolyzed	['haɪdrəlaɪzd]	水解
hypaconitine	['haɪpəkɔnɪtaɪn]	海帕乌头碱
hyphenated	['haɪfəneɪtɪd]	联用的
I		
identification	[aɪˌdentɪfɪ'keɪʃn]	检识

(continued)

Identification of Chinese Materia Medica	[aɪˌdentɪfɪˈkeɪʃn][əv][ˌtʃaɪˈnɪːz] [məˈtɪərɪə ˈmedɪkə]	中药鉴定学
ineffective constituent	[ˌɪnɪˈfektɪv][kənˈstɪtjuənt]	无效成分
injection	[ɪnˈdʒekʃn]	注射剂
Integrated Spectrum-Effect Fingerprint	[ˈɪntɪɡreɪtɪd][ˈspektrəm][ɪˈfekt][ˈfɪŋɡəprɪnt]	整合谱 - 效指纹图谱
isolation	[ˌaɪsəˈleɪʃn]	分离
L		
liposome equilibrium dialysis	[ˈlɪpəsəum][ˌiːkwɪˈlɪbriəm][daɪˈæləsɪs]	脂质体平衡透析
M		
mesaconitine	[ˈmezəkənɪtaɪn]	美沙乌头碱
metabonomics	[ˌmetəˈbɒnɒmɪks]	代谢组学
micro-dialysis	[ˈmaɪkrəu] [daɪˈæləsɪs]	微透析
multi-herb formula	[ˈmʌlti][hə:b][ˈfɔːmjələ]	复方
N		
Natural Medicinal Chemistry	[ˈnætʃrəl][məˈdɪsɪnl][ˈkemɪstri]	天然药物化学
Natural Products Chemistry	[ˈnætʃrəl][ˈprɒdʌkts][ˈkemɪstri]	天然产物化学
non-medicinal portion	[nʌn məˈdɪsɪnl][ˈpɔːʃn]	非药用部位
norephedrine	[nɔːreˈfedrɪn]	去甲基麻黄碱
Notoginseng Radix et Rhizoma	[nəuˈtɒdʒɪnseŋ][ˈreɪdɪks][et][raɪˈzəumə]	三七
Notoginseng Total Saponins	[nəuˈtɒdʒɪnseŋ][ˈtəutl][sæˈpɒnɪnz]	三七总皂苷
P		
Pharmaceutics of Chinese Materia Medica	[ˌfɑːməˈsjuːtɪks][əv][ˌtʃaɪˈnɪːz] [məˈtɪərɪə ˈmedɪkə]	中药药剂学
pharmacokinetics	[ˌfɑːməkəukiˈneitiks]	药代动力学
Pharmacology of Chinese Materia Medica	[ˌfɑːməˈkɒlədʒi][əv][ˌtʃaɪˈnɪːz] [məˈtɪərɪə ˈmedɪkə]	中药药理学
Pharmacopoeia	[ˌfɑːməkəˈpiːə]	药典
Phytochemistry	[faɪtəuˈkemɪstri]	植物化学
polysaccharide	[pɒlɪˈsækəraɪd]	多糖
precipitated	[prɪˈsɪpɪteɪtɪd]	沉淀
preparation	[ˌprepəˈreɪʃn]	制剂
processing	[ˈprəusesɪŋ]	炮制
Processing of Chinese Materia Medica	[ˈprəusesɪŋ][əv][ˌtʃaɪˈnɪːz][məˈtɪərɪə ˈmedɪkə]	中药炮制学
protein	[ˈprəutiːn]	蛋白质
pseudoephedrine	[ˌsjuːdəʊˈfedrɪn]	伪麻黄碱
Q		
qualitative	[ˈkwɒlɪtətɪv]	定性的

(continued)

quantitative	[ˈkwɔntɪtətɪv]	定量的
S		
Scutellaria Extract	[skjuːtəˈlærɪə][ˈekstrækt]	黄芩提取物
Scutellariae Radix	[skjuːtəˈlæriː][ˈreɪdɪks]	黄芩
self-assembled	[ˈself əˈsembld]	自组装
separation	[ˌsepəˈreɪʃn]	分离
spectroscopic	[ˌspektrəˈskɔpɪk]	光谱的
structure	[ˈstrʌktʃə]	结构
structure-activity relationship	[ˈstrʌktʃər][æˈktɪvɪtɪ][rɪˈleɪʃnʃɪp]	构效关系
T		
tablet	[ˈtæblət]	片剂
toxication	[ˌtɔksɪˈkeɪʃən]	中毒
V		
vinegar-frying	[ˈvɪnɪgə][ˈfraɪɪŋ]	醋炙

重 点 小 结

  中药化学是在中医药基本理论和临床实践经验的指导下，运用现代科学理论和技术研究中药化学成分的一门学科。其主要内容包括中药中各类化学成分的结构特征、理化性质、提取分离方法、检识方法、结构测定方法，以及生合成途径、结构改造、构效关系等方面的研究。

  绝大多数中药都含有很多成分，其中具有防病治病作用的成分被称为**有效成分**。相反那些不具有防病治病作用的成分则被称为无效成分。哪些成分有效，哪些成分无效，不是绝对的，取决于该成分所在的化学环境及科技的进步，例如：原来被认为是无效成分的蛋白质和多糖，后来研究表明某些中药所含的蛋白质、多糖是有效的。从中药中提取分离制备得到的以一个有效成分为主或结构相似的一组有效成分组成的混合物被称为**有效部位**。来自于某中药的任何一个单独的有效成分或有效部位都仅仅是组成该中药的一部分成分，不能完全代表该中药。能代表某中药全部药效的该中药中所有有效成分的总和称为**有效物质基础**。

  中药化学的核心任务就是阐明中药的有效物质基础。每一味药都具有自己独特的有效物质基础，与其性味归经功能主治等特性相对应。因此中药化学的研究是在中医药基本理论和临床用药经验指导下进行的，是针对代表该中药药性的有效成分进行研究的，因此与天然产物化学、植物化学、天然药物化学等相近学科有所不同。

  中药化学既是研究中药的基础，又可以将研究成果直接应用到新药开发、制药工业等产业中去，是沟通中医药基本理论与中药产业的桥梁。①通过研究中药的有效物质基础，可以深入了解中药的四气五味、归经等药性与其有效物质基础之间的关系，从而赋予药性理论科学的内涵；通过研究中药的有效物质基础，可以了解炮制方法的作用机制，且更好地完善炮制工艺；研究中药的有效物质基础，可以探寻中药复方的配伍规律，挖掘新的复方。②中药化学的发展，可以促进中药新药的研发，例如扩大药源，将原来的非药用部位经研究后得到合理应用，甚至发现新的药用资源；利用中药化学的知识分离纯化制备有效部位或有效成分，可以开发质量可控性强、用量少、携带方便的新型现代中药制剂；中药质量标准的制定更离不开中药化学的知识。③中药化学与中药相关学科均有密切关系，例如中药鉴定学中，中药的理化鉴定主要是应用中药化学的知识；中药炮制学的炮制原理、炮制工艺的研究都离不开中药化学的知识；中药药剂学中各种剂型的制备，中药原料药的提取、净化，辅料的理化性质等均需要中药化学的知识；中药药理学在研究中药的药效时，药物的制备及保存等也需要对药物的主要成分理化性质等进行充分的了解，也需要中药化学的知识。

随着科技的不断进步，有关中药化学的研究，在中药有效物质基础挖掘、中药新药研发、中药质量控制等方面均取得了一些新的进展。

目 标 检 测

题库

一、单选题

1. 指导中药化学研究的理论不包括（　　）
 A. 中药的质地
 B. 中药的四气五味
 C. 中药的归经
 D. 中药的升降浮沉
 E. 中药的毒性

2. 中药化学的核心任务是（　　）
 A. 测定有效成分的含量
 B. 阐明中药的有效物质基础
 C. 测定有效成分的结构
 D. 阐明药性理论的科学内涵
 E. 阐明中药的炮制机制

3. 关于有效成分和无效成分的描述错误的是（　　）
 A. 中药中具有防病治病作用的成分被称为有效成分
 B. 中药中不具有防病治病作用的成分被称为无效成分
 C. 有效成分与无效成分是绝对的
 D. 有效成分与无效成分是相对的
 E. 某些中药中的多糖是有效成分

4. 关于有效成分描述错误的是（　　）
 A. 是指单一成分
 B. 是指结构清楚的单一成分
 C. 是指结构清楚有某种药理作用的单一成分
 D. 是从某中药中提取分离出来的有某种药理作用的单一成分
 E. 是能代表某中药药效的单一成分

5. 关于有效部位描述错误的是（　　）
 A. 以某个有效成分为主
 B. 是结构相似的一组有效成分
 C. 是从某中药中提取分离制备出来的
 D. 是从某中药中提取分离制备出来的混合物
 E. 是某中药的药用部位

6. 关于中药有效物质基础描述错误的是（　　）
 A. 是从该中药中分离得到的所有有效成分

B. 是该中药所含有的所有有效成分

C. 是能代表该中药药效的所有有效成分

D. 是一组有效成分

E. 包括多个有效成分

7. 不属于中药化学研究内容的是（　　）

A. 生合成途径　　　　　　　　B. 理化性质　　　　　　　　C. 提取分离方法

D. 结构测定方法　　　　　　　E. 含量测定方法

8. 关于中药化学的应用描述错误的是（　　）

A. 促进中药药性理论的研究　　　　　　B. 阐明中药的有效物质基础

C. 促进生合成途径的研究　　　　　　　D. 促进中药新药的研发

E. 阐明中药的炮制机制

二、多选题

1. 中药化学的研究对象包括（　　）

A. 中药提取物　　　　　　　　B. 中药材　　　　　　　　C. 中药饮片

D. 中成药　　　　　　　　　　E. 中药复方

2. 指导中药化学研究的理论包括（　　）

A. 中药的禁忌　　　　　　　　B. 中药的四气五味　　　　　C. 中药的归经

D. 中药的升降浮沉　　　　　　E. 中药的毒性

3. 关于有效成分和无效成分的描述正确的是（　　）

A. 中药中具有防病治病作用的成分被称为有效成分

B. 中药中不具有防病治病作用的成分被称为无效成分

C. 有效成分与无效成分不是绝对的

D. 有效成分代表该中药的药效

E. 有效成分代表该中药的部分药效

4. 关于有效成分描述错误的是（　　）

A. 是一组结构相似的成分

B. 是结构清楚的单一成分

C. 是指结构清楚有某种药理作用的单一成分

D. 是从某中药中提取分离出来的有某种药理作用的单一成分

E. 是能代表某中药药效的单一成分

5. 关于有效部位描述错误的是（　　）

A. 以某个有效成分为主　　　　　　　　B. 是结构相似的一组有效成分

C. 是某中药的总提物　　　　　　　　　D. 是某中药的炮制品

E. 是某中药的药用部位

6. 关于中药有效物质基础描述错误的是（　　）

A. 是从该中药中分离得到的所有有效成分

B. 是从该中药中鉴定出的所有有效成分

C. 是能代表该中药药效的所有有效成分

D. 是一组有效成分

E. 包括多个有效成分

7. 不属于中药化学研究内容的是（　　）

   A. 原植物鉴定　　　　　　　B. 结构鉴定　　　　　　　　　　C. 分离方法

   D. 检识方法　　　　　　　　E. 含量测定方法

8. 关于中药化学的应用描述正确的是（　　）

   A. 促进中药药性理论的研究　　　　　　　B. 阐明中药的有效物质基础

   C. 促进生合成途径的研究　　　　　　　　D. 促进中药新药的研发

   E. 阐明中药的炮制机制

三、思考题

1. 从理论基础、研究对象、研究内容、研究方法等方面分析中药化学与植物化学的异同。
2. 请简述中药化学的应用。

（高增平）

Chapter 2   General Methods for Chemical Investigation of Chinese Herbs

 学习目标

知识要求：

1. 掌握 中药化学成分的提取与分离方法的原理及应用范围。

2. 熟悉 中药化学成分的结构鉴定方法和分类方法。

3. 了解 中药化学成分的生物合成途径。

能力要求：

学会中药化学成分 3 种主要提取方法和 6 种主要分离方法的实际操作步骤，重点掌握溶剂提取法、超临界流体萃取法、结晶法及色谱法的原理及应用；学会采用 4 种波谱方法对中药化学成分的结构进行研究。

Chinese herbs are from various natural sources including plants, animals and minerals, etc. They can be a whole, a part of, the extract of an organism or pure compounds from an organism. With new technology development in the areas of separation technology (分离技术), spectroscope (波谱方法), and microplate-based ultrasensitive (基于微孔板的超灵敏的) *in vitro* assays (体外实验), researches on Chinese herbs are becoming more and more fruitful. Many novel and active compounds or their structural analogues isolated from Chinese herbs can be potential drug candidates.

1 Biosynthetic (生物合成的) Pathways and Classification of Chemical Constituents from Chinese Herbs

Biosynthetic pathways give rise to two classes of metabolites (代谢物), primary and secondary. Primary metabolites (DNA, RNA, fat, α-amino acids (氨基酸), chlorophyll (叶绿素) in green plants, etc.) are essential to the metabolic functions of the cells. Secondary metabolites [antibiotics (抗生素), alkaloids (生物碱), pheromones (信息素), terpenoids (萜类), etc.] generally support the function and survival of the whole organism. Unlike primary metabolites, secondary metabolites are an expression of the individuality of the species and only found in specific organisms or groups of organisms. They are important tools against herbivores and microbes. Some of them are also function as signal molecules to attract pollinating arthropods or seed-dispersing animals. Secondary metabolism provides most of the pharmacologically active compounds, which are often the targets for pharmaceutical research. Therefore, the biosynthetic pathways for secondary metabolites are the focus of this chapter.

1.1 Biosynthetic Pathways

The secondary metabolites are always small molecules (molecular weight <2000 amu approximately), Some of them are produced during idiophase (繁殖期), have defense mechanisms, and participate in regulatory processes.

There are five main important biosynthetic pathways of secondary metabolites, which are summarized in Table 2-1.

Table 2-1　Main biosynthetic pathways of secondary metabolites

Precursor (前体)	Biosynthetic pathway	Secondary metabolites
CH_3CO-S-CoA (乙酰辅酶A)	Acetate pathway (乙酸途径)	Fatty acids, polyketides (聚酮), quinones (醌类)
Mevalonic acid (甲戊二羟酸)	Mevalonate and deoxyxylulose phosphate pathway (甲戊二羟酸和磷酸脱氧木酮糖途径)	Terpenoids and steroids (甾体)
Shikimic acid (莽草酸)	Shikimate pathway (莽草酸途径)	Aromatic (芳香族的) amino acids, simple benzoic acids, and phenylpropanoids (苯丙素)
Amino acids	Amino acid pathway (氨基酸途径)	Alkaloids, and other nitrogen compounds
	Combined pathway (复合途径)	Chalcones (查耳酮), flavanones (二氢黄酮), terpenoid alkaloids

1.2 Classification of Chemical Constituents

The chemical constituents in Chinese herbs can be classified according to their molecular skeleton [i.e. open-chain aliphatic (脂肪族的) compounds versus cyclic-aliphatic compounds, aromatic or benzenoid (苯类的) compounds versus heterocyclic (杂环的) compounds], physiological activity (i.e. hormones, vitamins, antibiotics, and mycotoxins), or functional groups (i.e. acids versus bases). The main types of chemical constituents in Chinese herbs are summarized below.

1.2.1 Saccharides(糖类)

Saccharides are defined as polyhydroxyaldehydes (多羟基醛) or polyhydroxyketones (多羟基酮), or compounds that upon hydrolysis produce any of the above. They are also called carbohydrates (碳水化合物) because most of them are in the form of $C_n H_{2n} O_n$ or $C_n(H_2O)_n$.

1.2.2 Glycosides(苷类)

Glycosides are defined as the organic compounds that are formed by dehydration(脱水) reaction between a hydroxyl (羟基) group of hemiacetal (半缩醛) or hemiketal (半缩酮) from sugar or sugar derivatives (衍生物) and a group from non-sugar. The non-sugar moiety of a glycoside is called aglycone (苷元) or genin (配基). Glycosides play important roles in living organisms. Many plants store chemicals in the form of glycosides.

1.2.3 Quinones

Quinones are a group of compounds that have quinonoid groups [unsaturated cyclodione (不饱和环二酮)]. They can be divided into four subtypes: benzoquinones (苯醌), naphthoquinones (萘醌), phenanthraquinones (菲醌) and anthraquinones (蒽醌). Quinones, especially anthraquinones, are a major class of active constituents from Chinese herbs. They typically form strong-color pigments covering the entire visible spectrum.

1.2.4 Phenylpropanoids

Phenylpropanoids represent a large group of natural products that contain in their structure one or several C_6-C_3 units (a phenyl ring attached to a three-carbon side chain). They are widely distributed in Chinese herbs and many of them have various pharmacological activities. Examples include coumarins(香豆素) and lignans(木脂素).

1.2.5 Flavonoids(黄酮)

Flavonoids are a group of naturally occurring phenolic (酚的) compounds, which occur both in free form and glycosides. The classic definition of flavonoids was described as a derivative of 2-phenylchromone (2-苯基色原酮). Now, flavonoids are also described as the natural products with skeleton (骨架) of C_6-C_3-C_6 system.

1.2.6 Tannins(鞣质)

Tannins are defined as polyphenols that can precipitate proteins from aqueous solution. Tannins react with proteins to form water-insoluble copolymers. This reaction has been used by industry to transform animal skins to leathers.

1.2.7 Alkaloids

Alkaloids are a naturally occurring large group of physiologically active nitrogen-containing organic compounds from organisms (mainly are plants). In most alkaloids, there is a complex heterocyclic ring system and the nitrogen atom is part of the rings. Most of alkaloids are biosynthetically derived from amino acids.

1.2.8 Terpenoids

Terpenoids are regarded as derivatives of mevalonic acid (MVA), whose structures may be divided into isoprene units, hence these compounds are also called isoprenoids. Actually, terpenoids are also collectively called terpenes (萜烯). Terpenoids are lipophilic (亲脂性的) and are rich in volatile (易挥发的) oils. Terpenoids can be classified into monoterpenes (单萜), sesquiterpenes (倍半萜), diterpenes (二萜), sesterterpenes (二倍半萜), triterpenes, tetraterpenes(四萜), and polyterpenes (多萜) according to the number of isoprene units.

1.2.9 Steroids

Steroids are compounds that contain a cyclopentanoperhydrophenanthrene (环戊烷骈多氢菲) nucleus. They are widely distributed in nature. Cholesterol (胆固醇) typifies the fundamental structure of steroids, further modifications to the side chain help to create a wide range of natural products, such as sterols (甾醇), cardiac glycosides (强心苷), bile acids (胆汁酸), etc.

1.2.10 Saponins(皂苷)

Saponinsare a group of glycosides which, even at low concentration, produce a frothing in aqueous solution and upon hydrolysis they yield an aglycone known as a sapogenin (皂苷元), either steroid or triterpenoid. The name saponin comes from the Latin "*sapo*" (soap) and plant materials containing saponins were originally used for cleaning clothes.

2 General Methods for Chemical Investigation of Chinese Herbs

Chinese herbs are complex matrices containing a lot of secondary metabolites with different functional groups and properties. The compounds of interest need to be isolated from the rest of compounds, possibly represent only a very small proportion of the total biomass and maybe spread throughout the organism, and possibly bound with other molecules. Thus, it seems a formidable task to approach the phytochemical (植物化学的) investigation of a Chinese herb.

Prior to any separation and purification (纯化), organic compounds have to be extracted (or released) from the herb. Since chemical compounds are very diverse and present distinct physicochemical properties (e.g. polarity, solubility, stability etc.), the question to address is how to extract these compounds efficiently from the herb. Particular procedures can be used to remove unwanted interfering compounds and to enrich the extract with desired compounds.

Various extraction methods are available for the initial and bulk laboratory scale extraction of natural compounds from Chinese herbs (solid–liquid extraction mainly).

2.1　Extraction Methods

The choice of extraction methods depends on the compounds to be isolated and the nature of the source material. Prior to the choosing of an extraction method, it is necessary to establish the target of the extraction. The ideal extraction procedure should be exhaustive (i.e. extract as much of the desired compounds or as many compounds as possible), fast, simple and reproducible if it is to be performed repeatedly. The selection of a suitable extraction method mainly depends on whether or not the desired compounds are known. If a Chinese herb is being investigated for the first time, it is very important to perform a preliminary test before the formal and complete study of chemical constituents of the herb. There are many different extraction methods including solvent extraction, steam distillation (水蒸气蒸馏) and supercritical fluid extraction (SFE, 超临界流体萃取) and so on.

2.1.1　Solvent Extraction

Solvent extraction is widely used for initial and intermediate purification prior to purification by chromatography, crystallization (结晶法), or precipitation (沉淀法). It is easy to handle, potentially high-throughput and maybe adaptable to continuous operation. It relies on the principle of either "liquid-liquid" or "solid-liquid" extraction.

The extraction procedure can be divided into the following steps. The solvent first diffuses into the cells, then dissolves the metabolites and subsequently effuses out of the cells containing the extracted compounds. In general, extractions can be facilitated by grinding (to destroy the cells in order to release compounds) and high temperature (to help dissolve the compounds). After evaporation of the organic solvents or freeze-drying of the aqueous solutions, dried crude extracts can be obtained. Solvent removal should be performed immediately after extraction to minimize the loss of unstable compounds in solution.

Solvent extraction follows the principle of 'like dissolves like', namely, nonpolar solvents dissolve lipophilic compounds [e.g. alkanes, fatty acids, pigments (色素), waxes, sterols, some terpenoids, alkaloids, coumarins, etc.] and polar solvents dissolve polar compounds (e.g. glycosides, tannins, saponins, some alkaloids, etc.).

(1) Selection of a Suitable Solvent

Successful development of a solvent-extraction depends on a large degree of the selection of the appropriate solvent. Important factors for solvent selection include solubility (溶解度), toxicity (毒性), solute selectivity, viscosity (黏度), boiling point, operational hazards (操作的危险性), flammability (易燃性), volatility (挥发性) and price. Final choice should be an optimization (最优化) and compromise (综合) among these factors. The physicochemical properties of some commonly used solvents are listed in Table 2-2.

Table 2-2   Physicochemical properties of commonly used solvents

Solvents	Boiling point (℃)	Polarity index	Dielectric constant (20℃)	Viscosity	Toxicity (PDE*)
Chloroform (三氯甲烷)	61	25.9	4.8	0.57	Class 2 (0.6mg/d)
Pyridine (吡啶)	115	30.2	12.9	0.97	Class 2 (2.0mg/d)
Hexane (正己烷)	69	0.9	1.9	0.33	Class 2 (2.9mg/d)
Acetonitrile (乙腈)	82	46.0	37.5	0.37	Class 2 (4.1mg/d)
Dichloromethane (二氯甲烷)	40	30.9	9.1	0.44	Class 2 (6.0mg/d)
Toluene (甲苯)	111	9.9	2.4	0.59	Class 2 (8.9mg/d)
Xylene (二甲苯)	138	7.4	2.3	0.65	Class 2 (21.7mg/d)
Methanol (甲醇)	65	76.2	32.6	0.60	Class 2 (30.0mg/d)
Ethyl ether (乙醚)	35	11.7	4.3	0.23	Class 3 (low toxic potential)
n-Butanol (正丁醇)	118	60.2	18.2	2.95	Class 3 (low toxic potential)
i-Propanol (异丙醇)	82	54.6	18.3	2.37	Class 3 (low toxic potential)
Ethyl acetate (乙酸乙酯)	77	23.0	6.0	0.45	Class 3 (low toxic potential)
Methyl acetate (乙酸甲酯)	57	29.0	6.7	0.38	Class 3 (low toxic potential)
Tetrahydrofuran (四氢呋喃)	66	21.0	7.6	0.55	Class 3 (low toxic potential)
Acetone (丙酮)	56	35.5	20.6	0.32	Class 3 (low toxic potential)
Ethanol (乙醇)	78	65.4	22.4	1.20	Class 3 (low toxic potential)
Petroleum ether (石油醚)	30–60	0.6	1.8	0.30	no adequate toxicological date
Water	100	100.0	79.7	1.00	no toxicity

* PDE: Permitted Daily Exposure

Molecular polarity depends on the difference in electronegativity (电负性) between atoms in a compound and the asymmetry (不对称性) of the structure. Polarity underlies a number of physical properties such as surface tension, and melting- or boiling-points. Generally, there is a direct relationship between the polarity of a molecule and the numbers and types of polar or non-polar covalent bonds (共价键) that are presented in a molecule.

There are three kinds of solvents: water, polar organic solvents (i.e. methanol, ethanol and acetone) and non-polar organic solvents (immiscible with water). The polarities with decreasing order are:

$$H_2O > MeOH > EtOH > Me_2CO > n\text{-}BuOH > EtOAc > Et_2O > CHCl_3 > CH_2Cl_2 > cyclohexane > hexane \approx$$

petroleum ether(Pet.et)

Water is not often used in the initial extraction even if the aim is to extract water-soluble compounds (i.e. glycosides, quaternary alkaloids, tannins). Instead, polar organic solvents such as methanol or ethanol are often used in the extraction of water-soluble compounds, because organic solvents break up the compartmental structures and subsequently make it easier for the desired water-soluble compounds. Also, these organic solvents are much easier to evaporate than water. Moreover, organic solvents prevent microbial growth, one of the major problems related to the isolation of water-soluble compounds.

High toxic solvents and those harmful to the environment [i.e. benzene, toluene and carbon tetrachloride (四氯化碳)] should not be used. Ethyl ether should generally be avoided as it is highly flammable and can lead to the formation of explosive peroxides.

Petroleum ether is mostly used to defat plant material as it selectively disolves waxes, fats and other lipophilic compounds. Chloroform is more toxic than dichloromethane. Chloroform, dichloromethane and methanol may produce artifacts (人工产物) to complecate the isolation. Acetone may also give rise to artifacts under acidic conditions.

An aqueous-alcoholic mixture is the most commonly used solvent for extraction. The solubility of compounds in different solvents is listed in Table 2-3.

Table 2-3　Solubility of compounds in different solvents

Compounds		Water	Polar organic solvent	Non-polar organic solvent
Free form alkaloids		–	+	+
Alkaloid salts		+	+	–
Glycosides		+	+	+/– or –
Aglycones		–	+	+
Volatile oils		–	+/–	+
Saccharides	mono-, oligo-	+	+/–	–
	poly-	+	–	–
Organic acids	large molecule	–	+	+
	small molecule	+	+	–
Amino acids		+	+	–
Proteins, enzymes		+	–	–
Tannins		+	+	–
Pigments	Hydrophilic (亲水的)	+	+	–
	Lipophilic	–	+	+
Fats		–	–	+

(2) Extraction Protocols

① Maceration (浸渍)

Maceration is a simple but widely used protocol. The procedure is leaving the pulverized (粉碎的) materials in a suitable solvent in a closed container at room temperature to soak. Occasional or constant stirring of the mixture by using mechanical shakers or mixers can increase the speed of the extraction. The extraction ultimately stops when the equilibrium is obtained between the liquid and the pulverized material. This method is suitable for initial and bulk extractions.

Maceration doesn't usually cause degradation of thermolabile (热不稳定的) compounds because it is performed at room temperature. The main disadvantages of this method are time-consuming (a few hours to several weeks), solvent-consuming and the potential of loss of compounds. Some compounds may not be extracted efficiently by using this method if they are poorly soluble at room temperature.

② Percolation (渗漉)

In percolation, the pulverized material is soaked initially with a solvent in a percolator [a cylindrical (圆柱形的) or conical (圆锥形的) container with a tap at the bottom]. Additional solvent is then added on top of the material and allowed to percolate slowly (drop-wise) out of the bottom of the percolator. Filtration of the extract is not needed because there is a filter at the outlet of the percolator (Figure 2-1). Percolation is suitable for both initial and large-scale extraction.

Successive percolations can be performed to extract materials exhaustively by repeatedly refilling fresh solvent and pooling all extracts together. To ensure the percolation is complete, the percolate can be tested for the presence of desired compounds with specific reagents.

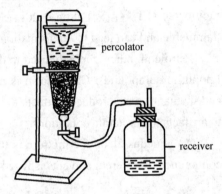

Figure 2-1　Percolation structure diagram

Both the contact time between the solvent and the materials (i.e. the percolation rate) and the temperature of the solvent can affect the extraction yield. A higher temperature will improve extraction but may lead to decomposition of labile compounds. The disadvantages include that large volumes of solvents are required and the process can be time-consuming.

③ Decoction (煎煮)

Decoction is a traditional method that relies principally on the use of hot water to obtain preparations that are used externally or internally. Boiling water improves extraction of chemical compounds. Its main disadvantage is that thermolabile compounds may be degraded. In addition, it is difficult to concentrate (浓缩) the extract by evaporation because the boiling point of water is 100℃.

④ Reflux (回流)

For reflux extraction, materials are immersed (浸渍) in a solvent in a round-bottomed flask that is connected to a condenser (Figure 2-2). The solvent is heated until it reaches its boiling point. When the vapor is condensed, the solvent is recycled back to the flask. The main disadvantage is that thermolabile compounds may be degraded.

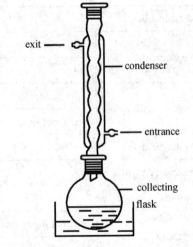

Figure 2-2　Reflux extraction structure

⑤ Successive Reflux (连续回流)

Successive reflux, especially Soxhlet extraction (索氏提取), is used widely in the extraction of Chinese herbs because it is easy to do. This method is suitable for both initial and bulk extraction. The pulverized material is placed in a cellulose mesh in the extraction chamber. The extraction chamber is placed on the top of the collection flask but underneath the condenser. A suitable solvent is added to the flask and the collection flask is heated with water bath. When an adequate level of condensed solvent has accumulated in the extraction chamber, it will be siphoned into the collection flask beneath via the small side tube (Figure 2-3).

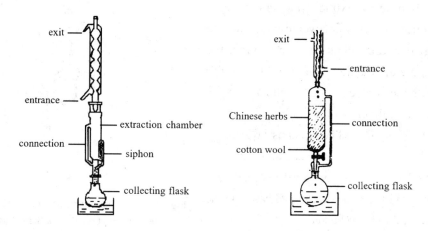

Figure 2-3　Successive reflux extraction structure diagram

Its main advantages include: it is a continuous process, it is less time-consuming and solvent-consuming than maceration or percolation or reflux. However, its main disadvantage is that the extract is constantly heated at the boiling point of the solvent. Heating may damage thermolabile compounds and/ or induce the formation of artifacts.

Ultrasound-assisted (超声辅助的) and pressurized (加压的) solvent extraction methods can also be used for extraction of Chinese herbs. The principles are similar to the above solvent extraction.

(3) Affecting Factors

① Grinding (粉碎度)

Grinding means fragmentation of the material into smaller particles. It can improve the subsequent extraction by making the sample more homogenous, increasing the surface area, and facilitating the penetration of solvent into the cells. Though generating suitable particle sizes through grinding is important for an effective extraction, grinding may cause potential problems for the extraction. For example, grinded seeds or fruits which are rich in fats and volatile oils may clog the sieves during the extraction process and the heat generated may damage thermolabile compounds.

② Temperature

Generally, high temperature increases the penetration of solvent into the material cells and improves compound solubility, therefore enhances the extraction speed and yield. However, high temperature may also lead to decomposition of labile compounds. Thus, temperature below 100℃ is recommended to avoid the loss/degradation of thermolabile compounds (e.g. the volatile compounds).

③ Concentration (浓度)

The extraction efficiency depends on the concentrations of the target compounds in the extract and in the source material. In order to increase the concentration differences, several methods such as stirring, refreshing the solvent and percolation can be used.

④ Duration (时间)

The contact duration between the solvent and the source material (i.e. the percolation rate) can also affect extraction yields. But once the equilibrium (平衡) is obtained between the extract and the source material, extended incubation is not warranted.

2.1.2　Steam Distillation

Steam distillation is a similar process as reflux and is commonly used for extraction of volatile oils. The material (dried or fresh) is covered with water in a flask connected to a condenser. Upon heating, the vapors (the mixture of volatile oil and water) condense and the distillate [separated into two immiscible (不互溶的) layers] is collected in a graduated receiver connected to the condenser. The aqueous layer is re-circulated into the flask, while the volatile oil is collected separately (Figure 2-4). The optimum extraction conditions (e.g. distillation rate) have to be determined based on the nature of the material to be extracted.

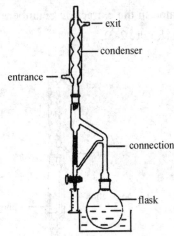

Figure 2-4　Steam distillation for volatile oils (when the density of oils is less than that of water)

In steam distillation, coarsely fragmented or crushed material is preferred over fine powdered material. Certain amount of glycerol can be added to the water to facilitate the extraction of tough materials (e.g. barks, seeds, roots, etc.). Xylene may be added to the graduated receiver to trap the distilled volatile oils produced.

2.1.3　Supercritical Fluid Extraction

Supercritical fluid extraction (SFE) is a general extraction strategy for a wide range of small lipophilic compounds from Chinese herbs. It is an environment-friendly alternative to the use of organic solvents for extraction, offering many advantages including less solvent usage, controllable selectivity, cleaner extracts and less thermal degradation compared to conventional solvent-extraction and steam-distillation methods.

In this method, a supercritical fluid (SCF, 超临界流体) is used to extract organic compounds. SCF is a phase state that a homogeneous fluid formed at temperature and pressure above the critical point (临界点) defined as the highest temperature and pressure at which the substance can exist in vapor-liquid equilibrium. The density of SCF is similar to its liquid, but has the penetration power of gas to make it become an effective and selective solvent. The solubility power of a SCF may vary near its critical point by small pressure and temperature changes.

Supercritical carbon dioxide (CO_2) is the most preferred SCF because of its particularly attractive properties including nontoxic, nonflammable, noncorrosive (无腐蚀性的), chemically inert (惰性的), low critical temperature (31.4℃), moderately low critical pressure (7.37MPa), easily accessible, cost-effective and environmental friendly (Figure 2-5). But supercritical CO_2 is lipophilic and only suitable for extraction of non-polar to slightly polar compounds. Modifiers can be added to the supercritical CO_2 to increase the polarity. Commonly used modifiers are methanol, ethanol and acetone. Little work has been done using modified supercritical CO_2 systems for highly polar compounds.

The example below is to extract the volatile oils from Aucklandiae Radix (木香) by using SFE method (Figure 2-6).

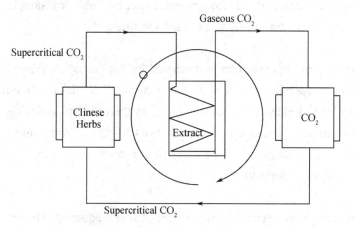

Figure 2-5   CO₂ supercritical fluid extraction

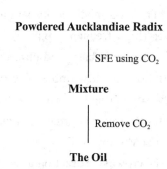

Powdered Aucklandiae Radix

| SFE using CO_2

Mixture

| Remove CO_2

The Oil

Figure 2-6   Extraction of volatile oils from Aucklandiae Radix

2.1.4   Other Extraction Methods

(1) Sublimation (升华法)

Sublimation is the process of transition of a compound from the solid phase to the gas phase without going through an intermediate (中间体) liquid phase. Sublimation is a technique used to purify compounds. A solid is typically placed in a sublimation apparatus and heated. The solid volatilizes and condenses as a purified compound on a cooled surface leaving non-volatile impurities behind. Once the heating ceases, the purified compound may be collected from the cooling surface (Figure 2-7).

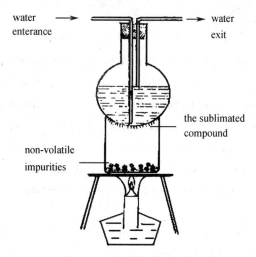

Figure 2-7   Normal pressure sublimation structure

(2) Absorption (吸收法)

Absorption is a method usually used to extract rare essential oils (精油), such as rose oil, jasmine oil, etc. The essential oils, especially the ones with low boiling points, are absorbed by using the sorbent matrix of lipophilic resin. Normally, flowers containing essential oils are wrapped up by two layers of fat or soaked in warm fats (50–60℃), and essential constituents are absorbed by the fats, the fats absorbing essential oil are used for medical and perfume industry.

(3) Grinding in a Suitable Solvent

Mechanical grinders are used to shred plants to various particle sizes to help dissolution. Grinding (i.e. fragmentation of the plant into smaller particles) improves subsequent extraction by rendering sample more homogenous, increasing surface area, and facilitating penetration of solvent into cells.

(4) Ultrasonic Extraction (超声提取)

This is a modified maceration method where the extraction is promoted by the use of ultrasound waves (high-frequency pulses, 20kHz). The powdered material is placed in a vial. The vial is placed in an ultrasonic bath, and ultrasound is applied to induce a mechanical stress on the cells by producing cavitations in the sample. The cellular breakdown increases the solubilization (溶解) of compounds in the solvent and improves extraction yields. The efficiency of the extraction depends on the solvent, instrument frequency, the duration and temperature of sonication.

(5) Microwave Extraction

Microwave extraction uses microwave energy(wavelength between 1mm–1m or frequency between 3×10^6–3×10^5Hz) to produce elevated temperature and pressure conditions in the sample and solvent to increase compound solubilization and improve extraction yield. Microwave extraction is effective in increasing extraction yield and protecting compound integrity. The method is suitable for rapid extraction of large amount samples.

(6) Enzymatic (酶的) Extraction

Enzymatic extraction method uses enzymes to degrade the cell walls of a Chinese herb with water acting as the solvent. This makes compounds coming out from cell much easier and improves extraction yields. The costs of this extraction method are estimated to be much higher than that of conventional solvent extraction method.

2.2　Isolation Methods

Isolation of compounds with high purity from Chinese herbs is the most important, but difficult and time-consuming step. It is difficult to apply any single separation technique to isolate individual compounds from the crude extract of Chinese herbs. Hence, isolation is often performed in steps. Initially, the crude extract is separated into several fractions containing compounds of similar polarities or molecular sizes. Secondly, to design/develop an isolation protocol based on the particular features of the molecule, such as solubility (hydrophobicity or hydrophilicity), acid–base properties, stability, charge and molecular size. Generally used isolation methods are summarized below.

2.2.1　Solvent Partitioning

Depending on the chemical and physical properties of desired compounds, a crude extract is generally partitioned in two immiscible solvents in a separatory funnel. The two phases may be adjusted to different pH for better separation of the desired compounds, such as alkaloids, phenols, etc.

(1) Acid and Alkali (碱) Treatment

For the acidic or basic compounds, acid and alkali treatment can be applied in partitioning. The pH values of aqueous layer are typically 3, 7, and 10.The pH value is one of the most important variables (particularly for weak bases and acids) for partition coefficients (分配系数) because it affects the solubility of compounds in solvents. Some compounds are weak acids or bases, and the pH can be used to control and even reverse the distribution coefficient. It is necessary to adjust the aqueous solution or suspension with mineral acid or alkali (a buffer can also be used), followed by the addition of organic solvent and solvent extraction, then the acid or alkali compounds can be separated from other compounds. After the organic and aqueous phases are separated, TLC can be used to identify the presence of desired compounds. This experiment can also provide information on the stability of compounds at various pH values.

The preparation of Coptidis Rhizoma Extract (total alkaloids) is an example of using this method (Figure 2-8).

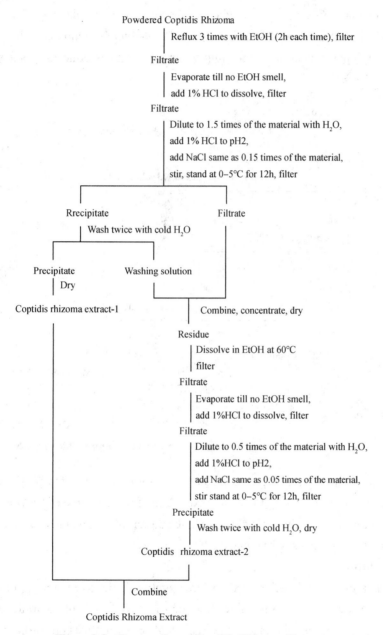

Figure 2-8   Preparation of Coptidis Rhizoma Extract

(2) Solvent Partitioning

Solvent partitioning method involves the use of two immiscible solvents in a separatory funnel, and the compounds are distributed in two solvents according to their different partition coefficients. Normally one of the solvents chosen is water while the other is hydrophobic (疏水的) organic solvent. This method can be used to separate different classes of natural compounds. It is relatively easy to operate and highly effective. It is usually used as the first step for medium to large scale separation of compounds from crude extract of Chinese herb.

In general, the crude extract of Chinese herb is suspended inappropriate amount of water. The suspension is then partitioned with cyclohexane, chloroform ($CHCl_3$), ethyl acetate (EtOAc), and n-butanol (n-BuOH), successively. The cyclohexane partitioning step is sometimes referred to as "defatting" because it yields a fraction containing non-polar compounds such as lipids, chlorophylls, etc. Low polar compounds are present in the $CHCl_3$ soluble fraction, and polar compounds probably up to monoglycosides are present in the EtOAc soluble part. The n-BuOH fraction contains polar compounds, mainly glycosides. Evaporation of the remaining water layer leaves polar glycosides and sugars as a viscous gum (Figure 2-9).

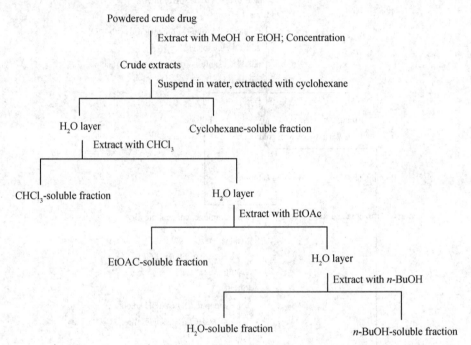

Figure 2-9   A general partitioning scheme by using immiscible solvents

The efficiency of the partitioning can be increased by doing repeated partitioning using small volumes of solvents compared to using the combined volume for a one-time extraction. It is worth noting that solvent partitioning doesn't always yield a clear separation of compounds. Overlapping compounds profile in successive fractions is usually found.

2.2.2   Precipitation

Precipitation is a classic separation method. Precipitation is the formation of a solid from a liquid phase that occurs particularly if an insolublecompound is introduced into a solution and the density happens to be greater (otherwise the precipitate will float or form a suspension). Precipitation can be accelerated if the solution becomes supersaturated with the target compound.

There are three types of precipitations: solvent precipitation, acid-base precipitation and reagent precipitation. These methods all can be applied to purify natural products.

2.2.3   Crystallization

The process of crystallization is generally used at the final stages of purification or used to produce crystals for structure determination by single-crystal X-ray diffraction analysis.

Solvent selection is the most important in crystallization. A suitable solvent should be easy soluble in a hot solution and insoluble in a cold solution for a sample to be purified, while for the impurities, this solvent should be all soluble in a hot and cold solution or all insoluble in a hot and cold solution (Figure 2-10). The commonly used solvents include methanol, ethanol, acetone, ethyl acetate, chloroform, ethyl ether and so on. Solvent mixtures can provide an easy way of tailoring solubility to a desired level. For example, for two-solvent crystallization, if the desired compound is soluble in solvent-1 at the boiling point, then solvent-2 can induce crystallization when added to a saturated solution of the desired compound in solvent-1.

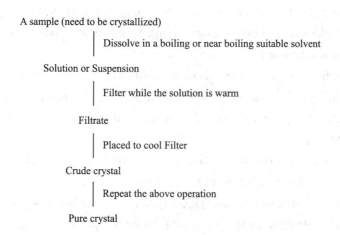

Figure 2-10　Procedure of crystallization and Recrystallization

As a general rule, good single crystals are produced from unstirred solutions slowly. These conditions limit nucleation, while high degree of super-saturation results in rapid formation of large number of nuclei and tends to yield unsuitable crystals for X-ray analysis.

2.2.4　Membrane Separation

Membrane separation plays an important role in isolation of compounds based on the molecular size of the separated compounds. The widely used membrane processes include microfiltration (微滤), ultra-filtration (UF,超滤), nanofiltration (纳滤), reverse osmosis (RO，反相渗透), electrolysis (电解), dialysis (透析), electrodialysis (电渗析). All processes except dialysis and electrodialysis are pressure driven. The advantage of membrane separation is that it operates without heating samples.

(1) Microfiltration

Microfiltration is a membrane filtration process which removes small particles from a fluid (liquid & gas) through a microporous (多微孔的) membrane. A typical microfiltration membrane pore size range is 0.2–10 micrometres (μm). It can be used as a pretreatment technique for Chinese herbal solution.

(2) Ultrafiltration

Ultrafiltration is a variety of membrane filtration in which hydrostatic (静力学的) pressure forces a liquid against a semi-permeable membrane. Suspended solids and solutes of high molecular weightcompounds are retained, while water and low molecular weight solutes pass through the membrane. The size of the membrane is about 0.001–0.02μm. It is used for separation and concentration of low molecular compounds from Chinese herbs, removing high molecular compounds in the solution such as tannins, polysaccharides, proteins and so on.

(3) Nanofiltration

Nanofiltration is a relatively new membrane filtrationtechnique used most often to remove low molecule or ionic impurity (杂质) from large molecular compounds in water. The nominal pore size of the membrane is typically about 1 nanometre (nm). It is a cross-flow filtrationtechnique which ranges somewhere between UF and RO.

(4) Dialysis

Dialysis works on the principles of the diffusion of solutes across a semipermeable (半透性的) membrane, in which small size molecules can pass through, and large size compounds will be retained inside. It is useful to purify and concentrate large molecular compounds such as saponins, polysaccharides (多糖), peptides (肽) and proteins to remove inorganic compounds and monosaccharides (单糖).

2.2.5 Fractionation(分馏法)

Mixtures of liquids are separated by fractional distillation based on different boiling points. The more difference in boiling points between two liquids, the easier for them to separate by fractionation, and if the difference is more than 100℃, no fractional distillation apparatus is needed.

2.2.6 Chromatography

Chromatography is the most popular methodfor separating and analyzing chemical constituents of Chinese herbs. It involves the distribution of a compound between two phases—a mobile phase (流动相) that is passed through a stationary phase (固定相). Separation is based on the compounds' properties that enable them to distribute between the two phases. As mobile phase carrying the solute passes through the stationary phase, the solutes are in constant dynamic equilibrium between the two phases. The stationary phase can be a solid or a liquid and the mobile phase can be a liquid or a gas, to form liquid chromatography (LC) and gas chromatography (GC), respectively. Chromatography can be classified in many ways. Classical chromatographic techniques include: thin-layer chromatography (TLC), preparative thin-layer chromatography (PTLC), open-column chromatography (CC), flash chromatography (FC). Modern chromatography techniques include: high-performance thin-layer chromatography (HPTLC), vacuum liquid chromatography (VLC), droplet countercurrent chromatography (DCCC), high-performance liquid chromatography (HPLC), hyphenated techniques (e.g., HPLC-PDA, LC-MS, LC-NMR, LC-MS-NMR). Details about the chromatography methods and their applications in the separation of natural compounds from Chinese herbs are introduced below according to the principles of chromatography.

(1) Adsorption Chromatography (吸附色谱)

Adsorption chromatography is one of the most popular chromatography techniques that involve partitioning of compounds between the surface of a solid stationary phase and a liquid mobile phase. The dynamic equilibrium of solutes as they switch between the stationary and mobile phases (the processes of sorption and desorption, respectively) is specific for each compound and is affected by competition that exists between solutes and solvents. This is a purely physical process involving the formation of no chemical bonds, but only the relatively weak forces of hydrogen bonds, Van der Waals forces, electrostatic forces, charge transfer forces and dipole-dipole interactions (Figure 2-11).

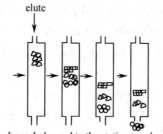

elute

○ Loosely boumd to the stationary phase

△ Midllely boumd to the stationary phase

▭ Stringly bound to the statinary phase

Figure 2-11　Separation principle of adsorption chromatography

① Adsorbent (吸附剂)

In theory, almost any inert material can be used as an absorbent. The provisos are that it is insoluble in the mobile phase and does not react with either the sample or the mobile phase. Commonly used adsorbents include silica gel (硅胶), alumina, polyamide (聚酰胺), and activated charcoal (活性炭).

② Eluent (洗脱剂)

In adsorption chromatography, the eluent is a mobile phase. Generally, the more polar adsorbents, the stronger adsorption (吸附) for polar compounds. On the other hand, the more polar eluent, the stronger ability for elution, so the polarity of eluents should be decreased if the adsorption of adsorbent is decreased. Commonly used eluents are various organic solvents or their mixtures.

③ Application

The commonly used adsorbents and their application are listed in Table 2-4.

Table 2-4　Commonly used adsorbents and their application

Adsorbent		Eluent	Main applications	Notes
Silica gel		Single organic solvent or solvent mixtures	Neutral and acidic constituents, such as phenols, anthraquiones, glycosides, terpenoids, steroids, etc.	Activated by heating at 105℃ for 30 minutes to remove water
Alumina	basic	Single organic solvent or solvent mixtures	Basic constituents, such as alkaloids	To remove resin (树脂), chlorophyll and other lipophilic impurities
	neutral		Basic and neutral constituents	
	acidic		Seldom used for acidic constituents	
Polyamide		Organic solvents without water H_2O-EtOH (MeOH)	Flavonoids, anthraquinones, tannins, organic acids, etc.	Normal-phase chromatography Reversed-phase chromatography
Activated charcoal		H_2O-EtOH (MeOH)	Water-soluble compounds	To absorb lipophilic impurities from water solution

(2) Partition Chromatography (分配色谱)

Partition chromatography employs the separation principle of liquid-liquid extraction with the advantages of chromatography. Separation is based on the distribution constant (Ko) of a compound between two phases. A stationary phase can be a liquid that is coated onto a solid support, for example a

29

column of cellulose coated with water, or functional groups are coated onto a solid support, such as C_{18} silica, C_8 silica, CN (cyano) silica. Separation is carried out on a stationary phase with an immiscible / organic mobile phase. The mobile phase is a moving phase, which usually uses a solvent system in which the composition of solvents changes during the separation [gradient elution (梯度洗脱）]. By using two or more solvents, the proportions of them change during a run, and it is possible to separate solutes with widely different retention times. The mobile phase change can occur at a number of set intervals (step gradient) or continuously throughout the run (continuous gradient).

Based on the polarity of stationary phase and mobile phase, there are two kinds of partition chromatography: normal-phase chromatography (正相色谱) and reversed-phase chromatography (反相色谱). If the stationary phase has larger polarity than the mobile phase, this is normal-phase chromatography. An example of this is a silica gel column with its polar silanol groups and a mobile phase of an organic solvent. When the stationary phase has less polarity than the mobile phase, this is the reversed-phase chromatography. For example, a water-acetonitrile (or methanol) is mobile phase and the alkyl-bonded silica packing, e.g. with C_8 or C_{18} groups covering the silica surface is the stationary phase. The reversed-phase chromatography is widely used as a form of HPLC.

(3) Ion Exchange Chromatography (离子交换色谱)

Ion exchange chromatography (IEC) is used for isolation of charged or ionizable compounds, such as acids, bases, and amphoteric compounds. This involves a stationary phase that consists of an insoluble matrix and the surface of which carries a charged group, either negative or positive. These charged groups are associated with a counter-ion of the opposite charge. The principle of separation lies in the ability of the sample ions to exchange with the counter-ions and bind to the stationary phase.

Separation occurs due to the difference among sample compounds in the degree and strength of interaction with the exchange sites. Once the sample compounds are bound, they can be eluted selectively from the binding site by either adjustment of ion strength or changes of the pH value of the mobile phase.

① Selection of Ion Exchange Resin

Ion exchange resins are used in the form of water-insoluble particles or beads which are covalently bonded to negatively or positively charged-groups. The support matrices can be synthetic polymers, silica or polysaccharides.

The charge and nature of the functional group on the stationary phase determine the type of ion-exchange resin, and they are classified into two types: anion (阴离子) exchangers and cation (阳离子) exchangers. Compounds bear a negative charge, such as a carboxylate anion. They can be purified by using anion exchangers. Both strong and weak anion exchangers are available.

The selection of an ion exchange resin is empirical and often based on what is available in the lab or from local suppliers. If the charge of the solute to be separated is known, the choice of ion-exchanger type will be obvious. For example, when designing an isolation process for a compound with a carboxyl group, strong anion exchange packing materials (SAX) should be investigated first; when designing an isolation process for a basic compound with an amine group, a strong cationic exchange resin (SCX) should be explored first. Because the structure of the desired compound is often unknown, the best approach to select resin is through the use of probe columns.

② Elution

Water is the most commonly used solvent in IEC. There are two strategies for eluting bound solutes from an ion-exchange column: changes in ionic strength or changes in pH value. Useful buffers are listed in Table 2-5.

Table 2-5　Useful buffers for IEC

Buffer	pH range	Buffer	pH range
Citrate	2.0-6.0	Triethanolamine (Tris)	6.7-8.7
Phosphate	2.0-3.0, 7.1-8.0	Borate	8.0-9.8
Formate	3.0-4.5	Ammonia	8.2-10.2
Acetate	4.2-5.4		

The use of mixture of organic solvent and water, such as MeOH-H_2O, in the elution step can help to minimize backbone interactions. The backbone interactions result from the adsorption of the hydrophobic portions of compounds onto the hydrophobic portions of the resin support. The degree of interaction obviously depends on the nature of the sample ions and of the functional groups on the ion-exchange resin. Sample ions that react strongly with the stationary phase ions are powerfully retained and will elute more slowly, while weakly binding solute will be eluted more rapidly.

(4) Macroporous Resin (大孔树脂) Chromatography

Macroporous resin is a fused mass of polymer micro-spheres. The micro-spheres confer on the polymer a relatively high surface area together with a high porosity. The separation principle of macroporous resin chromatography depends on the physical adsorption of the resin and the size of compounds. Both the pore size and surface diffusion play important roles in the process of solute transfer to the adsorbent. Generally, the polarity of the stationary phase is lower than that of the mobile phase, and the polar compound is easier to be eluted out from column. For example, glycosides are always eluted from the column first and their aglycones last. Polar solvents have lower ability to elute components, so water is the weakest solvent to elute.

In general, the crude extract of Chinese herbs is dissolved in water and applied to the column, then elute with increasing amount of methanol or ethanol in water. The adsorption capacity can be affected by pH, temperature and salt concentration.

There are many types of macroporous resins, such as Amerlite, Diaion, GDX, AB-8, X-5, NKA-9, SIP, etc. They can be used for desalting from biological samples, casein non-phosphorylated peptides, and taurine at industry manufacturing scale with good hydrolysate recoveries. While salt is completely rinsed off with deionized water (去离子水), and hydrolysates are retained and can be subsequently desorbed using alcohol.

Macroporous resins can be easily regenerated by immersing and washing them with EtOH, 1mol/L HCl and 1mol/L NaOH. Therefore, the macroporous resin chromatography method is very popular in purification and isolation of Chinese herbal extracts.

(5) Gel Filtration Chromatography (凝胶过滤色谱)

Gel filtration chromatography (GFC) is similar to the size-exclusion chromatography (SEC) and gel-permeation chromatography (GPC), but aqueous solutions are used instead. In the gel filtration chromatography, the stationary phase comprises non-adsorbing porous particles for which the pore size is strictly controlled. When the mobile phase flows through these particles, solutes carried in the mobile phase may flow in and out of the pores. Compounds that are larger than the pore size cannot enter the pores and will be eluted at the first peak in the chromatogram, a phenomenon called "total exclusion". Smaller compounds that can enter the pores will have an average retention time in the particles that depends on the compounds' size and shape. As a result, compounds are eluted in the order of decreasing sizes in the gel filtration chromatography. The largest ones are eluted at first, and the smallest are eluted at last (Figure 2-12).

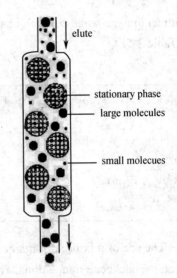

Figure 2-12   Basic mechanism of GFC

Sephadex G gels are manufactured by crosslinking of water-soluble dextran (葡聚糖) with epichlorohydrin (环氧氯丙烷). Sephadex G gels are hydrophilic. They swell in water and are usually defined by the amount of solvent picked up by dry beads upon swelling. For example, Sephadex G-15 picks up 1.5 ml of water per gram of dry beads, whereas the G-100 picks up 10 ml/g. The highly crosslinked G-10 and G-15 are well-suited for the separation of constituents from Chinese herbs. Their use is limited to separating compounds in aqueous solutions. Thus, they are ideal for fractioning water-soluble mixtures such as polysaccharides and proteins.

Sephadex LH-20 (羟丙基葡聚糖凝胶) is a hydroxypropylated form of Sephadex G-25. This derivative has added lipophilicity that allows it swell sufficiently in organic solvents to be conditioned for the fractionation of organic-soluble compounds. Therefore, Sephadex LH-20 is a preferred gel and widely used in separation of natural products.

When a single solvent is used, the separation mainly occurs by gel filtration mode. If a solvent mixture is used, the gel will take up predominantly the polar component of the solvent mixture. This result in a two-phase system with stationary and mobile phases of different compositions, separation takes place by virtue of size exclusion. Additional adsorption mechanisms, such as hydrogen bonding, also aid the separation process.

Sephadex gels have two important advantages: they are usually inert and do not adsorb compounds irreversibly; and the Sephadex gels can be used multiple times without the need of regeneration.

(6) Affinity Chromatography (亲和色谱)

Affinity chromatography is a method based on specific and reversible molecular interactions between biologically active compounds. There are several variants involved even when the matrix-bound ligand does not originate exclusively from biological matters (Table 2-6). Immunoaffinity chromatography (IAC, 免疫亲和色谱) is one type of affinity chromatography. It utilizes antibody and antigen interaction to achieve specific extraction purpose. Because of its high affinity and selectivity, IAC with immobilized antibody is a very popular method for purification of proteins.

Table 2-6   Variants of affinity chromatography

Chromatographic method	Basis of the separation effect	Examples
Biospecific affinity (biosorption)	Specific adsorption (biospecific recognition)	Biologically active compounds, including cell fragments, viruses, and cells
Dye-ligand	Specific interaction of biomacromolecules with triazine and triphenylmethane dyes	Enzymes (dehydrogenases, kinases, esterases, peptidases), nucletic acids, nucleic acid binding proteins
Metal chelate	Complex formation between a matrix-bound metal chelate and the substance to be separated by exchange of low-molecular-weight metal-bound ligands	Peptides, proteins, nucleic acids
Charge transfer adsorption	Interaction between electron-accepting and electron-donating groups	Amino acids, peptides, nucleotides
Hydrophobic interaction	Formation of contacts between a polar groups in aqueous solution	Various proteins and nucleic acids
Covalent (chemisorption)	Formation of convalent disulfide bonds that can be cleaved again under mild conditions	Thiol groups containing peptides and proteins, mercurated polynucleotides

2.2.7   Other Separation Methods

Electrophoresis (电泳) is the motion of dispersed particles under the influence of a spatially uniform electric field. Electrophoresis is caused by the presence of a charged interface between the particle surface and the surrounding fluid. Capillary electrochromatography (CEC) is a hybrid separation technique that combines capillary HPLC with capillary zone electrophoresis, and its main advantage is an enormous number of theoretical plates that can be achieved, which is useful for increasing the separation efficiency.

2.3   Structure Determination Methods

In most cases, extraction and isolation of Chinese herbs are followed by the purity confirmation of an isolated compound and structure determination.

The definition of pure compound means that the amount of any impurity does not exceed some arbitrarily set acceptable level. It is important to know the capability and sensitivity of analytical instrument. TLC and HPLC are commonly used methods to detect the purity of a compound isolated from Chinese herb. In addition, the melting point can classically be used to characterize organic compounds and to confirm the purity.

2.3.1   General Procedure of Structure Determination

Structure determination of compounds is time consuming, and sometimes can be the "bottleneck" in Chinese herbal research. A comprehensive and systematic approach involving a variety of physical, chemical and spectroscopic techniques are required. Information on the chemistry of the family of Chinese herbs under investigation could sometimes provide some hints regarding the possible chemical class of the unknown compound. The structure elucidation procedure and methods are listed in Table 2-7.

Table 2-7 Structure elucidation procedure and methods

Procedure	Method
Preliminary judgment of compound type	Literature research
	Behavior of samples during process of extraction and isolation
	Physical and chemical properties
	Spectroscopic characteristics
Confirmation of molecular formula	Element analysis, mass spectrum (质谱) to determine molecular mass, HR-MS to determine molecular formula
	Isotope abundance ratio to get molecular formula
Determination of functional groups, fragment or bone of molecules	Spectroscopic data (UV, IR, MS, NMR)
	Quality and quantity analysis of functional groups
Determination of planar structure of molecules	Total analysis of data above
	Compared with literature or model compound
Determination of absolute configuration of molecules	CD or ORD spectrum, NOESY or 2D-NMR information
	X-ray diffraction analysis; synthesis or chemical communication

2.3.2 Spectroscopic Methods

One classical method for establishing structure of natural compounds is based on a stepwise degradation of the unknown molecule into smaller and known compounds followed by a logical restructuring step. The degradation usually requires a substantial amount of the initial compound. It is worth noting that during the degradation some structural information, especially information related to stereochemistry (立体化学) of the broken bonds is sometimes lost.

Modern spectroscopic methods such as ultraviolet-Visible spectroscopy (UV-Vis, 紫外–可见光谱), infrared spectroscopy (IR, 红外光谱), mass spectrometry (MS, 质谱), and nuclear magnetic resonance (NMR, 核磁共振) spectroscopy are very powerful tools to establish structures of organic compounds from Chinese herbs.

(1) Ultraviolet–Visible Spectrometry (UV-Vis, 紫外 –可见光波谱)

UV–Vis spectrum is one of the most readily accessible information pertaining to molecular structure. It is plotted as absorbance versus wavelength (λ: 200-400nm for UV, 400-800nm for Vis). The wavelengths of maximal absorbance (λ_{max}) and the extinction coefficient (ε) are characteristics of the chromophoric groups presented in a molecule. Some compounds that contain conjugated systems, such as flavonoids, isoquinoline alkaloids, anthraquinones and coumarins, to name a few, can be primarily characterized the chemical class by the characteristics of UV–Vis spectra.

Figure 2-13 is the UV spectrum of lasianthuoside A from *Lasianthus acuminatissimus* (长尾粗叶木).

(2) Infrared Spectrometry (IR)

Infrared (IR) radiation refers broadly to the electromagnetic spectra between the visible and microwave regions. Of the greatest practical use, is the limited portion between 4000cm^{-1} and 400cm^{-1} (Table 2-8). IR spectra provide information about the presence or absence of functional groups, but they are not as useful or informative as NMR or MS spectra.

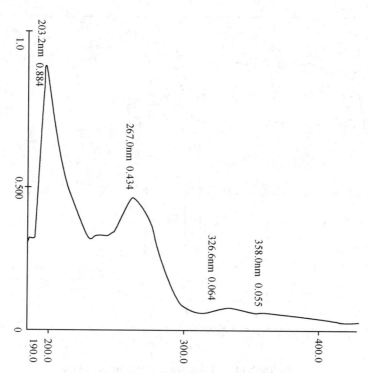

Figure 2-13　UV spectrum of lasianthuoside A

Table 2-8　IR absorption regions using hooke's law

Bond type	Absorption region (cm^{-1})	
	Observed	Calculated
C—O	1300–800	1113
C—C	1300–800	1128
C—N	1250–1000	1135
C=C	1900–1500	1657
C=O	1850–1600	1731
C≡C	2150–2100	2101
C—D	2250–2080	2225
C—H	3000–2850	3032
O—H	3800–2700	3553

Figure 2-14 is the IR spectrum of lasianthuoside A from *Lasianthus acuminatissimus*.

(3) Mass Spectrometry (MS)

The principles of MS is that when a compound is ionized, the ions are separated on the basis of their mass/charge ratios, and the ions representing each mass/charge ratio is recorded as a spectrum. Microgram amounts of compounds are usually enough for several MS experiments even though only less than 1% of the amount undergoes ion formation by any single ionization (离子化) technique.

In most cases, MS is the most sensitive method for obtaining some molecular information of

35

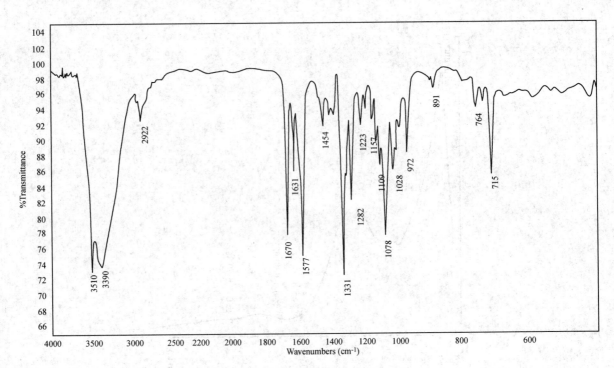

Figure 2-14   IR spectrum of lasianthuoside A

an unknown compound. It is useful for characterizing molecules that can be ionized to positively or negatively charge status under controlled conditions. It provides information about the molecular mass, molecular formula and fragmentation pattern. This information together with evidence from other spectrometry (e.g. UV, IR and NMR) can lead to the identification of the structure of a compound.

There are many ionization methods that work effectively on most of compounds. The most common ones are: electron impact (EI, 电子轰击), chemical ionization (CI, 化学电离), electrospray ionization (ESI, 电喷雾电离), Field desorption（FD, 场解吸）and fast atom bombardment (FAB, 快原子轰击). The mass analyzer used to separate the mixture of ions that are generated during the ionization step by m/z in order to obtain a spectrum is the heart of each mass spectrometer. There are several different types of MS with different characteristics, such as magnetic sector mass spectrometer (扇形磁场质谱仪), quadrupole mass spectrometer (四极质谱仪), ion trap mass spectrometer (离子阱质谱仪), time-of-flight mass spectrometer (飞行时间质谱仪), fourier transform mass spectrometer (傅里叶变换质谱仪), and tandem (串联的) mass spectrometry, to name a few.

The different properties of ionization methods and mass analyzers are listed in Table 2-9 and Table 2-10.

Table 2-9   Summary of ionization methods

Ionization method	Ions formed	Sensitivity	Advantage	Disadvantage
EI	M^+	ng–pg	Data base searchable Structure information Volatile and small molecular compounds	M^+ occasionally absent
CI	M+1, M+18 ,etc	ng–pg	M^+ usually present	Little structural information
FD	M^+	μg–ng	Non volatile compounds	Specialized equipment

(continued)

Ionization method	Ions formed	Sensitivity	Advantage	Disadvantage
FAB	M+1, M^+ cation	μg–pg	Non volatile compounds Sequencing information	Matrix interference Difficult to interpret
ESI	M^+, M^{++}, M^{+++}, etc.	ng–pg	Non volatile compounds interfaces W/LC Forms multiply charged ions	Little structural information

Table 2-10 Summary of mass analyzers

Mass analyzer	Mass range	Sensitivity	Resolution	Advantage	Disadvantage
Magnetic sector	1–15, 000	Low	0.0001	High resolution	Low sensitivity Very expensive High technical expertise
Quadrupole	1–5000	High	0.1	Easy to use Inexpensive High sensitivity	Low resolution Low mass range
Ion trap	1–5000	High	0.1	Easy to use Inexpensive High sensitivity Tandem MS (MS^n)	Low resolution Low mass range
Time of flight	Unlimited	High	0.0001	High resolution and mass range Simple design	
Fourier transform	Up to 70 kDa	High	0.0001	High resolution and mass range	Very expensive High technical expertise

EI-MS can be used to analyze volatile and small molecular compounds. CI-MS can be used to analyze volatile compounds. FAB-MS and ESI-MS can be used to analyze non volatile and polar compounds, such as glycosides, peptides, etc.

(4) Nuclear Magnetic Resonance (NMR)

Under appropriate conditions in a magnetic field, a compound can absorb electromagnetic radiation that is specific to the compound. Absorption is a function of certain nuclei existed in a molecule. NMR spectrum is a plot of frequencies of absorption peaks versus peak intensities that reveals information on the number and types of protons (质子) and carbons (and other elements like nitrogen, fluorine, etc.) presented in a molecule and the relationships among these atoms.

Simple NMR spectra are recorded in solutions, and Deuterated (deuterium = ^{2}H, often symbolized as D) solvents are preferred [e.g. deuterated (含重氢的) water, D_2O, deuterated acetone, $(CD_3)_2CO$, deuterated methanol, CD_3OD, deuterated dimethyl sulfoxide (DMSO), $(CD_3)_2SO$, and deuterated chloroform, $CDCl_3$]. In addition, solvents without hydrogen, such as carbon tetrachloride, CCl_4 or carbon disulphide, CS_2, may also be used. Tetramethylsilane (TMS) is often used as an internal standard for calibrating the chemical shifts of each proton. NMR techniques (^{1}H-NMR and ^{13}C-NMR) are powerful tools for molecular structure characterization.

① ¹H-NMR

¹H-NMR is the application of NMR to hydrogen-1nuclei of a molecule in order to determine the molecular structure. ¹H-NMR spectra of most organic compounds are characterized by chemical shifts (the range +14 to -4, δ) and by spin-spin coupling between protons (coupling constant, J). The proton integration curve reflects the abundance of individual protons in a molecule.

¹H-NMR spectrum of sibiscolacton from *Sibiraea angustata* (窄叶鲜卑花) is shown in Figure 2-15.

The Nuclear Overhauser Effect (NOE, 核的增益效应) is the change in the integrated NMR absorption intensity of a nuclear spin when the NMR absorption of another spin is saturated. NOE occurs through space, not through chemical bonds. Thus atoms that are in close to each other can give a NOE, the inter-atomic distances derived from the observed NOE can often help to confirm a precise molecular conformation. The NOE spectrum of lasianthuoactone is shown in Figure 2-16.

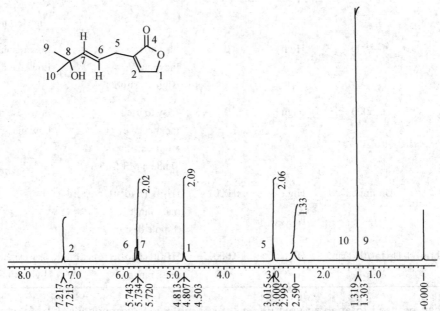

Figure 2-15 ¹H-NMR spectrum of sibiscolacton from *Sibiraea angustata*

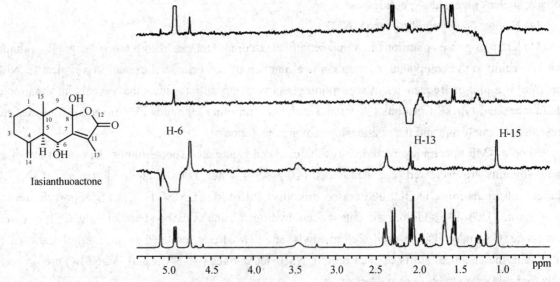

Figure 2-16 NOE spectrum of lasianthuslactone from *Lasianthus acuminatissimus*

② ^{13}C-NMR

^{13}C-NMR is the application of NMR spectroscopy to carbons. It allows the identification of carbon atoms in an organic molecule. ^{13}C-NMR detects only the ^{13}C isotope whose natural abundance is only 1.1%. Therefore, ^{13}C-NMR is much less sensitive than ^{1}H-NMR, it needs more sample than ^{1}H-NMR. On the other hand, ^{13}C-NMR spectra are proton decoupled to remove signal splitting. Also couplings between carbons can be ignored owing to the low natural abundance of ^{13}C. ^{13}C-NMR spectrum shows a single peak for each chemically non-equivalent carbon atom, which makes ^{13}C-NMR easier to distinguish than ^{1}H-NMR. The polarization transfer from ^{1}H to ^{13}C has an advantage of increasing the ^{13}C spectrum sensitivity because of carbon's nuclear overhauser effect. The ^{13}C-NMR spectrum of sibiscolacton is shown in Figure 2-17 and the data of NMR spectra are listed in Table 2-11.

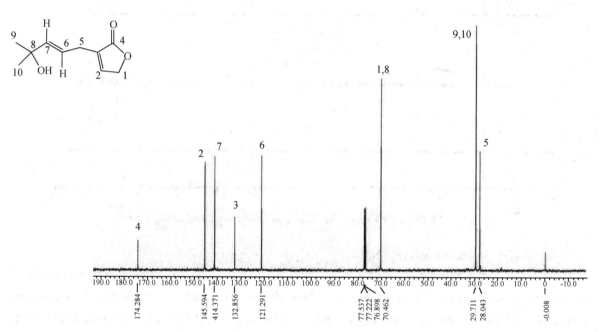

Figure 2-17　^{13}C-NMR spectrum of sibiscolacton from *Sibiraea angustata*

Table 2-11　Data ^{1}H-NMR (400 MHz) and ^{13}C-NMR (100 MHz) of sibiscolacton (in CDCl$_3$)

No.	δ_{H}	δ_{C}
1	4.81 (2H, m)	70.4
2	7.21(1H, dd, J= 2.0, 3.4)	145.5
3		132.9
4		174.2
5	3.01 (2H, m)	28.1
6	5.75 (1H, ddd, J= 2.5, 9.8, 15.4)	121.3
7	5.72 (1H, d, J= 15.4)	141.4
8		70.5
9	1.33 (3H, s)	29.7
10	1.32 (3H, s)	29.7

Distortion enhancement by polarization transfer (DEPT, 极化转移增强谱) sequence has become the preferred procedure for identifying the primary, secondary, and tertiary carbon atoms. The DEPT experiment differentiates among CH, CH_2, and CH_3 groups by variation of the selection of the angle parameter (the tip angle of the final ^1H pulse): 135° angle gives all CH and CH_3 in a phase opposite to CH_2. 90° angle gives only CH groups, the others being suppressed. 45° angle gives all carbons with attached protons (regardless of number) in phase. Signals from quaternary carbons and other carbons with no attached protons are absent due to the lack of attached protons. The DEPT spectrum of sibiscolacton is shown in Figure 2-18.

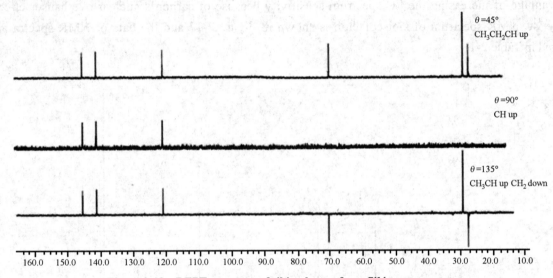

Figure 2-18   DEPT spectrum of sibiscolacton from *Sibiraea angustata*

③ Two-Dimensional NMR (2D-NMR)

2D-NMR is a set of NMR spectroscopy methods that provide data plotted in a space defined by two frequency axes rather than one. One axis always represents the nucleus detected during acquisition. The other one can represent the same nucleus (e.g. ^1H-^1H COSY), a different nucleus (e.g. ^1H-^{13}C COSY also called HMQC or HETCOR) or a coupling constant (e.g. *J*-resolved spectroscopy). 2D-NMR spectra provide more information about a molecule than 1D-NMR spectra and are especially useful in determining the structure of a molecule that is too complicated to work with using 1D-NMR.

a. ^1H-^1H COSY

The first and most popular 2D-NMR method is the homonuclear (同核) correlation spectroscopy (COSY,化学位移相关谱) sequence, such as ^1H-^1H COSY to identify proton spins that are coupled to each other. The ^1H-^1H COSY spectrum of sibiscolacton is shown in Figure 2-19, the correlation of protons could be observed.

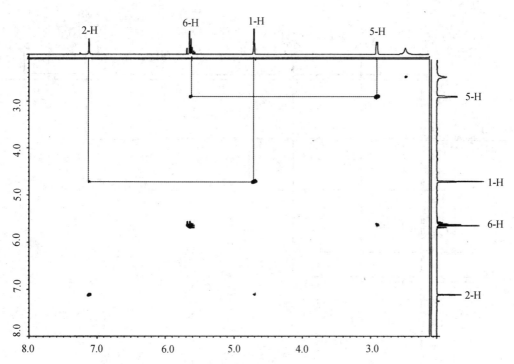

Figure 2-19 ^1H-^1H COSY of sibiscolacton from *Sibiraea angustata*

b. Total Correlation Spectroscopy (TOCSY, 全相关谱)

The TOCSY method is similar to the COSY experiment, in that cross peaks of coupled protons are observed. However, cross peaks are observed not only for nuclei that are directly coupled, but also between nuclei that are connected by a coupling chain. This makes it useful for identifying the larger interconnected networks of the spin couplings. This ability is achieved by inserting a repetitive series of pulses that cause isotropic mixing during the mixing period. Longer isotropic mixing times cause polarization to spread out through an increasing number of bonds. TOCSY is sometimes called "homonuclear Hartmann–Hahn spectroscopy" (HOHAHA).

c. Heteronuclear Correlation (HETCOR, 碳氢直接相关谱)

HETCOR is carbon detected ^{13}C-^1H COSY. This experiment correlates ^{13}C nuclei with directly attached protons, these are one-bond ($^1J_{CH}$) couplings.

d. Heteronuclear Multiple Quantum Correlation Spectroscopy (HMQC, 异核多量子相关谱)

HMQC is proton detected ^1H-^{13}C COSY. It detects correlations between two different nuclei that are separated by one bond. This method gives one peak per pair of coupled nuclei, whose two coordinates are the chemical shifts of the two coupled atoms.

The major difference between HETCOR and HMQC is that the HETCOR experiment is carbon detected, the HMQC method is proton detected. Due to the relative abundance and sensitivity differences between proton and carbon, the HMQC method is preferred than HETCOR.

e. Heteronuclear Single Quantum Correlation Spectroscopy (HSQC, 异核单量子相关谱)

HSQC gives an identical spectrum as HMQC. The two methods provide similar quality results for small to medium sized molecules, but HSQC is considered to be superior to larger molecules. The HSQC spectrum of sibiscolacton is shown in Figure 2-20.

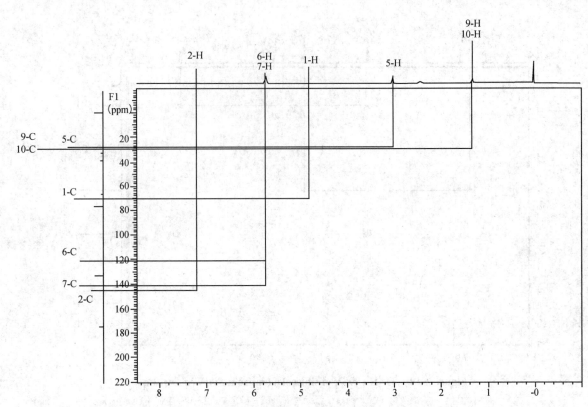

Figure 2-20   HSQC of sibiscolacton from *Sibiraea angustata*

f. Heteronuclear Multiple Bond Coherence (HMBC, 异核多键相关谱)

HMBC is proton detected long range $^1H-^{13}C$ heteronuclear correlation. It detects heteronuclear correlations over long ranges of about 2–4 bonds(including the coupling system separated by hetero atom). The difficulty of detecting multiple-bond correlations is that the HSQC and HMQC sequences contain a specific time–delay between pulses that allows the detection of only a range around a specific coupling constant. The interpretation of HMBC requires a degree of flexibility. It is because of that we do not always find what we expect to find. Some of the two-bond correlations ($^2J_{CH}$) or three-bond correlations ($^3J_{CH}$) are occasionally absent and four-bond correlations ($^4J_{CH}$) in frequently missing. The Key HMBC correlation and spectrum of sibiscolacton are shown in Figure 2-21 and Figure 2-22.

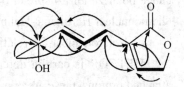

Figure 2-21   Key HMBC correlations of sibiscolacton

g. Nuclear Overhauser Effect Spectroscopy (NOESY, NOE差谱)

The nuclear overhauser cross relaxation between nuclear spins during the mixing period is used to establish correlations in NOESY. The spectrum obtained is similar to COSY, with diagonal and cross peaks, however the cross peaks connect resonances from nuclei that are spatially close rather than those that are through bond coupled to each other. One application of NOESY is in the study of large biomolecules such as in protein NMR.

h. Rotating-frame Overhauser Effect Spectroscopy (ROESY, 旋转 NOE差谱)

ROESY is similar to NOESY. The nuclear Overhauser effect difference experiment provides information about $^1H-^1H$ through space proximity. NOESY is used primarily with biological macromolecules. Both NOESY and ROESY experiments correlate protons that are close to each other in space (4.5 Å or less).

(5) Optical Rotary Dispersion (ORD, 旋光谱) and Circular Dichroism (CD, 圆二色谱)

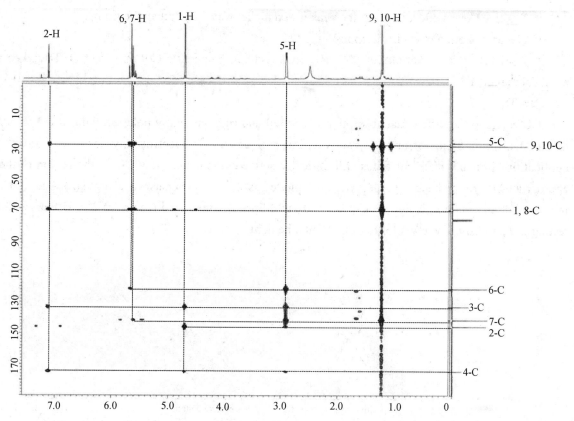

Figure 2-22　HMBC of sibiscolacton from *Sibiraea angustata*

① ORD

ORD is the variation in the optical rotation of an optical active compound with a change in the wavelength of light. ORD can be used to find the absolute configuration of the chiral (手性的) molecule. The ORD curve is a plot of molar rotation [*M*] versus wavelength (λ), and clockwise rotation is plotted positively, while counterclockwise rotation is plotted negatively, which is based solely on the index of refraction, because short wavelengths are rotated more than longer wavelengths. There are two kinds of ORD curves:

a. Chiral compound that lacks a chromophore (发色团) can give plain curves (Figure 2-23).

b. Chiral compounds containing a chromophore can give Cotton effect curves (Figure 2-24).

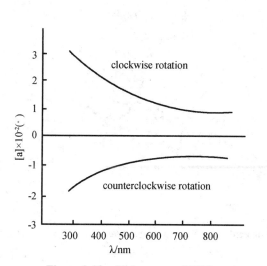

Figure 2-23　Plain curve of ORD

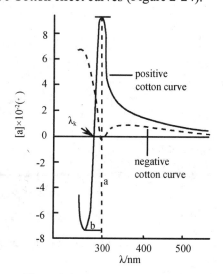

Figure 2-24　Cotton curve of ORD

• Positive Cotton effect is where the peak is at a higher wavelength than the trough
• Negative Cotton effect is the opposite
• Optically pure enantiomers (对映体) always display opposite Cotton effect ORD curves of identical magnitude.

② CD

CD refers to the differential absorption of the left and right circularly polarizedlight. It is exhibited in the absorption bands of optically activechiral molecules. CD spectroscopy has a wide range of applications in many different fields. All optically active compounds show CD in the region of their appropriate absorption band. CD spectroscopyis plotted as $\Delta\varepsilon$ (ε_L-ε_R) versus wavelength (λ). And for CD, the transmitted radiation is not plane-polarized but elliptically polarized (Figure 2-25). Usually before testing CD spectroscopy, UV spectroscopy should be done.

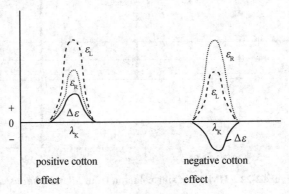

Figure 2-25   Cottoncurve of CD

(6) X-ray Crystal Diffraction Analysis (X射线单晶衍射分析)

The X-ray crystal diffraction analysis is the most powerful tool for determination of molecular structure, because it allows us to "see" atom positions in 3D space. This technology is particularly suitable for determination, confirmation, and establishment of conformation and configuration of complete molecular structures, especially those that are structurally novel or have a great deal of stereochemistry. Figure 2-26 is the solid structure of sibiraic acid from *Sibiraea angustata*.

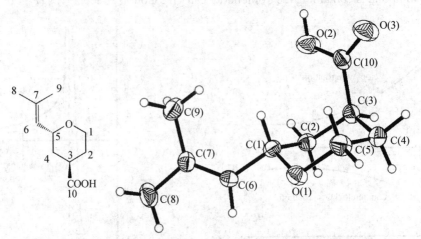

Figure 2-26   Solid structure of sibiraic acid from *Sibiraea angustata*

词 汇 表

An Alphabetical List of Words and Phrases

A		
absorbent	[ædˈsɔːbənt]	吸附剂
absorption	[əbˈzɔːpʃn]	吸收法
acetone	[ˈæsɪtəun]	丙酮
acetonitrile	[ˌæsɪtəuˈnaɪtril]	乙腈
activated charcoal	[ˈæktɪveɪtɪd][ˈtʃɑːkəul]	活性炭
adsorption	[ædˈsɔːpʃən]	吸附
adsorption chromatography	[ædˈsɔːpʃən][ˌkrəuməˈtɔgrəfi]	吸附色谱
affinity chromatography	[əˈfɪnəti][ˌkrəuməˈtɔgrəfi]	亲和色谱
aglycone	[æglìːˈkəun]	苷元
aliphatic	[ˌæləˈfætɪk]	脂肪族的
alkali	[ˈælkəlaɪ]	碱
alkaloid	[ˈælkəlɔɪd]	生物碱
amino acid	[əˈmiːnəu][ˈæsɪd]	氨基酸
anion	[ˈænaiən]	阴离子
asymmetry	[eɪˈsɪmətri]	不对称性
anthraquinone	[ˌænθrəˈkwɪnəun]	蒽醌
antibiotic	[ˌæntɪbaɪˈɔtɪk]	抗生素；抗生的
aromatic	[ˌærəˈmætɪk]	芳香族的
artifact	[ˈɑːtɪfækt]	人工产物
Aucklandiae Radix		木香
B		
benzenoid	[ˈbenzənɔɪd]	苯类的
benzoquinone	[ˌbenzəuˈkwɪnəun]	苯醌
bile acids	[baɪl][ˈæsɪdz]	胆汁酸
biosynthetic	[ˌbaɪəsɪnˈθetɪk]	生物合成的
C		
carbohydrate	[ˌkaːbəuˈhaɪdreɪt]	碳水化合物
cardiac glycoside	[ˈkaːdɪæk][ˈglaɪkəsaɪd]	强心苷
cation	[ˈkætaɪən]	阳离子
chalcone	[ˈkælkəun]	查耳酮
chemical ionization (CI)	[ˈkemɪkəl][ˌaɪənaɪˈzeɪʃn]	化学电离
chiral	[ˈtʃɪrəl]	手性的
chloroform	[ˈklɔːrəfɔːm]	三氯甲烷
chlorophyll	[ˈklɔːrəfɪl]	叶绿素

(continued)

cholesterol	[kəuˈləstərəl]	胆固醇，胆甾醇
chromatography	[ˌkrəuməˈtɔgrəfi]	色谱法
chromophore/chromophoric group	[ˈkrəuməfɔ:]/[ˌkrəuməˈfɔrɪk][gru:p]	发色团，生色团
circular dichroism (CD)	[ˈsə:kjulə][ˈdaɪkrəuɪzm]	圆二色谱
compromise	[ˈkɔmprəmaɪz]	综合
concentrate	[ˈkɔnsəntreɪt]	浓缩（液）；v. 浓缩
concentration	[ˌkɔnsenˈtreɪʃən]	浓度
conical	[ˈkɔnɪkl]	圆锥形的
correlation spectroscopy	[ˌkɔrəˈleɪʃn][spekˈtrɔskəpi]	化学位移相关光谱
coumarin	[ˈku:mərɪn]	香豆素
covalent bond	[kəuˈveɪlənt][bɔnd]	共价键
critical point	[ˈkrɪtɪkəl][pɔɪnt]	临界点
crystallization	[ˌkrɪstəlaɪˈzeɪʃn]	结晶
cyclodione		环二酮
cyclopentanoperhydrophenanthrene	[saɪkləupentəˈnəupəhaɪdrəu fəˈnænθri:n]	环戊烷骈多氢菲
cylindrical	[səˈlɪndrɪkl]	圆柱形的
D		
decoction	[dɪˈkɔkʃən]	煎煮
dehydration	[ˌdi:haɪˈdreɪʃn]	脱水
deionized water	[di:ˈaɪənaɪzd][ˈwɔ:tə]	去离子水
derivative	[dɪˈrɪvətɪv]	衍生物
deuterated	[ˈdju:təreɪtɪd]	含重氢的
dextran	[ˈdekstræn]	葡聚糖
dialysis	[daɪˈælɪsɪs]	透析
dichloromethane	[daɪklɔ:rəˈmeθeɪn]	二氯甲烷
distortion enhancement by polarization transfer (DEPT)	[dɪˈstɔ:ʃn][ɪnˈhɑ:nsmənt] [baɪ] [ˌpəulərɪˈzeɪʃn][trænsˈfə:]	极化转移增强谱
diterpene	[daɪtəˈpi:n]	二萜
duration	[djuˈreɪʃn]	时间
E		
electrodialysis	[ɪˌlektrəudaɪˈælɪsɪs]	电渗析，电泳
electrolysis	[ɪlekˈtrɔɪsɪs]	电解
electron impact (EI)	[ɪˈlektrɔn][ˈɪmpækt]	电子轰击
electronegativity	[ɪˈlektrəuˌnegəˈtɪvətɪ]	电负性
electrophoresis	[ɪˌlektrəfəˈri:sis]	电泳
electrospray ionization (ESI)	[elektrəuˈspreɪ][ˌaɪənaɪˈzeɪʃn]	电喷雾电离
eluent	[ˈelju:ənt]	洗脱剂

(continued)

enantiomer	[ɪˈnæntɪəumə]	对映体
enzymatic	[ˌenzaɪˈmætɪk]	酶的
epichlorohydrin	[epɪklɔːrəˈhaɪdrɪn]	环氧氯丙烷
equilibrium	[ˌiːkwəˈlɪbriːəm]	平衡
essential oil	[ɪˈsenʃl][ɔɪl]	精油
ethanol	[ˈeθənɔl]	乙醇
ethyl acetate	[ˈeθɪl][ˈæsɪteɪt]	乙酸乙酯
ethyl ether	[ˈeθɪl][ˈiːθə]	乙醚
F		
fast atom bombardment (FAB)	[fɑːst][ˈætəm][bɔmˈbɑːdmənt]	快原子轰击
field desorption (FD)	[fiːld][dɪˈsɔːpʃən]	场解吸
flammability	[ˌflæməˈbɪlɪti]	易燃性
flavanones	[ˈfleɪvənəunz]	二氢黄酮
flavonoid	[ˈfleɪvənəuɪd]	黄酮
fourier transform mass spectrometer	[ˈfɔːrɪə][trænsˈfɔːm][mæs][spekˈtrɔmɪtə]	傅里叶变换质谱仪
fractionation	[ˌfrækʃəˈneɪʃən]	分馏法，分别
G		
gel Filtration Chromatography	[dʒel][fɪlˈtreɪʃən][ˌkrəuməˈtɔɡrəfi]	凝胶过滤色谱
genin	[ˈdʒenɪn]	苷元
glycoside	[ˈɡlaɪkəˌsaɪd]	苷类
gradient elution	[ˈɡreɪdɪənt][ɪˈluːʃən]	梯度洗脱
grinding	[ˈɡraɪndɪŋ]	粉碎度
H		
hemiacetal	[ˌhemɪˈæsɪtæl]	半缩醛
hemiketal	[ˌhemɪˈkiːtəl]	半酮缩醇
heterocyclic	[ˌhetərəˈsaɪklɪk]	杂环的
heteronuclear correlation (HETCOR)	[ˌhetərəˈnjuːklɪə][ˌkɔːrəˈleɪʃn]	碳氢直接相关谱
heteronuclear multiple bond correlation (HMBC)	[ˌhetərəˈnjuːklɪə][ˈmʌltɪpl][bɔnd][ˌkɔːrəˈleɪʃn]	异核多键相关谱
heteronuclear multiple quantum coherence (HMQC)	[ˌhetərəˈnjuːklɪə][ˈmʌltɪpl][ˈkwɔntəm][kəuˈhɪərəns]	异核多量子相关谱
heteronuclear single quantum correlation spectroscopy (HSQC)	[ˌhetərəˈnjuːklɪə][ˈsɪŋgl][ˈkwɔntəm][ˌkɔːrəˈleɪʃn][spekˈtrɔskəpɪ]	异核单量子相关谱
hexane	[hekˈseɪn]	正己烷
homonuclear	[ˌhɔməˈnjuːklɪə]	同核
hydrophilic	[ˌhaɪdrəˈfɪlɪk]	亲水的
hydrophobic	[ˌhaɪdrəfəuˈbɪk]	疏水的

(continued)

hydrostatic	[ˌhaɪdrəʊˈstætɪk]	静力学的
hydroxyl	[haɪˈdrɒksɪl]	羟基
I		
idiophase	[ˌɪdɪˈɔfeɪs]	繁殖期
immerse	[ɪˈmə:s]	浸渍
immiscible	[ɪˈmɪsəbl]	不能混合的，不互溶的
immunoaffinity chromatography	[ɪmjunəʊˈfɪnɪtɪ][ˌkrəʊməˈtɒɡrəfɪ]	免疫亲和色谱
impurity	[ɪmˈpjʊərəti]	杂质
inert	[ɪˈnə:t]	惰性的
infrared spectrometry (IR)	[ˌɪnfrəˈred][spekˈtrɒmɪtrɪ]	红外光谱
intermediate	[ˌɪntəˈmi:dɪət]	中间体
ion exchange chromatography	[ˈaɪən][ɪksˈtʃeɪndʒ][ˌkrəʊməˈtɒɡrəfɪ]	离子交换色谱
ionization	[ˌaɪənaɪˈzeɪʃn]	离子化，电离化
ion trap mass spectrometer	[ˈaɪən][træp][mæs][spekˈtrɒmɪtə]	离子阱质谱仪
i-propanol	[ˌaɪsəˈprəʊpənɒl]	异丙醇
L		
Lasianthus Acuminatissimus	[ˈleɪʃnθəs][əkjuˌmɪnəˈtɪsɪməs]	长尾粗叶木
lignan	[ˈlɪɡnæn]	木脂素
lipophilic	[ˌlɪpəˈfɪlɪk]	亲脂性的
M		
maceration	[ˌmæsəˈreɪʃən]	浸渍
macroporous Resin	[ˈmækrəˈpɔ:rəs][ˈrezɪn]	大孔树脂
magnetic sector mass spectrometer	[mæɡˈnetɪk][ˈsektə][mæs][spekˈtrɒmɪtə]	扇形磁场质谱仪
mass spectrometry	[mæs][spekˈtrɒmɪtrɪ]	质谱
mass spectrum	[mæs][ˈspektrəm]	质谱
metabolite	[meˈtæbəlaɪt]	代谢物
methanol	[ˈmeθənɒl]	甲醇
methyl acetate	[ˈmeθɪl][ˈæsɪteɪt]	乙酸甲酯
mevalonic acid (MVA)	[ˌmevəˈləʊnɪk][ˈæsɪd]	甲戊二羟酸
microfiltration	[ˌmaɪkrəʊfɪlˈtreɪʃn]	微滤
microplate-based ultrasensitive	[maɪkrəʊˈpleɪt][beɪst][ˈʌltrəˈsensɪtɪv]	基于微孔板的超灵敏性
microporous	[ˌmaɪkrəʊˈpɔ:rəs]	多微孔的
mobile phase	[ˈməʊbaɪl][feɪz]	流动相
monosaccharide	[ˌmɒnəʊˈsækəraɪd]	单糖
monoterpene	[ˌmɒnəˈtə:pi:n]	单萜
N		
nanofiltration	[nænɔ:fɪltˈreɪʃn]	纳米过滤

Chapter 2 General Methods for Chemical Investigation of Chinese Herbs

(continued)

naphthoquinone	['næfθəkwɪ'nəun]	萘醌
n-butanol	['bjutənəul]	正丁醇
noncorrosive	['nɒnkə'rəusɪv]	无腐蚀性的
normal-phase chromatography	['nɔːml][feɪz][ˌkrəumə'tɒgrəfi]	正相色谱
nuclear magnetic resonance	['njuːklɪə(r)][mæg'netɪk]['rezənəns]	核磁共振
nuclear overhauser effect (NOE)	['njuːklɪə(r)][ˌəuvə'hɔːzə][ɪ'fekt]	核的增益效应
nuclear overhauser effect spectroscopy (NOESY)	['njuːklɪə(r)][ˌəuvə'hɔːzə][ɪ'fekt][spek'trɒskəpi]	NOE 差谱
O		
operational hazard	[ˌɒpə'reɪʃənl]['hæzəd]	操作的危险性
optical rotary dispersion (ORD)	['ɒptɪkəl]['rəutəri][dɪs'pɜːʃn]	旋光谱
optimization	[ˌɒptɪmaɪ'zeɪʃən]	最优化
P		
Partition Chromatography	[pɑː'tɪʃn][ˌkrəumə'tɒgrəfi]	分配色谱
partition coefficient	[pɑː'tɪʃn]['kəuɪ'fɪʃnt]	分配系数
peptide	['peptaɪd]	肽
percolation	[ˌpɜːkə'leɪʃn]	渗漉
petroleum ether	[pɪ'trəulɪəm]['iːθə]	石油醚
phenanthraquinone	[fɪnənθrækwɪ'nəun]	菲醌
phenolic	[fɪ'nɒlɪk]	酚的
phenylchromone	[fenɪlk'rəumnəun]	苯基色原酮
phenylpropanoid	[fenɪl'prɒpənɔɪd]	苯丙氨酸，苯丙素
pheromone	['ferəməun]	信息素
phytochemical	[ˌfaɪtəu'kemɪkəl]	植物化学的
pigment	['pɪgmənt]	色素
polyamide	[pɒlɪ'æmaɪd]	聚酰胺
polyhydroxyaldehyde	[pɒlɪhaɪdrɒksɪ'əːldɪhaɪd]	多羟基醛
polyhydroxyketone	[pɒlɪhaɪ'drɒksaɪktəun]	多羟基酮
polyketide	[pɒ'laɪkɪtaɪd]	聚酮
polysaccharide	[ˌpɒlɪ'sækəraɪd]	多糖
polyterpene	['pɒlɪ'tɜːpiːn]	多萜
precipitation	[prɪˌsɪpɪ'teɪʃn]	沉淀
pressurized	['preʃəraɪzd]	加压的
proton	['prəutɒn]	质子
pulverize	['pʌlvəraɪz]	粉碎，把……弄碎
purification	[ˌpjuərɪfɪ'keɪʃn]	纯化
pyridine	[ˌpɪrə'daɪnə]	吡啶

49

(continued)

Q		
quadrupole mass spectrometer	[ˈkwɔdrəpəul][mæs][spekˈtrɔmɪtə]	四极质谱仪
quinone	[kwɪˈnəun]	醌类
R		
reflux	[ˈriːflʌks]	回流
resin	[ˈrezɪn]	树脂
reverse osmosis	[rɪˈvəːs][ɔzˈməusɪs]	反相渗透
reversed-phase chromatography	[rɪˈvəːst][feɪz][ˌkrəuməˈtɔgrəfi]	反相色谱
Rotating-frame Overhauser Effect Spectroscopy (ROESY)	[rəuˈteɪtɪŋ][freɪm][ˌəuvəˈhɔːzə][ɪˈfekt][spekˈtrɔskəpi]	旋转 NOE 差谱
S		
saccharide	[ˈsækəraɪd]	糖类
sapogenin	[səˈpudʒənɪn]	皂苷元
saponin	[ˈsæpənɪn]	皂苷
semipermeable	[ˈsemɪˈpəːmɪəbl]	半透性的
separation technology	[ˌsepəˈreɪʃn][tekˈnɔlədʒi]	分离技术
Sephadex LH-20		羟丙基葡聚糖凝胶
sesquiterpene	[ˌseskwɪˈtəːpiːn]	倍半萜
sesterterpene	[sestəˈtəːpiːn]	二倍半萜
shikimic acid/shikimate	[ʃɪˈkɪmɪk][ˈæsɪd] / [ˈʃɪkɪmeɪt]	莽草酸
Sibiraea Angustata		窄叶鲜卑花
silica gel	[ˈsɪlɪkə][dʒel]	硅胶
skeleton	[ˈskelɪtn]	骨架
solubility	[ˌsɔljuˈbɪləti]	溶解度
solubilization	[ˌsɔljubɪlaɪˈzeɪʃən]	溶解
Soxhlet extraction		索氏提取
spectroscope	[ˈspektrəskəup]	波谱方法
stationary phase	[ˈsteɪʃənəri][feɪz]	固定相
steam distillation	[stiːm][ˌdɪstəˈleɪʃn]	水蒸气蒸馏
stereochemistry	[ˌstɪərɪəˈkemɪstrɪ]	立体化学
steroid	[ˈstɪərɔɪd]	甾体，甾族化合物，类固醇
sterol	[ˈsterəul]	固醇，甾醇
sublimation	[ˌsʌblɪˈmeɪʃn]	升华法，升华物
supercritical fluid	[ˌsjuːpəˈkrɪtɪkəl][ˈfluːɪd]	超临界流体
supercritical fluid extraction	[ˌsjuːpəˈkrɪtɪkəl][ˈfluːɪd][ɪkˈstrækʃn]	超临界流体提取
T		
tandem	[ˈtædəm]	串联的

(continued)

tannin	['tænɪn]	鞣质
terpenes	[təˈpiːnɪz]	萜烯
terpenoid	[ˈtəːpənɔɪd]	萜类
tetrachloride	[ˌtetrəˈklɔːraɪd]	四氯化碳
tetrahydrofuran	[tetrəhaɪdrəˈfjuərən]	四氢呋喃
tetraterpene	[tetreɪtəˈpiːn]	四萜
thermolabile	[ˌθəːməuˈleɪbɪl]	不耐热的
time-of-flight mass spectrometer	[taɪm][əv][flaɪt] [mæs][spekˈtrɒmɪtə]	飞行时间质谱仪
toluene	[ˈtɒljuiːn]	甲苯
total correlation spectroscopy (TOCSY)	[ˈtəutəl][ˌkɒrəˈleɪʃn][spekˈtrɒskəpi]	全相关谱
toxicity	[tɒkˈsɪsɪtiː]	毒性
U		
ultrafiltration	[ˌʌltrəfɪlˈtreɪʃən]	超滤
ultrasonic extraction	[ˌʌltrəˈsɒnɪk][ɪkˈstrækʃn]	超声波提取
Ultrasound-assisted	[ˈʌltrəsaund][əˈsɪstɪd]	超声辅助的
ultraviolet spectroscopy (UV)	[ʌltrəˈvaɪələt][spekˈtrɒskəpi]	紫外光谱
ultraviolet-visible spectrometry	[ʌltrəˈvaɪələt][ˈvɪzɪb(ə)l][spekˈtrɒmɪtri]	紫外－可见光波谱
unsaturate	[ʌnˈsætʃərɪt]	未饱和的，不饱和的
V		
viscosity	[vɪˈskɒsəti]	黏性，黏度
vitro assays	[ˈvɪtrəu][əˈseɪz]	体外实验
volatile	[ˈvɒlətaɪl]	易挥发的
volatility	[ˌvɒləˈtɪləti]	挥发性
X		
X-ray crystal diffraction analysis	[ˈeksˌreɪ][ˈkrɪst(ə)l][dɪˈfrækʃn][əˈnælɪsɪs]	X 射线单晶衍射分析
xylene	[ˈzaɪliːn]	二甲苯

重 点 小 结

中药化学成分的生物合成途径有：乙酸－丙二酸途径、甲戊二羟酸和脱氧木酮糖磷酸途径、莽草酸途径、氨基酸途径和复合途径。

中药化学成分按照结构母核分类，主要有：糖类、苷类、醌类、苯丙素类、黄酮类、鞣质类、生物碱类、萜类、甾体类和皂苷类等。

中药中有效成分的提取分离常用的溶剂有：石油醚、环己烷、二氯甲烷、三氯甲烷、乙醚、乙酸乙酯、正丁醇、丙酮、乙醇、甲醇和水等。

中药化学成分的提取方法有：溶剂法、水蒸气蒸馏法、超临界流体萃取法、升华法、吸收法等。其中，溶剂法是最常用的一种，提取原理是"相似相溶"。常用溶剂包括水、亲水性有机溶剂（乙醇、甲醇和丙酮）和亲脂性有机溶剂（石油醚、环己烷、三氯甲烷、乙醚、乙酸乙酯和正丁醇等）。溶剂提取法的操作方法包括：浸渍法、渗漉法、煎煮法、回流提取法和连续回流提取法。浸渍法适用于热不稳定成分的提取或含大量淀粉、果胶、黏液质的中药提取，但效率较低；渗漉法同样适用于热不稳定成分的提取，提取效率高于浸渍法，但溶剂消耗量较大、费时较长；煎煮法简单易行，但含挥发性成分或热不稳定成分的提取不宜用；回流提取法可使用有机溶剂，但溶剂消耗较大，不适用于热不稳定成分的提取；连续回流提取法弥补了回流提取法中溶剂消耗量较大的不足，但耗时较长，也不适用于提取热不稳定成分。超声、微波等常用于辅助溶剂提取法。

常用的分离方法包括溶剂分离法、沉淀法、结晶法、膜分离法、分馏、色谱法等。溶剂分离法又包括酸碱溶剂法和系统溶剂萃取法，常用于粗提物的初步分离；沉淀法可以根据被分离组分在不同溶剂中溶解度的不同采用溶剂沉淀法，也可以根据被分离组分的结构特点选择专属性沉淀试剂进行沉淀法分离；结晶法主要用于含杂质较少的最后纯化阶段；色谱法是应用最广泛的分离方法，根据分离原理，色谱法可分为：吸附色谱法、分配色谱法、离子交换色谱法、大孔树脂色谱法、凝胶过滤色谱法、免疫亲和色谱法和细胞膜色谱法等。吸附色谱法应用较广，利用吸附剂对被分离组分的吸附能力差异而达到分离的目的。常见的吸附剂有硅胶、氧化铝、聚酰胺和活性炭等。分配色谱法是利用被分离组分在固定相与流动相之间的分配系数差异来实现分离，根据固定相和流动相的极性不同分为正相分配色谱和反相分配色谱。离子交换色谱适合分离带电荷或可电离的化合物，如酸性、碱性或两性化合物。大孔树脂是吸附性与分子筛原理相结合的分离材料，它的吸附性是范德华力或产生氢键的结果，分子筛作用是由大孔吸附树脂的多孔性决定的。凝胶色谱法是利用分子筛原理分离物质的一种方法，物质分子按由大到小的顺序先后流出。

为了顺利测定化合物的结构，获得准确的波谱信息，在进行结构测定前需进行纯度检查，可根据熔距的大小判断化合物的纯度，也常用色谱法（TLC法和HPLC法）检查化合物的纯度。紫外光谱（UV）、红外光谱（IR）、质谱（MS）和核磁共振光谱（NMR）四大波谱技术可用于鉴定中药化学成分的结构，旋光谱、圆二色谱和X-单晶衍射等技术可用于确定化学成分的立体结构。其中，核磁共振谱（1D, 2D-NMR）可以用于绝大多数化合物的平面结构及立体结构鉴定，是最为重要的结构鉴定方法。质谱技术是根据化合物分子经离子化、裂解产生的各种碎片离子，获得化合物结构信息的最灵敏的方法，主要提供分子质量、分子式和断裂模式等信息。红外光谱主要提供化合物官能团信息，如羟基、羰基等。紫外光谱只用于不饱和共轭体系的初步判断。

目 标 检 测

题库

一、单选题

1.下列溶剂中，毒性最小的是（　　　）
　　A. 三氯甲烷　　　　B. 吡啶　　　　　C. 二氯甲烷　　　　D. 甲苯　　　　E. 甲醇
2.下列哪种提取方法最适合生物碱的提取（　　　）
　　A. 酸提碱沉　　　　　　　B. 碱提酸沉　　　　　　　　C. 水提醇沉
　　D. 醇提水沉　　　　　　　E. 有机溶剂提取

3. 确定化合物的分子式和分子量可采用（　　　）
   A. UV　　　　　　B. IR　　　　　　C. HR-MS　　　　D. ^{1}H-NMR　　E. ^{13}C-NMR

4. 水蒸气蒸馏法主要用于提取（　　　）
   A. 强心苷　　　B. 生物碱　　　C. 糖类　　　D. 黄酮苷　　　E. 挥发油

5. 下列哪种波谱不是吸收光谱（　　　）
   A. 紫外　　　　B. 红外　　　C. 氢谱　　　D. 碳谱　　　E. 质谱

6. 与水能分层的有机溶剂是（　　　）
   A. 正丁醇　　　B. 乙醇　　　C. 甲醇　　　D. 丙酮　　　E. 异丙醇

7. 有关氧化铝性质叙述错误的是（　　　）
   A. 氧化铝是一种极性吸附剂　　　　　B. 分为碱性、中性、酸性三种
   C. 碱性适合分离碱性成分　　　　　　D. 酸性适合分离酸性成分
   E. 中性适合分离酸性、碱性、中性成分

8. 对凝胶过滤色谱（Sephadex G）叙述不正确的是（　　　）
   A. 大分子被阻滞，流动慢；小分子阻滞小，流动快
   B. 凝胶过滤色谱的原理是分子筛
   C. 适合分离蛋白质、多糖等
   D. 常以吸水量大小决定凝胶分离范围
   E. 凝胶吸水量小时，用于分离分子量较小的物质

9. 从中药水煎液中萃取有效成分不能使用的溶剂是（　　　）
   A. 乙醚　　　B. 三氯甲烷　　　C. 丙酮　　　D. 正丁醇　　　E. 乙酸乙酯

10. 结晶法成败的最关键步骤是（　　　）
    A. 控制好温度　　　　　B. 选择合适溶剂　　　　　C. 除尽杂质
    D. 做成饱和溶液　　　　E. 适当时间

二、多选题

1. 常用的溶剂提取方法有（　　　）
   A. 浸渍法　　　　　　　　B. 渗漉法　　　　　　　　C. 煎煮法
   D. 回流提取法　　　　　　E. 连续回流提取法

2. 水能较容易地提取出的有效成分有（　　　）
   A. 挥发油　　　B. 甾醇　　　C. 鞣质　　　D. 糖类　　　E. 蜡

3. 利用有机溶剂提取中药成分时，一般采用（　　　）
   A. 浸渍法　　　　　　　　B. 渗漉法　　　　　　　　C. 煎煮法
   D. 回流提取法　　　　　　E. 连续回流提取法

4. 中药成分结构研究时采用的主要方法有（　　　）
   A. HPLC　　　B. MS　　　C. GC　　　D. UV　　　E. NMR

5. 常见的生物合成途径有（　　　）
   A. 醋酸－丙二酸途径　　　　B. 甲戊二羟酸途径　　　　C. 莽草酸途径
   D. 氨基酸途径　　　　　　　E. 复合途径

6. 下列溶剂或基本结构相同的化合物按极性增大的排序，正确排列的是（　　　）
   A. 石油醚、苯、乙醚、三氯甲烷、乙酸乙酯、正丁醇、丙酮、乙醇、甲醇、水

B. 烷、烯、醚、酯、酮、醛、胺、醇和酚、酸

C. 正丁醇、石油醚、水

D. 水、乙醚、胺

E. 石油醚、三氯甲烷、乙酸乙酯、正丁醇、乙醇、水

7. 适用于热不稳定成分的提取方法有（　　　）

A. 浸渍法　　　　　　　　　　B. 渗漉法　　　　　　　　　　C. 煎煮法

D. 回流提取法　　　　　　　　E. 超声提取法

8. 超声波提取法是采用超声波辅助溶剂进行提取，其特点为（　　　）

A. 超声波产生高速、强烈的空化效应和搅拌作用

B. 破坏有效成分的结构

C. 破坏植物药材的细胞，使溶剂渗透到药材细胞中

D. 缩短提取时间，提高提取率

E. 延长提取时间，提高提取率

9. 二氧化碳超临界流体萃取法的适用范围有（　　　）

A. 适用于对热不稳定物质的提取

B. 适用于脂溶性成分的提取

C. 适用于水溶性成分的提取

D. 加入夹带剂，改变萃取介质的极性，适用于水溶性成分的提取

E. 加入夹带剂，改变萃取介质的极性，适用于脂溶性成分的提取

10. 结晶法选择溶剂的原则是（　　　）

A. 沸点不能太高，不与结晶化合物发生反应

B. 结晶化合物加热溶解，放冷析出结晶

C. 杂质化合物加热溶解，放冷不析出结晶

D. 首选常见溶剂为水、乙醇、甲醇、丙酮等

E. 选择单一溶剂不能结晶，可选用混合溶剂如乙醇 – 水

三、简答题

1. 简述 ^{1}H-NMR 谱在中药化学成分结构研究中的作用。

2. 简述正相分配色谱和反相分配色谱的概念及其应用范围。

（李　斌）

Chapter 3　Saccharides and Glycosides

PPT

 学习目标

知识要求：

1. 掌握　糖和苷的定义及主要理化性质；掌握苷的提取分离及检识方法。

2. 熟悉　糖和苷的分类及结构研究的一般程序及方法。

3. 了解　枸杞子和苦杏仁中主要活性成分的结构特征及其饮片的质量控制标准。

能力要求：

学会应用 Molish 反应检识苷类化合物；学会应用苷键裂解的原理，结合具体苷类化合物的结构特征选择适合的提取分离方法，解决苷类化合物在提取分离过程中存在的技术问题。

1　Saccharides

1.1　Introduction

Saccharides (糖) maybe defined as polyhydroxyaldehydes (多羟基醛) or polyhydroxyketones (多羟基酮), or compounds that upon hydrolysis produce any of the above. They are also called carbohydrates (碳水化合物) or hydrates of carbon, because most of them are in the form of $C_nH_{2n}O_n$ or $C_n(H_2O)_n$. Some saccharides, such as methylpentose (甲基五碳糖), amino sugar (氨基糖), deoxy sugar (去氧糖), uronic acid (糖醛酸), and alcohol sugar (醇糖), are not in the form of $C_nH_{2n}O_n$ or $C_n(H_2O)_n$.

Saccharides are substances of universal occurrence and are abundant in plants, animals and microorganisms. For example, Ginseng Radix et Rhizoma, Astragali Radix (黄芪), Lycii Fructus (枸杞子), and many Chinese herbs contain a large number of saccharides, which have many biological activities such as anti-tumor, anti-aging, protection of liver and kidney, regulation of immune system. Saccharides are an essential structural component of living cells, a source of energy for the organism existing in forms of starch, cellulose, chitin, glycogen, and etc. Saccharides combine with non-sugar (or aglycone, 苷元) to form glycosides (苷). Many glycosides are active components of Chinese herbs, such as ginsenosides (人参皂苷), astragalosides (黄芪皂苷), and so on.

医药大学堂
WWW.YIYAODXT.COM

1.2　Structure and Classification

Monosaccharides（单糖）are sugars that cannot be further hydrolyzed. More than 200 natural monosaccharides have been found. They contain 3 to 8 carbon atoms, but five or six carbon monosaccharides are common, such as ribose ($C_5H_{10}O_5$) and glucose ($C_6H_{12}O_6$).

Monosaccharides have two of the most common functional groups, aldehyde（醛）and ketone（酮）. A monosaccharide containing aldehyde is known as an aldose（醛糖）. If it contains ketone, it is called ketose or keto sugar（酮糖）. When a monosaccharide contains carboxyl（羧基）or amino groups（氨基）, it is named as uronic acid or amino sugar respectively, such as glucuronic acid（葡萄糖醛酸）, and glucosamine（氨基葡萄糖）(2–amino–2–deoxy–D–glucose). A monosaccharide that lacks the usual numbers of hydroxyl groups（羟基）is often called a deoxy sugar, e.g. 2–deoxyribose（2– 去氧核糖）.

Monosaccharides may exist as open chain molecules (Fisher projection) or as cyclic compounds (Haworth projection).The ring structure of hemiacetal（半缩醛）or hemiketal（半缩酮）is formed by the intramolecular nucleophilic reaction（分子内亲核反应）of a hydroxyl group and a carbonyl group（羰基）. Many monosaccharides exist in an equilibrium condition（平衡条件）between open chain and cyclic forms. The cyclic monosaccharides commonly have a six-membered pyranose（吡喃糖）or a five-membered furanose（呋喃糖）structure. The formation of the ring or the cyclic structure is demonstrated below (Figure 3-1, Figure 3-2).

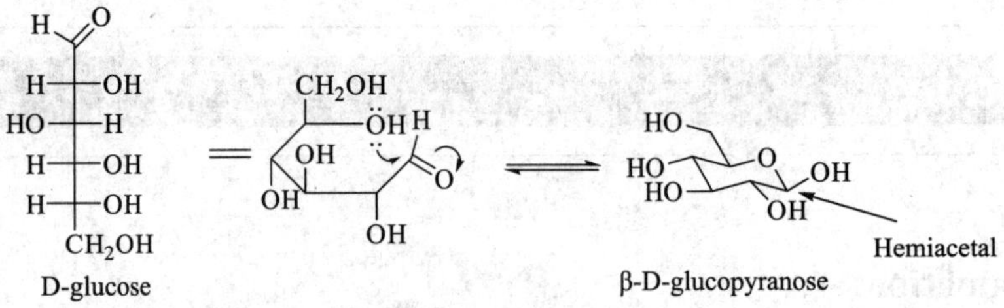

Figure 3-1　Cyclization of glucose

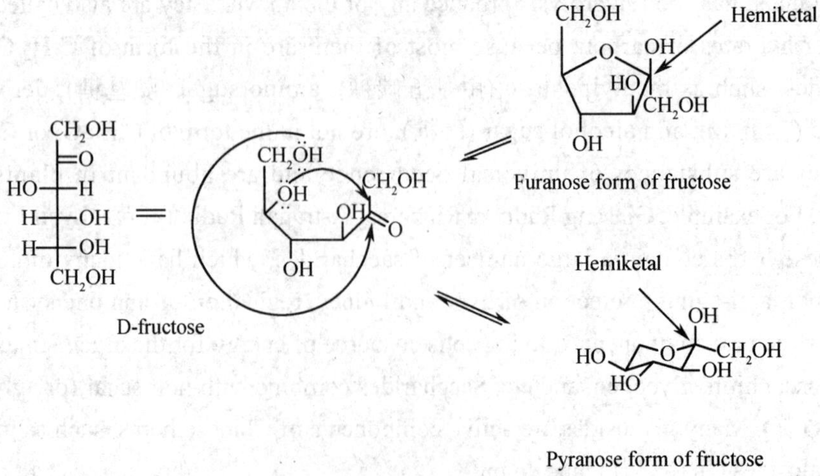

Figure 3-2　Cyclization of fructose

In the open chain form, if the hydroxyl group on the chiral carbon (手性碳) farthest from the carbonyl group is on the right hand, the monosaccharide has the same configuration (构型) as D-glyceraldehyde（D– 甘油醛）, e.g. D-glucose. In the same way, a monosaccharide will have the same configuration as L-glyceraldehyde if the hydroxyl group is on the left hand, e.g. L-rhamnose.

In the cyclic form, the terminal unit (the "—R" or —CH₂OH in Figure 3-3) in a Fisher formula (C-5 in pyranose or C-4 in furanose) can project upwards (D configuration) or downwards (L configuration). As a consequence of the formation of the ring structure, a new chiral center at C-1 forms and it is called anomeric carbon (端基碳) (Figure 3-3).

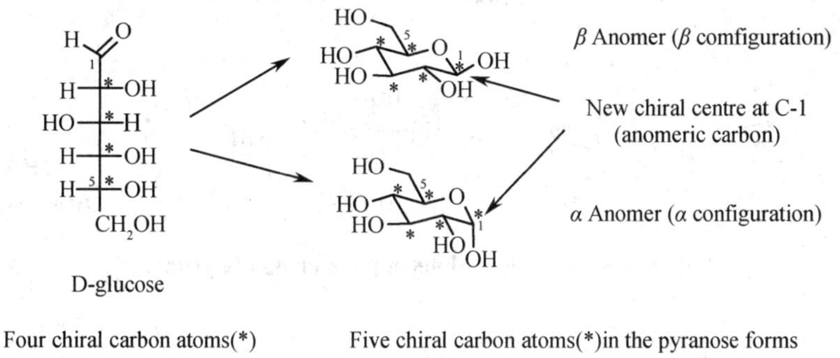

Figure 3-3 Chiral carbon atoms in glucose

Also during the formation of the ring structure, the reaction between the carbonyl group and the hydroxyl group can happen in two directions and consequently two anomers（端基异构体）are formed. When the direction of the terminal unit is the same as that of the hydroxyl group at the anomeric carbon, the configuration of the monosaccharide is *β*, e.g. *β*-D-glucose. Conversely, if the terminal unit is at the opposite direction as the hydroxyl group at the anomeric carbon, the configuration of the monosaccharide is α, e.g. α-L-rhamnose. A monosaccharide can have four configurations: α-D, β-D, α-L, and β-L. In reality, the absolute configurations of anomeric carbons of β-D and α-L are the same, and those of α-D and β-L are the same. Most of the monosaccharides exist as β-D or α-L format in nature. It is important to note that each sugar can exist as more than one optically active isomer (光学活性异构体). However, only one form is normally presented in plants. For example, glucose is usually the β-D-isomer and rhamnose is the α-L-isomer. Also, each monosaccharide can theoretically exist in both pyranose and furanose although one of the forms is usually favored. Glucose normally maintains the pyrano-configuration whereas fructose is usually the furano-form (Figure 3-4, Some hydroxyl groups are not drawn in the following sugar structural formula).

Furan ring of furanose is plane shaped and pyran ring of pyranose is boat and chair shaped. The chair configuration, which is the preferred configuration, includes C1 and 1C as shown below. Most of monosaccharides exist as C1 configuration, only few as 1C (i.e. D-glucose, L-rhamnose, Figure 3-5).

The hydroxyl group on the anomeric carbon in the cyclic structure of a monosaccharide is called hemiacetal (i.e. in glucose) or hemiketal (i.e. in fructose). If it is replaced by a –OR group, acetal or ketal is formed (Figure 3-6). R can be a non-sugar group or another sugar. When R is a non-sugar, the product is named as glycoside. The non-sugar group is called aglycone or genin (配基). The chemical bond between the anomeric carbon and the bridging atom in the non-sugar group is called glycosidic linkage (苷键). The bridging atom is named as glycosidic atom (苷原子).

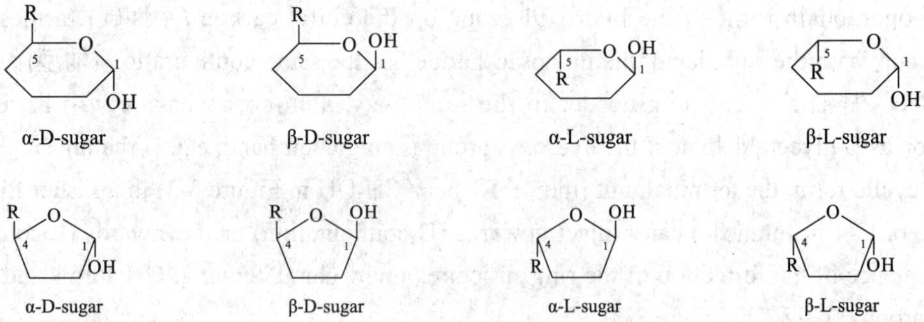

Figure 3-4   Configurations of a monosaccharide

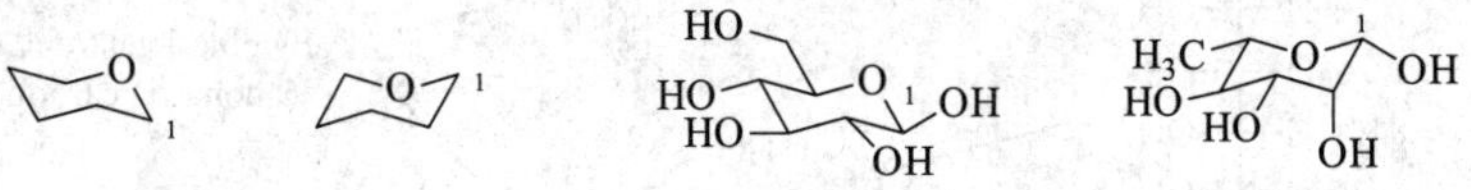

Figure 3-5   Configurations of pyran ring of pyranoses

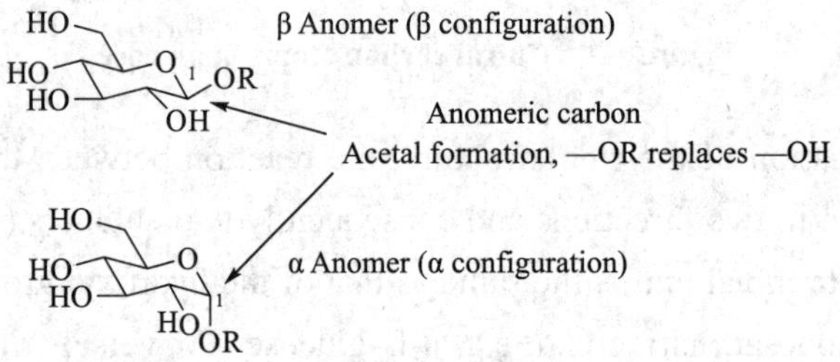

Figure 3-6   Acetal formation of glucopyranose

Saccharides are classified into monosaccharide, oligosaccharide (低聚糖) and polysaccharide (多糖) based on the number of simple sugars it can produce upon hydrolysis.

Monosaccharides are sugars that cannot be further hydrolyzed to simple sugars. They are the smallest units to form saccharides. The main monosaccharides and derivatives presented in plants are listed in Table 3-1.

Table 3-1   Main monosaccharides and derivatives presented in plants

Categories	Examples		
Pentoses (五碳糖)	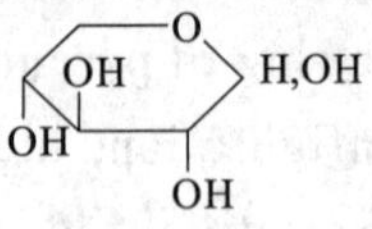 D-xylose	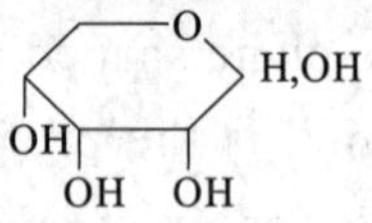 D-ribose	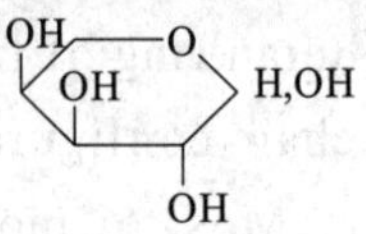 L-arabinose
Methylpentoses (甲基五碳糖)	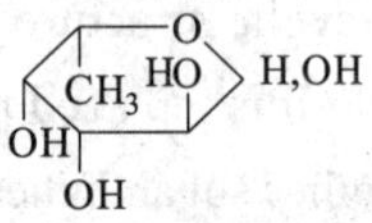 L-fucose	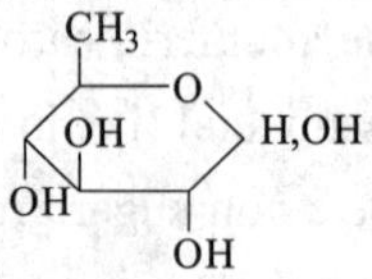 L-quinovose	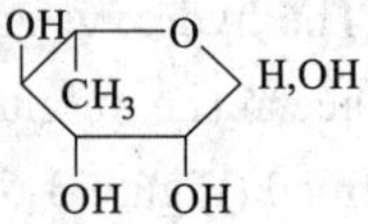 L-rhamnose

(continued)

Categories	Examples		
Aldohexose (己醛糖)	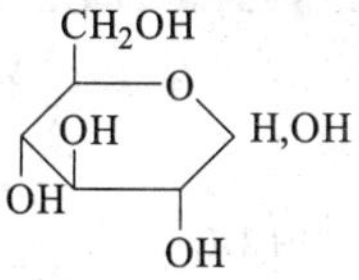 D-glucose	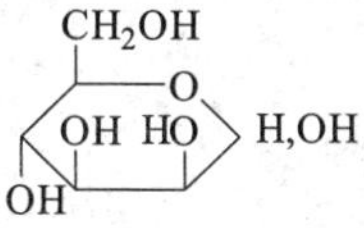 D-mannose	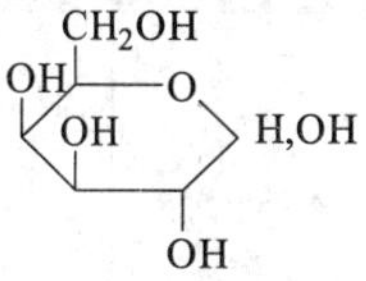 D-galactose
Ketohexose (己酮糖)	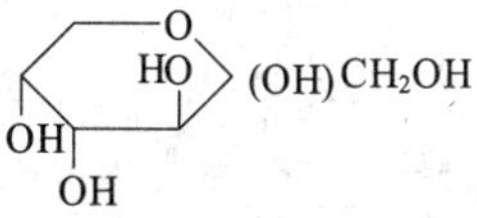 D-fructose	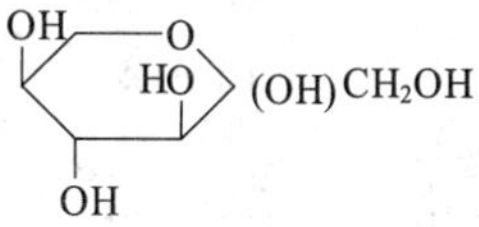 L-sorbose	
Ketoheptose (庚酮糖)	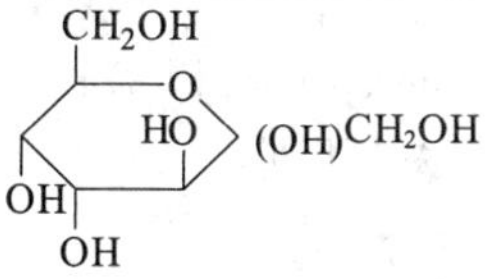 D-sedoheptulose		
Hexuronic acid (己糖醛酸)	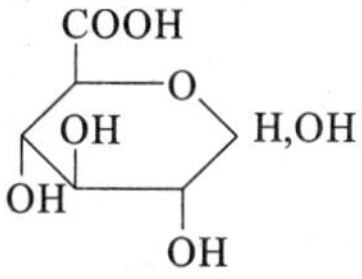 D-glucuronic acid	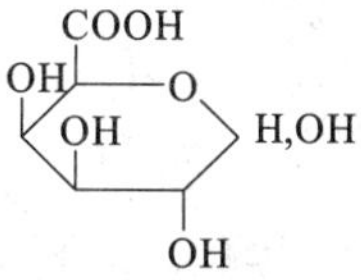 D-galacuronic acid	
Hexitol (己糖醇)	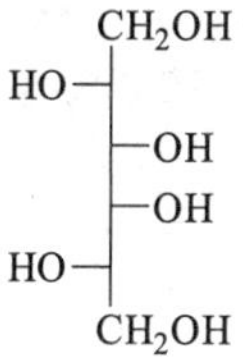 ducitol	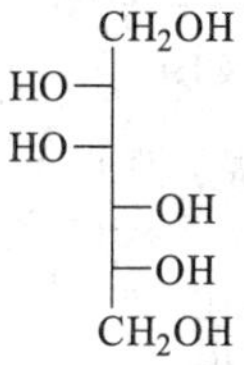 D-mannitol	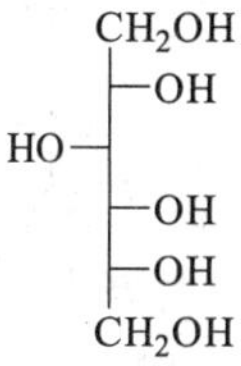 D-sorbitol
Special monosaccharides	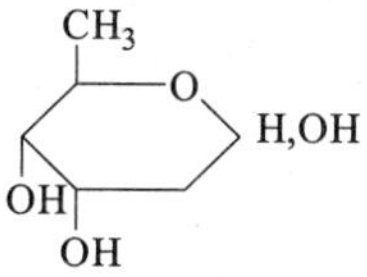 D-digitoxose	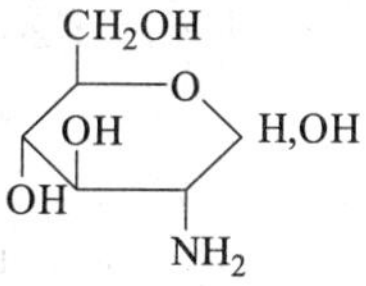 2-amino-2-deoxy-D-glucose	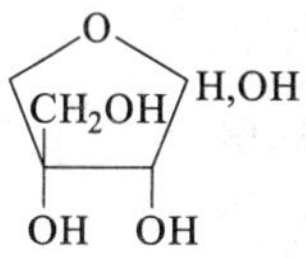 D-apiose

The saccharides that can be hydrolyzed to yield 2–9 molecules of monosaccharides are called oligosaccharide. Oligosaccharides containing 2–4 molecules of monosaccharides are the most common in plants. They are named as disaccharides (双糖), trisaccharides (三糖) and tetrasaccharides (四糖) respectively. Examples of di-, tri-, and tetrasaccharides from Chinese herbs are listed in Table 3-2. Based on whether a sugar molecule contains free hemiacetal hydroxyl group or not, oligosaccharides are grouped into reducing sugar (还原糖) (e.g. rutinose, sophorose, and neohesperidose) and non-reducing sugar (非还原糖）(e.g. sucrose).

59

Table 3-2   Examples of di-, tri-, and tetrasaccharides from Chinese herbs

Categories	Examples
Disaccharide (二糖)	sucrose, sophorose (槐糖), neohesperidose (新橙皮糖), rutinose (芸香糖), gentiobiose (龙胆二糖)
Trisaccharide (三糖)	raffinose (棉子糖)
Tetrasaccharide (四糖)	stachyose (水苏糖)

Polysaccharides are composed of ten or more monosaccharides by glycosidic linkages. The commonly found polysaccharides in plants include starch, cellulose, hemicellulose (半纤维素), fructans (果聚糖), gum (树胶), mucilage (黏液质), and pectin substance (果胶质). Glycogen (糖原), chitin (壳多糖，几丁质), heparin (肝素), chondroitin sulfate (硫酸软骨素), and hyaluronic acid (透明质酸) are polysaccharides commonly presented in animals. Polysaccharides are also found in fungi, such as Ganoderma (灵芝), Poria (茯苓), and Polyporus (猪苓) etc.

Some polysaccharides can dissolve in water, hence named as soluble polysaccharides. They serve as nutritional substances in living organisms, for example, starch, gum, and pectin. Most of the soluble polysaccharides are branched-chain polysaccharides and they become colloid when dissolved in water.

Polysaccharides that are insoluble in water are called insoluble polysaccharides (i.e. cellulose and chitin). They are in the line-chain form and serve as the main structural elements for many living organisms.

A number of the same monosaccharide units combine together, forming a homosaccharide (均多糖). The naming convention for homosaccharide is to add "-an" to the monosaccharide name, such as glucan, fructan, etc. Heterosaccharide (杂多糖) is composed of two or more different kinds of monosaccharides. The naming convention is to arrange the different monosaccharides in alphabetical order and add "-an" to the last monosaccharide name. For example, the name of "glucomannan" comes from glucose and mannose with an "an" at the end to represent the heterosaccharide composed of glucose and mannose.

The number of monosaccharides included in a polysaccharide is usually not exactly known. Consequently, it is difficult to define their chemical structures. Their molecular formulas are therefore represented by using the repeating units of monosaccharides and its derivatives with the number of the repeating units being added at the end. The abbreviated English names of these units are linked with " → ", and pyranose and furanose are designated as "p" and "f" respectively. An example of lentinan's (香菇多糖的) molecular formula is shown below (Figure 3-7).

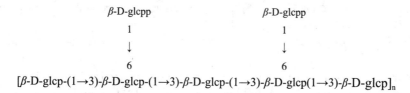

β-D-glcpp　　　　　　　　　β-D-glcpp

1　　　　　　　　　　　　　　1

↓　　　　　　　　　　　　　　↓

6　　　　　　　　　　　　　　6

$[\beta$-D-glcp-(1→3)-β-D-glcp-(1→3)-β-D-glcp-(1→3)-β-D-glcp(1→3)-β-D-glcp$]_n$

Figure 3-7　Lentinan's molecular formula

Polysaccharides have three-dimensional (3D) structures. The active centers of their 3D structures may contribute to the bioactivities of polysaccharides. Because the numbers of different kinds of monosaccharides that form polysaccharides are more than the amino acids that form proteins, structure elucidation for polysaccharides, especially heterosaccharides with branched-chain molecule, is much more difficult than that for proteins.

Many Chinese herbs, i.e. Ginseng Radix et Rhizoma, Astragall Radix, and Acanthopanacis Senticosi Radix et Rhizoma seu Caulis (刺五加), contain polysaccharides that have effect on tumor, immune system modulation, etc. Polysaccharide peptides (or proteins) that are the combination of peptides (or proteins) with polysaccharide side chains often have anti-tumor activities as well. Some products are used to treat infectious hepatitis, leukopenia, neurasthenia, etc.

Currently, dietary fibers attract great attention because of its effect on prevention of adiposity, hyperlipemia, coronary heart disease, diabetes, and colorectal cancer. The main components of dietary fibers are a variety of polysaccharides, oligosaccharides and other matters such as cellulose, hemicellulose, gum, mucilage, and pectic substance that cannot be digested and absorbed by the digestive system. Some examples of polysaccharides are listed in Table 3-3.

Table 3-3   Polysaccharides and related herbs

No.	Name	Biological source	Constituents	Uses
1	Guar gum (瓜尔豆胶)	*Cyamopsis tetragonolobus* (瓜尔豆) (Leguminosae) (豆科)	Guaran (瓜尔糖)	Binding agent (黏合剂), emulgent (乳化剂), disintegrating agent (崩解剂)
2	Algin (藻胶素)	*Macrocystis pyrifera* (巨藻) (Lessoniaceae) (巨藻科)	Alginic acid (褐藻酸)	Thickening and suspending agent (增稠悬浮剂)
3	Tragacanth (黄芪胶)	*Astragalus gummifer* (胶黄芪) (Leguminosae)	Tragacanthin (黄芪胶素), tragacanthic acid (黄芪酸), bassorin (西黄芪胶黏素)	Thickening agent, demulcent (调和剂)
4	Pectin (果胶)	*Citrus limon* (柠檬) *C. aurantium* (酸橙) (Rutaceae) (芸香科)	D-galactouronic acid, pectric acid	Adsorbent, thickening agent
5	Gum ghatti (印度果胶)	*Anogeissus latifolia* (宽叶榆绿木) (Combretaceae)(使君子科)	Two distinct polysaccharides	Emulgent, pharmaceutical aid (药物辅料)
6	Gum karaya (卡拉亚胶)	*Sterculia urens* (刺梧桐) (Sterculiaceae) (梧桐科)	A polysaccharide containing 8% acetyl and 37% uronic acid residues and no methoxyl group	Thickening agent, emulgent
7	Chitin (几丁质)	Shell of Lobster (龙虾) crab (蟹), cell walls of lower plants	2-Acetamide-2-deoxy-cellulose	Wound healing, adhesive to glass and plastics, sizing of rayon
8	Isapgol (车前子壳膳食纤维)	*Plantago ovata* (卵叶车前子) (Plantaginaceae) (车前草科)	Pentosan (戊聚糖), mucilage (胶浆), aldobionic acid (醛酸)	Demulcent (黏滑剂), laxative (通便剂), pharmaceutical aid
9	Psyllium (欧车前子壳膳食纤维)	*Plantago psyllium* (欧车前) (Plantaginaceae)	Mucilage, pentosans (戊聚糖)	Laxative (泻药), pharmaceutical aid
10	Agar (琼脂)	*Gelidium amansii* (石花菜) (Gelidiaceae)(石花菜科)	Agarose (琼脂糖), agaropectin (琼脂凝集素)	Laxative, bacteriological cultures
11	Carrageenan (卡拉胶)	*Chondrus cryspus.* (皱波角叉菜) *Gigartina sps.* (杉藻属植物)(Gigarginaceae)(杉藻科)	κ-carrageenan λ-carrageenan	Demulcent, antidiarrhrea, pharmaceutical aid
12	Inulin (菊粉)	*Inula helenium* (土木香) (Compositae)(菊科)	Fructo-furanose unit (呋喃果糖)	Source of fructose in foods and drinks

(continued)

No.	Name	Biological source	Constituents	Uses
13	Locust bean (槐豆)	*Ceratonia siliqua* (长角豆) (Leguminosae)	88% D-galacto-D-manoglycon (D– 半乳 –D– 甘露聚糖)	Thickener, pharmaceutical aid
14	Starch	*Zae mays* (玉米), *Oryza sativa* (水稻) (Gramineae) (禾本科)	Amylose and amylopectin (直链淀粉和支链淀粉)	Disintegrating agent, demulcent (消毒剂), nutritive (营养剂)
15	Echinacea (松果菊)	*Echinacea purpurea* (紫松果菊) (Compositae) (菊科)	Arabinogalactan (阿拉伯半乳聚糖)	Immunostimulant

1.3　Properties of Saccharides

Monosaccharides and low molecular weight saccharides (i.e. glucose, fructose and sucrose) are crystalline, sweet, and water-soluble. The high molecular weight polysaccharides, for example, starch, cellulose, gum, pectin, inulin, etc. are amorphous powder (无定形粉末), tasteless and relatively less soluble in water. In general, the larger the molecular weight is, the lower the solubility is in water.

In general, polysaccharides have hundreds or thousands molecules of monosaccharides yielding very large molecular weight. The physical and chemical properties of polysaccharides are very different from those of monosaccharides. For example, polysaccharides are not sweet, non-reducing, and insoluble in methanol, ethanol, and other organic solvents. Therefore, the method of water extraction and alcohol precipitation is often used to extract and purify polysaccharides.

2　Glycosides

2.1　Introduction

Glycosides are defined as the organic compounds that are formed by dehydration reaction (脱水反应) between a hydroxyl group of hemiacetal or hemiketal from sugar or sugar derivatives (糖衍生物)and a group from non-sugar. The non-sugar moiety (非糖部分) of a glycoside is called aglycone or genin.

In aglycone moiety, the atom linked to the anomeric carbon of the sugar is named as glycosidic atom. The chemical bond between the anomeric carbon and the glycosidic atom is called glycosidic linkage.

The sugar moiety in glycosides has two diastereoisomers (非对映异构体), named as anomers, and their corresponding configurations are designated as *α* or *β*. Consequently, the glycosidic linkages also have *α* and *β* configurations. In nature, the glycoside with D-sugar commonly exists as *β* configuration and the glycoside with L-sugar exists as *α* configuration. The naming conventions are to replace the "ose" suffix of the parent sugar with "oside", add the configurational prefix (*α* or *β* and D or L) immediately preceding the parental sugar name, and place the aglycone name in front of the sugar name. For example, the name for gastrodin (天麻素，天麻苷) is 4-hydroxymethylphenyl-β-D-glucopyranoside.

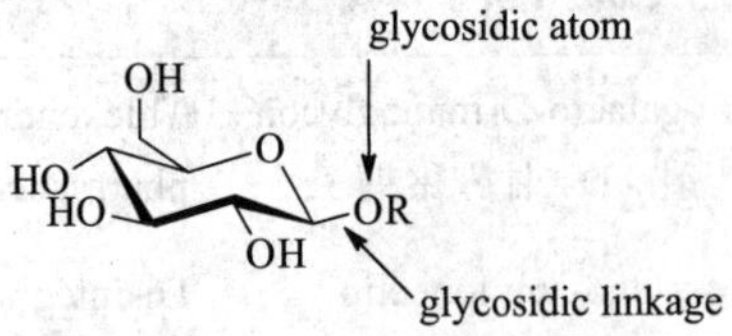

β-D-glucoside, R = aglycone group

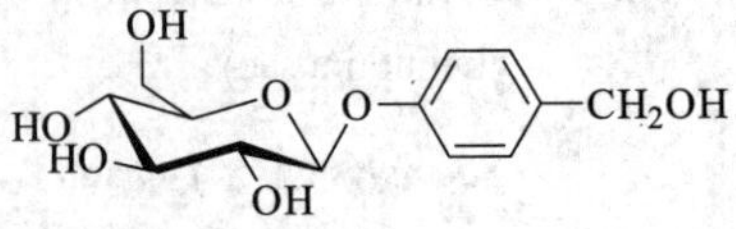

gastrodin
4-hydroxymethylphenyl-β-D-glucopyranoside

In nature, many secondary metabolic compounds, such as flavonoids, anthraquinones, phenylpropanoids, terpenoids, steroids, and alkaloids, may link sugar to form glycosides. Therefore, glycosides are extensively found in the plant kingdom. In general, glycosides and their hydrolysis enzymes exist in different cells of the same organ. When the organ is crushed, glycosides and hydrolysis enzymes are mixed together, and the enzyme can hydrolyze the glycoside into aglycone and sugar under suitable conditions like temperature, moisture, etc.

2.2 Structure and Classification

2.2.1 Structure

Glycosides are formed after the hydroxyl group on the anomeric carbon is replaced by a non-sugar moiety possessing a nucleophilic (亲核的) atom. The sugar groups in glycosides commonly include mono-, di-, or trisaccharide moieties. The glycosides containing moieties of more than tetrasaccharide occur most frequently in saponins and cardiac glycosides. The sugar group is common in the line-chain structure. However, most of the groups in the branched-chain are in saponins, e.g. ophiopogonin D (麦冬皂苷D) and lanatoside A (毛花洋地黄苷A).

Ordinarily, there are one or two glycosidic atoms in each glycoside molecule. It is rare that more than three glycosidic atoms exist in one glycoside molecule, for which an example found in astragaloside Ⅶ (黄芪苷Ⅶ) is shown below.

Glycosidic atoms commonly include oxygen, sulfur, nitrogen, and carbon. They are named as *O*-glycoside (*O*–苷), *S*-glycoside (*S*–苷), *N*-glycoside (*N*–苷) and *C*-glycoside (*C*–苷), respectively. *C*-glycoside exists less in nature. Puerarin (葛根素) is an example of *C*-glycoside.

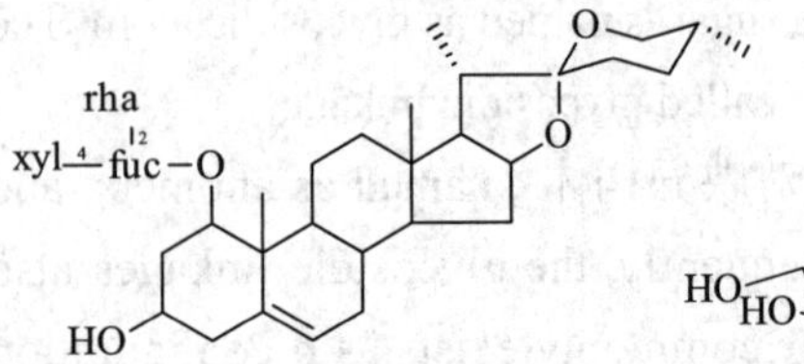

ophiopogonin D

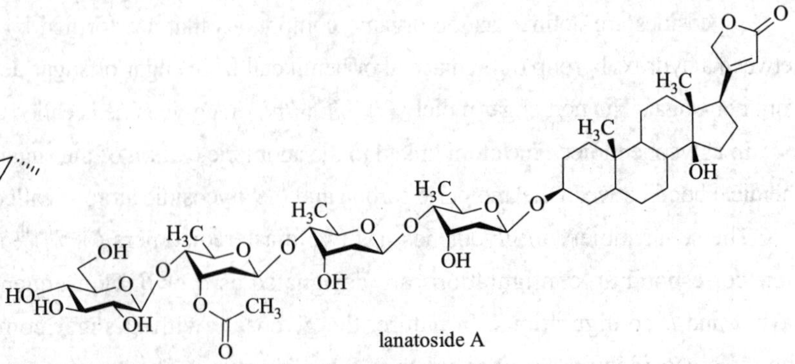

lanatoside A

astragaloside Ⅶ

puerarin

2.2.2   Classification

The classification of glycosides is complicated, because there are many kinds of glycosides in nature. The sugar groups from different glycosides have similar physical and chemical characteristics, but their aglycones may have different structures and bioactivities. Some classification methods are discussed here.

(1) Classification Based on Glycosidic Atom

Glycosides can be classified into four groups based on the glycosidic atoms: oxygen glycoside (氧苷), sulfur glycoside (硫苷), nitrogen glycoside (氮苷), and carbon glycoside (碳苷).

① Oxygen Glycosides

In oxygen glycosides (*O*-glycosides), if the oxygen, the glycosidic atom comes from alcohol, phenol, carboxyl, or *α*-OH nitrile (腈), the subsequent glycoside is alcoholic glycoside (醇苷), phenolic glycoside (酚苷), ester glycoside (酯苷), or cyanogenic glycoside (氰苷), respectively. Alcoholic glycosides and phenolic glycosides are common in Chinese herbs.

a. Alcoholic Glycosides: The alcoholic hydroxyl group from aglycone reacts with a hydroxyl group of hemiacetal or hemiketal from sugar to form alcoholic glycoside. Many alcoholic glycosides from Chinese herbs are active. For example, the geniposide (京尼平苷) from Gardeniae Fructus (栀子) has lapactic and cholagogue actions; the ranunculin (毛茛苷), a *β*-D-glucoside of protoanemonin (原白头翁素) from *Ranunculus japonicus* (毛茛) has the action of antibacteria and desinsection (杀虫); the rhodioloside (红景天苷) from Rhodiolae Crenulatae Radix et Rhizoma (红景天) has the adaptogen action.

geniposide   ranunculin   rhodioloside

b. Phenolic Glycosides: The dehydration reaction between the phenolic hydroxyl group in the aglycone and the sugar hemiacetal hydroxyl group forms phenolic glycoside. Phenolic glycosides are commonly phenol glycosides, naphthol glycosides (萘酚苷), anthracenol glycosides (蒽酚苷), coumarin glycosides (香豆素苷), flavonoid glycosides (黄酮苷), and lignan glycosides (木脂素苷). Many Chinese herbs contain phenolic glycosides with different bioactivities. For example, gastrodin in Gastrodiae Rhizoma (天麻) has sedative effect. Arbutin (熊果苷) in *Arctostaphylos uva-ursi* (熊果) is used as a urethra antiseptic. Esculin (秦皮甲素) in Fraxini Cortex (秦皮) has antibacterial activity. Sennoside (番泻苷) A in Rhei Radix et Rhizoma (大黄) is a purgative compound. Rutin (芦丁) is used in the treatment of softening vessels and preventing cardiovascular diseases.

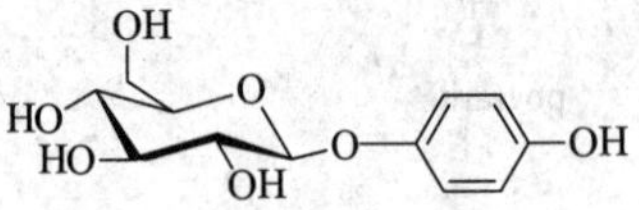

arbutin

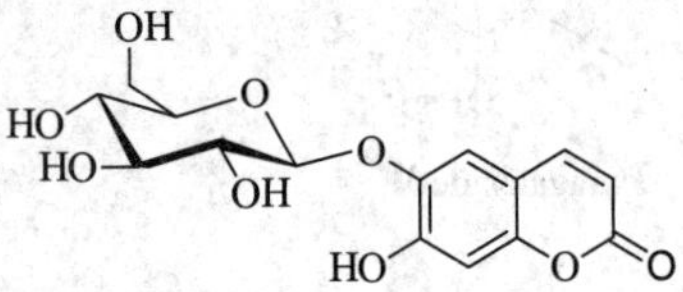

esculin

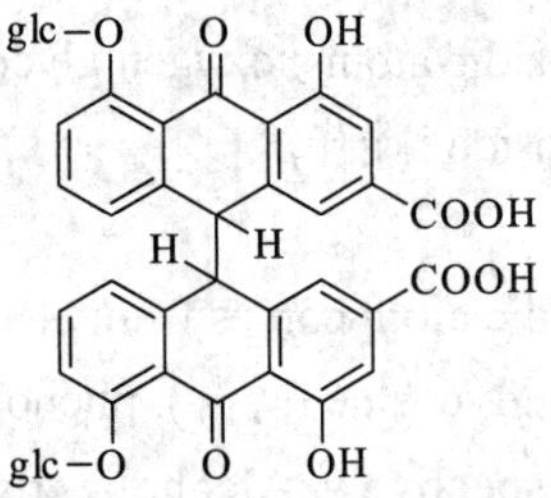

sennoside A

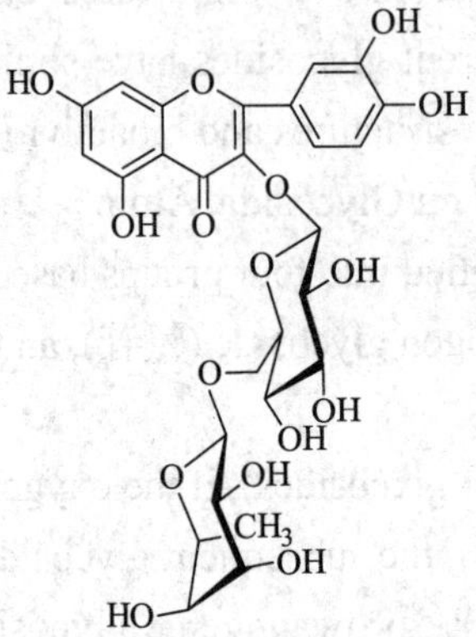

rutin

c. Ester Glycosides: The sugar hemiacetal hydroxyl group may react with a carboxyl group of aglycone to form ester glycoside. The glycosidic linkage that has chemical properties of acetal and ester can be hydrolyzed by both dilute acid and dilute base. For example, tuliposide (山慈菇苷) A and B, which are antifungal compounds, can be hydrolyzed by acid to yield cyclization aglycones, tulipalin (山 慈菇内酯) A and B, respectively (Figure 3-8). Ester glycosides are found in diterpenoid glycosides, and more common in triterpenoid saponins.

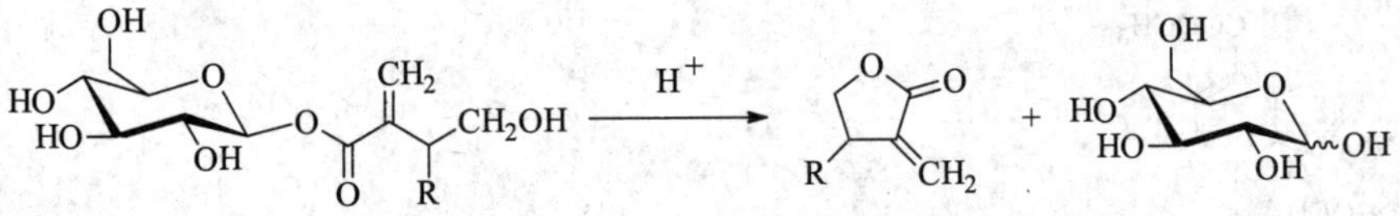

R=H   tuliposide A
R=OH   tuliposide B

R=H   tulipalin A
R=OH   tulipalin B

Figure 3-8   The hydrolysis reaction of tuliposide A and B

d. Cyanogenic Glycosides: The hydroxyl group in α-hydroxyl-nitrile (e.g. mandelonitrile，苯乙醇腈) reacts with the sugar hemiacetal hydroxyl group to form cyanogenic glycoside.

Amygdalin (苦杏仁苷) from Armeniacae Semen Amarum (苦杏仁) can be hydrolyzed to produce mandelonitrile or prunasin (野樱苷), unstable intermediate compounds, and then degraded into hydrocyanic acid (氢氰酸, both active and toxic compound) and benzoic aldehyde (苯甲醛). The processes of decomposition of amygdalin under different conditions are shown in Figure 3-9.

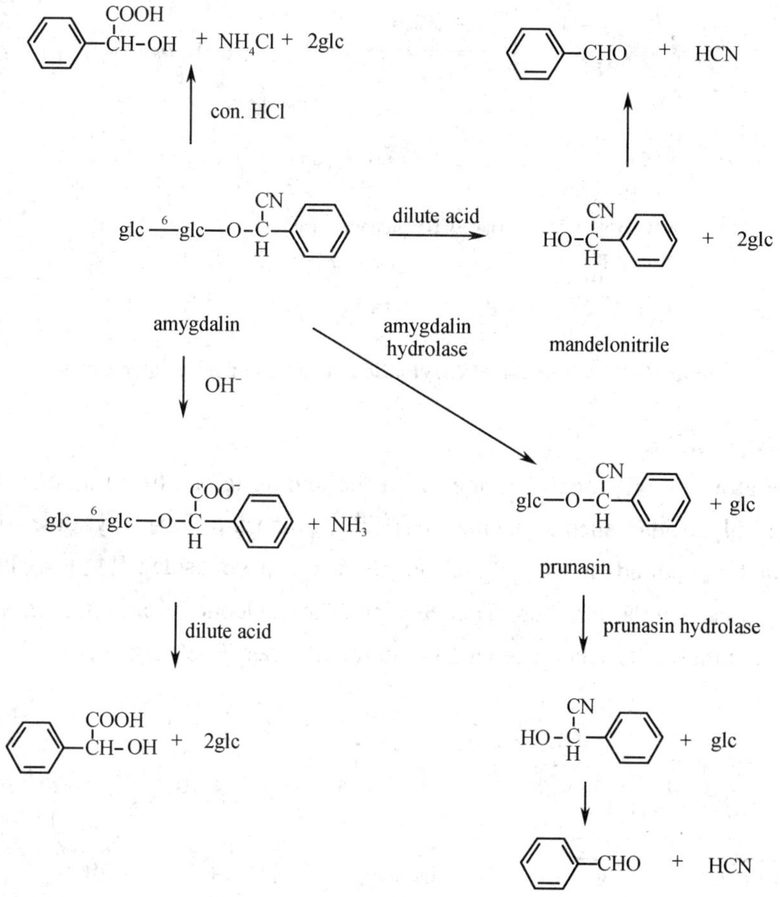

Figure 3-9   Processes of decomposition of amygdalin under different conditions

② Sulfur Glycosides

Sulfur glycosides are the products of the sulfhydryl (thiol) group (巯基) in aglycone joined with the hemiacetal hydroxyl group in sugar. Sulfur glycosides exist mainly in Cruciferae (十字花科), for example, glucoraphenin (萝卜苷) in radish, sinigrin (黑芥子苷) in *Brassia nigra* (黑芥), sinalbin (白芥子苷) in Sinapis Semen (芥子).

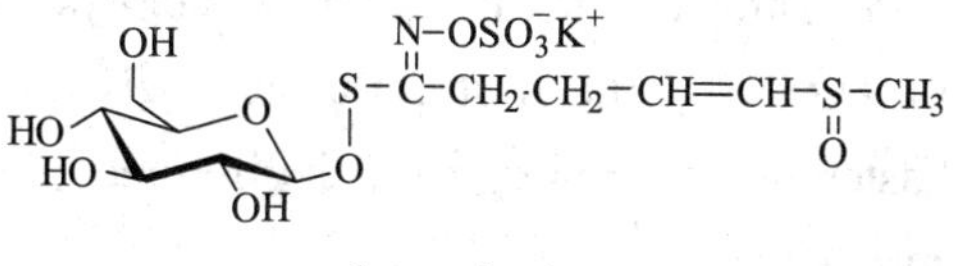

glugoraphenin

Sulfur glycosides are always accompanied by the appropriate hydrolytic enzyme, for example, thio-glucosidase (硫葡萄糖苷酶) is known as myrosinase (芥子酶). Whenever fresh tissues are crushed in aqueous solution, the hydrolysis of sulfur glycosides takes place yielding D-glucose and a labile aglycone. The labile aglycone is spontaneously rearranged with the loss of sulfate to yield an isothiocyanate (异硫氰酸酯). The isothiocyanates have no free sulfhydryl group which is different from other glycosides. The reaction of enzymatic hydrolysis of sulfur glycosides is shown in Figure 3-10.

67

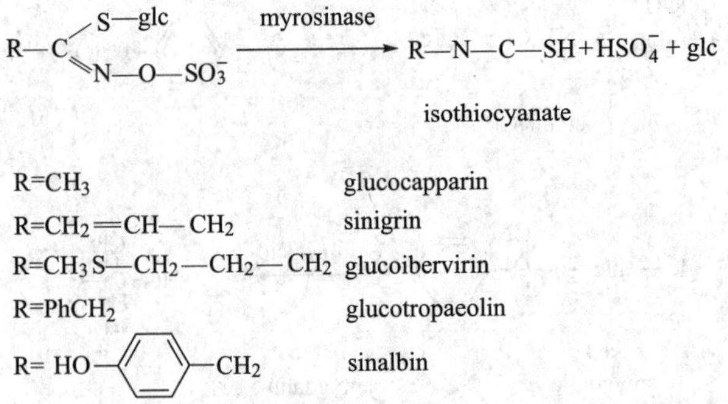

$$R-C \overset{S-glc}{\underset{N-O-SO_3^-}{\diagup}} \xrightarrow{\text{myrosinase}} R-N-C-SH+HSO_4^- + glc$$

isothiocyanate

R=CH₃   glucocapparin

R=CH₂═CH—CH₂   sinigrin

R=CH₃S—CH₂—CH₂—CH₂ glucoibervirin

R=PhCH₂   glucotropaeolin

R= HO—⟨benzene⟩—CH₂   sinalbin

Figure 3-10　Reaction of enzymatic hydrolysis of sulfur glycosides

③ Nitrogen Glycosides

The nitrogen atom in aglycone combines with the anomeric carbon of a sugar to form nitrogen glycoside. Nitrogen glycosides, such as adenosine (腺苷), guanosine (鸟苷), cytidine (胞苷), and uridine (尿苷) are important compounds in the field of biochemistry. Crotonoside (巴豆苷) which exists in Crotonis Fructus (巴豆) has similar structure as adenosine. The aglycone of crotonoside is highly toxic and can inhibit protein synthesis. Its subcutaneous LD_{50} in rabbits was 50–80 mg/kg.

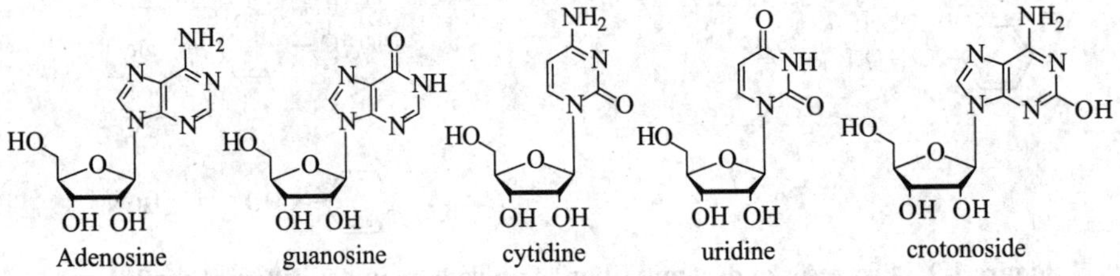

Adenosine　　　guanosine　　　cytidine　　　uridine　　　crotonoside

④ Carbon Glycosides

When a carbon atom in aglycone combines with the anomeric carbon of a sugar directly, a carbon glycoside is formed. Aglycones of *C*-glycosides are commonly found in flavonoids and anthraquinones. For example, vitexin (牡荆素), a *C*-glycoside of flavonoids, exists in plants of Verbenaceae (马鞭草科) and Moraceae (桑科). Vitexin is one of the active chemicals found in many cultivated species of Crataegi Fructus (山楂). Recently, this compound was also found in *Trollius chinensis* (金莲花). Vitexin has many medical effects, such as anti-tumor, anti-inflammation, anti-spasmolysis and anti-hypotension. Another example of *C*-glycoside is aloin (芦荟苷), the first anthrone *C*-glycoside found in Aloe (芦荟) with lapactic activity. It is a pair of diastereomer (非对映体) with different optical activity (旋光性) and circular dichroism（圆二色性）(Figure 3-11).

In the above chemical structures, the carbon atoms in aglycones link with anomeric carbons of sugars. This is because the hydrogen atom on the carbon is activated by the hydroxyl group at the *ortho*-position (*o*-position) or *para*-position (*p*-position). The anomeric carbon of sugar always links to *meta*-position (*m*-position) of two or three phenolic hydroxyl groups in aromatic ring structures.

(2) Other Classification Methods

Other methods used to classify glycosides are based on their glycosidic hydrolysis, sugar groups, aglycone groups, sources, and therapeutic applications.

Glycosides that exist in plants naturally are known as primary glycosides (原生苷). Glycosides that are produced by hydrolysis from primary glycosides are called secondary glycosides (次生苷). For

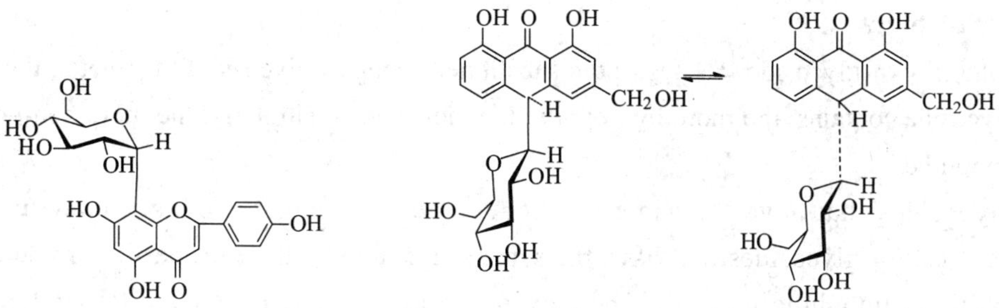

vitexin

aloin or barbaloin

Figure 3-11　Disatereomer of aloin

example, amygdalin exists in almond as a primary glycoside; once hydrolyzed, it yields prunasin as a secondary glycoside.

　　The classification of glycosides can also base on the sugar groups, such as glucoside (葡萄糖苷), xyloside (木糖苷), and 2-deoxy-glucoside(2–去氧–葡萄糖苷). Similarly, when the sugars are fructose or galactose, the glycosides are called fructosides (果糖苷) or galactosides (半乳糖苷), respectively.

　　The classification of glycosides can also base on the structure of aglycones, therefore, anthraquinone, flavonoid, iridoid (环烯醚萜), lignan or steroid glycosides are consequently named.

　　The classification of glycosides can also base on their physicochemical properties or physiological activities, for example, saponins have "soap-like" propertie, and cardiac glycosides have effect on heart muscles.

　　If the classification is based on the number of monosacchride group in glycoside, then monosaccharide-, disaccharide-, trisaccharide-, or tetrasaccharide-glycosides are named. According to the number of glycosidic atoms in glycoside, the monodesmosidic-(单糖链的), bidesmosidic-(双糖链的), tridesmosidic-(三糖链的), or tetradesmosidic-(四糖链的) glycosides are also named.

　　Sometimes, the source of glycosides is used as a basis for classification, for example ginsenoside, rhodioloside, gastrodin, etc.

2.3　General Physicochemical Properties

The physical, chemical, and therapeutic properties of glycosides are mostly dictated by aglycones.

2.3.1　Exterior Characteristics

Glycosides of small molecular weight are solid crystals. The ones with large molecular weight are amorphous powder. The color of glycosides depends on the structure of their aglycones. The color of aglycones depend on the size of conjugated system and the number of auxochromes (助色团) in its structure. Glycosides are also usually tasteless besides bitter or sweet. For example, ginseng saponin is bitter and liquorice saponin (甘草皂苷) is sweet. A few glycosides such as saponins and cardiac glycosides can cause irritation on mucosal membranes.

2.3.2　Optical Activities

Glycosides have optical activities, normally levorotary (左旋) effect. Hydrolyzed glycosides, which are mixtures of aglycones and sugars, normally show dextrorotation (右旋) because the sugar is dextrorotated. The magnitude of glycosides' optical rotations is in connection with the structure of aglycones and sugars, and the nature of chemical connections between them.

2.3.3　Solubility

The solubility of glycosides relates to the substituted group in glycoside. In general, the more polar groups a glycoside contains, the more hydrophilic the molecule is; similarly, the more non-polar groups, the more lipophilic.

For glycosides that have the same aglycones, the more sugar groups it contains, the more hydrophilic it is. For glycosides that have the same sugar moiety, their properties are determined by the hydrophilic or lipophilic groups in the aglycone. Aglycones generally are lipophilic and sugars are hydrophilic.

Monosaccharide glycosides with large molecular aglycones (i.e. steroids or triterpenes) are soluble in low polar organic solvents because the ratio of the hydrophilic moiety (e.g. sugar) to the lipophilic moiety (e.g. non-sugar) is low. For example, ginsenoside Rh₂ (人参皂苷Rh₂) is soluble in diethyl ether and insoluble in water. Some glycosides such as digitoxin (洋地黄毒苷) have trisaccharide and are insoluble in water due to three deoxysugars in the molecule.

In general, glycosides are soluble in water, methanol, ethanol and n-butanol containing water, and insoluble in non-polar solvents such as petroleum ether, benzene, chloroform, and diethyl ether. However, C-glycosides have low solubility in polar or non-polar solvents. Aglycones are usually insoluble in water and soluble in organic solvents.

2.3.4　Cleavage of Glycosidic Linkages

Glycosides are easily hydrolyzed into sugar and aglycone by dilute acids or enzymes. Phenolic glycosides and ester glycosides are also easily hydrolyzed by dilute alkali solutions. In order to retain the integrity of the constituents in Chinese herbs, it is necessary to avoid the hydrolysis of glycosides during extraction and isolation processes. In most cases, the dilute acid or alkali is not used to mix with Chinese herbs during extraction and isolation. On the other hand, the methods to cleave glycosidic linkages can be used to study the structures of glycosides. There are many methods to cleave glycosidic linkages, i.e. acidic hydrolysis, alkaline hydrolysis, enzymatic hydrolysis, methylation (甲基化) or acetylation (乙酰化) hydrolysis, and oxidative cleavage (氧化裂解), just to name a few.

(1) Acidic Hydrolysis

In general, glycosidic linkages are hydrolyzed easily by dilute acids, including hydrochloric acid (盐酸), sulphuric acid (硫酸), acetic acid (乙酸) and formic acid (甲酸) in aqueous or dilute alcohol. The first step is the protonation (质子化) of the glycosidic atom. The second step is the cleavage of glycosidic linkage to form the aglycone and sugar intermediate with carbonium ion (正碳离子). The third step is the dissolution of the intermediate in the aqueous solution. And the last step is the removal of the hydrogen ion to form sugar. The reaction processes are demonstrated below (Figure 3-12).

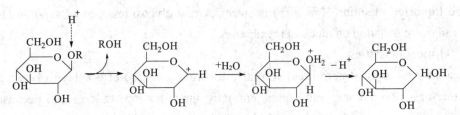

Figure 3-12　Mechanism of acidic hydrolysis of a glycoside

Based on the hydrolysis mechanism, it is conceivable that the easiness of acidic hydrolysis depends on the electron cloud density (电子云密度) and the spatial position (空间位置) of the glycosidic atom. Any factor that benefits the protonation of the glycosidic atom is favorable to acidic hydrolysis. This regularity is further elaborated on below.

① On the basis of glycosidic atoms, the order of acidic hydrolysis with increasing difficulties is *N*-glycoside, *O*-glycoside, *S*-glycoside, and *C*-glycoside as the *N*-atom in the *N*-glycoside has the highest electron cloud density that promotes hydrolysis reaction. The *C*-atom on *C*-glycosides, however, has no free lone-pair electrons and is difficult to be protonated. Consequently, acid hydrolysis of *C*-glucosides needs heat treatment for a long time. It is worth noting that some *N*-glycosides with *N*-atom in amide (酰胺) or pyrimidine ring (嘧啶环) are also difficult to be hydrolyzed by acid solutions because the cloud density of the free lone-pair electrons on *N*-atom is low, which is the result of electron-withdrawing (吸电子) and conjugation effect (共轭效应) of amide.

② The acidic hydrolysis for furanosides（呋喃糖苷）(e.g. fructoside and riboside) is easier than that for pyranoside (吡喃糖苷) (e.g. glucoside and rhamnoside) because the furanose moiety has higher internal energy due to its plane structure.

③ In general, ketoside (酮糖苷) is more easily hydrolyzed in acidic solutions than aldosides (醛糖苷) because most of ketosides are furanosides.

④ The larger the group on C-5 in pyranosides, the more difficult to hydrolyze, because of the increased sterohindrance for protonation of the glycosidic atom. The order of acidic hydrolysis with increasing difficulties is pentosides (五碳糖苷), methylpentosides (甲基五碳糖苷), hexosides (六碳糖苷), heptosides (七碳糖苷), and hexuronic acid glycosides (六碳糖醛酸苷).

⑤ Different groups (e.g. —NH₂ and —OH) on C-2 in sugar moiety compete at various degrees with the glycosidic atom for protonation because they provide with induction effect of electron-withdrawing that results in low electron cloud density of the glycosidic atom. The order of acidic hydrolysis with increasing difficulties is 2, 3-deoxysugar glycosides, 2-deoxysugar glycosides, 3-deoxysugar glycosides, 2-hydroxylsugar glycosides (2-羟基糖苷), 2-aminosugar glycosides (2- 氨基糖苷).

⑥ The aromatic glycosides are hydrolyzed much more easily than the aliphatic (脂肪族的) glycosides (e.g. terpenoid glycosides and sterol glycosides) because of some electron donor groups (供电子基团) on the aromatic glycosides. For example, some phenolic glycosides (anthraquinone glycosides and coumarin glycosides) can be hydrolyzed into aglycones and sugars by heating in water instead of acidic solutions.

To avoid degradation (most cases are dehydration) of aglycones when hydrolysis takes place under acidic conditions, a water-insoluble organic solvent (i.e. chloroform, etc.) is added to the acidic aqueous solution so that once the aglycone is yielded it can be dissolved into the organic solvent immediately for protection. This method is named as two-phase hydrolysis.

(2) Alkaline Hydrolysis

In general, glycosidic linkages are not easily hydrolyzed in alkali solution because the acetal structure of glycosidic bond is stable. However, four types of glycosides can be hydrolyzed easily in alkali solutions, they are ester glycosides (e.g. tuliposide A), phenolic glycosides (e.g. salicin) (水杨苷), enolic glycosides (烯醇苷) (e.g. triglochinin) (海韭菜苷), and glycosides with the electrophilic group at *β* position (e.g. picrocrocin) (藏红花苦苷).

salicin   triglochinin   picrocrocin

(3) Enzymatic Hydrolysis

In most cases, enzymes are used to hydrolyze glycosides that are unstable or cannot be hydrolyzed easily by acid or alkali. The conditions of enzymatic hydrolysis are mild (at 30–40℃) therefore aglycones usually can maintain their integrity structure throughout the enzymatic hydrolysis. Furthermore, enzymatic hydrolysis has high specificity (专属性) and is a gradual process. These characteristics provide significant advantages over acidic or alkali hydrolysis.

Enzyme has high specificity, for example, α-glycosidase only hydrolyzes α-glycosides and β-glycosidase only hydrolyzes β-glycosides. Some enzymes have specificities toward aglycones and/or sugars. For example, maltase (麦芽糖酶) is a α-glucosidase that only hydrolyzes α-glucosides. Emulsin (苦杏仁苷酶), however, is an example of a β-glycosidase with low specificity. It can hydrolyze β-glycosides including glucosides and other glycoside of hexoses. Due to the difficulty to obtain a specific enzyme, at present, most of the enzymes used to hydrolyze glycosides are still non purified mixed enzymes, such as emulsin, which is a kind of mixed enzyme.

Enzymatic hydrolysis is a gradual process. Therefore, secondary glycosides can be obtained from the primary glycosides through this gradual process. It is conceivable that information regarding the type of sugar, the configuration of glycosidic linkage, and the sequence of sugars can be revealed stepwise through enzymatic hydrolysis.

It is worth noting that Chinese herbs that contain glycosides usually contain the specific enzyme that can hydrolyze the glycoside. Therefore, during the harvest, storage, extraction, and isolation processes, special care needs to be exercised to avoid hydrolysis of the glycoside. After harvest, Chinese herbs can be treated with high temperature, sun-exposure, accelerated desiccation (快速干燥) to inhibit the activity of glycosidases (苷酶). Chinese herbs should be kept in cool and dry places to help maintain the structure integrity of glycosides.

High concentration methanol or ethanol, or boiling water should be used during extraction of glycosides to avoid enzymatic hydrolysis. For fresh plants, the aqueous solution of ammonia sulfate (硫酸铵) can be used to grind with the plant to degrade glycosidases. Calcium carbonate (碳酸钙) can also be used to incubate with the plant prior to extraction to ensure that glycosidases are degraded.

(4) Methylation and Hydrolysis

Hemiacetal or hemiketal exists in the cyclic structure of a sugar or sugar moiety in glycosides. The hydroxyl group of a hemiacetal or hemiketal is the most active group of all hydroxyl groups in a sugar. When glucose is heated in methanol containing hydrogen chloride, only the hydroxyl group at anomeric carbon is methylated to form methyl-glucosides (葡萄糖甲苷), which are also called monomethyl acetals (Figure 3-13).

Methylation can be used to determinate the linkage positions between monosaccharides in glycosides. In general, glycosides can be treated with different methylation methods, such as Haworth, Purdie, Kuhn, and Hakomori to obtain permethylated (全甲基化的) glycosides. The permethylated

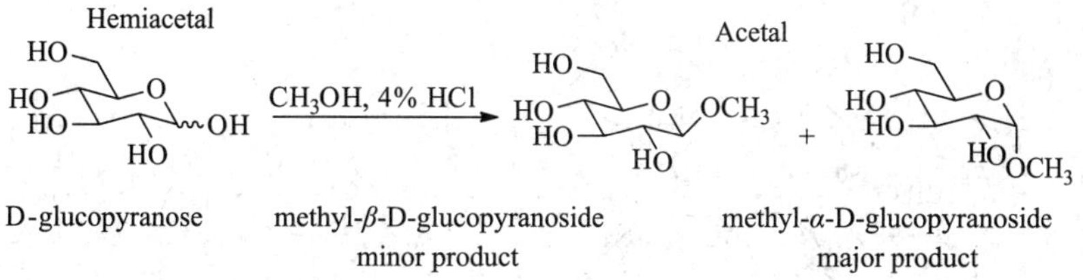

Figure 3-13 Reaction of methylation at the hydroxyl of anomeric carbon in a glucopyranose

glycoside is then alcoholyzed (醇解) by 6%–9% HCl-CH$_3$OH to yield various partially methylated monosaccharides and permethylated monosaccharides. These products can be identified by using the thin layer chromatography (TLC) or gas chromatography (GC) along with reference standards (对照品). Where permethylated monosaccharide is formed, the corresponding monosaccharide is usually located at the end of the sugar moiety. Where the free hydroxyl group is located on the partial methylated monosaccharides, it is the position that monosaccharides form linkage between them. The gas chromatography hyphenated mass spectrometry (GC-MS) can be used to detect the partial methylated monosaccharides as well. The alcoholysis reaction of permethylated glycosides is demonstrated below (Figure 3-14).

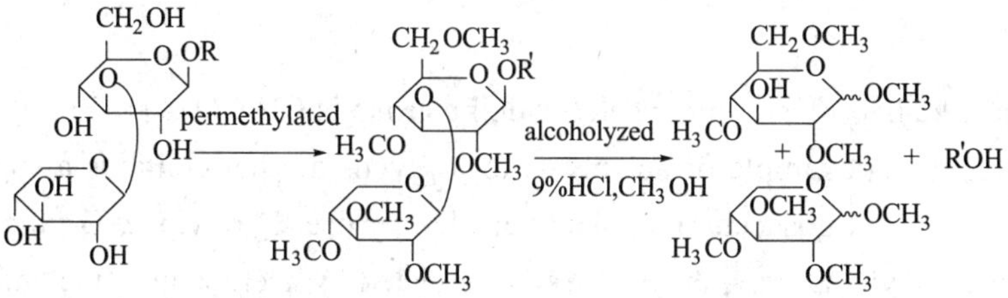

Figure 3-14 Permethylation and alcoholysis reaction of a glycoside

In the above example, after the permethylated glycoside is alcoholyzed, the products are identified by TLC and GC as 2, 3, 4-tri-O-methylpyranxyloside and 2, 4, 6-tri-O-methylpyranglucoside in addition to the aglycone. The former is permethylated xyloside, therefore it can be concluded that xylose is at the tail end in the sugar moiety. The latter is a partial methylated glucose that has one hydroxyl at C-3, so it is evidence that the hydroxyl at C-3 in glucose links to C-1 in xylose.

It is important to point out that the methylation methods for determination of the linkage position only apply to glycosides that contain mono- or disaccharides, not tri-, tetra- or even higher order polysaccharides. In addition, please also note that alcoholyzation may damage the structures of glycosides.

(5) Acetylation and Hydrolysis

Acetylation and hydrolysis are used to identify the linkages among sugar moieties that contain more than two monosaccharides in glycosides. This process is illustrated in Figure 3-15 through acetolysis (乙酰解) reaction that includes acetylation and hydrolysis. Some glycosidic linkages in glycosides can be disintegrated by the acetolysis reaction to produce peracetylated monosaccharides and oligosaccharides. TLC and GC can detect these acetylated products and the results will reveal the sugar moiety composition and the linkage position between the two sugar units. The reagents for acetolysis reaction consist of acetic anhydride (乙酸酐) and a mixture of different acids, such as sulfuric acid, perchloric acid (高氯酸) or Lewis acid , such as zinc chloride (氯化锌), boron trifluoride (三氟化硼), etc. The mechanisms are

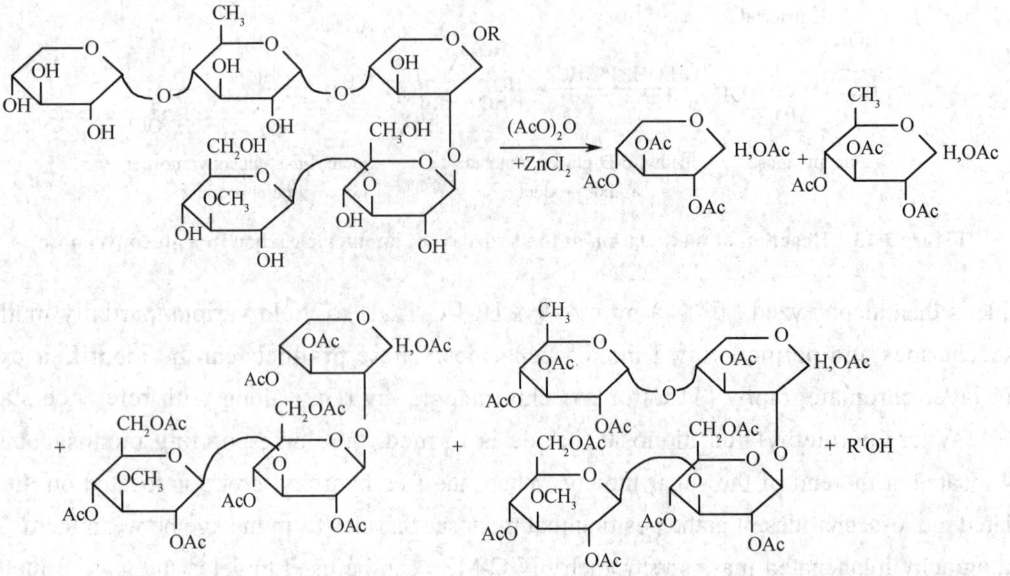

Figure 3-15 shows the acetylation and alcoholysis reaction scheme.

$$(AcO)_2O + ZnCl_2$$

R=aglycone. Ac = $CH_3\overset{\overset{O}{\|}}{C}$—

Figure 3-15 Acetylation and alcoholysis reaction of a glycoside with five monosaccharide units

similar to those of acidic hydrolysis, but the electrophilic group is CH_3CO^+.

Figure 3-15 shows an example of acetolysis of a glycoside that contains a sugar moiety of five monosaccharide units (an oligosaccharide). They are D-oxylose, D-oxylose, D-glucose, D-quinovose, and D-glucose-3- methoxyl（D–葡萄糖–3–甲醚）. Acetylated by acetic anhydride and zinc chloride, the sugar moiety forms peracetylated monosaccharide, trisaccharide, and tetrasaccharide. The linkages among monosaccharides are concluded in comparison with reference standards.

One of the factors that affect the rate of acetolysis reaction is the position of glycosidic linkage. If a hydroxyl group that can be acetylated is at *o*-position of a glycosidic linkage, the rate of acetolysis reaction will be slow because the electron cloud density of the glycosidic atom is low due to the electro-negativity（电负性）of the hydroxyl. Information from acetolysis of disaccharides showed that the order of acetolysis reaction with increased difficulties is $1 \rightarrow 6$, $1 \rightarrow 4$ or $1 \rightarrow 3$, $1 \rightarrow 2$ glycosidic linkages.

The operation of acetolysis is simple. Dissolve glycosides in solvent that contains acetic anhydride and acetic acid glacial（冰醋酸）. Add concentrated sulfuric acid to 3%–5% and leave it for 1–10 days at room temperature for the reaction to complete. Afterwards, put the reaction mixture in an ice-water bath （冰水浴）, and adjust to pH 3–4 using the sodium bicarbonate（碳酸氢钠）solution. Extract sugar acetate with chloroform, and the different peracetylated monosaccharides and oligosaccharides can be separated by column chromatography (CC).

(6) Oxidative Cleavage

The reaction of oxidative cleavage（氧化裂解）is also named as Smith degradation（Smith 降解）. It is used to cleave the chemical bonds between two vicinal hydroxyl groups in sugar moiety of the glycoside while avoiding damaging the structure of aglycone. The sugar moiety are cleaved into small compounds that are used to identify the types of sugars. In general, hexose, methylpentose, and pentose form glycerol（甘油）, propylene glycol（丙二醇）, and ethylene glycol（乙二醇）, respectively.

Oxidative cleavage has three steps as shown below (Figure 3-16):

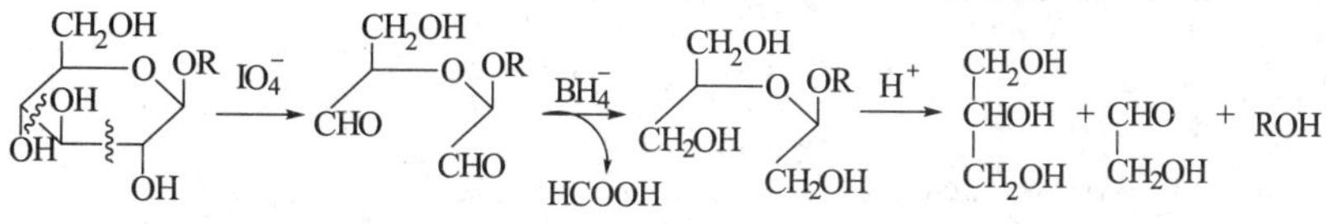

CH₂OH ... D-glucoside, R=aglycone group ... glycerol glycollicaldehyde

Figure 3-16　Oxidative cleavage of a glycoside

The first step is periodate (过碘酸) oxidation of sugar to form aldehyde by sodium periodate (过碘酸钠) in aqueous or dilute alcohol at room temperature. Sodium borohydride (四氢硼酸钠) then reduces the dialdehyde (丙二醛) to form a dialcohol (二醇). The last acid hydrolysis step takes place and forms glycerol (or propylene glycol or ethylene glycol), hydroxyl aldehyde (羟基乙醛), and aglycone under pH 2 at room temperature.

Smith degradation plays an important role in the study of glycosidic structure in the past, but it is rarely used nowadays. It is a suitable method for hydrolysis of *C*-glycosides that is difficult to hydrolyze by acid. Some glycosides (i.e. ginsenosides) with unstable aglycones may be kept in the original state during Smith degradation. However, the aglycones that have vicinal alcoholic hydroxyls can also be degraded (Figure 3-17).

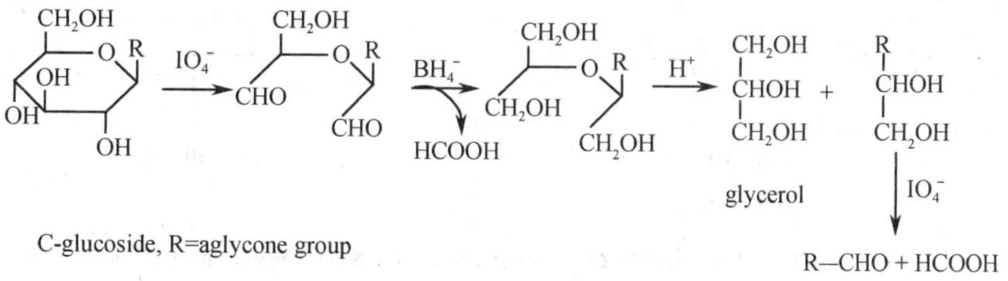

C-glucoside, R=aglycone group

Figure 3-17　Oxidative cleavage of a *C*-glycoside

2.3.5　Chemical Tests

Saccharides and glycosides have sugar moiety for which the same chemical tests (i.e. Molish, Fehling, and Tollen reactions) can be conducted. These reactions will be discussed in the identification section.

3　Extraction and Isolation Methods

3.1　Extraction Methods

3.1.1　Extraction of Saccharides

In general, water or dilute alcohol is used to extract monosaccharides and oligosaccharides from powdered crude drugs (药材). Before the extraction, enzyme activities should be inhibited by suitable methods, such as treatment with boiling water. Calcium carbonate is usually added to water or dilute alcohol during the extraction process as calcium carbonate inhibits enzyme activity and also neutralizes acid to keep the solution neutral.

The extraction of monosaccharides and oligosaccharides from Chinese herbs is illustrated as follows (Figure 3-18).

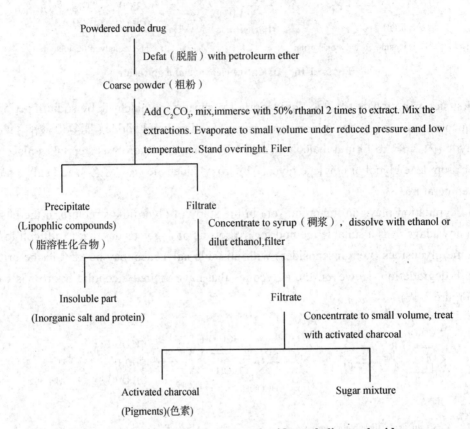

Figure 3-18 Extraction of monosaccharides and oligosaccharides

Polysaccharides and large molecular oligosaccharides are extracted with water. In addition, dilute base or salt aqueous solution and DMSO can also be used to extract polysaccharides from Chinese herbs based on the chemical properties of the polysaccharides. The aqueous extracts contain polysaccharides along with other water soluble constituents. The polysaccharides can be purified from the extracts by adding ethanol, methanol or acetone to precipitate. The extraction procedures are shown below (Figure 3-19, Figure 3-20).

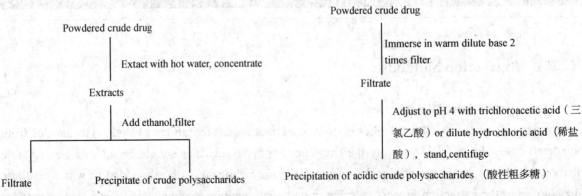

Figure 3-19 Extraction of polysaccharides　　　　**Figure 3-20　Extraction of acidic polysaccharides**

To avoid the cleavage of glycosidic linkages, acid and base should be used carefully and the extracts should be neutralized, concentrated, precipitated quickly no matter what type of acid or base used.

3.1.2　Extraction of Glycosides

Glycosides are easily hydrolyzed by enzymes, therefore, methanol, ethanol, or boiling water is generally used for extraction of glycosides. Also it is important to keep neutral conditions during the extraction of glycosides to avoid glycosides being degraded by acid or base.

If a secondary glycoside is the interest of the extraction from Chinese herbs, the hydrolysis of primary glycoside should be controlled through fine adjustment of acid, base, or enzyme. The selective hydrolysis or fermentation is generally used to obtain high yield of secondary glycoside.

The extraction method of gradually increasing polarity of solvent is employed in rough extraction of glycosides. Glycosides with different polarities are extracted into different fractions by solvents of different polarities.

The procedures for glycoside extraction and isolation are illustrated below (Figure 3-21).

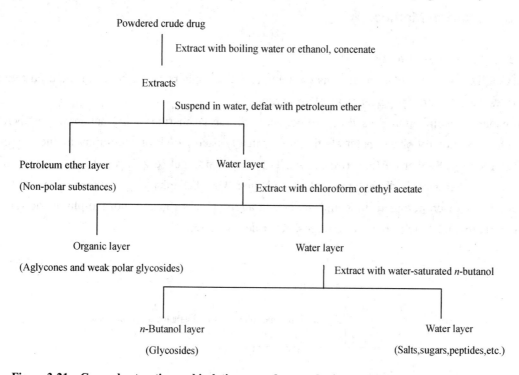

Figure 3-21　General extraction and isolation procedure to obtain total glycosides from crude drugs

In the above procedure, macroporous resin can also be used to collect total glycosides instead of partitioning with water-saturated *n*-butanol.

3.1.3　Extraction of Aglycone

The generally used method to extract aglycone is to hydrolyze Chinese herbs that contain glycosides with acid or enzymes. Afterwards, the mixture is neutralized and extracted with lipophilic organic solvent to obtain the total aglycones. Alternatively, total glycosides can be extracted first and then hydrolyzed by acid or enzymes to yield aglycones and sugars. The aglycones are subsequently extracted with lipophilic organic solvents.

Selecting a hydrolysis method that avoids the destroy of aglycone structure will ensure high yield of aglycones. The first extraction method discussed above is shown below (Figure 3-22).

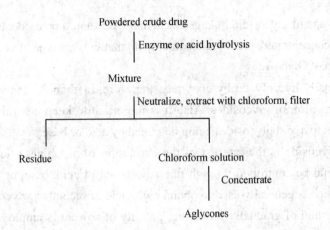

Figure 3-22   General extraction and isolation procedure to obtain total aglycones

3.2   Isolation Methods

3.2.1   Saccharides Isolation

Crystallization, precipitation, chromatography, and electrophoresis methods can be used to isolate saccharides based on their physicochemical properties.

In general, precipitation is used first to collect total polysaccharides. Chromatography is then used for isolation. Stationary phase materials that are typically used for chromatography include Sephadex gel (Sephadex G), Sepharose (e.g. Bio-gel A), Polyacrylamide gel (e.g. Bio-gel P), carboxyl methyl Sephadex (CM-Sephadex), diethylaminoethyl Sephadex (DEAE-Sephadex), activated charcoal (shown in Figure 3-23), macroporous resin, cellulose, etc. In addition, silica gels of normal-phase and reversed-phase chromatography are also used for oligosaccharides isolation.

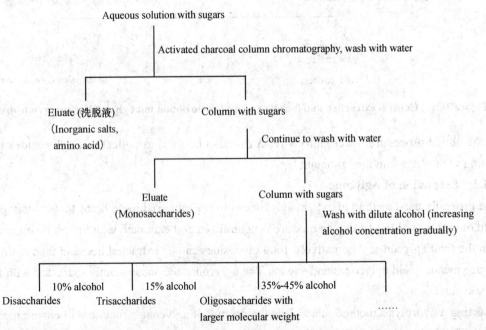

Figure 3-23   Isolation procedure of saccharides by using activated charcoal CC

Precipitation method is commonly used to separate polysaccharides with different molecular weights. The higher the concentration of methanol (or ethanol, acetone) is used, the lower the molecular weights of the polysaccharides are precipitated. If a polysaccharide is acidic, it also needs to be precipitated under acidic condition. The small molecular components precipitated together with polysaccharides can be removed by dialysis.

Electrophoresis is used to separate acidic polysaccharides by moving them to two conductors under electrical field. Ultracentrifugation (超速离心) is also used to separate polysaccharides based on that different molecular weights yield different sedimentation rates (沉积速率).

3.2.2　Glycosides Isolation

The isolation of glycosides is a difficult task because glycosides' polarities can vary in a wide range depending on the differences in their aglycones and sugars. General chromatography isolation methods for glycosides are shown below (Figure 3-24).

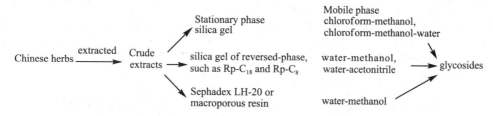

Figure 3-24　General chromatography methods for the isolation of glycosides

4　Identification

4.1　Physicochemical Identification

One of the ways to identify glycosides is to identify their sugar moiety. Therefore, it is important to remove free sugars in the sample before identification of glycosides. The general procedure is shown in Figure 3-25.

4.1.1　Molish Reaction

Molish reaction is commonly used to identify the existence of sugars or glycosides in Chinese herbs. The method is: Add 1ml test solution in a test tube; Add 1–3 drops of 5% α-naphthol (α-萘酚), vortex and mix; Drop concentrate sulfuric acid slowly down the side of the tube. If a purple ring forms between two layers, it indicates that the sample may contain sugar or glycoside. However, it should be noted that both C-glycosides and glycuronides show negative results in Molish reaction.

4.1.2　Fehling and Tollen Reactions

A positive result of the Fehling or Tollen reaction indicates the existence of reducing sugars. The sugar moiety in glycosides do not have reducing property. Therefore, glycosides show negative in Fehling or Tollen reactions. Only when glycosides are hydrolyzed to sugars with reducing properties, the Fehling and/or Tollen reaction results will be positive. After a negative result in either of the two reactions, filter

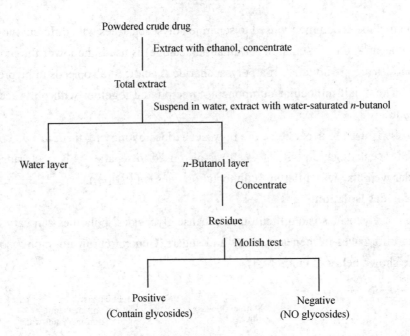

Figure 3-25　Identification procedure for glycosides by Molish reaction

the solution, hydrolyze the filtrate with acid, and add Fehling or Tollen reagent again. If the reaction becomes a positive result, it indicates the existence of glycosides in the sample (Table 3-4).

Table 3-4　Chemical Identifications of Carbohydrates and Glycosides

Sample	Molish	Tollen	Fehling
Reducing sugar (e.g. monosaccharide or some oligosaccharides)	+	+	+
Non-reducing sugar (e.g. polysaccharides or some oligosaccharides)	+	−	−
Glycosides	+	−	−
The hydrolysis products of glycosides with reducing sugar moiety	+	+	+

　+：Positive result；−：Negative result

4.2　Chromatography Identification

Thin layer chromatography（TLC）is an easy, cheap, rapid, and widely used method for identification of organic compounds in Chinese herbs. The stationary phases of TLC are usually silica gel and reversed-phase silica gel, or cellulose. Paper chromatography (PC) is rarely used nowadays.

For the identification of glycosides with strong polarities, strong polar solvent mixtures containing water, such as n-butanol-acetic acid-water (4 : 1 : 5, upper layer) (BAW), chloroform- methanol-water (65 : 35 : 10, lower layer), ethyl acetate-n-butanol-water (4 : 5 : 1, upper layer), etc., are commonly used as the mobile phase for silica gel TLC. For glycosides with low polarities, low polar solvent mixtures, such as chloroform-methanol, chloroform-acetone, etc., are used. If the stationary is reversed phase (e.g. C_{18} or C_8 reversed-phase silica gel), the mobile phase can be acetonitrile-methanol-water or methanol-water.

Glycosides identification does not have a universal method or chromatography condition or procedure because different glycosides have different properties.

5   Structure Determination

The structure determination procedures for polysaccharides and glycosides include determining the composition of monosaccharides, the order of monosaccharides, the position of glycosidic linkages, the configuration of glycosidic linkages, and the structure of aglycones.

Structure determination should be conducted on a pure compound. TLC or high performance liquid chromatography (HPLC) is generally used to test the purity of compounds. Electrophoresis may also be used to determine the purity of oligosaccharides or polysaccharides. It is worth pointing out that the purity of a polysaccharide cannot be estimated like that for small molecules based on their measured molecular weight versus theoretical molecular weight. In essence, "pure" polysaccharide refers to a mixture of polysaccharides in a certain molecular weight range, whose purity only represents the average distribution of similar chain length. The narrower the range is, the higher the purity is.

5.1   Determination of Physical Constants

Physical constants such as melting point, optical rotation, molecular weight (MW), are important indexes for a pure compound.

The optical rotation of polysaccharides is related to the type of monosaccharide in the molecule, the mode of glycosidic linkage connection and the molecular weight, especially to the configuration of sugar moiety (a or β). Generally, the optical rotation of polysaccharide with a-D-configuration is larger (mostly positive), but the optical rotation of a-L-configuration and β-D-configuration is smaller, or even negative.

5.2   Determination of Molecular Formula and Molecular Weight

In the past, the molecular composition was determined by qualitative and quantitative element analysis. At present, MS methods, such as field desorption ionization MS (FD-MS), field ionization MS (FI-MS), fast atom bombardment MS (FAB-MS), liquid secondary ion MS (LSI-MS), and electrospray ionization MS (ESI-MS) are widely used to determine the molecular weight of monosaccharides, oligosaccharides, and their glycosides.

High performance gel chromatography with refractive index detector is used to determine the molecular weight of polysaccharides by comparing the data to standard curves of various polysaccharides of known molecular weights and their elution volumes on gel column. Other methods, such as ESI-MS, centrifugation-sedimentation, light scattering, viscosity, and permeate pressure, are also used to determine the molecular weight of polysaccharides. In recent years, matrix-assisted laser desorption ionization and time of flight MS (MALDI-MS or MALDI-TOF-MS) provide advanced tools for molecular weight determination of polysaccharides.

High resolution FAB-MS (HR-FAB-MS) or HR-ESI-MS can be used to determine not only the molecular weight, but also molecular formula of glycosides.

5.3 Identification of Aglycones and Saccharides

Glycosides can be completely hydrolyzed by dilute acid or enzyme into aglycone and sugar(s), and these constituents can be further identified. Information of the types of monosaccharides and the ratio of each monosaccharide in the hydrolysis products should be obtained.

5.3.1 Structure Determination of Aglycone

Structure determination should be conducted on aglycones with high purity. The structure determination of various aglycones will be discussed in later chapters.

5.3.2 Identification of Saccharide Types

Traditionally, saccharide types in a glycoside can be identified by PC, TLC, HPLC, and GC. Before analysis by GC, the saccharide should be acetylated using methods described in this chapter. The acetylic products are analyzed by GC using allose (阿洛糖) or mannitol or inositol (肌醇) as an internal standard and known monosaccharides as control.

In general, saccharides in glycosides are identified by 1D-NMR and 2D-NMR. The values of ^{1}H-NMR and ^{13}C-NMR chemical shifts for some monosaccharides and their methyl-glycosides are listed in Tables 3-5 and Table 3-6.

Table 3-5 ^{1}H-NMR chemical shift values (δ) for some monosaccharide and its methyl-glycosides

Sugar (glycoside)	H-1	H-2	H-3	H-4	H-5	H-6	
β-D-glucose	4.64	3.25	3.50	3.42	3.46	3.72	3.90
α-D-glucose	5.23	3.54	3.72	3.42	3.84	3.76	3.84
β-D-galactose	4.53	3.45	3.59	3.89	3.65	3.64	3.72
α-D-galactose	5.22	3.78	3.81	3.95	4.03	3.69	3.69
β-D-mannose	4.89	3.95	3.66	3.60	3.38	3.75	3.91
α-D-mannose	5.18	3.94	3.86	3.68	3.82	3.74	3.84
β-L-rhamnose	4.85	3.93	3.59	3.38	3.39	1.30	
α-L-rhamnose	5.12	3.92	3.81	3.45	3.86	1.28	
β-L-fucose	4.55	3.46	3.63	3.74	3.79	1.26	
α-L-fucose	5.20	3.77	3.86	3.81	4.20	1.21	
Methyl-β-D-glucoside	4.27	3.15	3.38	3.27	3.36	3.82	3.62
Methyl-α-D-glucoside	4.70	3.46	3.56	3.29	3.54	3.77	3.66
Methyl-β-D-galactoside	4.20	3.39	3.53	3.81	3.57	3.69	3.74
Methyl-α-D-galactoside	4.73	3.72	3.68	3.86	3.78	3.67	3.61
Methyl-β-D-mannoside	4.47	3.88	3.53	3.46	3.27	3.83	3.63
Methyl-α-D-mannoside	4.66	3.82	3.65	3.53	3.51	3.79	3.65
Methyl-β-L-rhamnoside	4.16	3.74	3.72	3.89	3.55	3.77	
Methyl-α-L-rhamnoside	4.52	3.43	3.57	3.85	3.82	3.57	
Methyl-β-L-fucoside	4.21	3.14	3.33	3.51	3.88	3.21	
Methyl-α-L-fucoside	4.67	3.44	3.53	3.47	3.59	3.39	

Table 3-6 ^{13}C-NMR chemical shift values (δ) for some monosaccharides and their methyl-glycosides

Sugar (glycoside)	C-1	C-2	C-3	C-4	C-5	C-6
β-D-glucose	96.8	75.2	76.7	70.7	76.7	61.8
α-D-glucose	93.0	72.4	73.7	70.7	72.3	61.8
β-D-galactose	97.4	72.9	73.8	69.7	75.9	61.8
α-D-galactose	93.2	69.3	70.1	70.3	71.3	62.0
β-D-mannose	94.5	72.1	74.0	67.7	77.0	62.0
α-D-mannose	94.7	71.7	71.2	67.9	73.3	62.0
β-L-rhamnose	94.4	72.2	73.8	72.8	72.8	17.6
α-L-rhamnose	94.8	71.8	71.0	73.2	69.1	17.7
β-L-fucose	97.2	72.7	73.9	72.4	71.6	16.3
α-L-fucose	93.1	69.1	70.3	72.8	67.1	16.3
β-L-arabinose	93.4	69.5	69.5	69.5	63.4	—
α-L-arabinose	97.6	72.9	73.5	69.6	67.2	—
β-D-xylose	97.5	75.1	76.8	70.2	66.1	—
α-D-xylose	93.1	72.5	73.9	70.4	61.9	—
Methyl-β-D-glucoside	104.0	74.1	76.8	70.6	76.8	61.8
Methyl-α-D-glucoside	100.0	72.2	74.1	70.6	72.5	61.6
Methyl-β-D-galactoside	104.5	71.7	73.8	69.7	76.0	62.0
Methyl-α-D-galactoside	100.1	69.2	70.5	70.2	71.6	62.2
Methyl-β-D-mannoside	102.3	71.7	74.5	68.4	77.6	62.6
Methyl-α-D-mannoside	102.2	71.4	72.1	68.3	73.9	62.5
Methyl-β-L-rhamnoside	102.4	71.8	74.1	73.4	73.4	17.9
Methyl-α-L-rhamnoside	102.1	71.2	71.5	73.3	69.5	17.9
Methyl-β-L-fucoside	97.2	72.7	73.9	72.4	71.6	16.3
Methyl-α-L-fucoside	93.1	69.1	70.3	72.8	67.1	16.3

5.3.3   Determination of the Saccharide Numbers

The number of saccharides in a glycoside can be calculated based on the differences of the molecular weights between the glycoside and its aglycone according to their MS. It can also be inferred from the NMR based on the numbers of signals from the anomeric proton or carbon of the saccharides. In addition, 2D-NMR spectra can provide additional data to confirm the number of saccharide.

5.4   Determination of Linkage Sequence and Position of Monosaccharides

5.4.1   Sequence

Traditionally, partial hydrolysis methods such as dilute acidic hydrolysis, methylation and hydrolysis, acetylation and hydrolysis, and alkaline hydrolysis were used to analyze saccharide linkage sequences. Nowadays, spectrometric methods are generally used.

NMR spectrum provides the most useful information for the determination of saccharide linkage sequence. Glycosylation shift (GS, 苷化位移), chemical shift change of carbons in saccharide due to glycosylation, heteronuclear multiple quantum coherence (HMQC) and heteronuclear multiple bond correlation (HMBC) are used to identify the sequence of monosaccharides in glycosides.

Different carbons in a compound have different carbon spin relaxation times (T_1) in the ^{13}C-NMR spectrum. In glycosides, T_1 values for the outside saccharides are higher than that in the inside saccharides. This information can be used to determinate the saccharide sequence in glycosides.

In MS spectrum, the fragmentation mechanisms and the peaks of glycosyl fragment (糖基片段) are used as bases for the determination of saccharide sequence in glycosides. Because glycosides have no volatility, a conversion step using peracetolyzation, permethylation, or trimethylsilylation (三甲基硅烷化) methods is needed to change glycosides into volatile derivatives in order to perform EI-MS. The fragment ions of these derivatives are as follows (Figure 3-26).

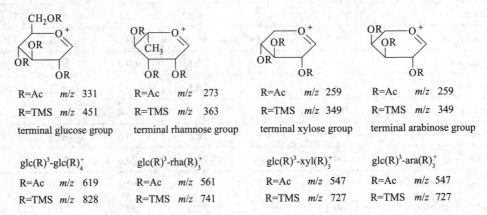

R=Ac *m/z* 331	R=Ac *m/z* 273	R=Ac *m/z* 259	R=Ac *m/z* 259
R=TMS *m/z* 451	R=TMS *m/z* 363	R=TMS *m/z* 349	R=TMS *m/z* 349
terminal glucose group	terminal rhamnose group	terminal xylose group	terminal arabinose group

glc(R)^3-glc(R)$_4^+$ glc(R)^3-rha(R)$_3^+$ glc(R)^3-xyl(R)$_3^+$ glc(R)^3-ara(R)$_3^+$

R=Ac *m/z* 619	R=Ac *m/z* 561	R=Ac *m/z* 547	R=Ac *m/z* 547
R=TMS *m/z* 828	R=TMS *m/z* 741	R=TMS *m/z* 727	R=TMS *m/z* 727

Figure 3-26　Fragment ions of glycoside derivatives

FD-MS and FAB-MS can also be used to identify the saccharide linkage sequence. For example, in FD-MS spectrum of ginsenoside Rb$_2$ (人参皂苷 Rb$_2$), besides *m/z* 1117 and *m/z* 1101 of [M+K]$^+$ and [M+Na]$^+$, high abundance fragment peaks, such as *m/z* 969, 939, 807, and 777, can be detected. The *m/z* 969 and *m/z* 939 correspond to [(M+Na)$^+$]-132 and [(M+Na)$^+$]-162, and indicate that arabinose and glucose, respectively, are at the end of 2 branched saccharide chains; similarly, *m/z* 807 and *m/z* 777 correspond to [(M+Na)$^+$]-132-162 and [(M+Na)$^+$]-162-162, which represent glucosyl-arabinosyl, and glucosyl-glucosyl, respectively.

5.4.2　Position of Saccharides

Currently, NMR, instead of chemical or enzyme degradation, is the most commonly used method for the determination of the linkage position between aglycone and saccharide.

^{13}C-NMR is an effective method to identify the linkage position between aglycone and saccharide. Glycosylation shift (GS) refers to the difference of chemical shifts before and after the formation of a glycoside at the *ipso*-carbon (the carbon that links with glycosidic atom) and *ortho*-carbon (the one adjacent to *ipso*-carbon) positions in an aglycone and at the anomeric carbon position in a saccharide. In general, different types of hydroxyl on aglycones yield different GSs during the formation of glycosides. For example, when an alcohol hydroxyl group is glycosidated, the signal of *ipso*-carbon moves to the down-field (4–10) and the signal of *ortho*-carbon moves to the up-field (−0.9~−4.6); while glycosidation of a phenol hydroxyl results in the *ipso*-carbon signal moves up-field and *ortho*-carbon signal moves down-field. It is very easy to identify which carbon in aglycone links with the saccharide based on the GS by comparing ^{13}C-NMR spectrum of aglycone with that of glycoside.

HMBC is widely used to identify the linkage positions between saccharide and aglycone. In HMBC spectrum, correlations between anomeric proton in saccharide and *ipso*-carbon in aglycone, or between the proton at *ipso*-carbon in aglycone and the anomeric carbon in saccharide will be detected. The position of linking between saccharide and aglycone can be easily determined by these correlations.

5.5   Determination of Configuration of Glycosidic Linkage

5.5.1 ^{1}H-NMR

At present, the commonly used method is to utilize the ^{1}H-NMR to analyze the coupling constant of the proton at the anomeric carbon in the sugar moiety of glycosides to determine the configuration of the glycosidic linkage. Compare with other protons in the sugar moiety of glycosides, the proton at the anomeric carbon is at lower fields, so it is easy to identify.

The H-2′ in some pyranoses (i.e. xylose, glucose, galactose etc.) is a-bond. When these sacchrides form glycosides with β-configurations, their H-1′ are a-bond too. The coupling constant (Jaa) between H-1′ and H-2′ is 6–9Hz. Conversely, when these sacchrides form glycosides with α-configurations, their H-1′ is e-bond. The coupling constant (Jae) between H-1′ and H-2′ is 2–3.5Hz. Therefore, the difference of the J values between H-1′ and H-2′ is used to determine the configuration of the glycosidic linkage. Examples of glucosides with perspective formulas and Newman projective types of structures are shown below (Figure 3-27).

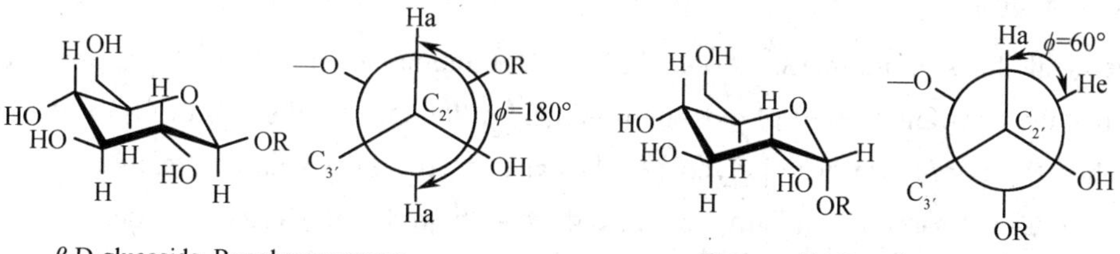

β-D-glucoside, R=aglycone group   α-D-glucoside, R=aglycone group

Figure 3-27   Configuration of glucosides

In the β-D-glucoside, the intersection angle (ϕ) between the a-bond H-1′ and H-2′ is 180°, $J = 6\sim9$Hz. In contrast in the α-D-glucoside of the above Newman projection, the intersection angle between H-1′ of e-bond and H-2′ of a-bond is 60°, $J = 2–3$Hz.

Some pyranoses, such as rhamnose and mannose, have an e-bond H-2′. The J values between H-1′ and H-2′ in α-configuration and β-configuration are the same. Therefore, the J values cannot be used to identify the configuration of glycosidic linkage. The Newman projection of rhamnose is demonstrated below (Figure 3-28).

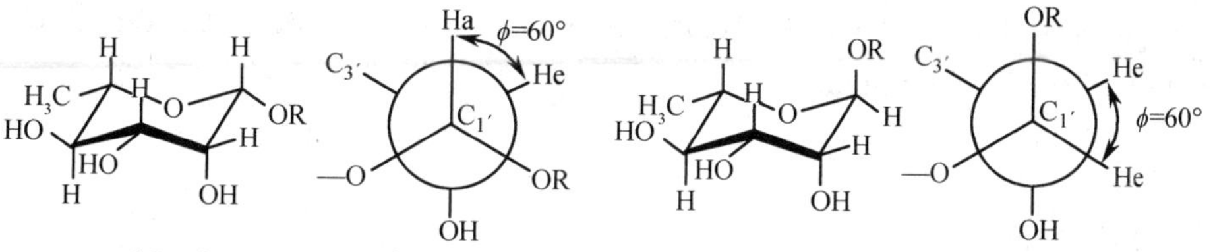

β-L-grhamnoside, R=aglycone group   α-L-rhamnoside, R=aglycone group

Figure 3-28   Conformation of rhamnosides

Please note that in the α-L-rhamnoside, the ϕ between the e-bond H-1′ and the e-bond H-2′ is at the same degree (60°) as in the β-L-rhamnoside between the a-bond H-1′ and the e-bond H-2′. Both J values are about 2Hz. Therefore it cannot be used to distinguish the configuration.

5.5.2 ^{13}C-NMR

The chemical shift of the anomeric carbon in saccharide and the coupling constant between the anomeric carbon and its proton are used to identify the configuration of glycosidic linkages. The concept is that the chemical shift of the anomeric carbon significantly increases after the formation of glycoside while that for other carbons remain almost unchanged. In some glycosides with α- or β-configurations, the chemical shifts of their anomeric carbons are different, so they can be used to identify the configuration of glycosidic linkages. Chemical shifts of some α- and β-glycosides are listed in Table 3-7.

Table 3-7　Chemical shifts of anomeric carbon in some α - and β -methylpyranosides

Configuration	Methylpyranoside							
	D-xyl	D-rib$^{\Delta}$	L-ara	D-glc	D-gal	D-man	D-fuc	L-rha
α	100.6	103.1	105.1	100.6	100.5	102.2	105.8*	102.6*
					101.3*	102.6*		
β	105.1	108.0	101.0	104.6	104.9	102.3	101.6*	102.6*
					106.6*	102.7*		

* C_5D_5N solvent　$^{\Delta}$ furanoside

The chemical shifts of anomeric carbons in D-methylmannoside and L-methlyrhamnoside cannot be used to identify the configuration of glycosidic linkage, but the chemical shifts of C-3 and C-5 have great difference when the configuration of glycosidic linkage is different. This is because both the chemical shifts of C-3 and C-5 in α-rhamnoside move up-field 1.5–3 than that in β- rhamnoside.

Moreover, the coupling constant between the anomeirc carbon and its proton may also be used to identify the configuration of glycosidic linkage (Table 3-8).

Table 3-8　J_{C1-H1} values of some methyl-glycosides

Configuration	Methyl-glycosides		
	D-glc	D-man	L-rha
α	170	166	168
β	159	156	158

In Table 3-8, the J_{C1-H1} values of the anomeric carbon in most methyl-α-pyranosides are about 170Hz while the J_{C1-H1} values are about 160Hz in most methyl-β-pyranosides. The 10Hz difference serves for the distinction of the configuration.

6　Examples of Chinese Herbs Containing Polysaccharides and Glycosides

6.1　Lycii Fructus (枸杞子)

6.1.1　Introduction

(1) Biological Source (基原)

Lycii Fructus is the dried ripe fruit of *Lycium barbarum* L. (枸杞). (Fam. Solanaceae) (茄科)

(2) Property (性), Flavor (味), and Channels Entered (归经)

Property and Flavor: Neutral (平); Sweet (甘).

Channels Entered: Liver, Kidney.

(3) Actions & Indications (功能与主治)

To nourish the liver and kidney, replenish essence and improve vision. For consumptive disease with deficiency of essence, dizziness and tinnitus, seminal emission, limp aching in the lower back and knees, impotence, internal heat wasting-thirst, blood deficiency and sallow complexion, blurred vision.

(4) Pharmacological Activities

The pharmacological activities associated with Lycii Fructus include hypoglycemic, lipotropic, immune-modulation, protection of hepatic function, anti-hypertension, anti-aging, anti-fatigue, antioxidant, etc. A wide range of health benefits, including cancer prevention and treatment, have been claimed for this fruit.

6.1.2　Main Chemical Constituents

Lycium barbarum grows from the southeast of Europe to China. It contains polysaccharides (LBP), carotenoids (类胡萝卜素), zeaxanthin (玉米素), glycerogalactolipids (甘油半乳糖脂), ascorbic acids (抗坏血酸), taurine (牛磺酸), flavonoids, etc.

(1) Polysaccharides and Glycoconjugates (复合糖)

The polysaccharides in *Gouqizi* are composed of two kinds of monosaccharides, namely glucose and fructose in molar ratios of 1：2.1. A new arabinogalactan-protein (阿拉半乳聚糖–蛋白) (LBP-Ⅲ), which is regarded as a potential neuroprotective agent in Alzheimer Dementia (AD), has been isolated from Lycii Fructus.

Many kinds of glycoconjugates, such as LbGp1, LbGp2, LbGp3, LbGp4, and LbGp5 have been isolated from Lycii Fructus. Their physicochemical properties and pharmacological activities are listed in Table 3-9.

Table 3-9　Properties and activities of some glycoconjugates from Lycii Fructus

Name	MW (kD)	Saccharide contents (%)	Saccharide types and ratio	N contents (%)	Activities
LbGp1	88	70	Ara：Gal：Glc=2.5：1.0：1.0	—	Pronounced immunoactivity
LbGp2	68.2	90.7	Ara：Gal =3：4	—	good immunoactivity and antioxidative activity
LbGp3	92.5	93.6	Ara：Gal=1：1	0.83	Pronounced immunoactivity

(continued)

Name	MW (kD)	Saccharide contents (%)	Saccharide types and ratio	N contents (%)	Activities
LbGp4	214.8	85.6	Ara : Gal : Rha : Glc=1.5 : 2.5 : 0.43 : 0.23	1.72	Pronounced immunoactivity
LbGp5	23.7	8.6	Rha : Ara : Xyl : Gal : Man : Glc=0.33 : 0.52 : 0.42 : 0.94 : 0.85 : 1	9.58	Pronounced immunoactivity

(2) Carotenoids

Eleven free carotenoids and seven carotenoid esters have been isolated from Lycii Fructus. Their contents have been analyzed by HPLC and shown in Table 3-10 and Table 3-11.

Table 3-10   Contents of all *trans* and *cis* forms of free carotenoids in Lycii Fructus

NO.	Carotenoids	Content (μg/g)
1	Neoxanthin (新叶黄素)	11.9 ± 0.0
2	9-or 9′-*cis*-zeaxanthin	30.4 ± 2.6
3	13-or 13′-*cis*-zeaxanthin	4.4 ± 0.7
4	15-or 15′-*cis*-zeaxanthin	29.6 ± 2.4
5	all-*trans*-zeaxanthin	1196.8 ± 13.1
6	9-or 9′-*cis*-zeaxanthin	5.1 ± 2.4
7	all-*trans*-β-cryptoxanthin (隐黄素)	48.1 ± 0.7
8	9-or 9′-*cis*-β-cryptoxanthin	5.1 ± 0.0
9	13-or 13′-*cis*-β-carotene (胡萝卜素)	48.1 ± 0.7
10	all-*trans*-β-carotene	15.0 ± 0.3
11	9-or 9′-*cis*-β-carotene	9.3 ± 0.2

Table 3-11   Contents of all *trans* and *cis* form of carotenoid esters in Lycii Fructus

NO.	Carotenoid esters	Content (μg/g)
1	zeaxanthin monopalmitate (玉米素单棕榈酸酯)	11.9 ± 0.3
2	zeaxanthin monopalmitate (isomer)	11.3 ± 0.1
3	β-cryptoxanthin monopalmitate	64.4 ± 0.0
4	zeaxanthin monopalmitate (isomer)	62.8 ± 0.2
5	β-cryptoxanthin monopalmitate (isomer)	32.9 ± 0.5
6	β-cryptoxanthin monopalmitate (isomer)	68.5 ± 0.5
7	zeaxanthin dipalmitate (玉米素二棕榈酸酯)	1143.7 ± 9.7

Zeaxanthin esters have been quantified based on their respective molecular masses using zeaxanthin as the calibration standard (校标). Total zeaxanthin has been determined after saponification (皂化) of the extracts. Lycii Fructus have been proved to be valuable zeaxanthin ester sources.

(3) Glycerogalactolipids

Fifteen glycerogalactolipids (1-15) have been isolated from Lycii Fructus. Their structures are as follows.

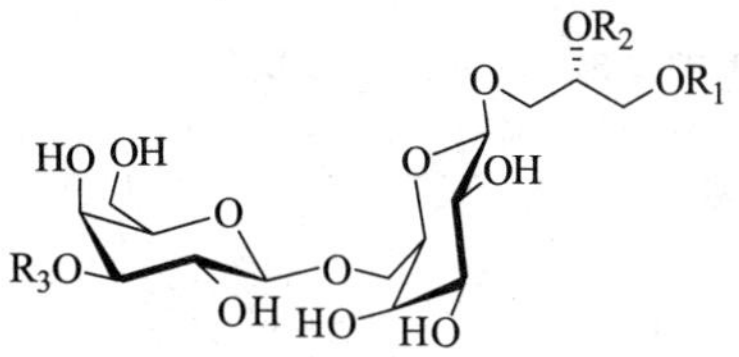

1. R_1 = palmitoyl, R_2 = R_3 = linolenoyl
2. R_1 = palmitoyl, R_2 = linolenoyl, R_3 = linoleoyl
3. R_1 = R_3 = palmitoyl, R_2 = linolenoyl
4. R_1 = R_3 = palmitoyl, R_2 = linoleoyl
5. R_1 = R_2 = R_3 = palmitoyl
6. R_1 = R_2 = palmitoyl, R_3 = H
7. R_1 = R_2 = linolenoyl, R_3 = H
8. R_1 = linolenoyl, R_2 = linoleoyl, R_3 = H
9. R_1 = palmitoyl, R_2 = linolenoyl, R_3 = H
10. R_1 = palmitoyl, R_2 = linoleoyl, R_3 = H
11. R_1 = palmitoyl, R_2 = oleoyl, R_3 = H
12. R_1 = stearoyl, R_2 = linoleoyl, R_3 = H

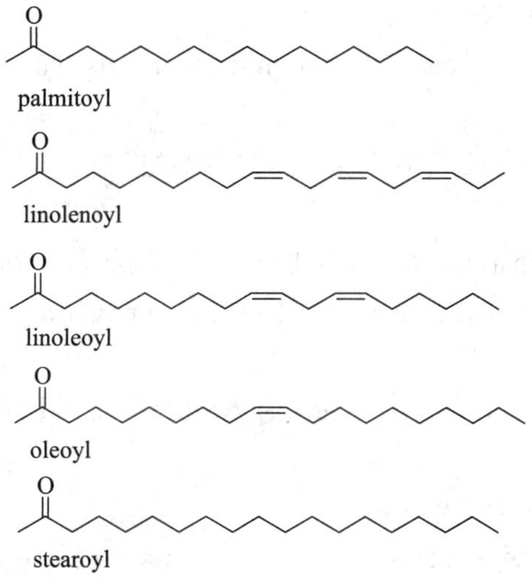

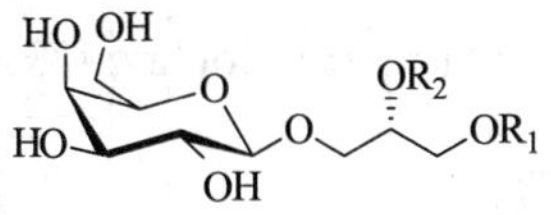

palmitoyl

linolenoyl

linoleoyl

oleoyl

stearoyl

13. R_1 = palmitoyl, R_2 = linolenoyl
14. R_1 = palmitoyl, R_2 = linoleoyl
15. R_1 = palmitoyl, R_2 = oleoyl

(4) Others

2-O-β-D-glucopyranosyl-L-ascorbic acid (AA-2βG) is a novel stable vitamin C analog. It is one of the main biologically active components of Lycii Fructus having selective suppression on cervical cancer Hela cells.

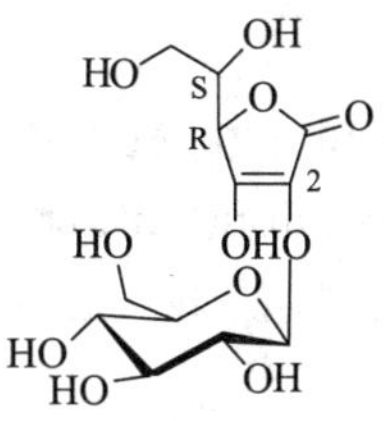

AA-2βG

Other chemicals found in Lycii Fructus include taurine, *p*-coumaric acid (对香豆酸), glucose, flavonoids, palmitic acid (棕榈酸) (C16：0), stearic acid (硬脂酸) (C18：0), oleic acid (油酸) (C18：1), linoleic acid (亚油酸) (C18：2), β-sitosterol（β– 谷甾醇）, daucosterol (蝙蝠葛甾醇), scopoletin (东莨菪内酯), and betaine (甜菜碱).

6.1.3　Quality Control Standards

(1) TLC Identification

Stationary Phase: Silica gel plate.

Standard: Authentic crude drug (对照药材).

Development System: Acetyl acetate - chloroform - formic acid (3 ：2 ：1).

Visualization: 365nm UV light.

(2) Tests

Water: Not more than 13.0%.

Total Ash: Not more than 5.0%.

Heavy Metals and Other Harmful Elements: Pb ≤5 ppm, Cd≤0.3 ppm, As≤2 ppm, Hg≤0.2 ppm, Cu≤20 ppm.

Extract (water): Not less than 55.0%.

(3) Assay

Polysaccharides: Not less than 1.80% (spectrophotometric method).

Betaine: Not less than 0.30% (Thin Layer Chromatography Scan method, TLCS).

6.2　Armeniacae Semen Amarum (苦杏仁)

6.2.1　Introduction

(1) Biological Source

Armeniacae Semen Amarum is the dried ripe seed of *Prunus armeniaca* L. var. *ansu* Maxim (山杏), *Prunus sibirica* L. (西 伯 利 亚 杏), *Prunus mandshurica* (Maxim.) Kochne (东北杏), or *Prunus armeniaca* L. (杏). (Fam. Rosaceae) (蔷薇科)

(2) Property, Flavor and Channels Entered

Property and Flavor: Mild warm (温热); Bitter; Slightly toxic (微毒).

Channels Entered: Lung, Large Intestine.

(3) Actions & Indications

Direct qi downward to suppress cough and relieve panting, and moisten the intestines to relax the bowels. For cough and panting, chest fullness, profuse sputum, and constipation caused by intestinal dryness.

(4) Pharmacological Activities

The pharmacological activities associated with Armeniacae Semen Amarum include anti-microbia, anti-mutage, anti-inflammation, anti-nociception, antioxidation, inhibitory activity against enzyme, cardio-protection, etc. Polyphenolic compounds in the extracts of Armeniacae Semen Amarum skin may be the effective components as antioxidant.

The toxicity of Armeniacae Semen Amarum is rooted mainly in amygdalin, which can be hydrolyzed by amygdalase to release hydrocyanic acid. The consumption of small amount of Armeniacae Semen Amarum containing amygdalin can inhibit the respiration center to stop coughing. Over consumption of containing high amount of amygdalin may cause intoxication in humans and animals.

6.2.2　Main Chemical Constituents

Nearly 570 compounds have been isolated from several Prunus species during the period of 1908 to June 2010. Armeniacae Semen Amarum contains mono- and polysaccharides, polyphenols, fatty acids, sterol derivatives, carotenoids, cyanogenic glucosides, and volatile components with specific fragrance.

The cyanogenic glucosides have bitter taste.

(1) Cyanogenic Glucosides

Cyanogenic glucosides are found in *P. armeniaca*. Amygdalin is the major component and it can release hydrocyanic acid under certain condition (Figure 3-29). Another cyanogenic glucoside presented in apricot seeds is prunasin, a metabolite of amygdalin.

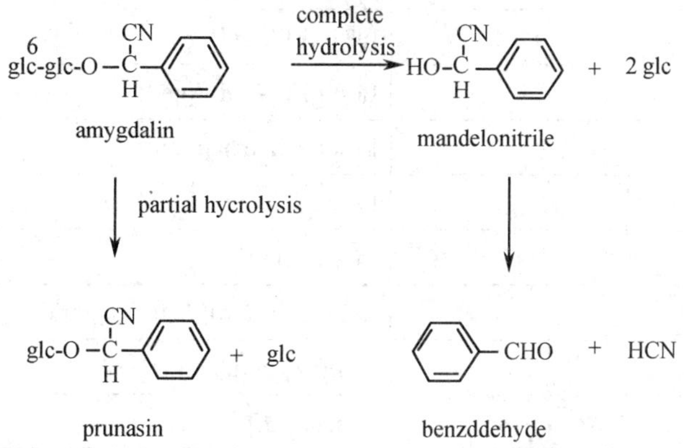

Figure 3-29   Hydrolysis of amygdalin

(2) Fatty Acids

Many fatty acids have been identified from Armeniacae Semen Amarum. These include oleic acid, linoleic acid, linolenic acid (亚麻酸), arachidonic acid (花生四烯酸), palmitic acid, stearic acid, and arachidic acid (花生酸), etc. The ansu apricot oil (安素杏油) from *P. armeniaca* L. var. *ansu* Maxim. is a natural source of antioxidants.

Additional components found in Armeniacae Semen Amarum include phthalic acid (邻苯二甲酸), 9-hexadecenoic acid (9– 十六烯酸), hexadecanoic acid (十六烯酸), 9, 12-octadecadienoic acid (9, 12–十八烯酸), 9-octadecenoic acid (9–十八烯酸), 10-octadecenoic acid (10–十八烯酸), eicosanoic acid (二十碳酸), and *b*-sitosterol and stigmasterol (豆甾醇), just to name a few.

6.2.3   Quality Control Standards

(1) TLC Identification

Stationary Phase: Silica gel plate.

Standard: Amygdalin (Chemical Reference Substance, CRS).

Development System: Chloroform-acetyl acetate-methanol-water (15：40：22：10) (Stand for 12h at 5-10℃ , lower layer).

Visualization: Spray the solution of 0.8% molybdophosphoric acid (磷钼酸)/ 15% sulphuric acid in ethanol, heat to 105℃ until spots are clear.

(2) Tests

Peroxide Value (过氧化值): Not more than 0.11.

(3) Assay

Amygdalin: Not less than 3.0% (HPLC method) for crude drug of Armeniacae Semen Amarum; Not less than 2.4% (HPLC method) for slices of Armeniacae Semen Amarum; Not less than 2.1% (HPLC method) for slices of stir-fried Armeniacae Semen Amarum.

词 汇 表

An Alphabetical List of Words and Phrases

A		
Acanthopanacis Senticosi Radix et Rhizoma seu Caulis		刺五加
accelerated desiccation	[æk'selərertɪd][ˌdesɪ'keɪʃn]	快速干燥
acetic acid	[ə'si:tɪk]['æsɪd]	乙酸
acetic acid glacial	[ə'si:tɪk]['æsɪd]['gleɪʃl]	冰醋酸
acetic anhydride	[ə'si:tɪk][æn'haɪdraɪd]	乙酸酐
acetolysis	[ˌæsɪ'tɔlɪsɪs]	乙酰解
acetylation	[əsetɪ'leɪʃən]	乙酰化作用
acidic crude polysaccharide	[ə'sɪdɪk][kru:d][ˌpɔlɪ'sækəraɪd]	酸性粗多糖
actions & indications	['ækʃnz][ˌɪndɪ'keɪʃnz]	功能与主治
adenosine	[ə'denəsi:n]	腺苷
agar	['eɪgɑ:]	琼脂
agaropectin	[ægərə'pektɪn]	琼脂凝集素
agarose	['ɑ:gərəus]	琼脂糖
aglycone	[ægli:'kəun]	苷元
alcohol sugar	['ælkəhɔl]['ʃugə]	醇糖
alcoholic glycoside	[ˌælkə'hɔlɪk]['glaɪkəsaɪd]	醇苷
alcoholyze	['ælkəhɔlaɪz]	醇解
aldehyde	['ældɪhaɪd]	醛
aldobionic acid	[ˌældəbaɪ'ɔnɪk]['æsɪd]	醛酸
aldohexose	[ˌældə'heksəus]	己醛糖
aldose	['ældəus]	醛糖
aldoside	['ældəsaɪd]	醛糖苷
algin	['ældʒɪn]	藻胶素
alginic acid	[æl'dʒɪnɪk]['æsɪd]	海藻酸
aliphatic	[ˌælə'fætɪk]	脂肪族的
allose	['æləus]	阿洛糖
aloe	['æləu]	芦荟
aloin	['æləuɪn]	芦荟苷
amide	['æmaɪd]	酰胺
amino group	['æmɪnəu][gru:p]	氨基
amino sugar	['æmɪnəu]['ʃugə]	氨基糖
ammonia sulfate	[ə'məunɪə]['sʌlfeɪt]	硫酸铵
2-aminosugar glycoside	[æmɪ'nəusugə]['glaɪkəusaɪd]	2-氨基糖苷

(continued)

amorphous powder	[ə'mɔːfəs]['paʊdə]	无定形粉末
amygdalin	[ə'mɪgdəlɪn]	苦杏仁苷
amylose and amylopectin	['æmɪləʊs][ənd][ˌæmələʊ'pektɪn]	直链淀粉和支链淀粉
Anogeissus latifolia		宽叶榆绿木
anomer	['ænəmə]	端基异构体
anomeric carbon	[æ'nəʊmerɪk]['kɑːbən]	端基碳
ansu apricot oil	['ænsjuː]['eɪprɪkɔt][ɔɪl]	安素杏油
anthracenol glycoside	[ænθ'reɪsenɔl]['glaɪkəʊsaɪd]	蒽酚苷
arabinogalactan	[æræbɪnɔgələk'tæn]	阿拉伯半乳聚糖
arabinogalactan-protein	[æræbɪnɔgələk'tæn]['prəʊtiːn]	阿拉半乳聚糖－蛋白
arachidic acid	[ɑːræ'kɪdɪk]['æsɪd]	花生酸
arachidonic acid	[ærəkɪ'dɔnɪk]['æsɪd]	花生四烯酸
arbutin	['ɑːbjutɪn]	熊果苷
Arctostaphylos uva-ursi		熊果
Armeniacae Semen Amarum		苦杏仁
ascorbic acid	[əs'kɔːbɪk]['æsɪd]	抗坏血酸
Astragali Radix	[æstrə'gæliː]['reɪdɪks]	黄芪
astragaloside	[æstrəgə'ləʊsaɪd]	黄芪苷
Astragalus gummifer		胶黄芪
authentic crude drug	[ɔː'θentɪk][kruːd][drʌg]	对照药材
auxochrome	['ɔːksəkrəʊm]	助色团
B		
bassorin	[bæ'sɔːrɪn]	黄芪胶糖
benzoic aldehyde	[ben'zəʊɪk]['ældɪhaɪd]	苯甲醛
betaine	['biːtəɪn]	甜菜碱
bidesmosidic	[ˌbaɪdɪs'mɔsɪdɪk]	双糖链的
binding agent	['baɪndɪŋ]['eɪdʒənt]	黏合剂
biological source	[ˌbaɪə'lɔdʒɪkəl][sɔːs]	基原
boron trifluoride	['bɔːrɔn][traɪ'fluəraɪd]	三氟化硼
Brassia nigra	['breɪzɪə]['nɪgrə]	黑芥
C		
calcium carbonate	['kælsɪəm]['kɑːbəneɪt]	碳酸钙
calibration standard	[ˌkælɪ'breɪʃn]['stændəd]	校标
carbohydrate	[ˌkɑːbə'haɪdreɪt]	碳水化合物
carbon glycoside	['kɑːbən]['glaɪkəsaɪd]	碳苷
carbonium ion	[kɑː'bəʊnɪəm]['aɪən]	正碳离子
carbonyl group	['kɑːbənɪl][gruːp]	羰基

(continued)

carboxyl	[kɑ:'bɔksɪl]	羧基
carotene	['kærəti:n]	胡萝卜素
carotenoid	[kə'rɔtənɔɪd]	类胡萝卜素
carrageenan	[ˌkærə'gi:nən]	角叉菜胶
Ceratonia siliqua		长角豆
C-glycosides	['glaɪkəsaɪdz]	碳苷
channels entered	['tʃænlz]['entə(r)d]	归经
chiral carbon	['tʃɪrəl]['kɑ:bən]	手性碳
chitin	['kaɪtɪn]	壳多糖，几丁质
chondroitin sulfate	[kən'drɔɪtɪn]['sʌlfeɪt]	硫酸软骨素
Chondrus cryspus		皱波角叉菜
circular dichroism	['sə:kjulə]['daɪkrəʊɪzm]	圆二色性
Citrus aurantium	['sɪtrəs][ɔ:rɔn'ti:ju:m]	酸橙
Citrus limon	['sɪtrəs]['laɪmən]	柠檬
coarse powder	[kɔ:s]['paudə(r)]	粗粉
Combretaceae	[kɔm'bretəsi:]	使君子科
Compositae	[kɔm'pɔzi:taɪ]	菊科
configuration	[kənˌfɪgɪə'reɪʃn]	构型
conjugation effect	[ˌkɔndʒu'geɪʃn][ɪ'fekt]	共轭效应
coumarin glycoside	['ku:mərɪn]['glaɪkəsaɪd]	香豆素苷
crab	[kræb]	蟹
Crataegi Fructus	[kræ'ti:gɪ]['frʌktəs]	山楂
Crotonis Fructus	['krəʊtʌnɪz]['frʌktəs]	巴豆
crotonoside	[krəʊtə'nəusaɪd]	巴豆苷
Cruciferae	[kru'saɪfərə]	十字花科
crude drug	[kru:d][drʌg]	药材
cryptoxanthin	['krɪptəuˌzænθɪn]	隐黄素
Cyamopsis tetragonolobus		瓜尔豆
cyanogenic glycoside	[saɪənəu'dʒenɪk]['glaɪkəsaɪd]	氰苷
cytidine	['saɪtədɪn]	胞苷
D		
daucosterol	[dɔ:'kɔstərɔl]	蝙蝠葛甾醇
defat	[dɪ'fæt]	脱脂
dehydration reaction	[ˌdi:haɪ'dreɪʃn][ri'ækʃn]	脱水反应
demulcent	[dɪ'mʌlsənt]	调和剂，消毒剂
deoxy sugar	[dɪ'ɔksɪ]['ʃugə]	去氧糖
2-deoxy-glucoside	[dɪ'ɔksɪ]['glu:kəsaɪd]	2– 去氧 - 葡萄糖苷

(continued)

2-deoxyribose	[diːˌɔksɪˈraɪbəus]	2– 去氧核糖
desinsection	[desɪnˈzekʃn]	杀虫
dextrorotation	[ˌdekstrəurəuˈteɪʃən]	右旋
D-galacto-D-manoglycon		D– 半乳糖 –D– 甘露聚糖
D-glucose-3- methoxyl	[ˈgluːkəus][ˈmetɔksɪl]	D– 葡萄糖 –3– 甲醚
D-glyceraldehyde	[ˌglɪsəˈrældɪhaɪd]	D– 甘油醛
dialcohol	[daɪˈælkəhɔl]	二醇
dialdehyde	[daɪˈældɪhaɪd]	丙二醛
diastereoisomer	[ˌdaɪəˌstɪərɪəuˈaɪsəmə]	非对映异构体
diastereomer	[daɪəˈstɪərɪəumə]	非对映体
digitoxin	[ˌdɪdʒɪˈtɔksɪn]	洋地黄毒苷
dilute hydrochloric acid	[daɪˈluːt][ˌhaɪdrəˈklɔrɪk][ˈæsɪd]	稀盐酸
disaccharide	[daɪˈsækəraɪd]	双糖
disintegrating agent	[dɪsˈɪntɪˌgreɪtɪŋ][ˈeɪdʒənt]	崩解剂
E		
Echinacea purpurea		紫松果菊
echinacea	[ˌekɪˈneɪsɪə]	松果菊
eicosanoic acid	[aɪkəuˈsænɔɪk][ˈæsɪd]	二十碳酸
electron cloud density	[ɪˈlektrɔn][klaud][ˈdensəti]	电子云密度
electron donor group	[ɪˈlektrɔn][ˈdəunə][gruːp]	供电子基团
electro-negativity	[ɪˈlektrəu][ˌnegəˈtɪvəti]	电负性
electron-withdrawing	[ɪˈlektrɔn][wɪðˈdrɔɪŋ]	吸电子
emulgent	[ɪˈmʌldʒənt]	乳化剂
emulsin	[ɪˈmʌlsɪn]	苦杏仁酶
enolic glycoside	[iːˈnɔlɪk][ˈglaɪkəsaɪd]	烯醇苷
equilibrium condition	[ˌiːkwɪˈlɪbrɪəm][kənˈdɪʃn]	平衡条件
esculin	[ˈeskjulɪn]	秦皮甲素
ester glycoside	[ˈestə][ˈglaɪkəsaɪd]	酯苷
ethylene glycol	[ˈeθəliːn][ˈglaɪkɔl]	乙二醇
F		
flavonoid glycoside	[ˈfleɪvənɔɪd][ˈglaɪkəsaɪd]	黄酮苷
flavor	[ˈfleɪvə]	味
formic acid	[ˈfɔːmɪk][ˈæsɪd]	甲酸
Fraxini Cortex		秦皮
fructan	[ˈfræktən]	果聚糖
fructo-furanose unit		呋喃果糖
fructoside	[ˈfrʌktəsaɪd]	果糖苷

(continued)

furanose	['fjuərənəus]	呋喃糖
furanoside	['fjuərænəsaɪd]	呋喃糖苷
G		
galactoside	[gə'læktəsaɪd]	半乳糖苷
Ganoderma	[gə'nɔdəmə]	灵芝
Gardeniae Fructus		栀子
Gastrodiae Rhizoma		天麻
gastrodin	[gæst'rɔdɪn]	天麻素，天麻苷
Gelidiaceae		石花菜科
Gelidium amansii		石花菜
genin	['dʒenɪn]	苷元，配基
geniposide	[dʒenɪ'pəusaɪd]	京尼平苷
gentiobiose	[ˌdʒenʃɪə'baɪəus]	龙胆二糖
Gigarginaceae		杉藻科
Gigartina sps.		杉藻属植物
ginsenoside	[gɪnse'nəusaɪd]	人参皂苷
ginsenoside Rb2		人参皂苷 Rb2
ginsenoside Rh2		人参皂苷 Rh2
glucoraphenin	[glu:'kɔræfnɪn]	萝卜苷
glucosamine	[glu:kəu'sæmi:n]	氨基葡萄糖
glucoside	['glu:kəsaɪd]	葡萄糖苷
glucuronic acid	[glu:kju'rɔnɪk]['æsɪd]	葡萄糖醛酸
glycerol	['glɪsərɔl]	甘油
glycerogalactolipid	[ˌglɪsərəuˌgəlæktə'lɪpɪd]	甘油半乳糖苷脂
glycoconjugate	[glɪkəukəndʒu'geɪt]	复合糖
glycogen	['glaɪkəudʒen]	糖原
glycosidase	[glaɪ'kəusɪdeɪs]	苷酶
glycoside	['glaɪkəsaɪd]	苷
glycosidic atom	[glaɪkəu'sɪdɪk]['ætəm]	苷原子
glycosidic linkage	[ˌglaɪkəu'sɪdɪk]['lɪŋkɪdʒ]	苷键
glycosylation shift (GS)	[ˌglaɪkəsɪ'leɪʃən][ʃɪft]	苷化位移
glycosyl fragment	['glaɪkəsɪl]['frægmənt]	糖基片段
Gramineae		禾本科
guanosine	['gwɑ:nəsɪn]	鸟苷
guar gum	[gwɑ:][gʌm]	瓜尔豆胶
guaran	['gɑ:ræn]	瓜尔糖
gum	[gʌm]	树胶

(continued)

gum ghatti	[gʌm]['gætɪ]	印度果胶
gum karaya	[gʌm][kə'raɪjə]	卡拉亚胶
H		
hemiacetal	[ˌhemɪ'æsɪtæl]	半缩醛
hemicellulose	[ˌhemɪ'seljuləus]	半纤维素
hemiketal	[ˌhemɪ'ki:təl]	半缩酮
heparin	['heperɪn]	肝素
heptoside	['heptəusaɪd]	七碳糖苷
9-hexadecenoic acid	[hekseɪ'desɪ'nəuɪk]['æsɪd]	9– 十六烯酸
heterosaccharide	[hetərəuzə'kærɪd]	杂多糖
hexadecanoic acid		十六烯酸
hexitol	['hekɪtɔl]	己糖醇
hexoside	[hek'səusaɪd]	六碳糖苷
hexuronic acid		己糖醛酸
hexuronic acid glycoside		六碳糖醛酸苷
homosaccharide		均多糖
hyaluronic acid	[ˌhaɪəlu'rɔnɪk]['æsɪd]	透明质酸
hydrochloric acid	[ˌhaɪdrəu'klɔrɪk]['æsɪd]	盐酸
hydrocyanic acid	[ˌhaɪdrəusaɪ'ænɪk]['æsɪd]	氢氰酸
hydroxyl aldehyde	[haɪ'drɔksɪl]['ældɪhaɪd]	羟基乙醛
hydroxyl group	[haɪ'drɔksɪl][gru:p]	羟基
2-hydroxylsugar glycoside	[haɪ'drɔksɪl'ʃugə] ['glaɪkəsaɪd]	2– 羟基糖苷
I		
ice-water bath	[aɪs]['wɔ:tə][bɑ:θ]	冰水浴
inositol	[ɪ'nəusɪtəul]	肌醇
intramolecular nucleophilic reaction	[ˌɪntə(:)mə'lekjulə][nju:klɪəu'fɪlɪk][ri'ækʃn]	分子内亲核反应
Inula helenium		土木香
inulin	['ɪnjulɪn]	菊粉
iridoid	[ɪərɪ'dɔɪdz]	环烯醚萜
isapgol	[ɪ'zæpgɔl]	车前子壳膳食纤维
isothiocyanate	['aɪsəuˌθaɪəu'saɪəneɪt]	异硫氰酸酯
K		
ketoheptose	[ˌki:təu'heptəus]	庚酮糖
ketohexose	[ˌki:təu'heksəus]	己酮糖
ketone	['ki:təun]	酮
ketose	['ki:təus]	酮糖

(continued)

keto sugar	['ki:təu]['ʃugə]	酮糖
ketoside	['ki:təusaɪd]	酮糖苷
L		
lanatoside A	[le'nætəsaɪd]	毛花洋地黄苷 A
laxative	['læksətɪv]	通便剂，泻药
Leguminosae		豆科
lentinan's	['lentɪnænz]	香菇多糖的
Lessoniaceae	[leˌsɔnɪ'eɪsiː]	巨藻科
levorotary	[ˌliːvə'rəutəri]	左旋的
lignan glycoside	['lɪgnæn]['glaɪkəsaɪd]	木脂素苷
linoleic acid	[lɪ'nəuliːk]['æsɪd]	亚油酸
linolenic acid	[lɪmə'lenɪk]['æsɪd]	亚麻酸
liquorice saponin	['lɪkərɪs]['sæpənɪn]	甘草皂苷
locust bean	['ləukəst][biːn]	槐豆
Lycii Fructus		枸杞子
Lycium barbarum L.		枸杞
M		
Macrocystis pyrifera		巨藻
maltase	['mɔːlteɪs]	麦芽糖酶
mandelonitrile	[ˌmændɪləu'naɪtraɪl]	苯乙醇腈
methylation	[meθɪ'leɪʃn]	甲基化作用
methyl-glucoside	['meθɪl]['gluːkəsaɪd]	葡萄糖甲苷
methylpentose	['meθɪlpəntəus]	甲基五碳糖
methylpentoside	[ˌmeθɪlpən'təusaɪd]	甲基五碳糖苷
mild warm	[maɪld][wɔːm]	温热
molybdophosphoric acid		磷钼酸
monodesmosidic	[ˌmɔnəu'dɪsməusaɪdɪk]	单糖链的
monosaccharide	[ˌmɔnəu'sækəraɪd]	单糖
Moraceae		桑科
mucilage	['mjuːsɪlɪdʒ]	黏液质
myrosinase	['maɪrəsɪneɪs]	芥子酶
N		
α -naphthol	['næfθɔl]	α – 萘酚
naphthol glycoside	['næfθɔl]['glaɪkəsaɪd]	萘酚苷
neohesperidose	[niːəuhespərɪ'dəus]	新橙皮糖
neoxanthin	[ˌniːəu'zænθɪn]	新叶黄素
neutral	['njuːtrəl]	中性；平

(continued)

N-glycosides	['glaɪkəsaɪdz]	*N*– 苷
nitrile	['naɪtraɪl]	腈
nitrogen glycoside	['naɪtrədʒən] ['glaɪkəsaɪd]	氮苷
non-reducing sugar	[nʌnrɪ'dju:ɡɪŋ]['ʃugə]	非还原糖
non-sugar moiety	[nʌn'ʃugə]['mɔɪətɪ]	非糖部分
nucleophilic	[ˌnju:klɪəu'fɪlɪk]	亲核的
nutritive	['nju:trɪtɪv]	营养剂
O		
9-octadecenoic acid		9– 十八烯酸
10-octadecenoic acid		10– 十八烯酸
9, 12-octadecadienoic acid	[ˌɔktə'dekɑ:dɪnəuɪk]['æsɪd]	9, 12– 十八烯酸
O-glycosides	['glaɪkəsaɪdz]	氧苷
oleic acid	[əu'li:ɪk]['æsɪd]	油酸
oligosaccharide	[ˌɔlɪɡəu'sækəraɪd]	低聚糖
ophiopogonin D	[ə'faɪɔpɔɡənɪn]	麦冬皂苷 D
optical activity	['ɔptɪkəl][æk'tɪvətɪ]	旋光性
optically active isomer	['ɔptɪkəlɪ]['æktɪv]['aɪsəmə]	光学活性异构体
Oryza sativa		水稻
oxidative cleavage	['ɔksɪdeɪtɪv]['kli:vɪdʒ]	氧化裂解
oxygen glycoside	['ɔksɪdʒən]['glaɪkəsaɪd]	氧苷
P		
palmitic acid	[pæl'mɪtɪk]['æsɪd]	棕榈酸
p-coumaric acid	['ku:mərɪn]['æsɪd]	对香豆酸
pectin	['pektɪn]	果胶
pectin substance	['pektɪn]['sʌbstəns]	果胶质
pentosan	['pentəsæn]	戊聚糖
pentose	['pentəus]	五碳糖
pentoside	['pentəsaɪd]	五碳糖苷
permethylated	[pə'meθɪleɪtɪd]	全甲基化的
perchloric acid	[pə'klɔ:rɪk]['æsɪd]	高氯酸
periodate	[pe'raɪɔdeɪt]	过碘酸
peroxide value	[pə'rɔksaɪd]['vælju:]	过氧化值
pharmaceutical aid	[ˌfa:mə'su:tɪkl][eɪd]	药物辅料
phthalic acid	['θælɪk]['æsɪd]	邻苯二甲酸
phenolic glycoside	[fɪ'nɔlɪk]['glaɪkəsaɪd]	酚苷
picrocrocin	[pɪ'krɔkrɔsɪn]	藏红花苦苷
Plantaginaceae		车前草科

(continued)

Plantago ovata	[plæn'teɪgəu]['əuvətə]	卵叶车前子
Plantago psyllium	[plæn'teɪgəu]['sɪljəm]	欧车前
polyhydroxyaldehyde	[pɔlɪhaɪdrɔksɪ'əɔːldɪhaɪd]	多羟基醛
polyhydroxyketone	[pɔlɪhaɪd'rɔksaɪktəun]	多羟基酮
Polyporus	[pɔlɪ'pɔrəs]	猪苓
polysaccharide	[pɔlɪ'sækəraɪd]	多糖
Poria	['pɔːrɪə]	茯苓
primary glycoside	['praɪmərɪ]['glaɪkəsaɪd]	原生苷
property	['prɔpəti]	性，药性
propylene glycol	['prəupɪliːn]['glaɪkɔl]	丙二醇
protoanemonin	[ˌprəutəuə'nemənɪn]	原白头翁素
protonation	[ˌprəutə'neɪʃən]	质子化
prunasin	['pruːnəsɪn]	野樱苷
Prunus armeniaca L.		杏
Prunus armeniaca L. var. *ansu* Maxim		山杏
Prunus mandshurica (Maxim.) Kochne		东北杏
Prunus sibirica L.		西伯利亚杏
psyllium	['sɪlɪəm]	欧车前子壳膳食纤维
puerarin	['pjuːrərɪn]	葛根素
pyranose	['paɪərənəus]	吡喃糖
pyranoside	[pɪ'rænəsaɪd]	吡喃糖苷
pyrimidine ring	[ˌpaɪə'rɪmɪdiːn][rɪŋ]	嘧啶环
R		
raffinose	['ræfɪnəus]	棉子糖
ranunculin	[rənʌn'kjulɪn]	毛茛苷
Ranunculus japonicus		毛茛
reducing sugar	[rɪ'djuːsɪŋ]['ʃugə]	还原糖
reference standards	['refrəns]['stændədz]	对照品
Rhei Radix et Rhizoma		大黄
Rhodiolae Crenulatae Radix et Rhizoma		红景天
rhodioloside	[rəuda'ɪələusaɪd]	红景天苷
Rosaceae		蔷薇科
Rutaceae		芸香科
rutin	['ruːtɪn]	芦丁
rutinose	[ruːtɪ'nəus]	芸香糖
S		
saccharide	['sækəraɪd]	糖

(continued)

salicin	[ˈsælɪsɪn]	水杨苷
saponification	[səˌpɒnɪfɪˈkeɪʃən]	皂化
scopoletin	[ˈskəupəletɪn]	东莨菪内酯
secondary glycoside	[ˈsekəndəri] [ˈglaɪkəsaɪd]	次生苷
sedimentation rate	[ˌsedɪmenˈteɪʃn][reɪt]	沉积速率
sennoside	[seˈnəusaɪd]	番泻苷
S-glycosides	[ˈglaɪkəsaɪdz]	S- 苷
shell of lobster	[ʃel][əv][ˈlɒbstə]	龙虾
sinalbin	[sɪnˈælbɪn]	白芥子苷
Sinapis Semen	[sɪˈnəpɪz][ˈsiːmən]	芥子
sinigrin	[ˈsɪnɪɡrɪn]	黑芥子苷
β-sitosterol	[saɪˈtɒstərəul]	*β*- 谷甾醇
slightly toxic	[ˈslaɪtli][ˈtɒksɪk]	微毒
Smith degradation	[smɪθ][ˌdegrəˈdeɪʃn]	Smith 降解
sodium bicarbonate	[ˈsəudiːəm] [ˌbaɪˈkɑːbənət]	碳酸氢钠
sodium borohydride	[ˈsəudiːəm][ˌbɔːrəˈhaɪdraɪd]	四氢硼酸钠
sodium periodate	[ˈsəudiːəm][peˈraɪədeɪt]	过碘酸钠
Solanaceae		茄科
sophorose	[sɔˈfɔrəus]	槐糖
spatial position	[ˈspeɪʃl][pəˈzɪʃn]	空间位置
specificity	[ˌspesɪˈfɪsəti]	专属性
stachyose	[ˈstækɪəus]	水苏糖
stearic acid	[stɪˈærɪk][ˈæsɪd]	硬脂酸
Sterculia urens		刺梧桐
Sterculiaceae		梧桐科
stigmasterol	[stɪɡˈmæstərəl]	豆甾醇
sugar derivative	[ˈʃuɡə][dɪˈrɪvətɪv]	糖衍生物
sulfhydryl (thiol) group	[sʌlfˈhaɪdrɪl] [ˈθaɪəul][ɡruːp]	巯基
sulfur glycoside	[ˈsʌlfə] [ˈglaɪkəsaɪd]	硫苷
sulphuric acid	[sʌlˈfjuərɪk][ˈæsɪd]	硫酸
sweet	[swiːt]	甘
syrup	[ˈsɪrəp]	稠浆
T		
taurine	[ˈtɔːriː(ː)n]	牛磺酸
tetradesmosidic		四糖链的
tetrasaccharide	[ˌtetrəˈsækəraɪd]	四糖
thickening and suspending agent	[ˈθɪk(ə)nɪŋ][ənd][səˈspendɪŋ] [ˈeɪdʒ(ə)nt]	增稠悬浮剂

(continued)

thioglucosidase	[ˌθaɪəʊˈgluːkəˌsaɪdeɪs]	硫葡萄糖苷酶
tragacanth	[ˈtrægəkænθ]	黄芪胶
tragacanthic acid	[ˈtrægəkænθɪk][ˈæsɪd]	黄芪酸
tragacanthin	[ˈtrægəkænθɪn]	黄芪胶素
trichloroacetic acid	[trɪkləˈrəusiːtɪk][ˈæsɪd]	三氯乙酸
tridesmosidic		三糖链的
triglochinin	[trɪgˈlɔtʃaɪnɪn]	海韭菜苷
trimethylsilylation	[traɪmeθəlsɪlɪˈleɪʃən]	三甲基硅烷化
trisaccharide	[traɪˈsækəraɪd]	三糖
Trollius chinensis		金莲花
tulipalin	[tjulɪˈpælɪn]	山慈菇内酯
tuliposide	[tjulɪˈpəusaɪd]	山慈菇苷
U		
ultracentrifugation	[ʌltrəsentrɪfjuˈgeɪʃn]	超速离心
uridine	[ˈjuərɪdiːn]	尿苷
uronic acid	[juəˈrɔnɪk][ˈæsɪd]	糖醛酸
V		
Verbenaceae		马鞭草科
vitexin	[vaɪˈteksɪn]	牡荆素
volatility	[ˌvɔləˈtɪləti]	挥发性
X		
xyloside	[ˈzaɪləsaɪd]	木糖苷
Z		
Zae mays		玉米
zeaxanthin	[zɪəˈzænθɪn]	玉米素
zeaxanthin dipalmitate	[zɪəˈzænθɪn] [daɪˈpaːmɪteɪt]	玉米素二棕榈酸酯
zeaxanthin monopalmitate	[zɪəˈzænθɪn] [mənəuˈpaːmɪteɪt]	玉米素单棕榈酸酯
zinc chloride	[zɪŋk] [ˈklɔːraɪd]	氯化锌

重 点 小 结

糖类是多羟基醛或多羟基酮及其衍生物的总称，大多数糖分子中氢和氧的比例是 2：1，具有

$C_nH_{2n}O_n$ or $C_n(H_2O)_n$ 的通式，因此也称为碳水化合物。根据糖水解后能生成最小结构单元的数目，糖可分为单糖、寡糖（低聚糖）和多糖。

单糖和部分低聚糖（聚合度小于4）是结晶，有甜味，易溶于水，难溶于乙醚等亲脂性有机溶剂；多糖无甜味、无定形粉末、无还原性，不溶于冷水，可溶于热水成胶体溶液，不溶于乙醇等有机溶剂，因此常采用水提取乙醇沉淀法从中药中制备总多糖。

苷类是糖或糖的衍生物与另一非糖物质通过糖的半缩醛或半缩酮羟基脱水缩合而成的一类化合物，苷也称配糖体，其中非糖物质称为苷元，也称配基；来自苷元，且与糖的端基碳连接成苷的原子称为苷原子；苷原子与端基碳之间的化学键称为苷键。

根据苷原子种类不同苷分为氧苷、硫苷、氮苷和碳苷。氧苷在自然界最常见，又可分为醇苷、酚苷、酯苷、氰苷；根据生理作用分类，如强心苷；根据物理性质分类，如皂苷；按苷中单糖的数目分类，如单糖苷、双糖苷、三糖苷等；按苷中连接糖链的数目分类，如单糖链苷、双糖链苷、三糖链苷等；按植物来源分类，如人参皂苷、薯蓣皂苷等。将原存在于有机体内的苷称为原生苷，原生苷经水解失去一部分糖的苷称为次生苷。

苷类一般为固体，连接单糖少的可形成结晶，糖基多的苷一般是无定形粉末，且常有吸湿性。苷类具有旋光性，多为左旋，水解后的混合物多为右旋。多数苷类化合物为亲水性成分，可溶于热水、甲醇、乙醇、含水正丁醇，难溶于三氯甲烷、石油醚等亲脂性强的有机溶剂。碳苷一般在水和有机溶剂中溶解度均比较小，但可溶于吡啶。

苷键的裂解包括酸水解、碱水解、酶催化水解、甲基化水解、乙酰化水解、氧化裂解（Smith降解）等。其中酸水解速度的规律为：① $N-$ 苷 $>O-$ 苷 $>S-$ 苷 $>C-$ 苷；②呋喃糖苷 $>$ 吡喃糖苷；③酮糖苷 $>$ 醛糖苷；④五碳糖苷 $>$ 甲基五碳糖苷 $>$ 六碳糖苷 $>$ 七碳糖苷 $>$ 糖醛酸苷；⑤ 2,3- 二去氧糖苷 $>2-$ 去氧糖苷 $>3-$ 去氧糖苷 $>2-$ 羟基糖苷 $>2-$ 氨基糖苷。Smith 降解具有较高选择性，一般裂解具有邻二醇羟基的碳碳键，且作用缓和，易得到原生苷元。

一般中药含有某种苷，就含有水解该苷的酶；为了提取原生苷，需抑制酶的活性，一般有三种方法：①溶剂法。70% 甲醇、乙醇或沸水提取。②碳酸钙法。提取前加入一定量的碳酸钙拌匀使酶失活。③硫酸铵法。提取时加入硫酸铵或新鲜植物采集后即与饱和的硫酸铵水溶液混合研磨，使酶沉淀。提取原生苷时应尽量避免采用酸或碱溶液提取；提取苷元一般采用两相酸水解法。

一般采用凝胶色谱分离纯化糖，也可测定糖的分子量；硅胶色谱分离纯化苷，包括正相硅胶和反相硅胶色谱。苷的检识常用 Molish 反应和 TLC 或 HPLC 等色谱法检识。

苷类化合物结构测定的一般程序为：①纯度测定。常采用色谱法（TLC 和 HPLC），同时测定物理常数，如熔点和熔距、旋光度。②分子量和分子式测定。高分辨质谱法（FAB-MS、ESI-MS、MALDI-TOF-MS）最常用。③苷元和糖的测定。苷元的测定在后续各章中叙述，糖的测定包括糖的种类和数目测定，常采用 1D，2D-NMR 法，通过比较单糖及其甲基苷的化学位移变化，确定糖的种类；糖的数目可以通过质谱法和 NMR 谱中糖的端基氢或碳的信号数目确定。④糖的连接顺序和连接位置测定。质谱中糖基的碎片离子峰或各种分子离子脱糖后的碎片离子峰，可以确定单糖的连接顺序。糖的连接位置包括苷元和糖之间、糖和糖之间的连接位置测定，HMBC 谱常用于确定苷元和糖之间连接位置。⑤苷键构型的确定。利用 ^{1}H-NMR 谱中端基质子的耦合常数判断苷键构型；^{13}C-NMR 谱中端基碳的化学位移也可判断苷键构型。

目 标 检 测

一、单选题

1. 苷原子来自于（ 　 ）
   A. 与苷元相连接的糖 　　　　　　B. 糖端基碳上半缩醛羟基 　　　　C. 糖的端基碳
   D. 与糖相连接的苷元 　　　　　　E. 以上都不是

2. 最难酸水解的苷类为（ 　 ）
   A. α- 羟基糖苷 　　　　　　　　　B. α- 氨基糖苷 　　　　　　　　　C. α- 去氧糖苷
   D. 6- 去氧糖苷 　　　　　　　　　E. 2,6- 二去氧糖苷

3. 药材的水提取液中缓缓加入无水乙醇，下列化合物先被沉淀的是（ 　 ）
   A. 小分子多糖 　　　　　　　　　B. 小分子低聚糖 　　　　　　　　C. 大分子多糖
   D. 大分子低聚糖 　　　　　　　　E. 单糖

4. 自然界中数量最多，且最常见的苷是（ 　 ）
   A. 氧苷 　　　　　　　　　　　　B. 硫苷 　　　　　　　　　　　　C. 氮苷
   D. 碳苷 　　　　　　　　　　　　E. 磷苷

5. 在天然苷类中，由 D 型糖衍生而成的苷多为（ 　 ）
   A. β-D- 糖苷 　　　　　　　　　　B. α-D- 糖苷 　　　　　　　　　　C. β-L- 糖苷
   D. α-L- 糖苷 　　　　　　　　　　E. 均不正确

6. 多糖分子量测定最常用柱色谱的固定相是（ 　 ）
   A. 硅胶 　　　B. 氧化铝 　　　C. 活性炭 　　　D. 聚酰胺 　　　E. 凝胶

7. 对多糖的描述正确的是（ 　 ）
   A. 结晶 　　　B. 有甜味 　　　C. 有还原性 　　　D. 可溶于水 　　　E. 可溶于乙醇

8. 能够产生氧化裂解反应的结构是（ 　 ）
   A. 邻二酚羟基 　　　　　　　　　B. 邻二醇羟基 　　　　　　　　　C. 邻二甲基
   D. 酚羟基 　　　　　　　　　　　E. 联苯

9. 只能使 α- 葡萄糖苷键水解的酶是（ 　 ）
   A. 麦芽糖酶 　　　　　　　　　　B. 苦杏仁苷酶 　　　　　　　　　C. 纤维素酶
   D. 均可 　　　　　　　　　　　　E. 均不是

10. 从植物药材乙醇提取液中使苷类沉淀析出而脂溶性杂质存留在母液中的方法是（ 　 ）
    A. 水提醇沉法 　　　　　　　　　B. 醇提水沉法 　　　　　　　　　C. 醇提醚沉法
    D. 铅盐沉淀法 　　　　　　　　　E. 酸提碱沉法

二、多选题

1. 苷键的裂解反应可使苷键断裂，其目的在于了解（ 　 ）
   A. 苷类的苷元结构 　　　　　　　　B. 所连接的糖的种类
   C. 所连接的糖的组成 　　　　　　　D. 苷元与糖的连接方式
   E. 糖与糖的连接方式和顺序

2. 关于苷类化合物的说法正确的有（　　　）

  A. 结构中均含有糖基　　　　　　B. 可发生酶水解反应　　　　　　C. 大多具有挥发性

  D. 可发生酸水解反应　　　　　　E. 大多具有升华性

3. 关于不同类型苷的酸水解速度，表达正确的有（　　　）

  A. N– 苷 > O– 苷 > S– 苷 > C– 苷

  B. 呋喃糖苷 > 吡喃糖苷

  C. 醛糖苷 > 酮糖苷

  D. 五碳糖苷 > 甲基五碳糖苷 > 六碳糖苷 > 七碳糖苷 > 糖醛酸苷

  E. 2– 去氧糖苷 > 2–NH_2 糖苷 > 2–OH 糖苷

4. 目前研究表明，构成枸杞子多糖的主要单糖是（　　　）

  A. 葡萄糖　　　　B. 半乳糖　　　　C. 鼠李糖　　　　D. 果糖　　　　E. 阿拉伯糖

5. 苦杏仁苷经过苦杏仁苷酶水解的最终产物包括（　　　）

  A. 野樱苷　　　　B. 苯甲醛　　　　C. 氢氰酸　　　　D. 龙胆双糖　　　　E. 葡萄糖

6. 糖与糖之间的苷键、糖与苷元之间苷键构型的判断可根据（　　　）

  A. 全甲基化后酸催化甲醇解　　　　　　B. 全乙酰化的乙酰解

  C. 酶水解　　　　　　　　　　　　　　D. Smith 降解

  E. ^{1}H-NMR 中 C_1–H 与 C_2–H 的耦合常数

7. 提取原生苷时，以下哪些措施是有利的（　　　）

  A. 提取过程避免与酸或碱接触　　　　　B. 新鲜原料采集后低温快速干燥

  C. 加入碳酸钙或硫酸铵　　　　　　　　D. 植物材料发酵一段时间后提取

  E. 70% 乙醇

8. 能够被碱水解的苷是（　　　）

  A. 酚苷　　　　　　　　　　B. 酯苷　　　　　　　　　　C. β– 吸电子基苷

  D. 烯醇式苷　　　　　　　　E. 碳苷

9. 苷类化合物的以下化学鉴别结果正确的是（　　　）

  A. Molish、Fehling 和 Tollen 反应均为阳性

  B. Molish、Fehling 和 Tollen 反应均为阴性

  C. Molish 反应阴性、Fehling 和 Tollen 反应均为阳性

  D. Molish 反应阳性、Fehling 和 Tollen 反应均为阴性

  E. 苷水解产物 Molish、Fehling 和 Tollen 反应均为阳性

10. 单糖是（　　　），是组成糖类及其衍生物的基本单元

  A. 多羟基醛　　　　　　　　B. 多羟基酮　　　　　　　　C. 多羟基酸

  D. 糖醛酸　　　　　　　　　E. 氨基糖

三、问答题

1. 某药材含有未知结构的苷类化合物，请设计其提取分离的工艺流程。

2. 请给出某苷类化合物（纯度 99% 以上）结构测定的一般程序及常用方法。

3. 请给出化学检识某中药中是否含有苷类化合物的实验流程图。

（吴锦忠）

Chapter 4   Quinones

 学习目标

知识要求:

1. 掌握 蒽醌类的分类、主要理化性质、检识反应及波谱特征，醌类化合物的酸性强弱规律及其在该类化合物提取分离中的应用。

2. 熟悉 醌类化合物的结构分类；大黄、丹参的主要有效成分结构特征、理化性质、提取分离方法。

3. 了解 醌类化合物分布和生理活性；紫草的主要有效成分结构特征、理化性质、提取分离方法。

能力要求:

学会应用不同的颜色反应检识不同类型的醌类化合物；学会应用蒽醌类化合物的理化性质，结合具体化合物的结构特征选择适合的提取分离方法，解决蒽醌类化合物在提取分离过程中存在的技术问题；学会根据理化反应、物理常数及波谱数据等信息解析出蒽醌类化合物的结构。

1 Introduction

Quinones (醌类) are a group of compounds that have quinonoid (醌式结构) nucleus, unsaturated cyclohexanedione (环己二酮) to be exact. They can be divided into four types: benzoquinones (苯醌), naphthoquinones (萘醌), phenanthraquinones (菲醌) and anthraquinones (蒽醌). Quinones, especially anthraquinones, are a major class of bioactive constituents from Chinese herbs.

Quinones are widely distributed in families of higher plants such as: Boraginaceae (紫草科), Lamiaceae (唇形科), Leguminosae (豆科), Liliaceae (百合科), Polygonaceae (蓼科), Rhamnaceae (鼠李科), Rubiaceae (茜草科), etc. They also present in lichens (地衣) and fungi. Quinones are commonly present in the roots, barks, leaves and heartwood of the plant, but they can also be found in the stalks, fruits and seeds.

Quinones have various bioactivities. Anthraquinones substituted with hydroxyl groups from Rhei Radix et Rhizoma have antibacterial action. Alizarin (茜草素) derivatives from Rubiae Radix et Rhizoma (茜草) exhibit hemostatic effect. Naphthoquinone pigments from Arnebiae Radix (紫草) show antibacterial, antiviral and hemostatic effects. Quinones from Salviae Miltiorrhizae Radix et Rhizoma (丹参) have sedative, antibacterial, antioxidant, anti-inflammatory and coronary artery dilating effects.

2   Structure Characteristics and Classification

2.1   Benzoquinones

Benzoquinones can be classified into *ortho* (邻)-benzoquinone (1, 2-benzoquinone) and *para* (对)-benzoquinone (1, 4-benzoquinone). Most of natural benzoquinones are *para*-benzoquinones, as *ortho*-benzoquinones are unstable.

para-benzoquinone   *ortho*-benzoquinone

Most of natural benzoquinones are yellow or orange crystals. For example, 2, 6-dimethoxy-1, 4-benzoquinone from *Ailanthus altissima* (臭椿) and embellin (信筒子醌) from *Embelia* (*E.*) *ribes* (白花酸藤果) and *E. oblongifolia* (多脉酸藤子) are both yellow crystals.

2, 6-dimethoxy-1, 4- benzoquinone   embellin

Ubiquinones (泛醌) that contain benzoquinone nucleus are a series of coenzymes, named coenzyme Q. They are involved in organism oxidation-reduction. The length of terpene (萜) chain in the structure varies according to species, and the value of n is between 7 to 10 in most organisms. Coenzyme Q_{10} is the redox carrier of human beings, and it has been used in the treatment of heart disease, hypertension and cancer.

coenzyme Q

2.2   Naphthoquinones

Naphthoquinones are classified into α-(1, 4)-naphthoquinones, β-(1, 2)-naphthoquinones, and *amphi*

(两边)-(2, 6)-naphthoquinone based on the position of the dione group. Most of natural naphthoquinones are α-(1, 4)-naphthoquinones, which are often orange or orange-red crystals.

α-(1, 4)-naphthoquinone   β-(1, 2)-naphthoquinone   *amphi*-(2, 6)-naphthoquinone

Naphthoquinones have various bioactivities. Juglone (胡桃醌) has antibacterial and anticancer effects, as well as sedative effect on central nerve system. Plumbagin (白花丹醌) relieves cough and reduces sputum besides antibacterial effect. Lapachol (拉帕醌) is a tumor inhibitor. Shikonin (紫草素) and alkannin (阿卡宁) have hemostatic, antibacterial, antiviral, anti-inflammatory and antitumor effects.

juglone   plumbagin   lapachol

shikonin   alkannin

2.3 Phenanthraquinones

Phenanthraquinones are classified into *ortho*- and *para*-phenanthraquinones.

ortho-phenanthraquinone   *para*-phenanthraquinone

Tanshinone (丹参酮) Ⅱ_A, tanshinone Ⅱ_B, hydroxy tanshinone Ⅱ_A, and methyl tanshinonate are *ortho*-phenanthraquinones. Neotanshinone (新丹参酮) A, B and C are *para*-phenanthraquinones. They are all isolated from the root of *Salvia miltiorrhiza* Bge (丹参).

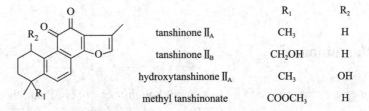

	R_1	R_2
tanshinone Ⅱ_A	CH_3	H
tanshinone Ⅱ_B	CH_2OH	H
hydroxytanshinone Ⅱ_A	CH_3	OH
methyl tanshinonate	$COOCH_3$	H

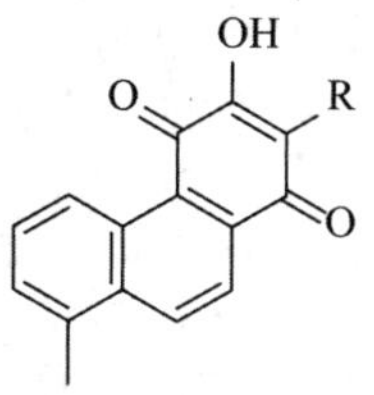

	R
neotanshinone A	$CH(CH_3)CH_2OH$
neotanshinone B	$CH(CH_3)_2$
neotanshinone C	CH_3

2.4   Anthraquinones

Anthraquinones are generally divided into two types according to the number of anthracene (蒽) nucleus they contain, i.e. single anthracene nucleus and double anthracene nucleus.

2.4.1   Single Anthracene Nucleus

(1) Hydroxyl Anthraquinones and Their Glycosides

Natural anthraquinones are 9, 10-anthraquinones. They are stable due to their conjugated system and the highest oxidation level at C-9 and C-10. The carbons of 9, 10-anthraquinone are numbered according to the structure of anthracene. In the structure of 9, 10-anthraquinone, positions 1, 4, 5, 8 are defined as α-positions, and positions 2, 3, 6, 7 are defined as β-positions, while positions 9 and 10 are defined as *meso* (中位)-positions.

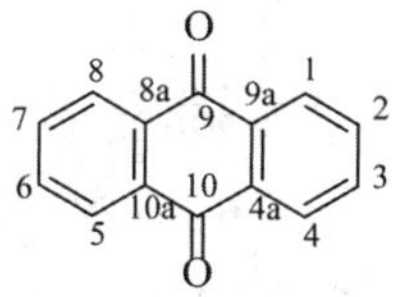

Natural anthraquinones are often substituted by hydroxyl, hydroxymethyl, methyl, methoxy and carboxyl groups on the aromatic rings. They exist in the forms of free and glycosides of anthraquinones. Most of anthraquinone glycosides are *O*-glycosides, but some are *C*-glycosides, such as barbaloin (芦荟苷).

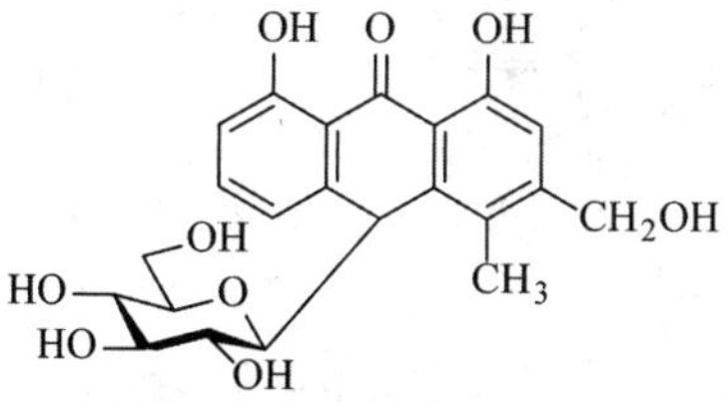

barbaloin

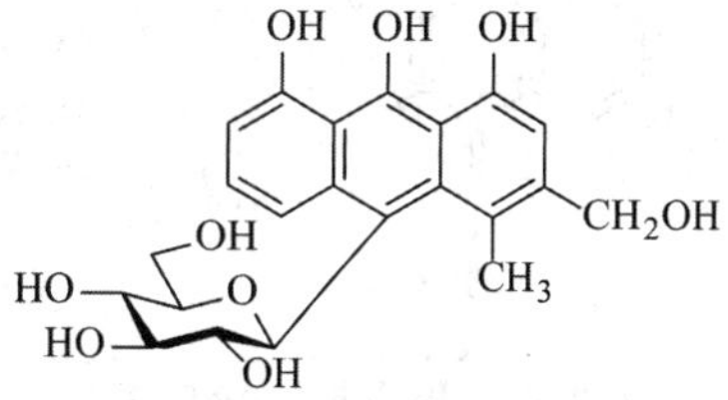

barbaloin
anthranol (蒽酚) tautomer (异构体)

Hydroxyl anthraquinones can be further divided into two subtypes based on the substituent positions of hydroxyl groups.

① Emodin Type

The hydroxyl groups of the Emodin type anthraquinones are distributed on two benzene rings. Most compounds in this group are yellow in color, e.g. chrysophanol (大黄酚), emodin (大黄素), physcion (大黄素甲醚) from Rhei Radix et Rhizoma.

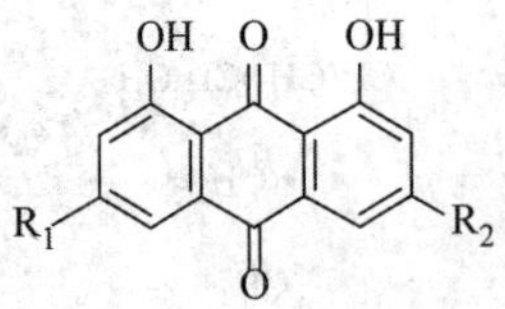

	R₁	R₂
chrysophanol	H	CH₃
emodin	OH	CH₃
physcion	OCH₃	CH₃
aloe-emodin	H	CH₂OH
rhein (大黄酸)	H	COOH

Most of the anthraquinone derivatives in Rhei Radix et Rhizoma link with glucose to form glycosides, most of which are monoglycosides and diglucosides.

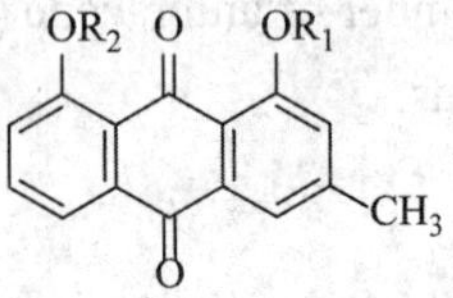

	R₁	R₂
chrysophanol-8-O-β-D-glycoside	H	glc
chrysophanol-1-O-β-D-glycoside	glc	H
chrysophanol-8-O-β-gentiobioside (龙胆双糖苷)	H	glc-(1 → 6)-glc

② Alizarin Type

The hydroxyl groups of the Alizarin type anthraquinones substitute on only one benzene ring. Compounds in this group are orange-yellow or orange-red, e.g. alizarin, purpurin (羟基茜草素), pseudopurpurin from Rubiae Radix et Rhizoma.

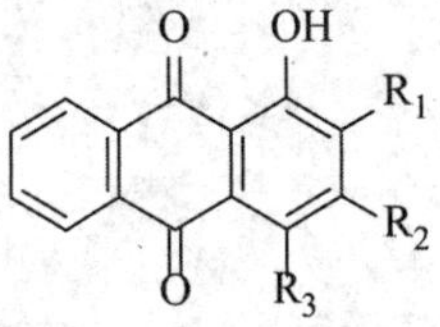

	R₁	R₂	R₃
alizarin	OH	H	H
purpurin	OH	H	OH
pseudopurpurin	OH	COOH	OH

(2) Anthranol, Anthrone (蒽酮) and Their Derivatives

In acidic condition, anthraquinones can be reduced to anthranol and its tautomer, i.e. anthrone (Figure 4-1).

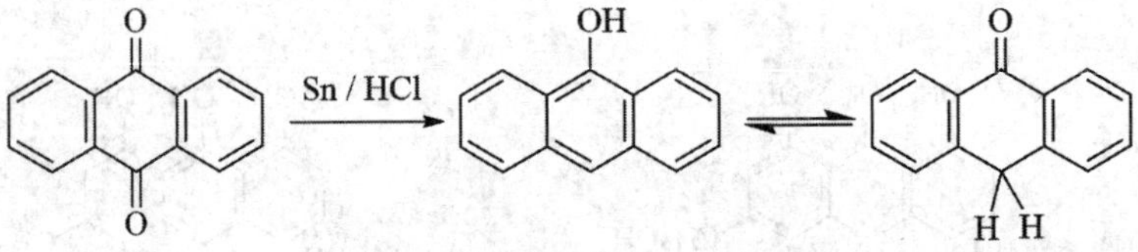

anthraquinone   anthranol   anthrone

Figure 4-1   The conversion of anthraquinone to anthranol and anthrone

Generally, the derivatives of anthranols and anthrones coexist with anthraquinones only in fresh plants. They are gradually oxidized into anthraquinones during collection and storage. For example, after more than two years of storage, anthranols can no longer be detected in Rhei Radix et Rhizoma. Derivatives of anthranol are stable if the *meso*-hydroxyl group is connected with saccharide to form glycosides as barbaloin.

2.4.2   Double Anthracene Nucleus

(1) Dianthrones (二蒽酮)

Dianthrones are condensation products of two anthrones through C-C bond. Most of dianthrones are connected with C₁₀-C₁₀', e.g. sennoside A, B, C, and D from Rhei Radix et Rhizoma and Sennae Folium (番泻叶).

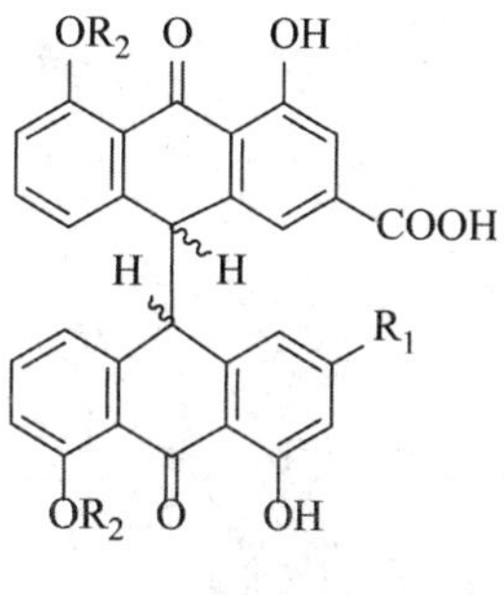

	R₁	R₂	C₁₀-C₁₀'	Absolute configuration
sennoside A	COOH	glc	*trans*	10*R*, 10'*R*
sennoside B	COOH	glc	*cis*	10*R*, 10'*S*
sennoside C	CH₂OH	glc	*trans*	10*R*, 10'*R*
sennoside D	CH₂OH	glc	*cis*	10*R*, 10'*S*
sennidin (番泻苷元) A	COOH	H	*trans*	10*R*, 10'*R*
sennidin B	COOH	H	*cis*	10*R*, 10'*S*
sennidin C	CH₂OH	H	*trans*	10*R*, 10'*R*
sennidin D	CH₂OH	H	*cis*	10*R*, 10'*S*

The C₁₀-C₁₀' bond easily breaks to yield anthrones. For example, sennoside A can be converted to rhein anthrone in intestine under the action of intestinal flora (Figure 4-2). Rhein anthrone can act on the large intestine and enhance the peristalsis.

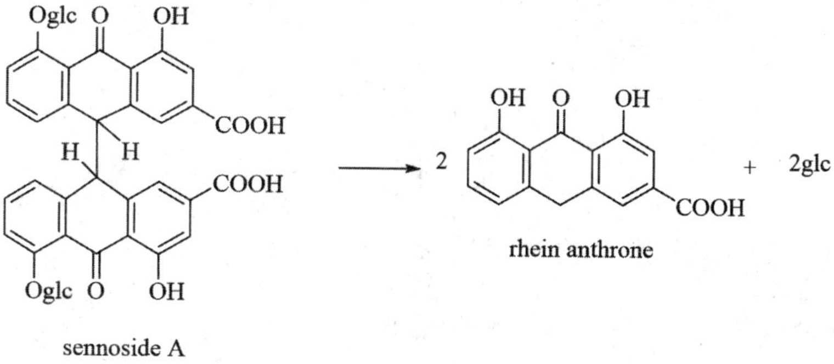

rhein anthrone

sennoside A

Figure 4-2   Decomposition of sennoside A

(2) Dimers of Anthraquinones

Dimers of anthraquinones are the condensation of two molecular anthraquinone. In nature, dimers of anthraquinone are composed of two moieties exact the same, e.g. skyrin (醌茜素) and cassiamine (山扁豆双醌).

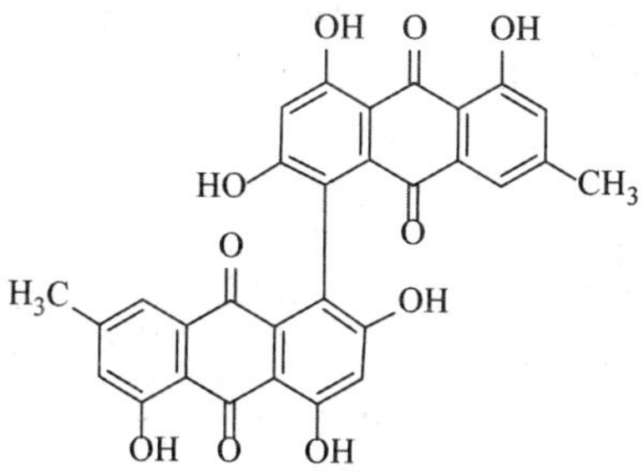

skyrin

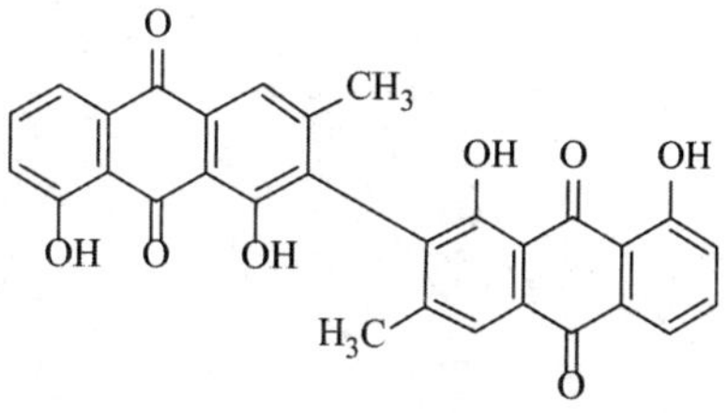

cassiamine

(3) Dehydrodianthrones (去氢二蒽酮类)

Dianthrones dehydrogenate again to form dehydrodianthrones, in which two anthrone rings are connected with a double bond. Dehydrodianthrones are often dark purple in color.

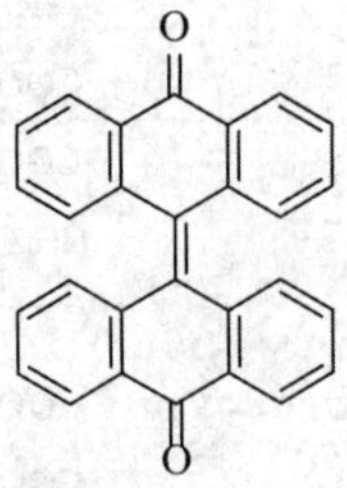

(structural diagram)

dehydrodianthrones

(4) Sunshine Anthrones (日照蒽酮类)

Dehydrodianthrones undergo further oxidation to yield sunshine anthrones, in which the α-positions of the two anthrone nucleus link to form a six-member ring. The polyhydroxyl derevatives of sunshine anthrone exist in plants of the genus of Hypericum (金丝桃属).

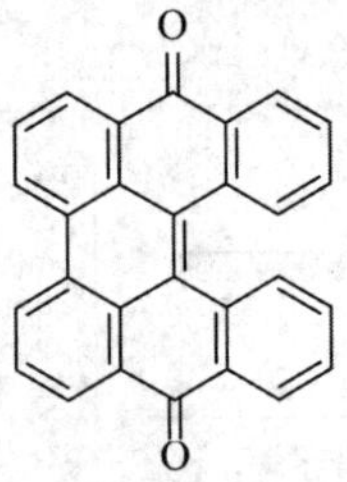

(structural diagram)

sunshine anthrone

(5) *Meso*-naphthodianthrones (中位萘二蒽酮类)

Meso-naphthodianthrones have the highest oxidation level in natural anthracene derivatives. They have highly fused poly-ring structures. For example, Hypericin (金丝桃) found in some plants from Hypericum is a *Meso*-naphthodianthrone and has antidepressant and antiviral effects.

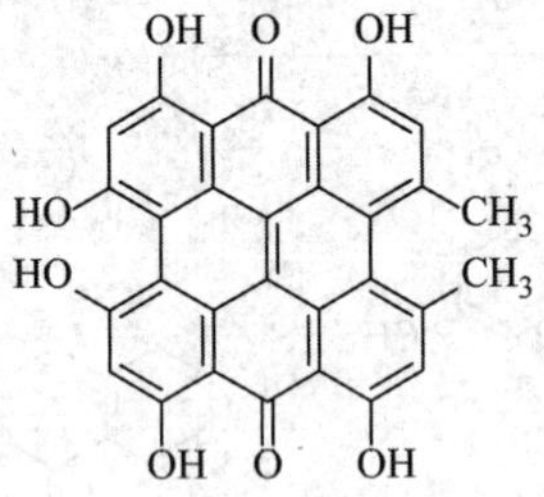

(structural diagram)

hypericin

3　Physical and Chemical Properties

3.1　Physical Properties

Generally, free quinones are crystals, but they are difficult to crystallize after linking with saccharides to form glycosides. Benzoquinones and naphthoquinones generally exist in free form in plants, while most of anthraquinones exist as glycosides. Most of quinones have color, and the color intensifies with increased number of auxochrome.

Anthraquinones in free form have sublimability. Benzoquinones and naphthoquinones with low molecular weight have volatility and can be extracted by steam distillation method.

Owing to their low polarity, free quinones are soluble in organic solvents, (e.g. methanol, ethanol, acetone, ethyl acetate, chloroform, or ethyl ether) and are insoluble in water. Glycosides of quinones are soluble in methanol, ethanol, and hot water, but their solubility in cold water is low. They are insoluble in organic solvents with low polar, such as chloroform, ethyl ether, etc. *C*-glycosides of anthraquinone dissolve neither in water nor in common organic solvents, but in pyridine easily.

3.2   Chemical Properties

3.2.1   Acidity

Most quinones have phenolic or enolic hydroxyl groups, as well as carboxyl group, so they are acidic. They can dissolve in alkaline solution and precipitate after acidifying.

The acidity of quinones varies with the number and location of carboxyl and hydroxyl group substituted. Generally, the acidity of carboxyl group is stronger than phenolic or enolic hydroxyl groups. For enolic hydroxyl group substitute on the quinone, due to the vinylogy (插烯规律), the acidity of this group is similar to that of carboxyl group. In the case of phenolic hydroxyl groups, the carbonyl on the quinone at the *para*-position of β-OH stabilize the phenoxy anoin due to electron withdraw effect. While for α-OH, the formation of hydrogen bond with its adjacent carbonyl reduces its acidity. The more acidic groups a qunione contains, the stronger the acidity is.

β-OH anthraquinone α-OH anthraquinone

Anthraquinones with the following groups have acidity in decreased order:

—COOH > two or more β-OH > one β-OH > two or more α-OH > one α-OH.

Alkaline solutions can be used to dissolve the above anthraquinones. Five percent sodium hydrogen carbonate is used to dissolve anthraquinones with carboxyl group, two or more β-OH. Five percent sodium carbonate is used to dissolve anthraquinones with one β-OH. One percent sodium hydroxide can dissolve anthraquinones with two or more α-OH. And 5% sodium hydroxide can dissolve anthraquinones with only one α-OH.

Anthraquinones can dissolve in concentrate sulfuric acid forming oxonium salt accompanied by color change. For example, emodin changes from orange-red to red in concentrate sulfuric acid. This reaction is used for color detection of anthraquinones.

3.2.2   Color Reactions

(1) Feigl Reaction

When heated under basic condition, quinones react quickly with formaldehyde and *o*-dinitrobenzene, producing purple compound. Interestingly, the structures of quinones do not change after this reaction.

They play as electron transmitters. The mechanism is shown in Figure 4-3.

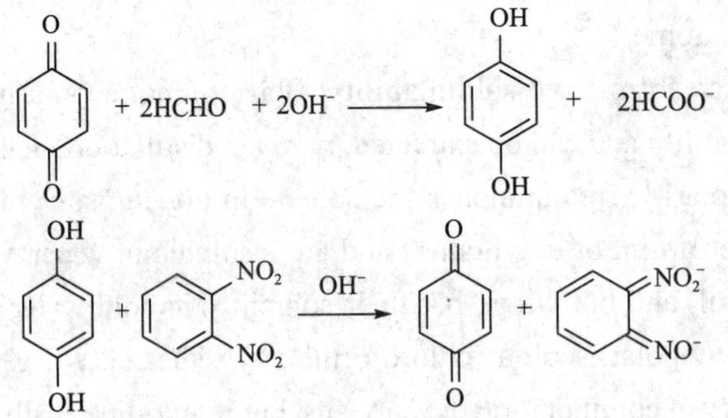

Figure 4-3   Mechanism of Feigl reaction

(2) Leucomethylene Blue (无色亚甲蓝) Reaction

Leucomethylene blue reaction is a special characteristic of benzoquinones and naphthoquinones. This reagent can be used as chromogenic (发色的) reagent PC or TLC, on which benzoquinones and naphthoquinones can be distinguished from anthraquinones with their blue spots.

(3) Kesting-Craven Reaction

The hydrogen on quinone ring of benzoquinones and naphthoquinones can react to some reagents with active methylene group in alkaline alcohol solution to produce blue-green or blue-purple products. Taking the reaction of naphthoquinone with diethyl malonate as an example, the product (1) is formed during the reaction, and then further electron transfer is carried out to form (2) and so on (Figure 4-4).

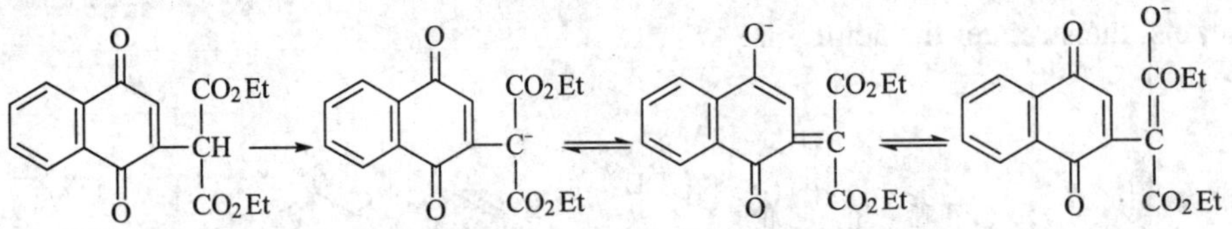

Figure 4-4   Mechanism of Kesting-Craven reaction

Anthraquinones cannot react with active methylene reagents, because there are benzene rings on both sides of the quinone ring and there is no position for the reagent to substitute. This reaction can be used to distinguish anthraquinones from benzoquinones and naphthoquinones.

(4) Reaction with basic solution

Hydroxylated quinones turn to deeper color in basic solutions, mostly to orange, red, purple and blue. The reaction between hydroxyl anthraqinones and basic solutions is defined as Bornträger reaction (Figure 4-5).

Anthranol, anthrone, and dianthrone show negative to Bornträger reaction until they are oxidized into hydroxyl anthraquinones.

(5) Complexation with Metal Ions

For anthraquinones with α-OH or *ortho*-diphenolic hydroxyl, they can form colorful complex with metal ions such as Mg^{2+}, etc. (Figure 4-6).

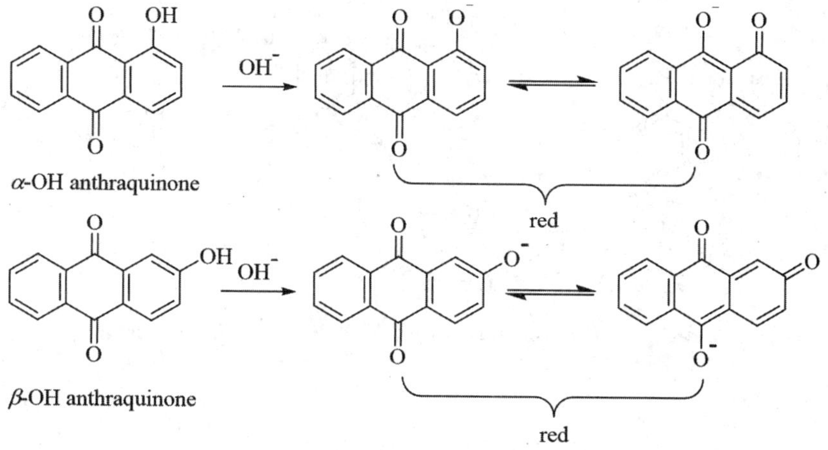

α-OH anthraquinone

β-OH anthraquinone

red

red

Figure 4-5　Mechanism of Bornträger reaction

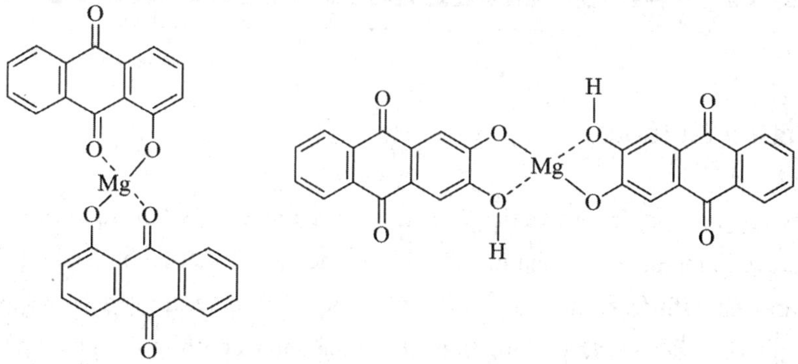

Figure 4-6　Mechanism of metal ion reactions

The color varies from orange-yellow and orange-red to purple-red, purple, or blue according to the structure of anthraquinones (Table 4-1).

Table 4-1　Structure of anthraquinones and Color of Mg-complex

Structure of anthraquinones	Color of Mg-complex
β-OH, or α- OH, or two OH on different rings	orange-yellow to orange
α,β-m-di-OH	orange-red to red
α,α-p-di-OH	purple-red to purple
α,β-O-di-OH	blue to violet

(6) p-Nitroso-N, N-Dimethylaniline (对亚硝基二甲苯胺) Reaction

Hydroxyl anthrones with active methylene group at C-10 condense with p-nitroso-N, N-dimethylaniline to produce colorful compounds (Figure 4-7). The color can be blue, green, violet, etc. Therefore, this reaction can be used to identify anthrones.

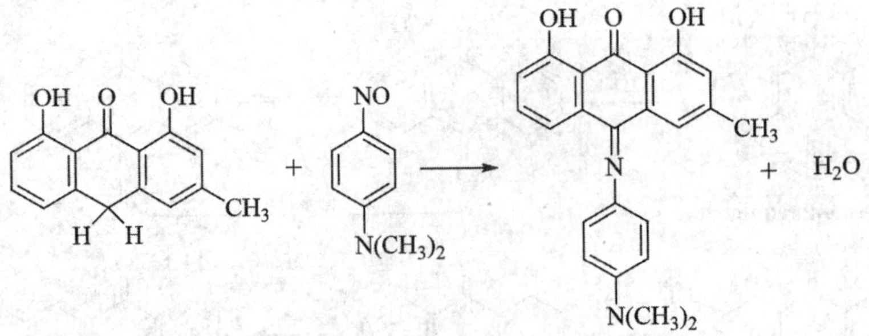

Figure 4-7　Mechanism of *p*-nitroso-*N*, *N*-dimethylaniline reaction

---

4　Extraction and Isolation Methods

4.1　Extraction Methods

Free quinones are low polar, but their glycosides are more polar. Both free quinones and their glycosides can dissolve in methanol or ethanol. Therefore, methanol or ethanol is generally used to extract total quinones. Quinones with free phenolic hydroxyl groups can be extracted with basic solutions, and subsequently precipitated after acidification. Benzoqinones and naphthoquinones with small molecular weight are volatile, so they can be extracted with steam distillation method.

4.2　Isolation Methods

4.2.1　Separation of Free Anthraquinones and Their Glycosides

The polarities of anthraquinones and their glycosides are different, so their solubility in organic solvents (i.e. $CHCl_3$ or Et_2O) is different. For example, free anthraquinones dissolve in $CHCl_3$, but anthraquinone glycosides do not. It's worth noting that hydroxyl anthraquinones and their glycosides usually exist in plants in the forms of salts with magnesium, potassium, sodium, or calcium, etc. In order to extract the total anthraquinone derivatives, acidification before extraction should be carried out.

4.2.2　Isolation of Free Anthraquinones

(1) pH Gradient Partition

The pH gradient partition method is commonly used to isolate free anthraquinones with different acidities. The procedure is shown in Figure 4-8.

(2) Column Chromatography

Column chromatography is an effective method to separate anthraquinones with similar structures. The commonly used adsorbent is silica gel. Anthraquinones that contain phenolic hydroxyl groups can also be isolated by polyamide as well. Due to the acidity of hydroxyl anthraquinones, alkaline aluminum oxide is not applied in the isolation.

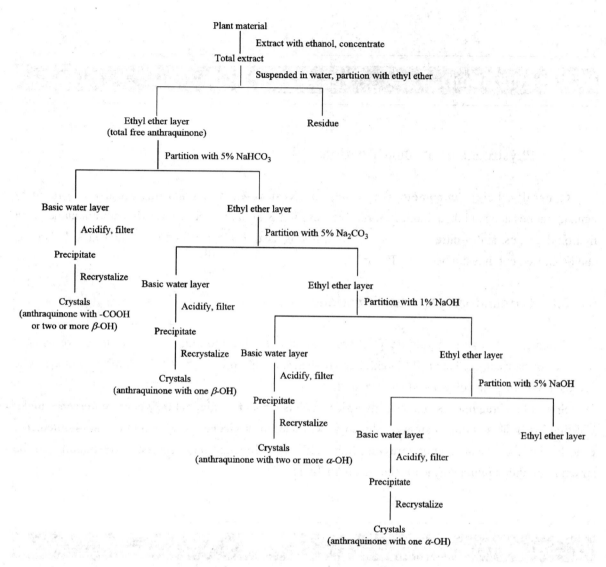

Figure 4-8　Procedure for pH gradient extraction

4.2.3　Isolation of Anthraquinone Glycosides

Anthraquinone glycosides can dissolve in water and organic solvents such as ethyl acetate and *n*-butanol. Therefore, ethyl acetate or *n*-butanol is commonly used in the partition anthraquinone glycosides from water and thus to separate them from water-soluble impurities. The chromatography method is used for further isolation to get pure anthraquinone glycosides.

Silica gel column chromatography is used in the isolation of anthraquinone glycosides. Sephadex LH-20 and reversed silica gel are also used for further separation for polar anthraquinone glycosides. For example, subject 70% methanol extract of Rhei Radix et Rhizoma to a Sephadex LH-20 column, elute with 70% methanol to obtain dianthrone glycosides (sennoside A, B, C and D), anthraquinone diglucosides, anthraquinone monoglucosides, free anthraquinones, successively.

5 Identification

5.1 Physicochemical Identification

Generally, Feigl, leucomethylene blue, and Kesting-Craven reactions are used to identify benzoquinones and naphthoquinones. Bornträger reaction is initially used to identify anthraquinones with hydroxyl groups, and *p*-nitroso-*N, N*-dimethylaniline is used to identify hydroxyl anthrones. Reactions can be carried out in test tubes or on PC or TLC.

5.2 Chromatography Identification

Silica gel TLC and polyamide TLC are usually used. Developing solvent systems are usually mixtures of benzene-methanol (9 : 1) and heptane-benzene-chloroform (1 : 1 : 1), etc. For anthraquinone glycosides, high polar solvent systems are used.

Spots of anthraquinones and their glycosides are visible under light, but they emit fluorescence under UV light. If basic solution is sprayed, the color will deepen or change. Magnesium acetate in methanol can also be used, heating after spraying, then different colors can be observed corresponding to the structure of anthraquinones (mentioned before in Table 4-1).

6 Structure Elucidation

After preliminary identification via color reactions, additional chemical experiments and spectrum analysis are required to determine the structure of quinones.

6.1 Chemical Methods

In order to determine the number of hydroxyl groups, or to protect these groups for further reaction of quinones, methylation and acetylation are applied.

6.1.1 Methylation

For hydroxyl groups with acidity, such as hydroxyl in carboxyl group and phenolic hydroxyl group, methylation can be carried easily. While for alcoholic hydroxyl group, strict condition is needed for methylation of the group. In the structure of quinone, β-OH is easier to react with methylation reagent than α-OH due to their difference in acidity. The difficulty of methylation also depends on the reagents and reactive conditions. Commonly used methylation reagents are listed in Table 4-2.

Table 4-2   Commonly used methylation reagents

Methylation reagents	Reaction groups
CH_2N_2/Et_2O	—COOH, β-OH, —CHO
CH_2N_2/Et_2O + MeOH	—COOH, β-OH, —CHO, one of two α-OH
$(CH_3)_2SO_4$ + K_2CO_3 + Et_2O	β-OH, α-OH
CH_3I + Ag_2O	—COOH, —CHO, phenolic-OH, alcoholic-OH

Since the number of methoxyl group produced in methylation reactions can be determined by NMR spectra, the number and type of hydroxyls can be deduced according to the spectra as well as the reagents used.

6.1.2   Acetylation

The reactivity of hydroxyl groups in acetylation depends on their basicity. Thus alcoholic hydroxyl group is the easiest to be acetylated, while α-OH is relatively difficult. The reactivity of commonly used acetylation reagents is listed in decrease order: $CH_3COCl>(CH_3CO)_2O>CH_3COOR>CH_3COOH$. The commonly used acetylation reagents and conditions are listed in Table 4-3.

Table 4-3   Acetylation reagents, reactive condition and the group of acetylation

Acetylation reagent	Reactive condition	Acetylated group
Glacial acetic acid (add little acetyl chloride)	cold-setting	alcoholic-OH
Acetic anhydride	heating shortly	alcoholic-OH, β-OH
	heating long-time	alcoholic-OH, β-OH, one of two α-OH
Acetic anhydride + boric acid	cold-setting	alcoholic-OH, β-OH
Acetic anhydride + concentrated H_2SO_4	overnight at room temperature	alcoholic-OH, β-OH, α-OH
Acetic anhydride + pyridine	overnight at room temperature	alcoholic-OH, β-OH, enolic-OH

Sometimes, for preventing α-phenolic hydroxyl from acetylation, acetic anhydride and boric acid can be used as acetylation reagent. The reaction is shown in Figure 4-9.

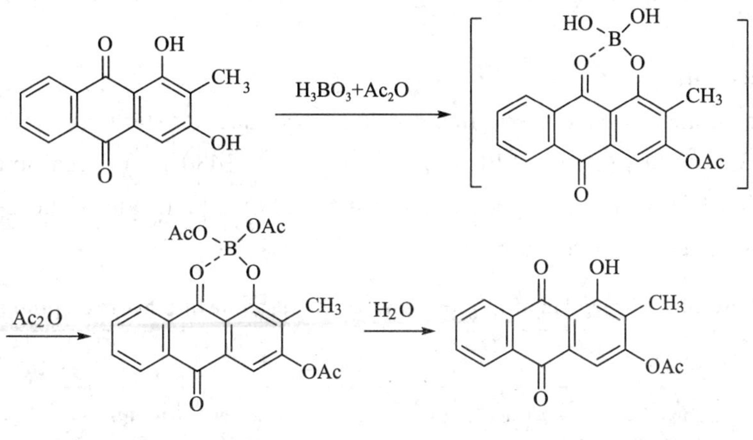

Figure 4-9   Acetylation reaction of acetic anhydride-boric acid

6.2 Spectroscopic Characters of Anthraquinones

6.2.1 UV Spectrum

Anthraquinones have four absorptions which are originated from benzene (1) and quinone (2) structure, respectively, as in Figure 4-10.

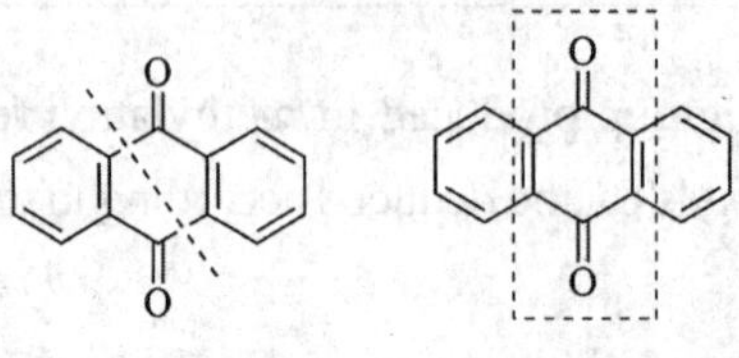

252 nm   325 nm   272 nm   405 nm
(1)   (2)

Figure 4-10   UV absorption bands of anthraquinone nucleus

UV spectra of hydroxyl anthraquinones are similar to that of anthraquinones. There are five main absorption bands: ~230nm (I), 240–260nm (II), 262–295nm (III), 305–389nm (IV), >400nm (V). The λ_{max} of band I will shift to longer wavelength with the increase of phenolic hydroxyl groups substituted, but the shift is not related to the substituted positions. The λ_{max} of band I and its relation to the number of phenolic hydroxyl groups are shown in Table 4-4.

Table 4-4 λ_{max} of band I and number of phenolic hydroxyl groups

The number of hydroxyl	Position of hydroxyls	λ_{max} (nm)
1	1-; 2-	222.5
2	1, 2-; 1, 4-; 1, 5-	225
3	1, 2, 8-; 1, 4, 8-; 1, 2, 6-; 1, 2, 7-	230 ± 2.5
4	1, 4, 5, 8-; 1, 2, 5, 8-	236

The intensity of band III is related to β-OH in anthraquinones. For anthraquinones with β-OH, the intensity of band III is above $\log\varepsilon$ 4.1. For anthraquinones without β-OH , the intensity of band III is below $\log\varepsilon$ 4.1.

6.2.2 IR Spectrum

Hydroxyl anthraquinones have absorption bands in the characteristic region of IR spectrum, such as $\nu_{C=O}$ (1675–1653cm^{-1}), ν_{OH} (3600–3130cm^{-1}), and ν_{Ar} (1600–1480cm^{-1}). Because carbonyl can form hydrogen bond with α-OH, which changes the dipole moment and the length of the C=O, the absorption of $\nu_{C=O}$ is closely related to the number and position of α-OH (Table 4-5).

Table 4-5   Absorption of $\nu_{C=O}$ and number and position of α-hydroxyl groups

α-OH		$\nu_{C=O}$ (cm^{-1})		$\Delta\nu_{C=O}$ (cm^{-1})
Number	Position	Free carbonyl	Bonded carbonyl	
0	—	1675–1653	—	—
1	1-	1675–1647	1637–1621	24–38

continued

α-OH		$\nu_{C=O}$ (cm^{-1})		$\Delta\nu_{C=O}$ (cm^{-1})
Number	Position	Free carbonyl	Bonded carbonyl	
2	1, 4- ; 1, 5-	—	1645–1608	—
	1, 8-	1678~1661	1626–1616	40-57
3	1, 4, 5-	—	1616–1592	—
4	1, 4, 5, 8-	—	1592–1572	—

6.2.3 ^{1}H-NMR Spectrum

The aromatic protons in anthraquinones can be divided into α-H and β-H according to their positions related to the quinone nucleus. The chemical shifts of them will be affected by substituent groups such as methyl, methoxyl, hydroxymethyl, phenyl hydroxyl, and carboxyl. They are shown in Table 4-6.

Table 4-6   Chemical shifts of protons in anthraquinones

Protons		δ_H	The changes of chemical shift in different position		
			ortho-	meta- （间）	para-
α-H		8.07	—	—	—
β-H		7.67	—	—	—
CH$_3$		2.1–2.9	–0.15	–0.10	–0.10
OCH$_3$		3.7–4.5	–0.45	–0.10	–0.40
CH$_2$OH	CH$_2$	≈4.6	+0.21	+0.10	+0.03
	OH	4.0–6.0			
Ar-OH	α-OH	11.6–12.6	–0.45	–0.10	–0.40
	β-OH	10.0–11.4			
COOH		10.0–13.0	+0.80	+0.25	+0.20

6.2.4 ^{13}C-NMR Spectrum

^{13}C-NMR spectrum has been also widely used in the structure elucidation for anthraquinones. The chemical shifts of 9, 10-anthraquinone and its derivatives in ^{13}C-NMR are shown in Figure 4-11. The chemical shifts are affected by the substituents. The substitution of hydroxyl or methoxyl groups leads the downfield shift of the carbon directly connected to the substituents, and upfield shift of the ortho- and para-carbons.

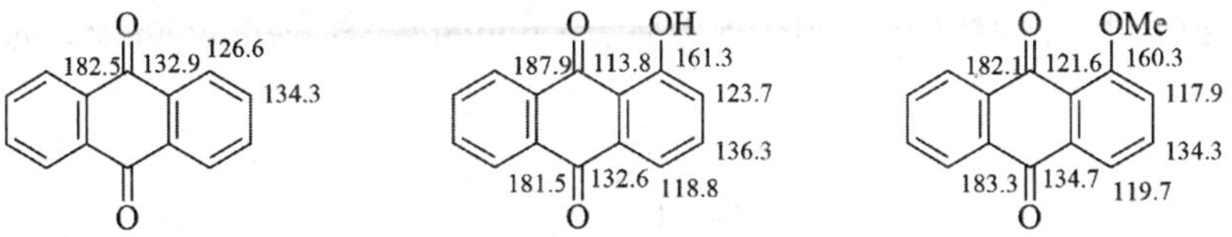

Figure 4-11   Chemical shifts of α-OH and α-OMe anthraquinones in ^{13}C-NMR

6.2.5   MS

Due to the stable structures of anthraquinones in free form, the molecular ion peaks of them are always the base peak in MS. Free anthraquinones lose CO successively producing fragments peaks at m/z 180 [M-CO] and 152 [M-2CO] with high abundance (Figure 4-12). Anthraquinone derivatives also fragment in the same way and produce similar fragment ion peaks.

m/z 208 m/z 180 m/z 152

Figure 4-12   Fragmentation ions of anthraquinones

The molecular ion peaks of anthraquinone glycosides are not easy to be detected in EI-MS. The base peak is often the aglycone ion. FD-MS, FAB-MS and ESI-MS are generally performed to obtain the information of the quasi-molecular ions of anthraquinone glycosides.

6.2.6   An Example of Structure Elucidation

Ophiohayatone-A was isolated from *Ophiorrhiza hayatana* O. (瘤果蛇根草) as a yellow powder with mp. 164–166℃. The HR-EI-MS showed a molecular ion at m/z 284.0685 corresponding to the molecular formula $C_{16}H_{12}O_5$.

The UV spectrum of ophiohayatone-A showed absorption peaks at 214, 278 and 337nm in MeOH. The IR absorption bands at 3407cm^{-1} and 1655cm^{-1} indicated the presence of hydroxyl and carbonyl groups. The molecular formula, UV, and IR suggested that it might be a free anthraquinone.

The ^{1}H-NMR spectrum in the aromatic region showed an ABX coupling system including protons at δ 8.04 (1H, d, J = 8.6Hz), 7.19 (1H, dd, J = 8.6, 2.4Hz) , and 7.48 (1H, d, J = 2.4Hz) assignable to H-5, H-6, and H-8, respectively. Two singlets at δ 8.13 and 7.52 were attributable to H-4 and H-1. Other signals in ^{1}H-NMR were a two-proton singlet of oxymethylene group (—CH$_2$O—) at δ 4.52 and a three-proton singlet of methoxyl group (—OCH$_3$) at δ 3.42. The above information indicated that ophiohayatone-A was a 2, 3, 7-trisubstituted anthraquinone.

The correlation between the methoxy proton signal at δ_H 3.42 and the carbon of oxymethylene (—CH$_2$O—) at δ_C 69.1 in HMBC experiment indicated that a methoxymethyl group (—CH$_2$OCH$_3$) was present in this compound. The HMBC spectrum also showed the correlation between H-4 (δ_H 8.13) and the carbon of oxymethylene (δ_C 69.1). This correlation in HMBC suggested that the methoxymethyl group attached at C-3 of ophiohayatone-A. Therefore, C-2 and C-7 should be substituted with hydroxyl groups according to the molecular formula observed in HR-EI-MS.

The up-field shift of signals for H-6, H-8 and H-1 from δ 7.67, 8.07, 8.07 to δ 7.19, 7.48, 7.52, respectively, could be attributed to the occurrence of hydroxyl groups on ophiohayatone-A. These results, as well as other correlations observed between protons and carbons in HMQC and HMBC, strongly supported the proposed structure of ophiohayatone-A as 2, 7-dihydroxy-3-methoxymethylanthraquinone.

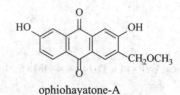

ophiohayatone-A

^{1}H-NMR (400 MHz) and ^{13}C-NMR (100 MHz) spectral data of ophiohayatone-A is listed in Table 4-7.

Table 4-7 ^{1}H-NMR (400 MHz) and ^{13}C-NMR (100 MHz) data of ophiohayatone-A (in acetone-d_6)

Position	δ_H	δ_C
1	7.52 (1H, s)	112.6
2	—	162.0
3	—	132.6
4	8.13 (1H, s)	129.9
5	8.04 (1H, d, J=8.6)	132.6
6	7.19 (1H, dd, J=8.6, 2.4)	121.7
7	—	163.8
8	7.48 (1H, d, J=2.4)	112.8
9	—	184.1
10	—	181.2
4a	—	134.8
8a	—	125.0
9a	—	135.9
10a	—	181.2
—CH$_2$—	4.52 (2H, s)	69.1
—OCH$_3$	3.42 (3H, s)	58.2

7 Examples of Chinese Herbs Containing Quinones

7.1 Rhei Radix et Rhizoma（大黄）

7.1.1 Introduction

(1) Biological Source

Rhei Radix et Rhizoma is the dried root and rhizome of *Rheum palmatum* L. (掌叶大黄), *R. tanguticum* Maxim. Ex Balf. (唐古特大黄) or *R. officinale* Baill. (药用大黄）(Fam. Polygonaceae).

(2) Property, Flavor and Channels Entered

Property and Flavor: Cold; Bitter.

Channels Entered: Spleen, Stomach, Large Intestine, Liver, Pericardium.

(3) Actions & Indications

To remove accumulation with purgation, clear heat and purge fire, cool the blood and remove toxin, expel stasis to unblock the meridian, drain dampness to abate jaundice. For accumulation, stagnation and constipation caused by excess heat, hematemesis caused by blood heat, red eyes and swollen throat, swelling abscess, deep-rooted boil and sore, abdominal pain caused by intestinal abscess, postpartum stasis and obstruction, blood-stasis amenorrhea, injuries from falls and fights, dampness-heat dysentery, jaundice and red urine, stranguria, edema, burn and scald.

(4) Pharmacological Activities

The pharmacological activities associated with Rhei Radix et Rhizoma include laxative, anti-tumor, anti-inflammatory, analgesic, antioxidant, antibiotic effects. It also protects the liver, gallbladder and kidney, lows blood lipids. Other effects of it include pancreatic secretion promotion, cardiotonic action, etc.

7.1.2　Main Chemical Constituents

Rhei Radix et Rhizoma distributes in most areas of China, mainly in Shanxi, Gansu, Sichuan, Yunnan, Qinghai provinces, and Tibet autonomous region. It contains anthraquinones and their glycosides, stilbene (二苯乙烯) glycosides, fatty acids, n-butyrophenones, polysaccharides, tannins, etc.

(1) Anthraquinones and Their Glycosides

Anthraquinones and their glycosides are main chemical constituents of Rhei Radix et Rhizoma. There are over 20 anthraquinones and their glycosides with the five main Emodin type anthraquinones mentioned before as aglycones. The glucose links to hydroxyl groups including phenolic and alcholic hydroxyl groups on the anthraquinone nucleus. The glucose can be further acylated with gallic acid (没食子酸) or malonic acid.

(2) Anthrones

The anthrones isolated from Rhei Radix et Rhizom are stereoisomers with laxative effects.

	R_1	R_2	R_3	R_4
rheinoside A	glc	glc	OH	H
rheinoside B	glc	OH	glc	H
rheinoside C	glc	glc	H	H
rheinoside D	glc	H	glc	H

(3) Dianthrones

Dianthrones isolated from Rhei Radix et Rhizom are palmidins (掌叶二蒽酮), rheidins (大黄二蒽酮) besides sennosides A, B, C, and D.

	R_1	R_2	R_3	R_4	R_5
palmidin A	CH_3	CH_2OH	OH	H	H
palmidin B	CH_3	CH_2OH	H	H	H
palmidin C	CH_3	CH_3	OH	H	H
rheidin A	CH_3	COOH	OH	H	H
rheidin B	CH_3	COOH	H	H	H
rheidin C	CH_3	COOH	OCH_3	H	H
sennosdie E/F	COOH	COOH	H	glc-oxalyl (草酰)	glc

(4) Stilbene and Their Glycosides

Nearly 30 stilbenes together with their glycosides have been isolated from Rhei Radix et Rhizom. Among them rhaponticin (土大黄苷) is the major one. The Chinese Pharmacopoeia stipulates that no rhaporntcin should be detected in Rhei Radix et Rhizoma under the specific experimental condition outlined in it. The stilbenes are classified into two main groups according to the configuration of the double bond. The sugar moiety can be glucose, xylose, etc, as well as their gallates.

	R$_1$	R$_2$	R$_3$
rhaponticin	OH	OCH$_3$	Oglc
rhapontigenin (土大黄苷元)	OH	OCH$_3$	OH
isorhapontigenin	OCH$_3$	OH	OH
deoxyrhapontigenin	H	OCH$_3$	OH
piceatannol (白皮杉醇)	OH	OH	OH
resveratrol (白藜芦醇)	H	OH	OH

trans-stilbene

cis-3, 5, 3′-trihydroxyl-4′methoxystilbene (*cis*-stilbene)

(5) Tannins

Over 40 tannins have been isolated from Rhei Radix et Rhizom. Most of them are dimers, trimers, even polymers condensed tannins (缩合鞣质).

7.1.3　Quality Control Standards

(1) TLC Identification

Stationary Phase: Silica gel H-CMC plate.

Standards: authentic crude drug; rhein.

Development System: Petroleum ether (30–60℃)-ethyl formate-formic acid (15 : 5 : 1).

Visualization: 365nm UV light and then fumigate with ammonium.

(2) Tests

Rhaponticin: No persistent bright purple fluorescence (UV 365nm).

Loss on Drying: Not more than 15.0%, 6 h at 105℃ .

Total Ash: Not more than 10.0%.

Water Soluble Extracts: Not less than 25.0% (heated extraction).

(3) Assay

Total of aloe-emodin, rhein, emodin, chrysophanol, physcion: Not less than 1.5% (HPLC).

7.2　Salviae Miltiorrhizae Radix et Rhizoma(丹参)

7.2.1　Introduction

(1) Biological Source

Salviae Miltiorrhizae Radix et Rhizoma is the dried root and rhizome of *Salvia miltiorrhiza* Bge. ﹝Fam. Labiatae (唇形科) ﹞.

(2) Property, Flavor and Channels Entered

Property and Flavor: Mild cold; Bitter.

Channels Entered: Heart, Liver.

(3) Actions & Indications

To activate blood and eliminate stasis, unblock the meridian to relive pain, clear heart-fire and relieve vexation, cool the blood and disperse abscesses. For chest impediment and heart pain, pain in the epigastrium and abdomen, lump in the abdomen causing distension and pain, hypochondriac pain, insomnia caused by vexation, menstrual irregularities, dysmenorrhea and amenorrhea, sore, ulcer, swelling and pain.

(4) Pharmacological Activities

The pharmacological activities associated with Salviae Miltiorrhizae Radix et Rhizoma include improving microcirculation, accelerating the flow rate of blood, inhibiting the function of platelet and blood coagulation, promoting fibrinolytic activity, lowering blood viscosity, improving the injuries due to cerebral ischemia in liver, kidney and lung. It also has effect of anti-tumor, anti-oxidation, anti-gastric ulcer, prevention of respiratory distress and inhibition of pulmonary fibrosis.

Tanshinones have inhibitory effects on liver, cervical, nasopharyngeal, lung, gastric cancer, as well as leukemia. Salvianic acids (丹酚酸) can protect the heart with coronary artery disease. Salvianic acid B can protect cardiomyocytes and cardiac microvascular endothelial cells, prevent and cure arteriosclerosis.

7.2.2　Main Chemical Constituents

S. miltiorrhiza widely grows in most areas of China, mainly in Sichuan, Shandong and Zhejiang provinces. Lipophilic tanshinones and hydrophilic salvianolic acids both are the major constituents of Salviae Miltiorrhizae Radix et Rhizoma. Other constituents are also identified such as fatty acids, sterols, terpenoids, flavonoids, saccharides, tannins and amino acids.

The typical liposoluble tanshinones have mentioned before. They belong to phenanthraquinones. While the hydrophilic salvianolic acids belong to phenylpropanoids.

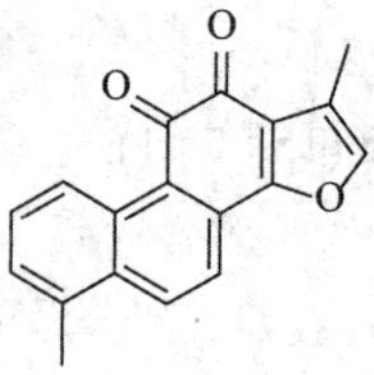

tanshinone I 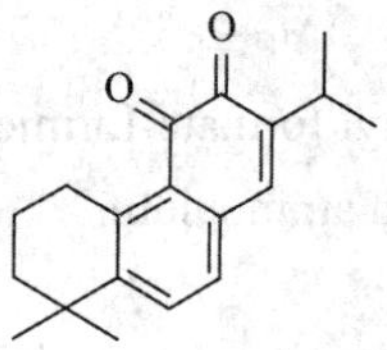　　　　miltiron　　　　cryptotanshinone　　　　tanshinlactone
　　　　　　　（次丹参醌）　　　　（隐丹参酮）　　　　　（丹参内酯）

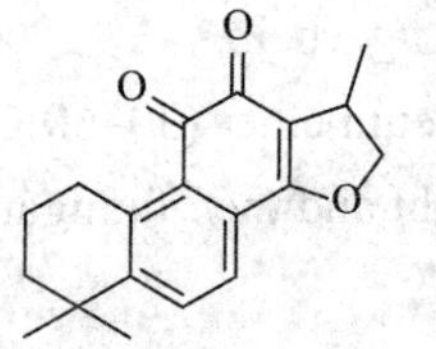

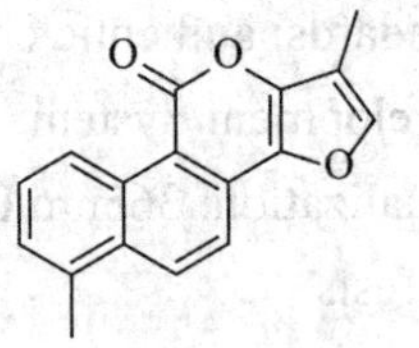

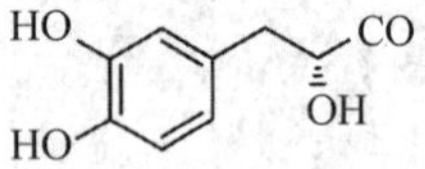

danshensu（丹参素） 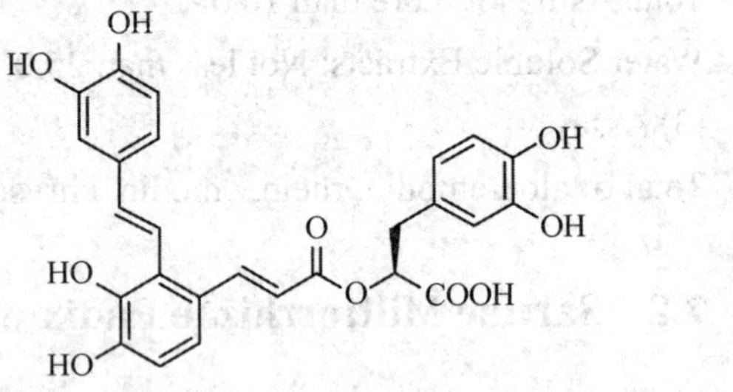　　　　　　　　salvianolic acid A

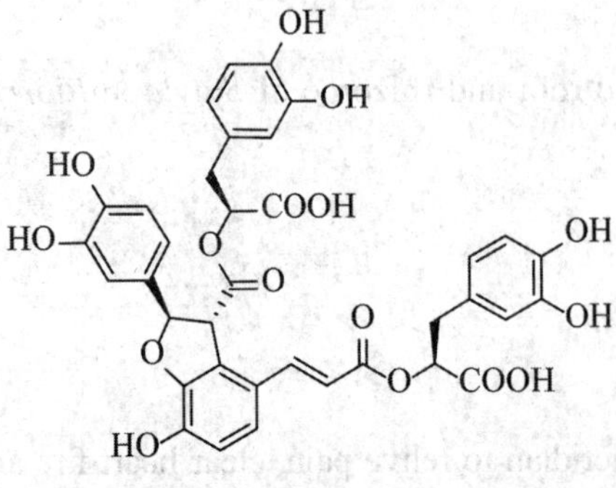

salvianolic acid B 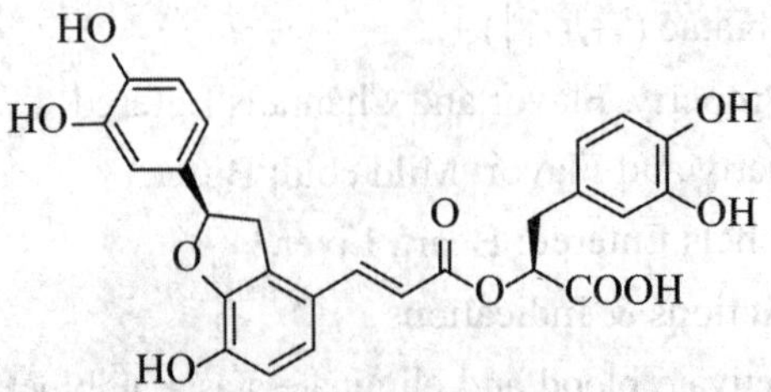　　　　　　　　salvianolic acid C

7.2.3 Quality Control Standards

(1) TLC Identification

Stationary Phase: Silica gel G plate (for tanshinone II_A), GF_{254} (for salvianolic acid B).

Standard: The test solution of authentic crude drug, tanshinone II_A, salvianolic acid B.

Development System: Petroleum-ethyl acetate (4 : 1) (for tanshinone II_A), toluene-chloroform-ethyl acetate-methanol-formic acid (2 : 3 : 4 : 0.5 : 2) (for salvianolic acid B) Visualization: Visible light (for tanshinone II_A); 254nm UV light (for salvianolic acid B).

(2) Tests

Water: Not more than 13.0%.

Total ash: Not more than 10.0%.

Acid-insoluble Ash: Not more than 3.0%.

Heavy Metals and Harmful Elements: Pb$\leqslant$5 ppm, Cd$\leqslant$0.3 ppm, As$\leqslant$2 ppm, Hg$\leqslant$0.2 ppm, Cu$\leqslant$20 ppm.

Water Soluble Extracts: Not less than 35.0% (cooled extraction).

Alcohol Soluble Extracts: Not less than 15.0% (heated extraction).

(3) Assay

Tanshinone II_A: Not less than 0.20% (HPLC).

Salvianolic acid B: Not less than 3.0% (HPLC).

7.3 Arnebiae Radix（紫草）

7.3.1 Introduction

(1) Biological Source

Arnebiae Radix is the dried root of *Arnebia euchroma* (Royle) Johnst. (新疆紫草) or *A. guttata* Bunge. (内蒙紫草)(Fam. Boraginaceae).

(2) Property, Flavor and Channels Entered

Property and Flavor: Cold; Sweet, salty.

Channels Entered: Heart, Liver.

(3) Actions & Indications

To clear heat and cool the blood, promote blood circulation and detoxify, promote rashes and eliminate plaques. For exuberant blood heat-toxin, dark purple macule and papule, unerupted measles, sore, ulcer, eczema, scald and burn.

(4) Pharmacological Activities

The pharmacological activities associated with Arnebiae Radix include antibiosis, antitumor, antivirus, anti-inflammatory, anti-anaphylaxis, liver protecting *via* transaminase lowering, promote burn and wound healing.

7.3.2 Main Chemical Constituents

Arnebia euchroma (Royle) Johnst. and *Arnebia guttata* Bunge grow in China and other countries and regions. Their roots contain naphthoquinones, benzoquinones, phenylpropionic acid, lignans, alkaloids, triterpenoid acids, sterols, flavonoids, polysaccharides, etc.

(1) Naphthoquinones

Naphthoquinones are the main bioactive constituents in Arnebiae Radix. They have the effects of antibiosis, antitumor and anti-inflammatory. They are also used as natural pigments in the industry of medicine, cosmetic, printing and dyeing. More than 30 naphthoquinones have been isolated from Arnebiae Radix with the nucleus of 5, 8-dihydroxy-1, 4-naphthoquinones linking with isohexene side chain. They are divided in two groups based on the absolute configuration of the chiral center on the side chain, i.e. shikonin-type (*R*) and alkannin-type (*S*).

		R
shikonin	alkannin	OH
deoxyshikonin	deoxyalkannin	H
methylshikonin	methylalkannin	OCH₃
acetylshikonin	acetylalkannin	OCOCH₃
propionylshikonin	—	OCOCH₂CH₃
isobutylshikonin	isobutylalkannin	OCOCH(CH₃)₂
isovalerylshikonin	isovalerylalkannin	OCOCH₂CH(CH₃)₂
β-hydroxy-isovalerylshikonin	β-hydroxy-isovalerylalkannin	OCOCH₂C(CH₃)₂OH
β-acetoxy isovalerylshikonin		OCOCH₂C(CH₃)₂OCOCH₃
α-methylbutylshikonin	α-methylbutylalkannin	OCOCH(CH₃)CH₂CH₃
β, β-dimethyl acryloylshikonin	β, β-dimethyl acryloylalkannin	OCOCH=CHCH(CH₃)₂
2, 3-dimethylpentenoyl shikonin	2, 3-dimethylpentenoyl alkannin	OCOCH₂C(CH₃)=C(CH₃)₂
ethylshikonin		OCH₂CH₃
cinnamoylshikonin		OCOCH=CHPh
3, 4-methylenedioxy-cinnamoylshikonin		OCOCH=CHPh(OCH₂O)
	β-methoxyacetyl alkannin	OCOCH₂OCH₃
	angelic acylalkannin	OCOC(CH₃)=CHCH₃

	R
amebin-5	H
amebin-6	OCOCH₃

(2) Naphthoquinone dimers

Naphthoquinone dimers have been isolated from the tissue culture of Arnebiae Radix. Naphthoquinones also form dimers under the conversion of enterobacteria.

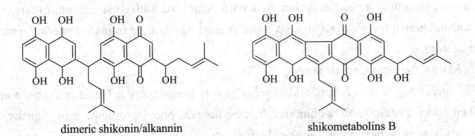

dimeric shikonin/alkannin   shikometabolins B

(3) Benzoquinones or *p*-dihydroxybenzene

Benzoquinones or *p*-dihydroxybenzene from Arnebiae Radix are always substituted with monoterpene side chain or skeleton derived from monoterpene.

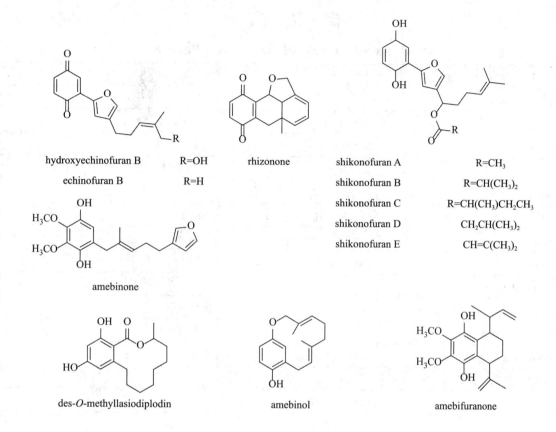

hydroxyechinofuran B   R=OH   rhizonone

echinofuran B   R=H

shikonofuran A   R=CH$_3$

shikonofuran B   R=CH(CH$_3$)$_2$

shikonofuran C   R=CH(CH$_3$)CH$_2$CH$_3$

shikonofuran D   CH$_2$CH(CH$_3$)$_2$

shikonofuran E   CH=C(CH$_3$)$_2$

amebinone

des-*O*-methyllasiodiplodin   amebinol   amebifuranone

(4) Lignans

Lignans from Arnebiae Radix belong to arylnaphthalene (芳基萘) type and benzofuran (苯骈呋喃) type, and always form esters with lactic acid.

(5) Alkaloids

Three alkaloids have been isolated from Arnebiae Radix belonging to pyrrolizidine (吡咯里西啶) type, which lead liver injury and cancer. So the alkaloids are the toxic constituents of Arnebiae Radix.

7.3.3　Quality Control Standards

(1) TLC Identification

Stationary Phase: Silica gel G plate.

Standard: authentic crude drug.

Development System: Cyclohexane-toluene-ethyl acetate-formic acid (5∶5∶0.5∶0.1).

Visualization: Visible light and then spray 10% NaOH to see spots again.

(2) Tests

Water: Not more than 15.0%.

(3) Assay

Total Hydroxyl Naphthoquinones: Not less than 0.80% (UV spectrophotometric method).

β, β-Dimethyl Acroloylalkannin: Not less than 0.30% (HPLC).

词 汇 表

An Alphabetical List of Words and Phrases

A		
Ailanthus altissima		臭椿
alizarin	[əˈlızərın]	茜草素，茜草色素
alkannin	[ˈɔːlkænın]	阿卡宁
amphi-	[ˈæmfiː]	〈构词成分〉两种，两边，在周围
anthracene	[ˈænθrəˌsiːn]	蒽
anthranol	[ˈænθrənɔl]	蒽酚
anthraquinone	[ˌænθrəˈkwınəun]	蒽醌
anthrone	[ˈænθrəun]	蒽酮
Arnebiae Radix		紫草
Arnebia euchroma (Royle) Johnst		新疆紫草
Arnebia guttata Bunge.		内蒙紫草
arylnaphthalene	[ærılˈnæfθəliːn]	芳基萘
B		
barbaloin	[bɑːˈbæləın]	芦荟苷
benzofuran	[ˈbenzɔːfrən]	苯骈呋喃
benzoquinone	[ˌbenzəuˈkwınəun]	苯醌
Boraginaceae		紫草科
C		
cassiamine	[ˈkæsıəmiːn]	山扁豆双醌
chromogenic	[krəuməˈdʒenık]	adj. 发色的
chrysophanol	[ˈkrısəfənəl]	大黄酚
condensed tannins	[kənˈdenst][ˈtænıns]	缩合鞣质
cryptotanshinone	[krıpˈtɔtənʃınən]	隐丹参酮
cyclohexanedione	[saıkləuˈheksəniːdıən]	环己二酮
D		
danshensu	[dænˈʃensʌ]	丹参素
dehydrodianthrones	[dıˌhaıdrəudaıˈænθrəunz]	去氢二蒽酮类
dianthrone	[daıˈænθrəun]	二蒽酮
dimethylaniline	[daıˌmeθılˈænılaın]	二甲基苯胺
E		
embellin	[ımˈbelın]	信筒子醌
Embelia (E.) ribes		白花酸藤果
Embelia oblongifolia		多脉酸藤子

(continued)

emodin	['emədɪn]	大黄素
G		
gallic acid	['gælɪk]['æsɪd]	没食子酸
gentiobioside	['dʒenti:əubaɪəsaɪd]	龙胆双糖苷
H		
hypericin	[haɪ'perɪsɪn]	金丝桃素
Hypericum	[haɪ'perɪkəm]	金丝桃属
J		
juglone	[dʒuː'gləun]	胡桃醌
L		
Labiatae		唇形科
Lamiaceae		唇形科
lapachol	['læpəkɔl]	拉帕醇，拉帕醌
Leguminosae		豆科
leucomethylene blue	[lju:kɔ'meθɪli:n] [blu:]	无色亚甲蓝
lichen	['laɪkən]	地衣
Liliaceae		百合科
M		
meso	['mesəu]	中位，内消旋
meso-naphthodianthrones		中位萘二蒽酮类
meta	['metə]	间（位）
miltiron	['mɪltɪrən]	次丹参醌
N		
naphthodianthrones		萘骈二蒽酮类化合物
naphthoquinone	['næfθəkwɪ'nəun]	萘醌
neotanshinone	['niːəutənʃɪnən]	新丹参酮
nitroso	[naɪ'trəusəu]	亚硝基
O		
Ophiorrhiza hayatana O.		瘤果蛇根草
ortho	['ɔːθəu]	邻（位）
oxalyl	['ɔksəlɪl]	草酰
P		
palmidin	['paːmɪdɪn]	掌叶二蒽酮
para	['pærə]	对（位）
phenanthraquinone	[fɪnənθrækwɪ'nəun]	菲醌
physcion	['fɪsʃn]	大黄素甲醚
piceatannol		白皮杉醇

(continued)

plumbagin	[plʌmbɪˈdʒɪn]	白花丹醌
p-nitroso-*N, N*-dimethylaniline		对亚硝基二甲苯胺
Polygonaceae		蓼科
purpurin	[ˈpəːpjurɪn]	羟基茜草素
pyrrolizidine	[pɪrəlɪˈzaɪdɪn]	吡咯里西丁
Q		
quinone	[kwɪˈnəun]	醌
quinonoid	[ˈkwɪnənɔɪd]	醌式结构
R		
resveratrol	[rezˈvɪərɪtrɔːl]	白藜芦醇
Rhamnaceae		鼠李科
rhaponticin	[ˈræpɔntɪsɪn]	土大黄苷
rhapontigenin	[ˈræpənˈtɪdʒənɪn]	土大黄苷元
rheidin		大黄二蒽酮
rhein	[raɪn]	大黄酸
Rheum officinale Baill.		药用大黄
Rheum palmatum L.		掌叶大黄
Rheum tanguticum Maxim. ex Balf.		唐古特大黄
Rubiaceae		茜草科
Rubiae Radix et Rhizoma		茜草
S		
Salviae Miltiorrhizae Radix et Rhizoma		丹参
Salvia miltiorrhiza Bge		丹参
salvianic acid	[ˈsælvɪənɪk][ˈæsɪd]	丹酚酸
Sennae Folium		番泻叶
sennidin	[seˈnaɪdɪn]	番泻苷元
shikonin	[ˈʃaɪkɔnɪn]	紫草醌，紫草素
skyrin	[skəˈrɪn]	醌茜素，天精
stilbene	[ˈstɪlbiːn]	二苯乙烯
sunshine anthrones	[ˈsʌnʃaɪn][ˈænθrəunz]	日照蒽酮类
T		
tanshinone	[ˈtænʃɪnən]	丹参酮
tanshinlactone	[ˈtænʃɪnˈlæktəun]	丹参内酯
tautomer	[ˈtɔːtəmə]	互变异构体
terpene	[ˈtəːpiːn]	萜
U		
ubiquinone	[juːˈbɪkwɪnəun]	泛醌
V		
vinylogy	[vaɪˈnɪlədʒɪ]	插烯规律

重 点 小 结

醌类是具有醌式结构（即不饱和环己二酮）的一类化合物，可分为苯醌、萘醌、菲醌和蒽醌。蒽醌可根据结构中的蒽核数目分为单蒽核类和双蒽核类。单蒽核类包括羟基蒽醌及其还原产物蒽酚和蒽酮，蒽酚或蒽酮的结构不稳定易被氧化变成蒽醌。羟基蒽醌又根据结构中的酚羟基是取代在双侧苯环上还是单侧苯环上进一步分为大黄素型和茜草素型。双蒽核类包括二蒽酮和蒽醌二聚体等类型。天然存在的蒽醌都是 9, 10- 蒽醌。在蒽醌的苯环上，1, 4, 5, 8 位称为 α- 位，2, 3, 6, 7 位称为 β- 位。

苯醌和萘醌多以游离形式存在，多为结晶性固体；蒽醌则多以成苷的形式存在，多为有色粉末。游离蒽醌具有升华性，小分子苯醌及萘醌具有挥发性。

醌类化合物结构中因多具有酚羟基、烯醇羟基及羧基，故多显酸性。羟基蒽醌的 α-OH 因与羰基形成氢键，故酸性弱于 β-OH，羟基蒽醌的酸性排序为：含 -COOH> 含 2 个以上 β-OH > 含一个 β-OH > 含二个 α-OH >含一个 α-OH，依次能溶于 5%NaHCO$_3$、5%NaHCO$_3$、5%Na$_2$CO$_3$、1%NaOH、5%NaOH，该性质可用于羟基蒽醌的提取、分离和检识。

醌类均可发生 Feigl 反应。苯醌和萘醌还可与无色亚甲蓝显色，当其醌核上有未被取代的位置时还能与活性亚甲基试剂发生 Kesting-Craven 反应。羟基蒽醌可与碱液呈红色，称为 Bornträger 反应。羟基蒽醌还可与醋酸镁形成有色络合物，其颜色与羟基位置及数目有关。羟基蒽酮可与对亚硝基二甲苯胺呈色。

醌类化合物的提取既可根据"相似相溶"原理选择溶剂，也可根据其酸性，使用碱溶酸沉法提取。对于酸性存在差异的游离蒽醌，可以采用 pH 梯度萃取法进行分离，从有机溶剂中依次用 5% NaHCO$_3$、5% Na$_2$CO$_3$、1% NaOH 及 5% NaOH 水溶液进行梯度萃取，可获得酸性不同的游离蒽醌。

羟基蒽醌的 UV 光谱一般具有 5 个谱带：230nm 左右（Ⅰ），240~260nm（Ⅱ），262~295nm（Ⅲ），305~389nm（Ⅳ），>400nm（Ⅴ），且如果带Ⅲ的吸收强度 logε>4.1，则说明结构中具有 β-OH。在蒽醌的 IR 谱中，$\nu_{C=O}$ 的数目和峰位与 α-OH 的数目和位置有关，可初步推断蒽醌的羟基取代情况。在蒽醌的 ^{1}H-NMR 谱中，α-H 因为处于羰基的负屏蔽区，较 β-H 位于低场。蒽醌苷元的 MS 中，分子离子峰常为基峰，并可产生连续失去 C=O 的碎片离子峰。

中药大黄中主要含有单蒽核的大黄素型羟基蒽醌及二蒽核的二蒽酮类成分；丹参中主要含有脂溶性的菲醌类成分和水溶性的酚酸类成分；紫草中主要含有萘醌类成分。

目 标 检 测

题库

一、单选题

1. α- 羟基蒽醌的下列颜色反应为阴性的是（　　　　）

A. Bornträger 反应　　　　　　　　　B. Feigl 反应

C. Kesting-Craven 反应　　　　　　　D. 乙酸镁

E. 三氯化铁

2. 可用于推测羟基蒽醌结构中是否具有 β-OH 的 UV 光谱特征是（　　）

    A. 带Ⅰ的吸收强度 $\log \varepsilon$ >4.1　　　　　　B. 带Ⅱ的吸收强度 $\log \varepsilon$ >4.1

    C. 带Ⅲ的吸收强度 $\log \varepsilon$ >4.1　　　　　　D. 带Ⅳ的吸收强度 $\log \varepsilon$ >4.1

    E. 带Ⅴ的吸收强度 $\log \varepsilon$ >4.1

3. 1,4- 萘醌 8 位引入羟基取代时，相应碳信号变化描述正确的是（　　）

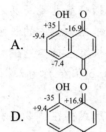

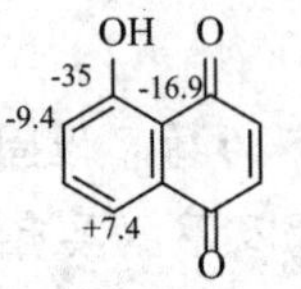

4. 下列化合物的生物合成途径为乙酸 – 丙二酸途径的是（　　）

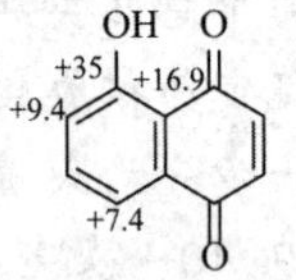

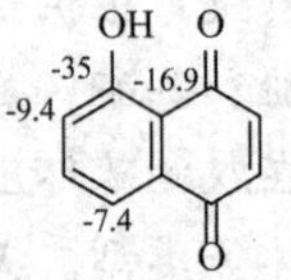

    A. 甾体皂苷　　　B. 蒽醌　　　C. 三萜皂苷　　　D. 香豆素　　　E. 糖

5. 检查羟基蒽醌类化合物常用（　　）

    A. 无色亚甲蓝溶液　　　　　　B. 异羟肟酸　　　　　　C. NaOH 溶液

    D. 变色酸 / 浓硫酸　　　　　　E. α– 萘酚

6. 羟基蒽醌类化合物在 UV 光谱下有几个吸收峰（　　）

    A. 5　　　　　B. 4　　　　　C. 3　　　　　D. 2　　　　　E. 1

7. 蒽醌类化合物取代基酸性强弱顺序为（　　）

    A. β-OH > α-OH > —COOH　　　　B. α-OH > β-OH > —COOH

    C. —COOH > α-OH > β-OH　　　　D. —COOH > β-OH > α-OH

    E. α-OH>—COOH > β-OH

8. 蒽醌类化合物可溶于 5%NaOH 反应结构中可能含有（　　）

    A. α-OH　　　B. β-OH　　　C. COOH　　　D. 均无　　　E. 均有

9. 中药丹参主要成分属于下列哪类化合物（　　）

    A. 黄酮　　　B. 菲醌　　　C. 苯醌　　　D. 蒽醌　　　E. 蒽酮

10. 无色亚甲蓝显色反应可用于检识（　　）

    A. 蒽醌　　　B. 香豆素　　　C. 黄酮　　　D. 萘醌　　　E. 苯酚

二、多选题

1. 丹参中所含有的最主要的脂溶性和水溶性的有效成分为（　　）

    A. 黄酮　　　B. 菲醌　　　C. 挥发油　　　D. 酚酸　　　E. 三萜

2. 在蒽醌的红外光谱中，α– 酚羟基与羰基形成氢键缔合，使（　　）

    A. 羰基吸收峰向低波数位移　　　　　　B. α– 酚羟基吸收峰向低波数位移

    C. 羰基吸收峰向高波数位移　　　　　　D. α– 酚羟基吸收峰向高波数位移

    E. 芳环骨架吸收峰向高波数位移

3. 关于大黄素描述正确的是（　　）

    A. 具有酸性　　　　　　B. 具有发泡性　　　　　　C. 蒽醌类化合物

    D. 萘醌类化合物　　　　E. 菲醌类化合物

4. 能溶于 5%NaHCO₃ 溶液的蒽醌类化合物，结构中可能有（　　　）

　　A. 1 个—COOH　　　　　　　　B. 2 个 *β*-OH　　　　　　　C. 1 个 *β*-OH

　　D. 2 个 *α*-OH　　　　　　　　　E. 1 个 *α*-OH

5. 可用于区别蒽醌和蒽酮的显色反应有（　　　）

　　A. 对亚硝基二甲苯胺反应　　　　B. Kesting-Craven 反应　　　C. Feigl 反应

　　D. FeCl₃ 反应　　　　　　　　　　E. Molish 反应

6. 大黄素 –8–*O*– 葡萄糖苷能够发生阳性反应的是（　　　）

　　A. Molish 反应　　　　　　　　　B. 对二甲氨基苯甲醛反应

　　C. 对亚硝基二甲苯胺反应　　　　D. Kesting-Craven 反应

　　E. Feigl 反应

7. 蒽醌类化合物包括（　　　）

　　A. 菲　　　　　B. 黄酮醇　　　　C. 蒽酮　　　　D. 蒽醌　　　　E. 蒽酚

8. 能溶于 5% 碳酸钠的有（　　　）

　　A. 大黄酸　　　　　　　　　　　　B. 2, 3– 二酚羟基蒽醌

　　C. 2, 4, 5– 三酚羟基蒽醌　　　　　D. 1, 4, 5– 三酚羟基蒽醌

　　E. 1, 2, 6– 三酚羟基蒽醌

9. 能溶于 5% 氢氧化钠的有（　　　）

　　A. 大黄酸　　　　　　　　　　B. 2, 3– 二酚羟基蒽醌　　　　C. 2,5– 二酚羟基蒽醌

　　D. 1, 4, 5– 三酚羟基蒽醌　　　E. 1, 2, 6– 三酚羟基蒽醌

10. 下列化合物能溶于 1% 氢氧化钠的是（　　　）

　　A. 大黄酸　　　　　　　　　　　B. 3, 6– 二酚羟基蒽醌

　　C. 1, 3, 7– 三酚羟基蒽醌　　　　D. 1– 酚羟基蒽醌

　　E. 1, 2, 6– 三甲氧基蒽醌

三、思考题

1. 已知中药大黄中含有蒽醌及其苷，其苷元为大黄酸、大黄素、大黄酚、芦荟大黄素、大黄素甲醚，设计一个提取分离流程图，从大黄中提取并分离大黄酸、大黄素、大黄酚、芦荟大黄素和大黄素甲醚。

2. 比较下列各化合物的酸性强弱，并说明理由。

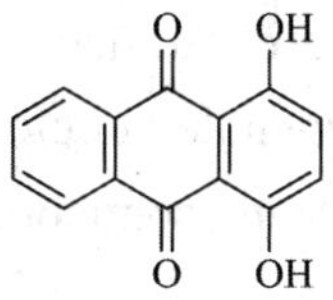

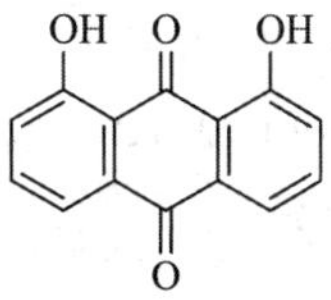

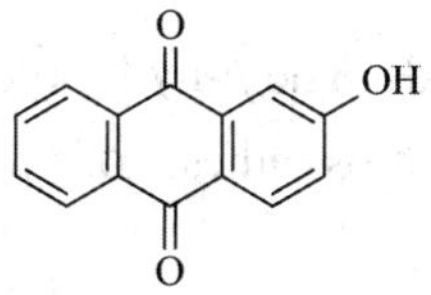

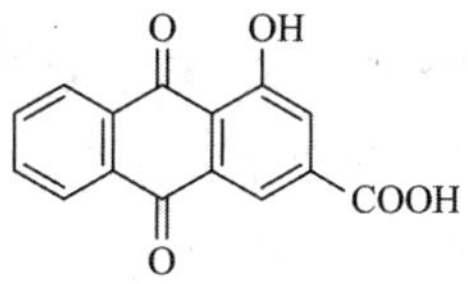

3. 从茜草中分离得到一橙色针状结晶，NaOH 反应呈红色，醋酸镁反应呈橙红色。光谱数据如下：UV 光谱 λ$_{max}$（MeOH）：213、277、341 和 424nm。IR 光谱 ν$_{max}$（KBr）：3400、1664、1620、1590 和 1300cm⁻¹。¹H-NMR（DMSO-d6）δ：13.32（1H, s）、8.06（1H, d, *J*=8.0Hz）、7.44（1H, d, *J*=3.0Hz）、7.21（1H, dd, *J*=8.0, 3.0Hz）、7.20（1H, s）、2.10（3H, s）。请推导该化合物可能的结构。

（曲　扬　何永志）

Chapter 5　Phenylpropanoids

 学习目标

知识要求：

1. **掌握**　苯丙素、香豆素、木脂素的定义；香豆素和木脂素的理化性质、提取分离及检识方法。

2. **熟悉**　香豆素、木脂素的结构分类及主要光谱特征。

3. **了解**　秦皮、五味子、连翘等中药中主要活性成分的结构特征及其质量控制标准。

能力要求：

学会根据香豆素类化合物和木脂素类化合物的存在状态及结构特点，选择适当方法进行提取分离及检识；学会根据香豆素和木脂素的结构特点解决在提取分离过程中存在的问题，并了解在操作过程中的注意事项。

1　Introduction

Phenylpropanoids (苯丙素) represent a large group of natural products that structurally contain one or more C_6–C_3 units (a phenyl ring attached to a three-carbon side chain). They present in many Chinese herbs and have various pharmacological activities. Generally, phenylpropanoids include simple phenylpropanoids (简单苯丙素), coumarins (香豆素), lignans (木脂素), lignins (木质素) and some other natural aromatic compounds.

The shikimate pathway is main biosynthetic pathway of phenylpropanoids. The *p*-hydroxyl (羟基)-cinnamic acid, also known as *p*-coumaric acid is the principal precursor. The biosynthesis of phenylpropanoids is shown in Figure 5-1.

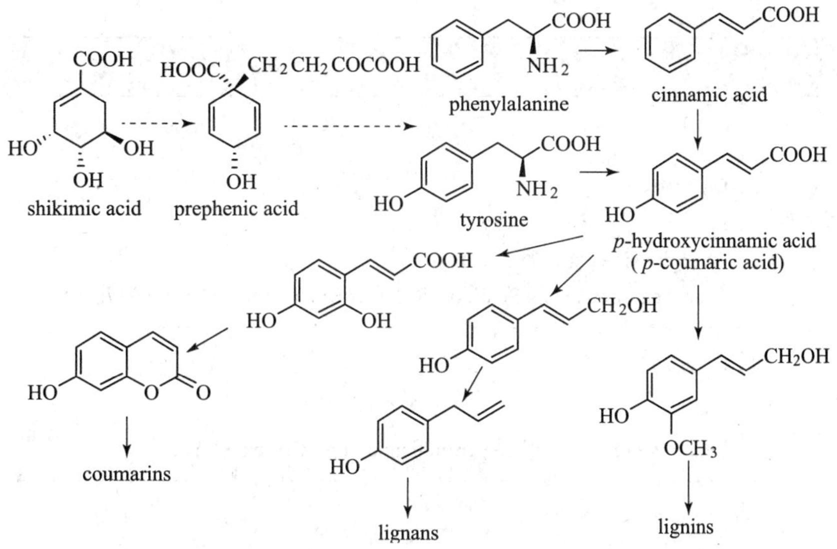

Figure 5-1　Shikimate pathway in phenylpropanoids biosynthesis

2　Simple Phenylpropanoids

2.1　Structure and Classification

Most of the simple phenylpropanoids are phenyl propane derivatives, such as phenylpropenes(苯丙烯), phenylpropyl alcohols (苯丙醇), phenylpropyl aldehydes (苯丙醛) and phenylpropionic acids (苯丙酸). Simple phenylpropanoids are common aromatic compounds in Chinese herbs. Some examples are shown in Table 5-1.

Table 5-1　Some examples of simple phenylpropanoids from Chinese herbs

Categories	Examples
Phenylpropenes	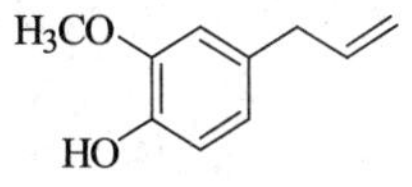 eugenol (丁香酚) from Caryophylli Flos (丁香)
	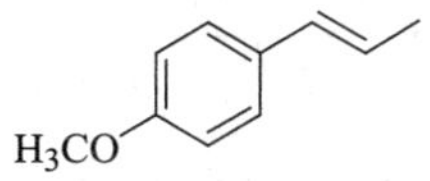 anethole (茴香醚) from Anisi stellati Fructus (八角茴香)
	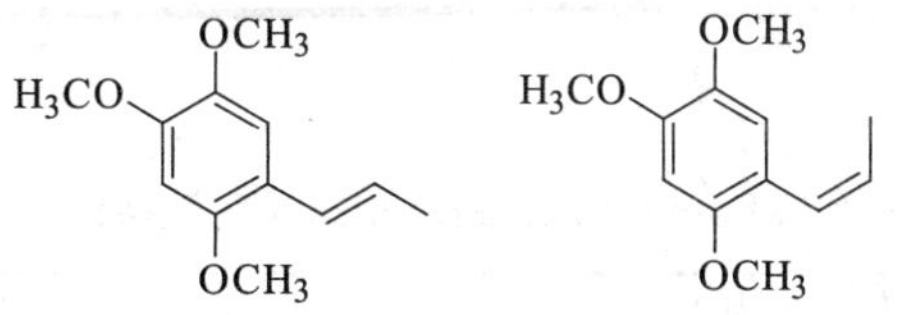 α-asarone（α-细辛醚）and β-asarone (β-细辛醚) from Asari Radix et Rhizome (细辛)

(continued)

Categories	Examples
Phenylpropyl lcohols	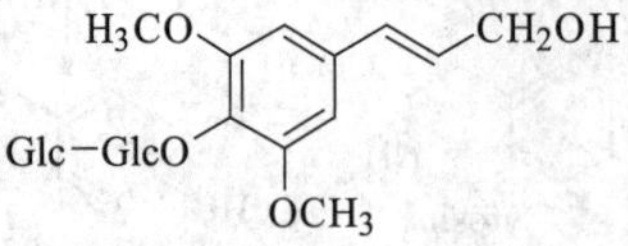 syringinoside (紫丁香酚苷) from Acanthopanacis Senticosi Radix et Rhzoma Seu Caults (刺五加)
Phenylpropyl aldehydes	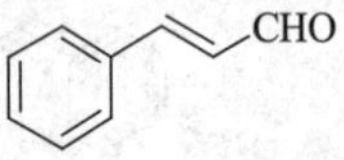 cinnamaldehyde (桂皮醛) from Cinnamomt Cortex (肉桂)
Phenylpropyl acids	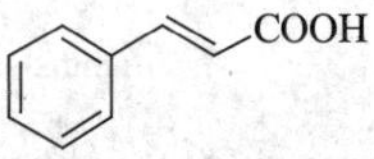 cinnamic acid (桂皮酸) from Cinnamomt Cortex and Foeniculi Fruitus (茴香)
	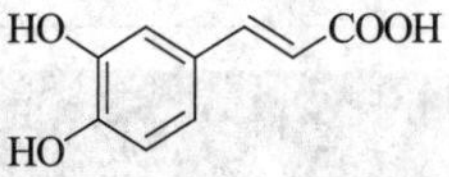 caffeic acid (咖啡酸) from Taraxaciherba (蒲公英), Cimicifug Rhizoma (升麻) and Crataegi Fruitus (山楂)
	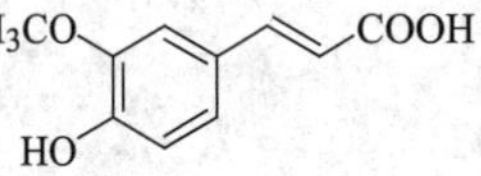 ferulic acid (阿魏酸) from Angelicae sinensis Radix (当归)
	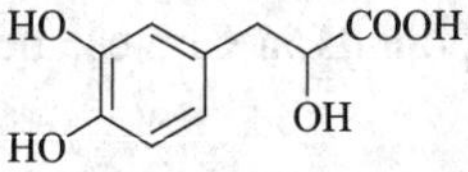 tanshinol (丹参素) from Salviae miltiorrhizae Radix et Rhizoma (丹参)
	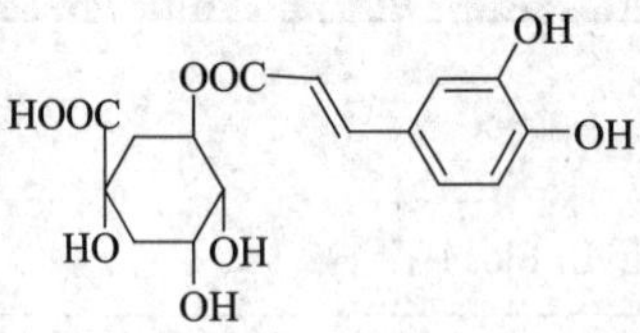 chlorogenic acid (绿原酸) from Lonicerae japonicae Flos (金银花)
	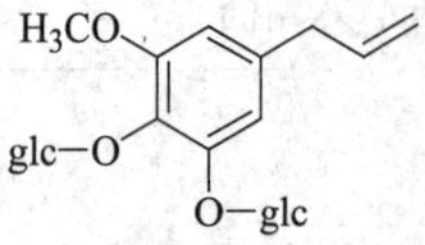 shashenoside (沙参苷 I) from Adenophorae Radix (南沙参)

2.2　Extraction and Isolation Methods

Simple phenylpropanoids can be extracted with organic solvent or water. Most of simple phenylpropenes, esters of phenylpropionic acids, phenylpropyl alcohols and aldehydes are volatile. They are the principle aromatic constituents of volatile oils and can be extracted by steam distillation method. Common isolation methods can be used to isolate simple phenylpropanoids, such as silica gel column chromatography and HPLC.

3　Coumarins

3.1　Introduction

Coumarins are a group of natural compounds with the skeleton of α-benzopyranone (苯骈-α-吡喃酮). Coumarins can be regarded as the lactones (内酯) formed by the loss of water from *cis-ortho*-hydroxycinnamic acid (顺式邻羟基桂皮酸). They are derived from *p*-hydroxycinnamic acids (对羟基桂皮酸) that have undergone *ortho* hydroxylation and subsequently formed lactone ring between the ortho hydroxyl and the carboxyl (羧基) after a *trans-* to *cis-* isomerization of the double bond on side chain. Oxygen-containing groups such as hydroxyl groups are often substituted on C-7. The 7-hydroxycoumarin （umbelliferone） (伞形花内酯) can be regarded as the mother nucleus of coumarins. And C-5, C-6, C-8 can also be substituted by oxygen-containing groups.

coumarin　　　　　umbelliferon　　　　　daphnin

The daphin (瑞香苷) (8-hydroxyl-7-*O*-β-D-glucosyl-coumarin) was the first coumarin isolated from *Daphne alpine* by Vauquelin in 1812. Its structure was confirmed in 1930. Coumarins are commonly found in higher plants, such as Umbeliferae, Lamiaceae, Rutacea (芸香科), Asteraceae (菊科), Fabaceae (豆科), Solanaceae, Thymelaeaceae(瑞香科), Orchidaceae (兰科), Araliaceae (五加科), etc. They may present in any organ of plants.

Coumarins are one type of important active constituents from Chinese herbs. The biological activities of coumarins include anti-tumor, antivirus, anti-inflammation, anti-oxidation, anticoagulation, and spasmolysis, etc.

3.2　Structure and Classification

Coumarins usually can be classified into four groups: simple coumarins (简单香豆素), furocoumarins (呋喃香豆素), pyranocoumarins (吡喃香豆素), and other coumarins.

Simple coumarins have no substituents present on α-pyrone ring and no other ring forming.

The furocoumarins or pyranocoumarins take shape by the isoprene (异戊烯基) groups on C-6 or C-8 forming the furan ring or pyran ring with the hydroxyl group on C-7. Bpth furocoumarins and pyranocoumarins can be classified into "linear type" (线型) and "angular type" (角型). The linear type contains furan ring or pyran ring that is formed by the isoprene group on C-6 and the hydroxyl group on C-7. The angular type contains furan ring or pyran ring that is formed by the isoprene group on C-8 and the hydroxyl group on C-7. The formation processes of furocomarins and pyranocoumarins are shown in Figure 5-2.

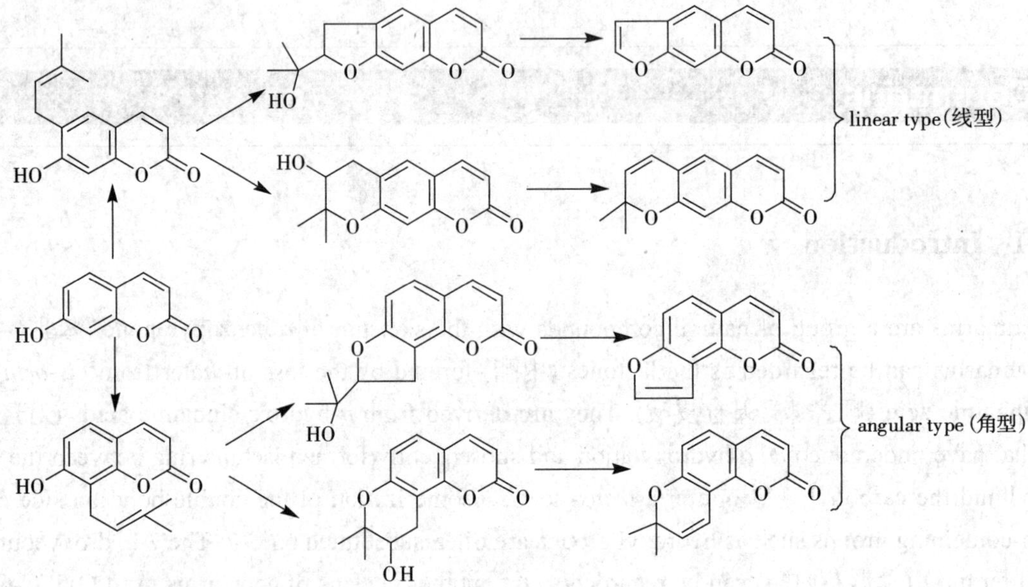

Figure 5-2　Formation processes of furocoumarins and pyranocoumarins

The examples of different types of coumarins from Chinese herbs are listed in Table 5-2.

Table 5-2　Examples of coumarins presented in Chinese herbs

Types	Examples	
Simple coumarins	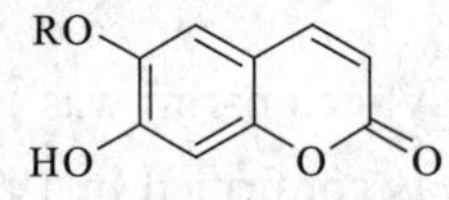 esculin (七叶苷): R=glc esculetin (七叶内酯): R=H Fraxini Cortex	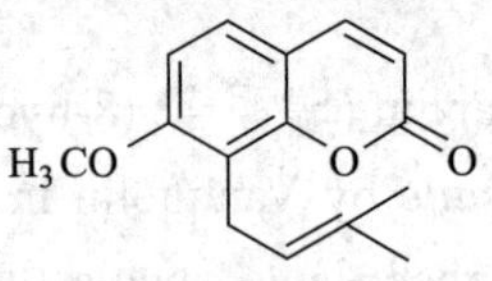 osthole (蛇床子素) Cnidii Fructus (蛇床子)
	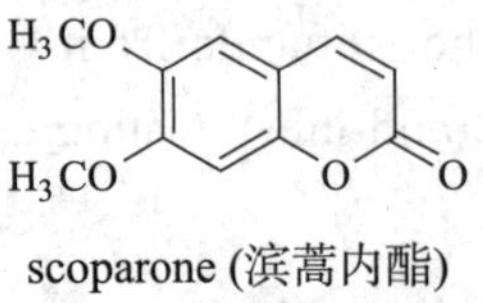 scoparone (滨蒿内酯) Artemisiae scopariae Herba (茵陈)	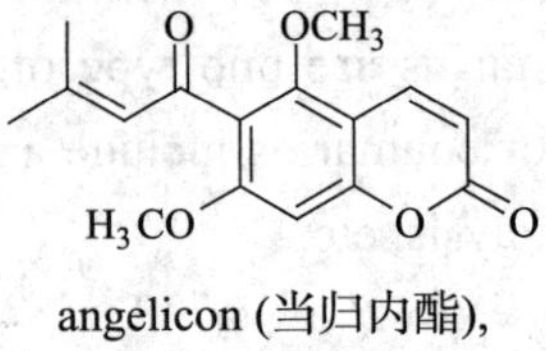 angelicon (当归内酯), Angelicae pubescentis Radix (独活)

(continued)

Types		Examples
Furo-coumarins	Linear type	psoralen (补骨脂素) Psoraleae Fructus (补骨脂) nodakenin (紫花前胡苷): R=glc nodakenetin (紫花前胡苷元): R=H Peucedani decursivi Radix (紫花前胡) bergapten (佛手柑内脂) *Heracleum hemsleyanum* (牛尾独活) imperatorin (欧芹属乙素) Angelicae dahuricae Radix (白芷)
	Angular type	angelin (当归素) Angelicae sinensis Radix pimpinellin (虎耳草素) isobergapten (异佛手柑内酯) *Heracleum hemsleyanum* columbianadin (哥伦比亚内酯) Angelicae pubescentis Radix daucoidin A (旱前胡甲素) *Ligusticum daucoides* (旱前胡)
Pyrano-coumarins	Linear type	decursidin (紫花前胡素) *l*-decursidinol (紫花前胡醇) pd-c-I (紫花前胡香豆素Ⅰ) *Peucedani decursivi Radix* (紫花前胡)
	Angular type	pteryxin (北美芹素) *d*-pracrutorin A (白花前胡丙素) praeroside Ⅱ（白花前胡苷Ⅱ) *Peucedanum pareruptorum* (白花前胡)

(continued)

Types	Examples		
Other coumarins	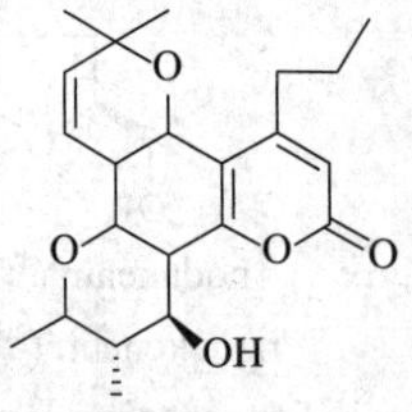 (+) calanolide A	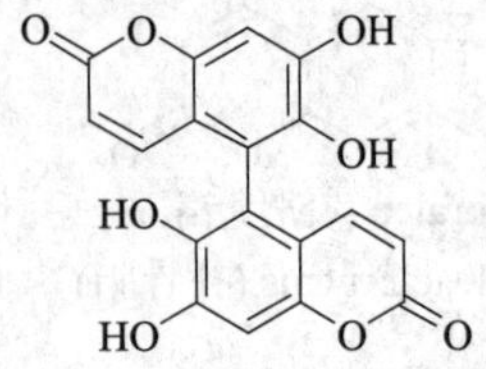 bisaesculetin (双七叶内酯)	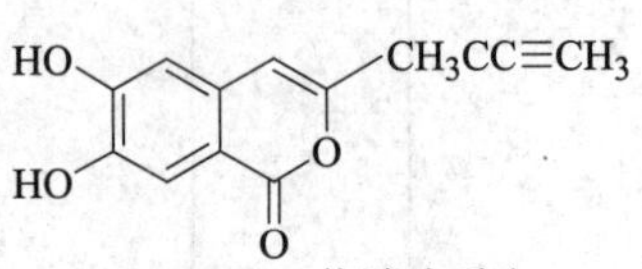 capillarin (茵陈内酯)

3.3   General Physicochemical Properties

3.3.1   Characteristics

Most of free form coumarins are colorless crystals with a sharp melting point. Some of them are liquid. Small molecular weight free form coumarins have aroma (芳香味), sublimability (升华性) and volatility. The glycosides of coumarin are powder or crystals, without sublimability and volatility. Most coumarins show blue or purple fluorescence (荧光) under UV light.

3.3.2   Solubility

Free form coumarins are generally soluble in organic solvents such as ethyl ether, chloroform, acetone, ethanol and methanol, but insoluble in cold water. In contrast, glycosides of coumarin can easily dissolve in water, ethanol and methanol, but insoluble in non-polar organic solvents such as ethyl ether, chloroform, etc.

3.3.3   Alkaline Hydrolysis of Lactone Ring

The lactone ring of coumarins can be opened in alkali solution to form salts of *cis*-adjacent hydroxy-cinnamic acid. The lactone ring can be formed again after acidified. However, if heated in alkaline aqueous solution for a long time, the cis-adjacent hydroxycinnamic acid (顺邻羟基桂皮酸) will be changed into *trans*-adjacent hydroxycinnamic acid (反式邻羟基桂皮酸) and the lactone ring will not be reformed after acidified. In addition, other ester groups (酯基) in coumarins will also be hydrolyzed when the lactone ring is opened (Figure 5-3).

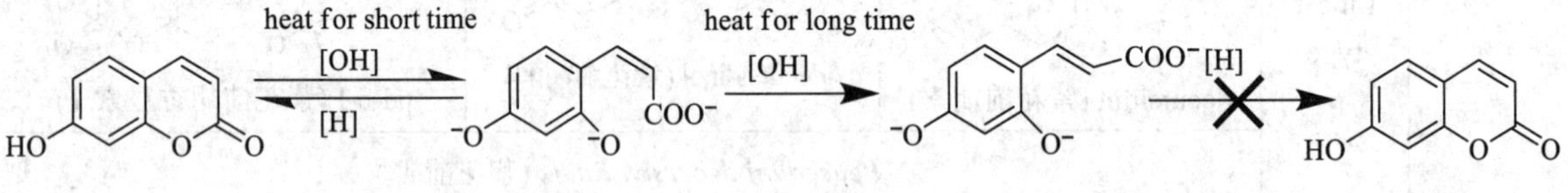

Figure 5-3   Alkaline hydrolysis of the lactone ring in coumarins

3.3.4   Reaction in Acidic Aqueous

The unsaturated side chain (不饱和侧链) such as isoprene groups on coumarins can form oxygen heterocyclic (氧杂环) like furan or pyran rings with vicinal hydroxyl group on coumarins (Figure 5-4). Coumarins with *o*-diol structure also can be rearranged under acidic conditions.

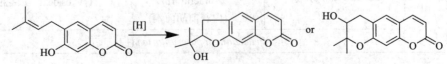

Figure 5-4   Cyclization of coumarins in acidic aqueous

3.3.5   Color Reactions

(1) Hydroxylamine-Ferric Chloride Reaction (异羟肟酸铁反应)

Hydroxylamine-ferric chloride (三氯化铁) reaction is the characteristic reaction of the lactone ring. The lactone ring of coumarins gives positive reaction with hydroxylamine hydrochloride (盐酸羟胺) in alkaline aqueous solution and then forms red complex with Fe^{3+} in acidic solution. The mechanism of this reaction is shown in Figure 5-5.

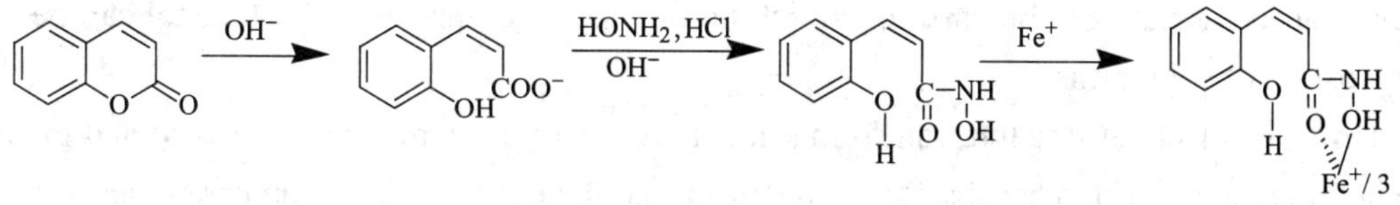

Figure 5-5   Mechanism of hydroxylamine-ferric chloride reaction of coumarins

(2) Phenolic Hydroxyl Groups Reaction

The coumarin with phenolic hydroxyl groups can react with $FeCl_3$ yielding green to blackish precipitate. The coumarin with phenolic hydroxyl groups also can react with diazotization reagents (重氮化试剂) producing red or purple color azodye (偶氮染料), if there is no substituted group on the *ortho*-position (邻位) or *para*-position (对位) of the phenolic hydroxyl group.

(3) Gibb's Reaction

Coumarins can be hydrolyzed by alkali (pH 9–10) to produce a hydroxyl group at the *para*-position of C-6. Then the hydroxyl group can react with 2, 6-dichlorobenzoquinone chlorine imine (2, 6-二氯苯醌氯亚胺)(Gibb's reagent) to show blue color, if there is no substituted group at C-6. Therefore, Gibb's reaction can be used to identify whether a coumarin has a substituted group at C-6. The mechanism of Gibb's reaction is shown in Figure 5-6.

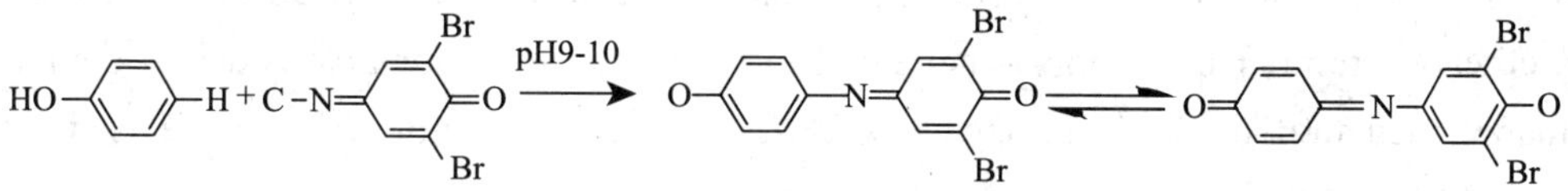

Figure 5-6   Mechanism of Gibb's reaction

(4) Emerson Reaction

Emerson reaction is similar to Gibb's reaction except the reagents used are 4-aminoantipyrine（4-氨基安替比林) and potassium ferricyanide (铁氰化钾). And the positive reaction shows color red. Emerson reaction can also be used to identify whether a coumarin has a substituted group at C-6. The mechanism of Emerson reaction is shown in Figure 5-7.

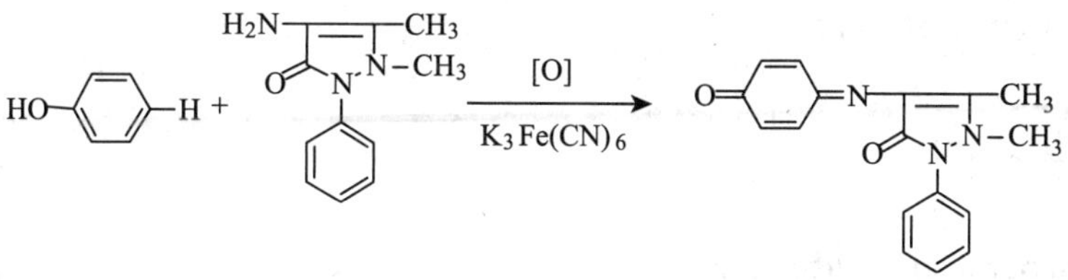

Figure 5-7   Mechanism of Emerson reaction

3.4 Extraction and Isolation Methods

3.4.1 Extraction Methods

(1) Solvent Extraction

Solvent extraction is the main method to extract coumarins. Ethanol is generally used to extract all free form coumarins and their glycosides from Chinese herbs. The total extract can be suspended in water. Subsequently acetyl acetate can be used to extract the free form coumarins and *n*-butanol can be used to extract glycosides of coumarins.

Coumarins with lactone structure can form salts of *cis*-adjacent hydroxycinnamic acid and dissolve in alkali solution to separate with other lipophilic impurities, and the lactone ring of coumarins can be reformed again after acidified. Therefore, free form coumarins can be extracted or purified by this treatment. Temperature and concentration of alkali solution should be strictly controlled to avoid isomerization (异构化) of the *cis*-adjacent hydroxycinnamic acid. In addition, some coumarins with acyl (酰基) substitutions on C-8 cannot form lactone ring again after being opened in alkali solution. Coumarins with an ester group, an allyl ether (烯丙醚) or an o-diol (邻二醇) may undergo hydrolysis or rearrangement during this treatment.

(2) Steam Distillation

Some small molecular weight free form coumarins can be extracted with steam distillation method due to their volatility. This method is not commonly used because high temperature and long processing time may damage the structures of coumarins.

3.4.2 Isolation Methods

Column chromatography, HPLC and preparative TLC (制备薄层色谱) are commonly used methods to separate coumarins.

Silica gel is generally used as adsorbent (吸附剂) to isolate coumarins. The commonly used elution systems for free form coumarins are cyclohexane (or petroleum ether)-ethyl acetate, cyclohexane (or petroleum ether)-acetone or chloroform-acetone. The elution systems for glycosides of coumarins are water-methanol, methanol- chloroform. Sephadex LH-20 column chromatography can be used to isolate a series of coumarins and their glycosides with different molecular weight.

HPLC is widely used for isolation of coumarins from Chinese herbs. For example, angelol-C (独活醇-C), angelol-L (独活醇-L), angelol-J (独活醇-J) were isolated from Chinese herb Angelicae Pubescentis Radix by normal-phase HPLC eluted with chloroform-methanol (50∶1) and reversed-phase HPLC eluted with methanol-water (6∶4).

The preparative TLC method can be used to isolate coumarins because most of coumarins can be easily located on the TLC plate for their fluorescence under UV light. Coumarins with low polarity can be isolated by cyclohexane (petroleum ether) -ethyl acetate system, while coumarins with high polarity can be isolated by chloroform-methanol system.

3.5 Identification

3.5.1 Physicochemical Identification

(1) Fluorescence

Most of coumarins emit blue or purple fluorescence under 365nm UV light. 7-Hydroxyl coumarins have strong blue fluorescence, and their fluorescence will be stronger in alkaline solution even change into green color. The fluorescence intensity of coumarins will decrease and turn into purple if the hydroxyl groups are etherified (醚化) or substituted by other groups，such as aesculetin dimethyl ether (七叶内酯二甲醚). When hydroxyl was introduced on C-8, fluorescence was reduced or even not observed. Coumarins with multiple alkoxyl (烷氧基) generally have yellowish green or brown fluorescence.

(2) Color Reactions

The lactone ring of coumarins can be identified by hydroxylamine-ferric chloride reaction. $FeCl_3$ can be used to identify the phenolic hydroxyl group on coumarins. Gibb's and Emerson reactions can be used to test whether C-6 of coumarins has been substituted.

3.5.2   Chromatography Identification

The common chromatography identification for coumarins is Silica gel TLC. The developing solvent systems used to separate free form coumarins are cyclohexane (or petroleum ether)-ethyl acetate (5∶1–1∶1), chloroform-acetone (9∶1–5∶1). The developing solvent systems used to separate coumarins glycosides are different ratios of chloroform-methanol. Most coumarins can be visible on the TLC plate under UV light (365nm). Also, spraying hydroxylamine-ferric chloride reagent on TLC plate will expose coumarins as red spots. In addition, polyamide chromatography (聚酰胺色谱) also can be used to identify coumarins.

3.6   Structure Determination

The structure determination of coumarins is achieved by combination of multiple spectroscopic data including UV, IR, NMR and MS.

3.6.1   UV Spectrum

Unsubstituted (未被取代) coumarins have maximum wavelength absorption at 274nm (log ε 4.03) and 311nm (log ε 3.72). The former is caused by benzene ring and the latter by α-pyranone (吡喃酮). When substituents are introduced, the position of absorption peak is often changed.

The absorption peak of coumarins with oxygen containing groups will shift toward the longer wavelength. For example, 7-hydroxyl, 7-methoxyl, or 7-O-glycosyl coumarins have maximum wavelength absorption at 217nm and 315–325nm. But alkyl substitution has little effect on it. The main absorptions of coumarins with phenolic hydroxyl will have a red-shift and the density will be enhanced in alkaline solution.

3.6.2   IR Spectrum

In IR spectrum, the lactone ring of coumarins produces strong absorption peaks at 1750–1700cm^{-1}, 1270–1220cm^{-1}, 1100–1000cm^{-1}, and the peak at 1750–1700cm^{-1} being the strongest one. The aromatic ring of coumarins produces three strong absorption peaks between 1660–1600cm^{-1}. These characteristics can distinguish coumarins from flavonoids, chromones (色原酮类) and lignan. The characteristic of furanocoumarins is a weak but very sharp double absorption peak at 3175–3025cm^{-1} that is caused by the furan ring C-H.

3.6.3   NMR Spectrum

(1) ^{1}H-NMR

Most of natural coumarins have no substituent (取代基) on C-3 and C-4. So the ^{1}H-NMR spectrum shows two well differentiated signals at δ_{H-4} 7.50–8.20 (d, J = 9.5Hz) and δ_{H-3} 6.10–6.50 (d, J = 9.5Hz).

These group peaks of H-4 and H-3 are typical signals with the most distinguishing characteristics of coumarins in ^{1}H-NMR.

The signals of H-5, H-6, H-8 in coumarins are similar to protons on general aromatic ring. The coumarins with a substitutent on C-7, the H-5 shows the double peak (d) (二重峰) (coupled with H-6, $J = 8.0$Hz), the H-6 shows the dd peak (coupled with H-5 and H-8, $J = 8.0$Hz, 2.0Hz), and the H-8 shows the d peak (coupled with H-6, $J = 2.0$Hz). The coumarins with substitutents on C-5 and C-7, there is only the *meta*-position (间位) coupling between H-6 and H-8 ($J = 2.0$Hz). The coumarins with substitutents on C-6 and C-7, such as linear type furocoumarins and pyranocoumarins, H-5 and H-8 are all single peak respectively. The coumarins with substitutents on C-7 and C-8, such as angle type furocoumarins and pyranocoumarins, H-5 and H-6 are *ortho*-position coupling relationship (偶合关系) ($J = 8.0$Hz).

(2) ^{13}C-NMR

There are nine carbon atoms in coumarin skeleton. The signals of C-2 and C-7 often appear at about δ 160.0. The signals of C-3 and C-4 often appear at δ 110.0–113.0 and δ 143–145, respectively. The signals of quaternary carbons of C-9 and C-10 appear at δ 149.0–154.0 and δ 110.0–113.0, respectively.

3.6.4　MS Spectrum

Most of coumarins have strong molecular ion peak in the EI-MS spectrum，and the molecular ion peak is often the base peak of simple coumarins. Losing CO, OH, H_2O, methyl or methoxyl group may yield a series of fragment ion peaks in EI-MS spectra of coumarins. In addition, a series of fragment ion peaks of substituent groups such as isopentene, acetoxyl group(乙酰氧基), 5 carbon unsaturated acyloxy (五碳不饱和酰氧基) and so on are characteristics of coumarins in EI-MS spectrum too.

The data of UV, IR, NMR and MS about several representative coumarins are shown in Table 5-3.

Table 5-3　UV, IR, NMR and MS data of several coumarins

Spectra	Data of coumarins		
	Esculetin	Psoralen	Isopsoralen (异补骨脂素)
UVλ_{MeOH} nm	352, 299, 257, 228, 208	328, 289, 245, 241	298, 247, 203
IR ν_{KBr} cm^{-1}	1665 (C=O), 1610, 1560, 1395, 1360, 1280, 950, 880, 850, 820, 635	1720 (C=O), 1630, 1580, 1545	1700 (C=O), 1618, 1540, 1480, 1445, 1270, 1120, 1038, 1040, 830, 740
^{1}H-NMR δ	^{1}H-NMR (CD$_3$OD): 6.22 (1H,d, J=9.5Hz, H-3), 6.79 (1H,s, H-5), 6.97 (1H,s, H-8), 7.82 (1H,d, J=9.5Hz, H-4)	^{1}H-NMR (CDCl$_3$): 6.35 (1H,d, J=10Hz, H-3), 6.82 (1H,dd, H-11), 7.45 (1H,s, H-8), 7.66 (1H,s, H-5), 7.68 (1H,d, J=2.3Hz, H-2'), 7.77 (1H,d, J=10Hz, H-4)	^{1}H-NMR (CDCl$_3$): 6.39 (1H,d, J=9.5Hz, H-3), 7.13 (1H,m, H-3'), 7.37 (1H,d, J=8.5Hz, H-5), 7.43 (1H,d, J=8.5Hz, H-6), 7.69 (1H,m, H-2'), 7.80 (1H, d, J=9.5Hz, H-4)

(continued)

Spectra	Data of coumarins		
	Esculetin	Psoralen	Isopsoralen (异补骨脂素)
^{13}C-NMR δ	^{13}C-NMR (CD$_3$OD): 164.3 (C-2), 112.5 (C-3), 146.0 (C-4), 113.0 (C-5), 144.6 (C-6), 152.0 (C-7), 103.6 (C-8), 150.5 (C-9), 112.8 (C-10)	^{13}C-NMR (CDCl$_3$): 160.9 (C-2), 114.6 (C-3), 144.0 (C-4), 119.8 (C-5), 124.8 (C-6), 156.4 (C-7), 99.8 (C-8), 152.1 (C-9), 115.4 (C-10), 106.3 (C-11), 146.9 (C-12)	^{13}C-NMR (CDCl$_3$): 160.7 (C-2), 141.1 (C-3), 144.4 (C-4), 123.8 (C-5), 108.8 (C-6), 157.4 (C-7), 116.9 (C-8), 148.5 (C-9), 113.5 (C-10), 145.6 (C-2′), 104.1 (C-3′)
EI-MS m/z	178(M$^+$), 150 (M-CO, 100%), 121, 104	186 (M$^+$), 158 (M-CO), 130 (M-2CO), 102 (M-3CO), 44 (O=C=O), 32 (O-CH=CH), 28 (CO)	186 (M$^+$), 158 (M-CO, 100%), 130 (158-CO), 129 (158-CHO), 102 (130-CO)

4 Lignans

4.1 Introduction

Lignans are typically dimeric C_6-C_3 derivatives, and mainly exist in woody tissues (木质组织) or resin of plants. Most of them are in free forms, but some exist as glycosides in plants. Lignans play important roles in a plant's defense system because their antimicrobial and antifungal actions.

Many lignans are effective constituents of Chinese herbs. For example, some lignans such as Schisantherin A, B, C and D (五味子酯甲、乙、丙和丁) can protect the liver, protect cranial nerves, anti-eclampsia, improve intelligence and physical strength. Arctiin (牛蒡子苷) and arctigenin (牛蒡子苷元) from Arctii Fructus (牛蒡子) have antibacterial, antiviral and anti-tumor activities. Phillygenol (连翘脂素) and phillyrin (连翘苷) are the main active compounds of Forsythiae Fructus (连翘) for antibacterial, antiviral, antipyretic and liver-protecting activities.

4.2 Structure and Classification

There are four C_6-C_3 monomers that make up lignans：cinnamic acid, cinnamaldehyde, cinnamyl alcohol (桂皮醇), propenyl benzene (丙烯苯) and allyl benzene (烯丙苯).

Because of the different condensation (缩合) positions of the C_6-C_3 monomer that makes up lignans and the dehydration condensation (脱水缩合) reaction of the oxygen-containing groups on the γ-carbon atom on the side chain, different types of lignans are formed. Some examples are shown in Table 5-4.

Table 5-4 Structures and categories of some lignans from Chinese herbs

Categories	Structures of some important lignans from Chinese herbs
Simple lignans （简单木脂素）	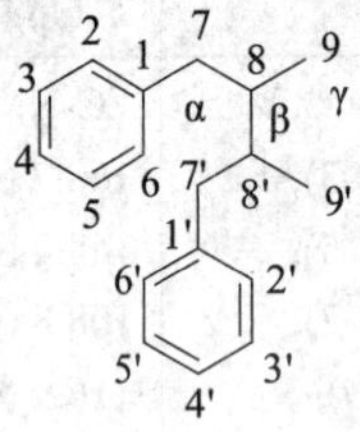 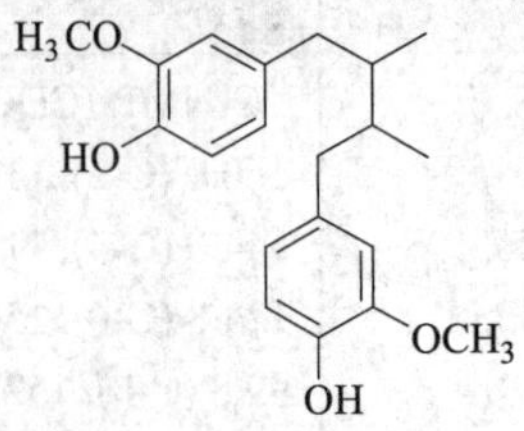 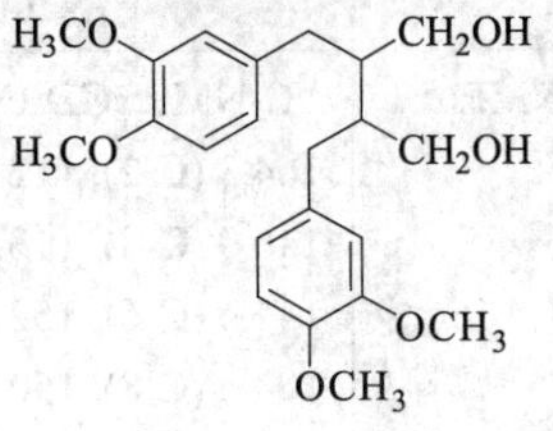 dihydroguaiaretic acid (DGA, 二氢愈创木脂酸) Ignum vitae resin (愈创木树脂)　　phyllanthin 　　　　　　　　　　　　　　　　　　*Phyllanthusnirui* (珠子草)
Monoepoxylignans （单环氧木脂素）	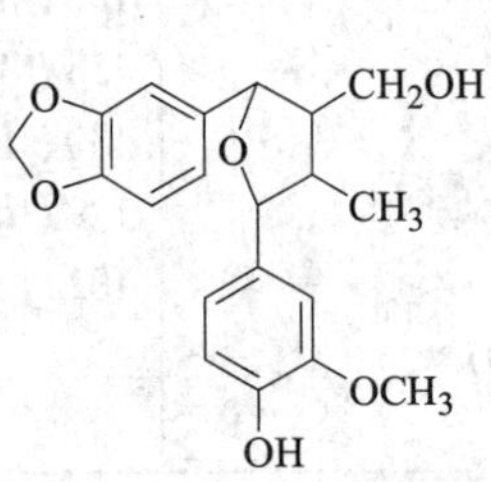 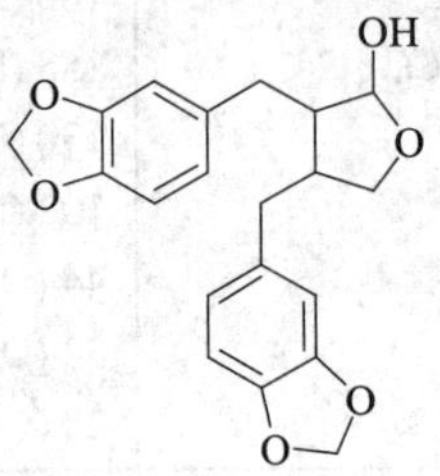 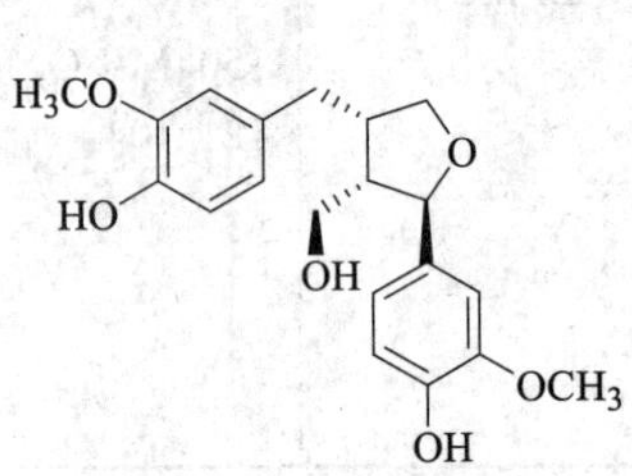 enshizhisu (恩施脂素)　　cubebin (毕澄茄脂素)　　lariciresinol (落叶松脂素) *Schisandra henryi* (翼梗五味子)　*Piper cubeba* (毕澄茄)　*Daphne tangatica* (陕甘瑞香)
Lignanolides （木脂内酯）	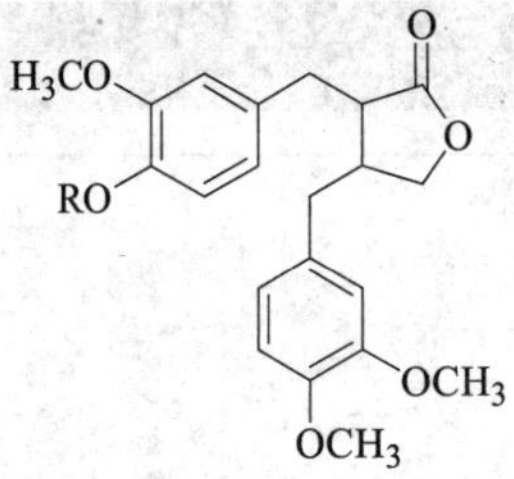 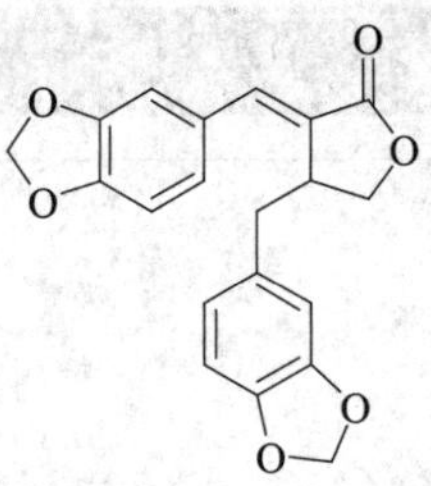 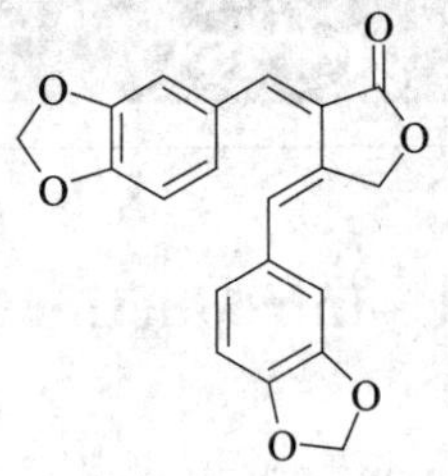 arctigenin: R=H　　taiwanin B (台湾脂素B)　　taiwanin A (台湾脂素A) arctiin: R=glc　　　　　　*Juniperus sabina* (自桧柏) Arctii Fructus
Cyclolignans （环木脂素）	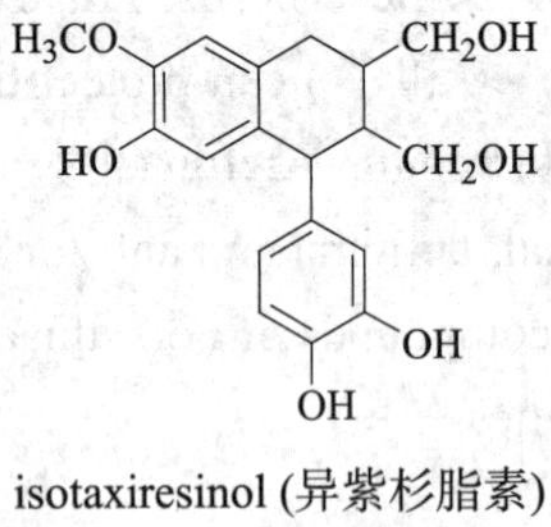 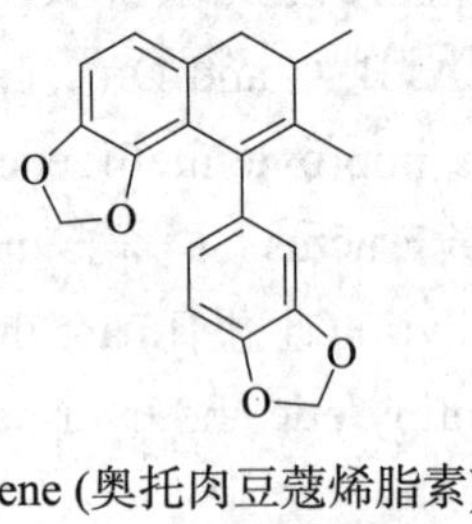 isotaxiresinol (异紫杉脂素)　　otoboene (奥托肉豆蔻烯脂素) *Taxus cuspidata* (中国紫杉)　　*Myristica otoba* (奥托肉豆蔻)
Cyclolignolides （环木脂内酯）	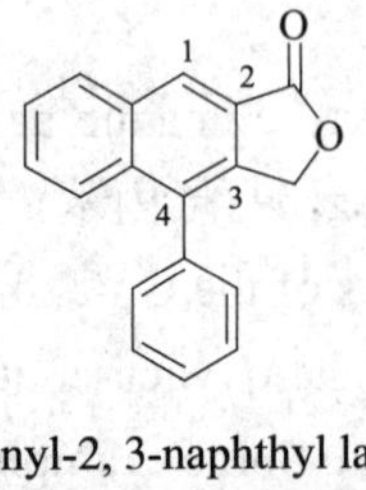 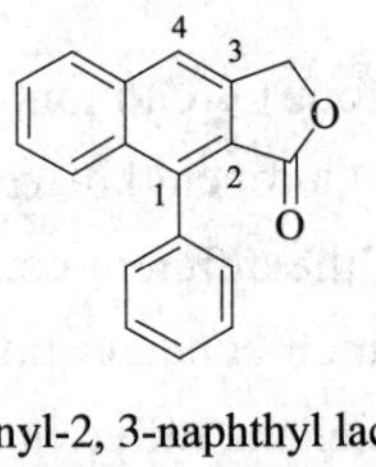 4-phenyl-2, 3-naphthyl lactone　　1-phenyl-2, 3-naphthyl lactone (4- 苯代 -2, 3- 萘内酯)　　　　(1- 苯代 -2, 3- 萘内酯)

(continued)

Categories	Structures of some important lignans from Chinese herbs
Cyclolignolides （环木脂内酯）	*1*-podophyllotoxin (*l*-鬼臼毒脂素): R=H *1*-podophyllotoxin-*β-O*-glc (*l*- 鬼臼毒脂素 -*β-O*-葡萄糖苷): R=glc *Podophyllum genus* (鬼臼) 　　helioxanthin 　　Polygalae Radix (远志)
Bisepoxylignans （双环氧木脂素）	enantiomer　　Ar-aryl　　enantiomer phillygenin (连翘脂素): R=H phillyrin: R=glc Forsythiae Fructus　　syringaresinol (丁香脂素) Senticosi Radix et Rhzoma Seu Caults
Dibenzocyclooctene lignans （联苯环辛烯型木脂素）	schisandrol (五味子醇): R=H schisandrin (五味子素): R=CH₃ Schisandrae chinensis Fructus (五味子)
Biphenylene lignans （联苯型木脂素）	magnolol (厚朴酚)　　honokiol (和厚朴酚) Magnoliae officinalis Cortex (厚朴)

(continued)

Categories	Structures of some important lignans from Chinese herbs
	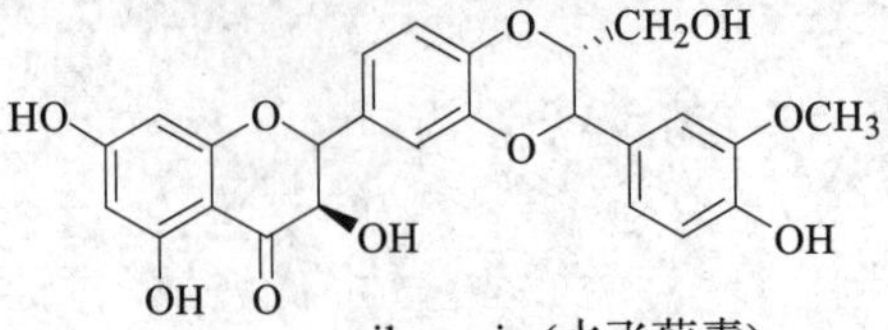 silymarin (水飞蓟素) Silybi Fructus (水飞蓟)
Other lignans	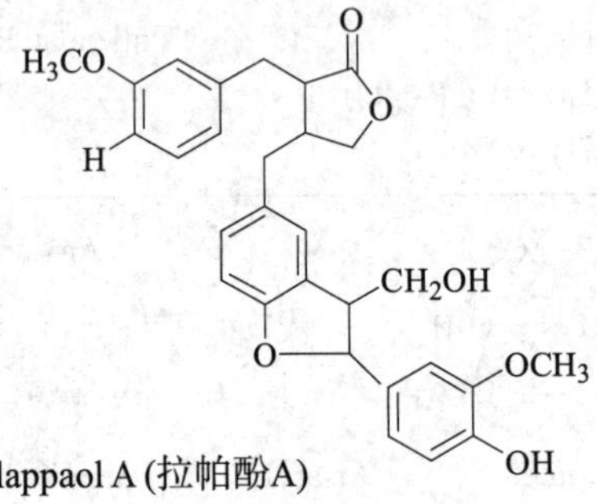 lappaol A (拉帕酚A) 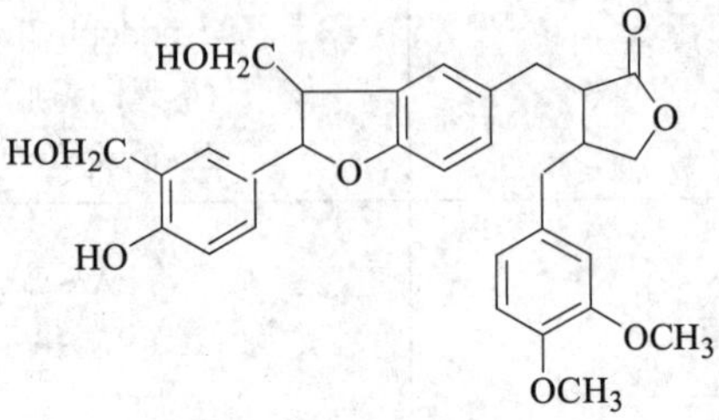　　　　lappaol B (拉帕酚B) *Arctium lappa* (牛蒡)

4.3　General Physiochemical Properties

4.3.1　Characteristics and Solubility

Most of lignans are colorless crystals. A few of them have sublimability such as dihydroguaiaretic acid. In general, most of lignans are free form and soluble in organic solvents such as ethyl ether, chloroform, methanol and ethanol, but unsoluble in water. Lignans with phenolic hydroxyl groups are soluble in alkaline aqueous solution.

4.3.2　Optical activity and isomerization

Most of lignans have optical activity and are easily changed in acidic solution. For example, when heated in HCl-EtOH solution, *d*-sesamin（*d*– 芝麻脂素）partially transfers into its stereoisomer (立体异构体) *d*-episesamin（*d*– 表芝麻脂素）which is also called *d*-asarinin（*d*– 细辛脂素）to reach balance. The reaction is shown in Figure 5-8.

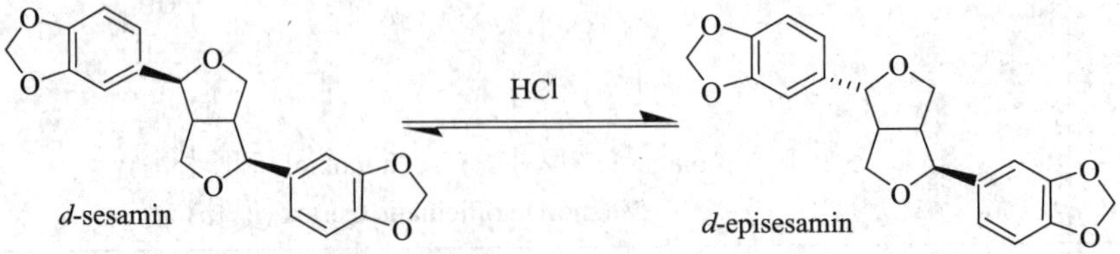

d-sesamin　　　　　　　　　　　　　　　　　*d*-episesamin

Figure 5-8　Isomerization of *d*-sesamin in acidic solution

The biological activities of some lignans are closely related to their optical activities. For example, podophyllotoxin has anticancer property, its tetrahydronaphthalene (四氢化萘) ring and lactone ring can be changed into *trans*-configuration (反式结构) (2*α*, 3*β*) named epipodophyllotoxin (表鬼臼毒素) treated by PCl₃. And epipodophyllotoxin exposed to alkaline solution, the lactone ring changes into its isomer with *cis*-configuration(顺式结构) (2*β*, 3*β*) named epipicropodophyllin (表鬼臼苦素). When podophyllotoxin is exposed to alkaline solution, the lactone ring changes into its isomer with *cis*-configuration (2*β*, 3*β*) named picropodophyllin (鬼臼苦素) (see Figure 5-9), and the anticancer activity is hence lost. Therefore, it is important to control the extraction and isolation conditions to avoid isomerization of lignans in acidic or alkali solutions.

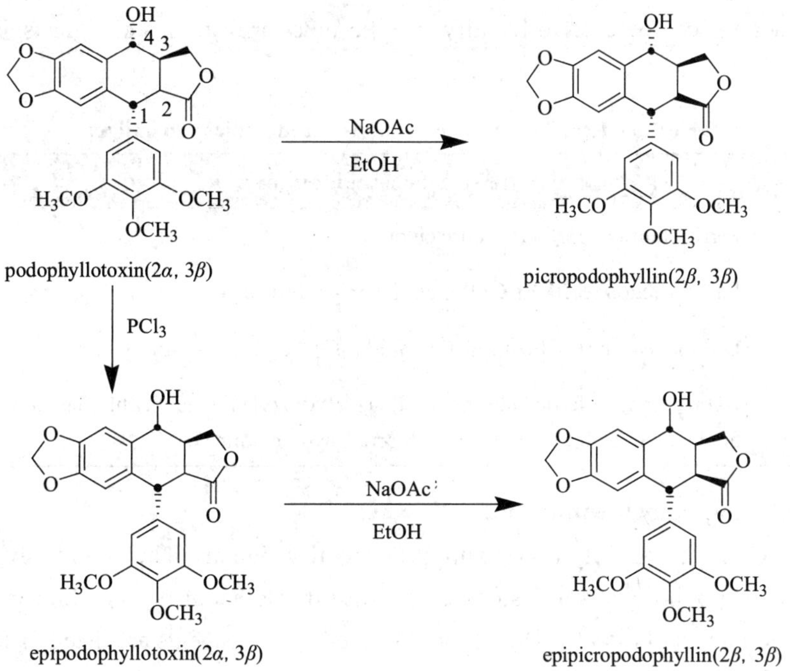

Figure 5-9　Isomerization of podophyllotoxin

4.4　Extraction and Isolation Methods

4.4.1　Extraction Methods

Solvent extraction is the most commonly method used for lignans. Usually the Chinese herbs can be extracted with ethanol and concentrated, then partitioned with petroleum ether, ethyl ether, ethyl acetate and so on, successively, and the different polarity parts can be obtained. Lignans often coexist with resinous substances in plants, and are easy to resinification in solvent treatment, which is a problem need to be solved in the process of extraction and separation.

The SFE method is more and more used for lignans extraction because it is environmental friendly and highly efficient.

Lignans with phenolic hydroxyl groups or lactone ring can be extracted with the alkali solution and followed by acid precipitation. But the concentration of alkali and the temperature of reaction should be carefully controlled to avoid isomerization and subsequent loss of biological activities.

4.4.2　Isolation Methods

The further separation of lignans must be used by chromatography methods. Silica gel and neutral alumina are generally used as adsorbents to separate lignans first. The common elution solvent systems are petroleum ether-ethyl ether and chloroform-methanol. Preparative HPLC and Sephadex LH-20 can also be used for further isolation.

4.5　Identification

4.5.1　Physicochemical Identification

Lignans have no a specific skeleton in structure, therefore there are no characteristic reactions for lignans. Some reactions can be used to identify specific functional groups of lignans. They are listed in Table 5-5.

Table 5-5　Reactions of functional groups identification of lignans

Functional groups	Reactions and Reagents	Color
Phenolic hydroxyl	Ferric chloride reaction：Ferric chloride	Dark green
Methylenedioxy（亚甲二氧基）	Labat reaction reaction：Gallic acid, con.-sulfuric acid	Blue-green
	Ecgrine reaction：Chromotropic acid (变色酸), con.-sulfuric acid	Blue-purple
Lactone ring	Hydroxylamine-ferric chloride reaction：Hydroxylammonium chloride, potassium hydroxide (氢氧化钾), ferric chloride, hydrochloric acid	Red

4.5.2　Chromatography Identification

Silica gel TLC is a commonly used method to identify lignans. The commonly used developing solvent systems are lipophilic solvents such as chloroform-methanol (9：1), chloroform-ethyl acetate (9：1), ethyl acetate-methanol (95：5). The commonly used spray reagents are listed in Table 5-6.

Table 5-6　Commonly used spray reagents for lignans on Silica gel TLC

Reagent	Procedure
1% anisaldehyde (茴香醛) -concentrated sulfuric acid solution	Heat for 5 minutes at 110℃
5%~10% phosphomolybdic acid (磷钼酸)-ethanol solution	Heat until spots are visible at 120℃
10% sulfuric acid-ethanol solution (硫酸乙醇溶液)	Heat for 5 minutes at 110℃
antimony butter reagent (三氯化锑试剂)	Heat for 10 minutes at 100℃, observe under UV light
iodine (碘) vapor	After fumigation, the spot should be yellow and brown (黄棕色) or observe fluorescence under UV light

4.6　Structure Determination

4.6.1　UV Spectrum

For most lignans, the two aromatic rings moieties are two isolated chromophores (发色团) with similar UV absorption peaks and additivity (加和性) of absorption intensity (吸收强度). In general, the UV spectra of lignans contain two peaks at 220–240nm (lg ε > 4.0) and 280–290nm (lg ε 3.5–4.0). The 4-phenylnaphthalene（4-苯基萘类化合物）compounds have unique features that differ from others.

They have a strong peak at 260nm (lgε > 4.5), and peaks at 225nm, 290nm, 310nm, 355nm.

4.6.2 IR Spectrum

The IR spectra of lignans usually contain absorptions for hydroxyl, methoxyl, methylenedioxy, aromatic ring and lactone ring. For example, hinokinin (扁柏脂素) has characteristic peaks of aromatic ring at 1600cm^{-1}, 1585cm^{-1}, and 1500cm^{-1}, methylenedioxy group at 936cm^{-1}, and five-membered lactone ring at 1760–1780cm^{-1}. Most benzodiazepine lignans have unsaturated lactone ring structure and show characteristic absorption at 1760cm^{-1}.

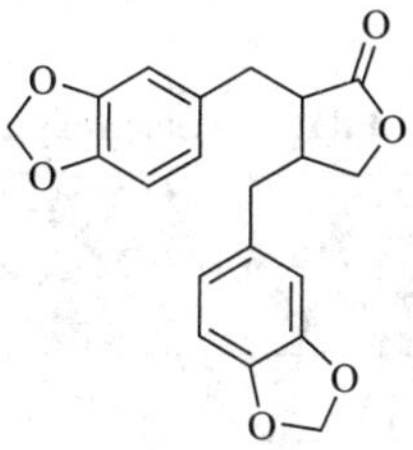

hinokinin

4.6.3 ^{1}H-NMR

Some ^{1}H-NMR signals can be used to differentiate certain functional group orientations in certain type of lignans. For example, the up and down direction of lactone ring in cyclolignolides can be distinguished by ^{1}H-NMR. The related data of ^{1}H-NMR are listed in Table 5-7.

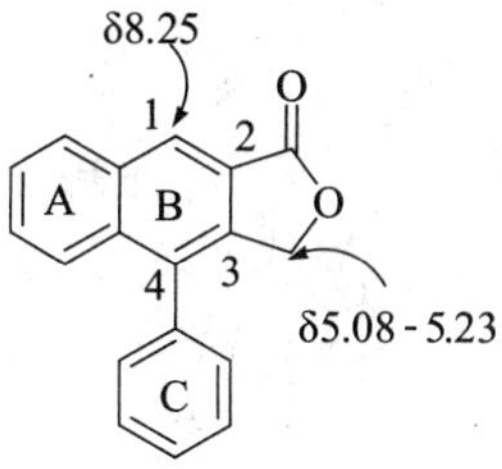

4-phenyl-2,3-naphthyl lactone
(4–苯代萘内酯)

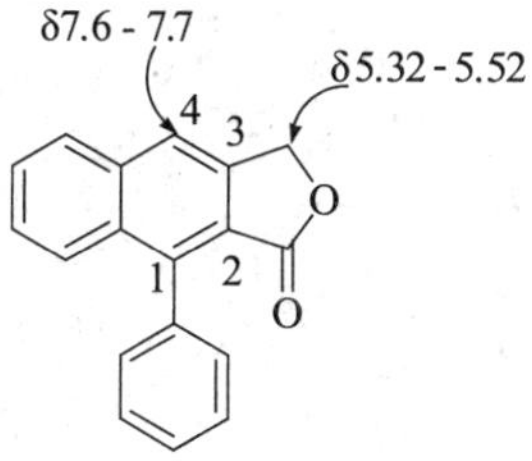

1-phenyl-2,3-naphthyl lactone
(1–苯代萘内酯)

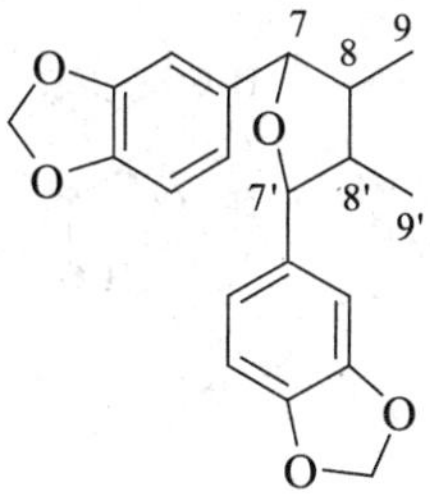

galbacin

Table 5-7 Characteristic signals of cyclolignolides in ^{1}H-NMR

The direction of lactone ring	The δ of H-1 or H-4	The δ of CH$_2$ in the lactone ring
Up	8.25	5.08-5.23
Down	7.60-7.70	5.32-5.52

Galbacin (加尔巴新) belongs to monoepoxylignans with symmetrical (对称的) structure. Its structure and partial data of ^{1}H-NMR (100MHz, CDCl$_3$) spectrum are listed in Table 5-8.

Table 5-8 Partial data of ^{1}H-NMR spectrum of galbacin

Data	Proton
1.05 (6H, d)	H-9 and H-9$'$
1.78 (2H, m)	H-8 and H-8$'$
4.61 (2H, d)	H-7 and H-7$'$
5.96 (4H, s)	H of methylenedioxy
6.82–6.93	H of aromatic ring

The coupling constants (偶合常数) (J) of H-7 and H-8 or H-7′ and H-8′ in ^{1}H-NMR can be used to identify the direction of the two aromatic rings in bisepoxylignans. The related data of ^{1}H-NMR are listed in Table 5-9.

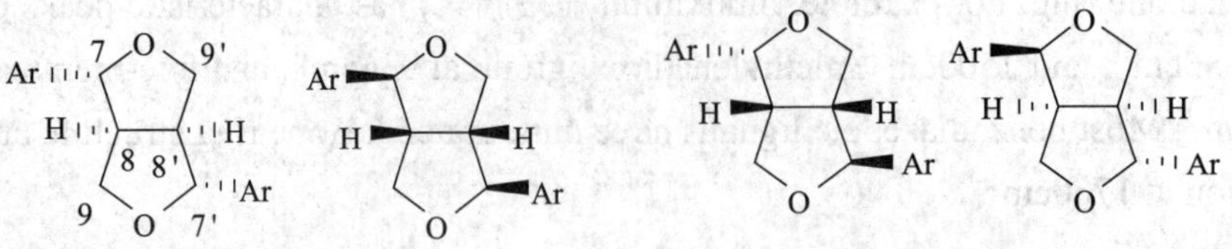

ipsilateral   opposite

Table 5-9   Related data of bisepoxylignans in ^{1}H-NMR

Direction of romatic ring	Configuration between H-7 and H-8	$J_{H7\text{-}H8}$	Configuration between H-7' and H-8'	$J_{H7'\text{-}H8'}$
Ipsilateral	trans	4-5Hz	trans	4-5Hz
Opposite	cis	4-5Hz	trans	7Hz

4.6.4   MS

Most of lignans show molecular ion peak in EI-MS spectrum. The benzyl (苄基) splitting often occurs in EI-MS spectra of lignans (Figure 5-10).

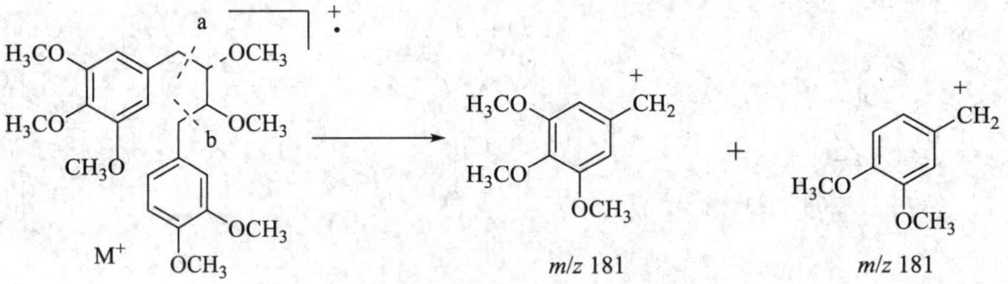

Figure 5-10   Benzyl splitting of lignans in EI-MS spectrum

Lignan glycosides usually show an ion peak of glycosyl fragment, such as [M-162]$^+$, in FAB-MS spectrum. An example of phyllanthostatin A is shown in Figure 5-11.

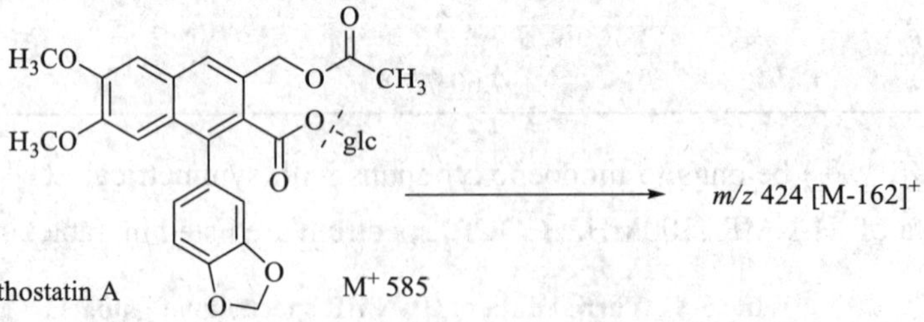

Figure 5-11   Ion of glycosyl fragment of phyllanthostatin A in FAB-MS spectrum

5 Examples of Chinese Herbs Containing Coumarins and Lignans

5.1 Fraxini Cortex（秦皮）

5.1.1 Introduction

(1) Biological Source

Fraxini Cortex is the dried branch skin or trunk skin of *Fraxinus rhynchophylla* Hance (苦枥白蜡树), *Fraxinus chinensis* Roxb (白蜡树), *Fraxinus szaboana* Lingelsh (尖叶白蜡树) or *Fraxinus stylosa* Lingelsh (宿柱白蜡树).(Fam. Oleaceae)（木犀科）

(2) Property, Flavor and Channels Entered

Property and Flavor: Cold; Bitter (苦), Astringent (涩).

Channels Entered: Liver, Gallbladder (胆), Large Intestine.

(3) Actions & Indications

To clear heat and dry dampness, astringe to check dysentery, check vaginal discharge and improve vision. For dampness-heat diarrhea and dysentery, red or white vaginal discharge, red painful swelling eyes and nebula.

(4) Pharmacological Activities

The pharmacological activities associated with Fraxini Cortex include mind-calming, anti-convulsion, anti-oxidation, anti-inflammation, antitussive, anti-tumor, anti-asthma, anti-influenza virus, anti-herpes virus, analgesic, expectorant, diuresis effects, promoting excretion of uric acid and so on.

5.1.2 Main Chemical Constituents

Main effective chemical constituents in Fraxini Cortex are coumarins and their glycosides. In addition, other phenolic compounds, tannins (鞣质) and bitter principle also present in this herb.

(1) Coumarins and Their Glycosides

Esculetin, esculin, fraxetin (秦皮素) and fraxin (秦皮苷) are the main effective compounds. *Fraxinus rhynchophylla* Hance contains esculetin and esculin. *Fraxinus chinensis* Roxb contains esculetin and fraxetin. *Fraxinus stylosa* Lingelsh contains esculetin, esculin, fraxetin. Other coumarins such as fraxidin (秦皮啶), isofraxidin (异秦皮啶), cichorin (菊苣苷), syringin (丁香苷), stylosin (宿柱白蜡苷) are also found in Fraxini Cortex.

Esculin: R=glc
Esculetin: R=H

Fraxin: R=glc
Fraxetin: R=H

The extraction and isolation schem of Esculin and Esculetin is shown in Figure 5-12.

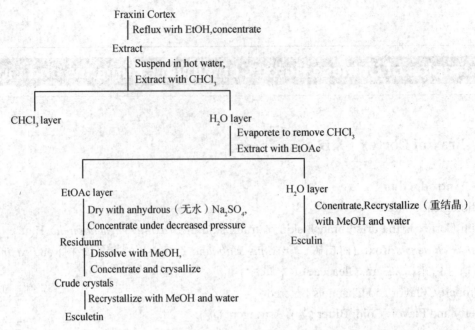

Fraxini Cortex
  │ Reflux wirh EtOH,concentrate
Extract
  │ Suspend in hot water,
  │ Extract with CHCl₃

CHCl₃ layer   H₂O layer
                       │ Evaporete to remove CHCl₃
                       │ Extract with EtOAc

EtOAc layer   H₂O layer
  │ Dry with anhydrous（无水）Na₂SO₄,   │ Conentrate,Recrystallize（重结晶）
  │ Concentrate under decreased pressure │ with MeOH and water
Residuum   Esculin
  │ Dissolve with MeOH,
  │ Concentrate and crysallize
Crude crystals
  │ Recrystallize with MeOH and water
Esculetin

Figure 5-12   Extraction and isolation scheme of Esculin and Esculetin

(2) Others

Mannitol (甘露醇), Scopoletin (东莨菪亭) and 2, 6-dimethoxy-*p*-benzoquinone（2, 6–二甲氧基对苯醌) are also found in *Fraxinus chinensis* Roxb. Caffeic acid, syringaldehyde (丁香醛), sinapaldehyde (芥子醛), triacontanoic acid (三十烷酸), *β*-sitosterol（*β*– 谷甾醇）, daucosterol (胡萝卜苷), ursolic acid (熊果酸), betulinic acid (白桦脂酸) were also isolated from Fraxini Cortex.

5.1.3   Quality Control Standards

(1) Fluorescence Identification

An easy method to identify Fraxini Cortex is to soak it in hot water. The solution emits blue fluorescence in daylight.

(2) TLC Identification

Stationary Phase: Silica gel plate (G or GF₂₅₄).

Standard: Esculetin, esculin, fraxetin.

Development System: Chloroform-methanol-formic acid (6 ∶ 1 ∶ 0.5).

Visualization: 365nm UV light for silica gel plate G, 254nm UV light for silica gel plate GF₂₅₄, spray Ferric chloride-Potassium ferricyanide reagent.

(3) Tests

Water: Not more than 7.0%.

Total ash: Not more than 8.0%.

Extract (ethanol): Not less than 8.0%.

(4) Assay

Esculetin and Esculin: The gross not less than 1.0% (HPLC).

5.2 Schisandrae Chinensis Fructus(五味子)

5.2.1 Introduction

(1) Biological Source

Schisandrae Chinensis Fructus is the dried ripe fruit of *Schisandra chinensis* (Turca) Baill (五味子) (Fam. Magnoliaceae) (木兰科).

(2) Property, Flavor and Channels Entered

Property and Flavor: Warm; Sour (酸), sweet.

Channels Entered: Lung, Heart, Kidney(肾).

(3) Actions & Indications

To astringe and secure, tonify qi and engender body fluid, tonify the kidney and calm the heart. For chronic cough, dyspnea of deficiency type, dream emission and spermatorrhea, chronic diarrhea, enuresis and frequent urination, spontaneous sweating and night sweating, thirst caused by fluid consumption, internal heat wasting-thirst, palpitation and insomnia.

(4) Pharmacological Activities

The pharmacological activities associated with Schisandrae Chinensis Fructus include protecting the liver and cranial nerves, calming the mind, improving intelligence and physical strength, exciting breath, reducing phlegm, enhancing immunity, promoting osteoblast, etc.

5.2.2 Main Chemical Constituents

Main effective constituents of Schisandrae Chinensis Fructus are lignans. The content of total lignans can be up to 18.1%–19.2% in it. Most of them are dibenzocyclooctene lignans, such as schisandrin (schisandrol A), deoxyschisandrin (去氧五味子素). Schisandrae Chinensis Fructus also contains volatile oils, triterpenes (三萜类), sterols (甾醇类), fatty acids, etc.

A series of lignans have been isolated from Schisandrae Chinensis Fructus. They mainly include schisandrin, deoxyschisandrin, γ-schisandrin (γ-五味子素), pseudo-γ-schisandrin(伪γ–五味子素), schisanhenol (五味子酚), gomisin A (五味子脂素A, 又称戈米辛A), schisantherin B (gomisin B) (五味子脂素 B, 又称五味子酯乙、华中五味子酯 B. 戈米辛 B), schisantherin A (gomisin C) (五味子酯甲 , 又称五味子脂素 C. 华中五味子酯 A. 戈米辛 C), tigloylgomisin H (巴豆酰五味子脂素H), benzoylgomisin H (苯甲酰五味子脂素H), isoschisandrin (异五味子素), angeloylgomisin H,Q,P (当归酰五味子脂素H、Q、P), gomisin D, E, F, G, H, J, K, N, O, P, Q, R, etc.

schisanhenol schisanhenol deoxyschisandrin schisandrin

schisanhenol γ-schisandrin

5.2.3 Quality Control Standards

(1) TLC Identification

Stationary Phase: Silica gel plate GF_{254}.

Standard: Authentic crude drug, deoxyschisandrin.

Development System: Petroleum ether (30–60℃)-ethyl formate-formic acid (15 : 5 : 1).

Visualization: 254nm UV light.

(2) Tests

Impurity: Not more than 1.0%.

Water: Not more than 16.0%.

Total Ash: Not more than 7.0%.

(3) Assay

Schisandrin: Not less than 0.40% (HPLC).

5.3 Forsythiae Fructus(连翘)

5.3.1 Introduction

(1) Biological Source

Forsythiae Fructus is the dried fruit of *Forsythia suspense* (Thunb.) Vahl (连翘). The nearly ripe and still greenish one is called *Qingqiao*. The fully ripe one is called *Laoqiao*. (Fam. Oleaceae)

(2) Property, Flavor and Channels Entered

Property and Flavor: Mild cold(微寒); Bitter.

Channels Entered: Lung, Heart, Small Intestine(小肠).

(3) Actions & Indications

To clear heat and remove toxin, disperse wind-heat, disperse swelling and dissipate binds. For abscesses and cellulitis, scrofula and acute mastitis, erysipelas, common cold caused by wind-heat, initial period of warm diseases, high fever with vexation and thirst, warm-heat entering ying, loss of consciousness, macula, heat strangury with slow pain.

(4) Pharmacological Activities

The pharmacological activities associated with Forsythiae Fructus include antibiosis, antiviral, antipyretic effects and protecting liver, etc. Forsythiaside (连翘脂苷) is the most important antibiosis active compound in Forsythiae Fructus.

5.3.2 Main Chemical Constituents

Forsythiae Fructus contains many different types of compounds including lignans such as forsythin (连翘苷), phenethyl alcohol glycosides like forsythiaside, volatile oils, flavonoids, alkaloids, organic acids and sterols, etc.

(1) Lignans and phenylethanoid glycosides

The main lignans of Forsythiae Fructus include phillygenin（forsythiaside）, phillyrin（forsythin）, pinoresinol (右旋松脂酚), arctigenin, arctiin, matairesinol (罗汉松脂素), matairesinoside (罗汉松脂苷), rengyol (连翘环己醇), forsythol (连翘酚）, and phenylethanoid glycosides such as forsythoside A, C, D, E (连翘脂苷A, C, D, E）and rengyoside A, B, C (连翘环己醇苷A, B, C）are also found in it.

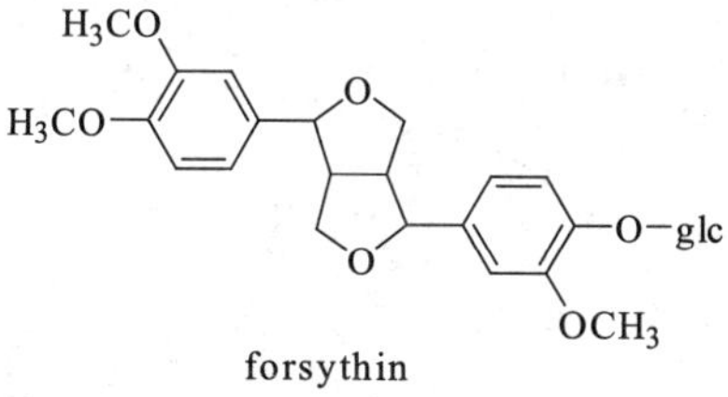

forsythin

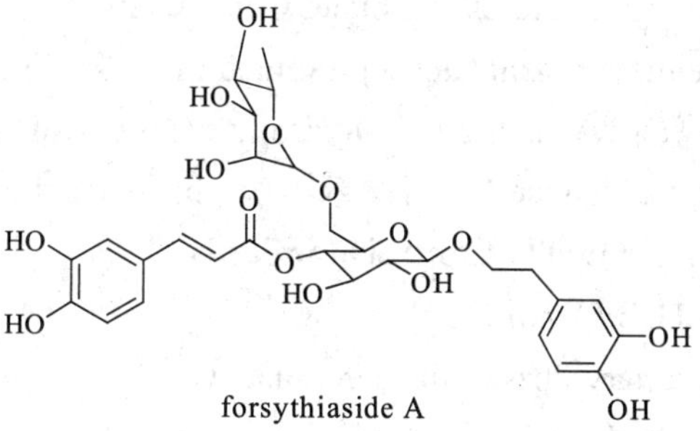

forsythiaside A

The extraction and isolation scheme for forsythin from Forsythiae Fructus and its leaves are shown in Figure 5-13 and Figure 5-14.

Forsythiae Fructus
　|　Extract with EtOH, concentrate
Extract
　|　Polyamide CC, gradient elute with EtOH-H₂O
Fractions contain forsythin
　|　Concentrate
Combined fractions
　|　Separate by preparation HPLC
Forsythin (Slight yellow powder)

Figure 5-13　Extraction and isolation of forsythin from Forsythiae Fructus

Leaves of Forsythiae Fructus
　|　Mix with few CaCO₃, boil with water, filter when hot, concentrate
Extract
　|　Extract with hot EtOH
Solution
　|　Add some calcined MgO, still 24h, filter
Precipitate
　|　Extract with EtOH, filter, concentrate, recrystallize with EtOH
Forsythin

Figure 5-14　Extraction and isolation of forsythin from the leaves of Forsythiae Fructus

(2) Volatile Oils

The main compounds in the volatile oils of Forsythiae Fructus include *α*-pinene（α-蒎烯）, *β*-pinene（β-蒎烯）, linalool (芳樟醇), phellandrene (水芹烯), camphene (莰烯), myrcene (月桂烯), *α*-terpinene（α-松油烯）, pinocarveol (松香芹醇), borneol (龙脑), myrcenol (月桂烯醇), piperitol (薄荷醇), etc.

(3) Flavones and Alkaloids

Flavones presented in Forsythiae Fructus include quercetin (槲皮素), isoquercetin (异槲皮素), astragalin (黄芪苷、紫云英苷), wogonin-7-*O*-glucoside (黄芩素–7–O– 葡萄糖苷), rutin etc. Alkaloids also have been found in Forsythiae Fructus, such as suspensine A, *l*-7'-*O*-methylegenine, *l*-egenine, *l*-bicuculline (荷包牡丹碱), etc.

(4) Organic Acids and Other Constituents

The main organic acids presented in Forsythiae Fructus include betulinic acid, ursolic acid, oleanolic acid (齐墩果酸), and 2α, 23-hydroxy ursolic acid, etc. β-sitosterol, n-dotriacontane (n-三十二烷), 4-hydroxy benzaldehyde (4-羟基苯甲醛) have also been found in Forsythiae Fructus.

5.3.3　Quality Control Standards

(1) TLC Identification

Stationary Phase: Silica gel plate G.

Standard: Authentic crude drug, forsythin.

Development System: Chloroform-methanol (8∶1).

Visualization: Spray the solution of 10% H_2SO_4 in ethanol, heat at 105℃ until spots are clear.

(2) Tests

Impurity: For *Qingqiao* it is not more than 3.0%, and for *Laoqiao* it is not more than 9.0%.

Water: Not more than 10.0%.

Total Ash: Not more than 4.0%.

(3) Assay

Forsythin: Not less than 0.15% (HPLC).

Forsythiaside A: Not less than 0.25% (HPLC).

词　汇　表

An Alphabetical List of Words and Phrases

A		
α-benzopyranone	[ˌbenzəuˈpɪrəˌnəun]	苯骈 α- 吡喃酮
absorption intensity	[əbˈzɔːpʃn] [ɪnˈtensəti]	吸收强度
Acanthopanacis Senticosi Radix et Rhzoma Seu Caults		刺五加
acetoxyl group	[əsˈtɔksɪl][gruːp]	乙酰氧基
acyl	[ˈæsɪl]	酰基
Adenophorae Radix		南沙参
additivity	[ˌædɪˈtɪvəti]	加和性
adsorbent	[ədˈzɔːbənt]	吸附剂
aesculetin dimethyl ether	[iːskjuˈletɪn] [daɪˈmiːθaɪl] [ˈiːθə]	七叶内酯二甲醚
alkoxyl	[ˈɔːlkɔksɪl]	烷氧基
allyl benzene	[ˈæləl] [ˈbenziːn]	烯丙苯
allyl ether	[ˈæləl] [ˈiːθə]	烯丙醚
4-aminoantipyrine	[ˌæmɪˈnəuæntɪpaɪərɪn]	4- 氨基安替比林
anethole	[ˈænəθəul]	茴香醚
Angelicae dahuricae Radix		白芷
Angelicae pubescentis Radix		独活
Angelicae sinensis Radix		当归

(continued)

angelicon	[ænˈdʒelɪkɔːn]	当归内酯
angelin	[ænˈdʒeliːn]	当归素
angelol	[ˌeɪndʒələˈlɔː]	独活醇
angeloylgomisin H、Q、P	[ˈændʒlɔɪlgəmɪsaɪn]	当归酰五味子脂素 H、Q、P
angular type	[ˈæŋgjələ] [taɪp]	角型
anhydrous	[ænˈhaɪdrəs]	无水
anisaldehyde	[ænaɪˈzældɪhaɪd]	茴香醛
Anisi stellati Fructus		八角茴香
antimony butter reagent	[ˈæntɪməni][ˈbʌtə][rɪˈeɪʒənt]	三氯化锑试剂
Araliaceae		五加科
arctigenin	[ˈɑːktɪdʒnɪn]	牛蒡子苷元
Arctii Fructus		牛蒡子
arctiin	[ɑːkˈtiːn]	牛蒡子苷
Arctium lappa		牛蒡
aroma	[əˈrəumə]	芳香味
Artemisiae scopariae Herba		茵陈
Asari Radix et Rhizome		细辛
asarinin	[ˈæsərinin]	细辛脂素
asarone	[ˈærərəun]	细辛醚
Asteraceae		菊科
astragalin	[æstrəˈgeɪlɪn]	黄芪苷、紫云英苷
astringent	[əˈstrɪndʒənt]	涩的
azodye	[əzəˈdaɪ]	偶氮染料
B		
benzyl	[ˈbenzaɪl]	苄基
benzoylgomisin H	[benˈzɔɪlgəmɪsiːn]	苯甲酰五味子脂素 H
bergapten	[bəˈgæpten]	佛手柑内脂
betulinic acid	[beˈtjulɪnɪk][ˈæsɪd]	白桦脂酸
bicuculline	[bɪkjuːˈkʌlaɪn]	荷包牡丹碱
biphenylene lignans	[baɪˈfiːnaɪləniː] [ˈlɪgnænz]	联苯型木脂素
bisaesculetin	[bɪˈsiːskjuˈletɪn]	双七叶内酯
bisepoxylignans	[biːzˈpɑːksi] [ˈlɪgnænz]	双环氧木脂素
bitter	[ˈbɪtə]	苦的
borneol	[bɔnɪˈɔl]	龙脑
C		
caffeic acid	[keˈfiːɪk][ˈæsɪd]	咖啡酸
camphene	[ˈkæmfiːn]	莰烯

(continued)

capillarin	[kəˈpɪləriːn]	茵陈内酯
5 carbon unsaturated acyloxy	[ˈkaːbən][ʌnˈsætʃəreɪtɪd][æsɪˈlɔksɪ]	五碳不饱和酰氧基
Caryophylli Flos		丁香
chlorogenic acid	[ˌklɔːrəuˈdʒenɪk][ˈæsɪd]	绿原酸
chromone	[ˈkrəuməun]	色原酮
chromophores	[ˈkrəuməfɔːs]	发色团
chromotropic acid	[krəuməuˈtrɔpɪk][ˈæsɪd]	变色酸
cichorin	[ˈsɪkəurɪn]	菊苣苷
cinnamaldehyde	[sɪnəˈmɔːldɪhaɪd]	桂皮醛
cinnamic acid	[səˈnæmɪk][ˈæsɪd]	桂皮酸
Cinnamomt Cortex		肉桂
cinnamylalcohol	[sɪˈnæmɪl][ˈælkəhɔl]	桂皮醇
Cimicifug Rhizoma		升麻
cis-adjacent hydroxycinnamic acid	[ˈsɪs][əˈdʒeɪsnt][haɪˈdrɔksiˌsəˈnæmɪk][ˈæsɪd]	顺邻羟基桂皮酸
cis-configuration	[sɪs][kənˌfɪgəˈreɪʃn]	顺式构型
cis-ortho-hydroxycinnamic acid		顺式邻羟基桂皮酸
Cnidii Fructus		蛇床子
columbianadin	[kəˈlʌmbɪənædɪn]	哥伦比亚内酯
condensation	[ˌkɔndenˈseɪʃn]	缩合
coumarins	[ˈkuːmərvns]	香豆素
coupling constant	[ˈkʌplɪŋ][ˈkɔnstənt]	偶合常数
coupling relationship	[ˈkʌplɪŋ][rɪˈleɪʃnʃɪp]	偶合关系
Crataegi Fruitus	[kræˈtɪːgɪl][ˈfruːtəs]	山楂
cubebin	[ˈkjuːbebɪn]	毕澄茄脂素
cyclolignans	[ˈsaɪkləuˈlɪgnænz]	环木脂素
cyclolignolide	[ˈsaɪkləuˈlɪgnɔːlɪd]	环木脂内酯
D		
n-dotriacontane	[dəutrɪəˈkɔnteɪn]	*n*-三十二烷
o-diol	[ˈdaɪəul]	邻二醇
daphin	[dæfˈnɪn]	瑞香苷
Daphne tangatica		陕甘瑞香
daucoidin A	[dɔːkəuˈɪdin]	旱前胡甲素
daucosterol	[dɔːkɔˈsterɔl]	胡萝卜苷
decursidinol		紫花前胡醇
decursidin	[diːˈkəːsaɪdɪn]	紫花前胡素
dehydration condensation	[ˌdiːhaɪˈdreɪʃn][ˌkɔndenˈseɪʃn]	脱水缩合

(continued)

deoxyschisandrin	[di:ɔksɪski:'zændərɪn]	去氧五味子素
diazotization reagent	[daɪˌæzətaɪ'zeɪʃən] [ri'eɪdʒənt]	重氮化试剂
dibenzocyclooctene lignans	[dɪ'benzəuˌsaɪkləu'ɔkti:n] ['lɪgnænz]	联苯环辛烯型木脂素
2, 6-dichlorobenzoquinone chlorine imine	['daɪklərəuˌbenzəkwɪ'nəun]['klɔ:rɪn] ['ɪmi:n]	2, 6- 二氯苯醌氯亚胺
2, 6-dimethoxy-*p*-benzoquinone	[ˌdaɪm'tɔ:kəsɪ] [ˌbenzəukwɪ'nəun]	2, 6- 二甲氧基对苯醌
dihydroguaiaretic acid	['daɪˌhɪdrɔ'gwaɪæ'rɪtɪk] ['æsɪd]	二氢愈创木脂酸
double peak (d)	['dʌbl] [pi:k]	二重峰
E		
enshizhisu	[ə:ntʃ'aɪði:θu]	恩施脂素
epipicropodophyllin	[ɪ'pəpɪkrɔpədɔ:fɪli:n]	表鬼白苦素
epipodophyllotoxin	[ɪ'pɪpədɔ:fɪlɔ:tɔ:ksɪn]	表鬼白毒素
episesamin	[ɪ'paɪsesəmɪn]	表芝麻脂素
esculin	['eskjulɪn]	七叶苷
esculetin	[ˌeskju'li:tɪn]	七叶内酯
ester groups	['estə][gru:ps]	酯基
etherify	[ɪ'θerɪfaɪ]	醚化
eugenol	['ju:dʒɪnɔl]	丁香酚
F		
Fabaceae（Leguminosae）		豆科
ferric chloride	['ferɪk] ['klɔ:raɪd]	三氯化铁
ferulic acid	[fə'ru:lɪk]['æsɪd]	阿魏酸
fluorescence	[flu:ə'resəns]	荧光
Foeniculi Fruitus		茴香
Forsythia suspense (Thunb.) Vahl		连翘
Forsythiae Fructus		连翘
forsythiaside	[fɔ:saɪ'θɪəsaɪd]	连翘脂素
forsythin	[fɔ:'saɪθɪn]	连翘苷
forsythol	[fɔ:'saɪθɔ:l]	连翘酚
forsythoside A, C, D, E	[fɔ:'saɪðəuzɪdə]	连翘脂苷 A、C、D、E
Fraxinus chinensis Roxb		白蜡树
Fraxinus rhynchophylla Hance		苦枥白蜡树
Fraxinus stylosa Lingelsh		宿柱白蜡树
Fraxinus szaboana Lingelsh		尖叶白蜡树
fraxetin	['fræksɪtɪn]	秦皮素
fraxidin	['fræksɪdɪn]	秦皮啶
fraxin	['fræksɪn]	秦皮苷

(continued)

furocoumarin	[furəuˈkəmərɪn]	呋喃香豆素
G		
galbacin	[gælˈbeɪsɪn]	加尔巴新
gallbladder	[ˈgɔːlˌblædə]	胆
gomisin	[ˈgɒmɪsiːn]	戈米辛
gomisin A	[ˈgɒmɪsiːn][eɪ]	五味子脂素 A、戈米辛 A
H		
helioxanthin	[ˈhiːlɪɒksænðiːn]	赛菊芋脂素
Heracleum hemsleyanum		牛尾独活
hinokinin	[hɪˈnəukiːnɪn]	扁柏脂素
honokiol	[ənəuˈkaɪəl]	和厚朴酚
4-hydroxy benzaldehyde	[haɪˈdrɒksɪ] [benˈzældɪhaɪd]	4-羟基苯甲醛
hydroxyl	[haɪˈdrɒksaɪl]	羟基
hydroxylamine hydrochloride	[haɪˌdrɒksɪləˈmiːn] [ˌhaɪdrəˈkləuraɪd]	盐酸羟胺
hydroxylamine-ferric chloride	[haɪˌdrɒksɪləˈmiːn][ˈferɪk] [ˈklɔːraɪd]	异羟肟酸铁
Hydroxylamine-Ferric Chloride Reaction	[haɪˌdrɒksɪləˈmiːn][ˈferɪk] [ˈklɔːraɪd] [riˈækʃn]	异羟肟酸铁反应
I		
ignum vitae resin		愈创木树脂
imperatorin	[ˌɪmpəˈrɑːtɔːrɪn]	欧芹属乙素
iodine	[ˈaɪədiːn]	碘
isobergapten	[ˈaɪsəuˈbərgæptən]	异佛手柑内酯
isofraxidin	[aɪsɒːfrækˈsaɪdɪn]	异秦皮啶
isomerization	[aɪsɒməraɪˈzeɪʃn]	异构化
isoprene	[ˈaɪsəpriːn]	异戊烯基
isopsoralen	[ˈaɪsəuˈpsɔrəlɪn]	异补骨脂素
isoquercetin	[ˈaɪsəuˈkwəˈsɪtɪn]	异槲皮素
isotaxiresinol	[ˈaɪsəuˈtæksɪˈrezɪnɔːl]	异紫杉脂素
isoschisandrin	[ˈaɪsəuˈskiːsəndrɪn]	异五味子素
J		
Juniperus sabina		自桧柏
K		
kidney	[ˈkɪdni]	肾
L		
lactones	[ˈlæktəunz]	内酯
lappaol		拉帕酚
lariciresinol	[ˈlɑːriˈsəˈrɪzɪnɔːl]	落叶松脂素

(continued)

lignanolides	['lɪgnænɔ:lɪdz]	木脂内酯
lignans	['lɪgnænz]	木脂素
lignins	['lɪgnɪnz]	木质素
Ligusticum daucoides		旱前胡
linalool	[lɪ'næləəul]	芳樟醇
linear type	['lɪnɪə] [taɪp]	线型
Lonicerae japonicae Flos		金银花
M		
Magnoliaceae		木兰科
Magnoliae officinalis Cortex		厚朴
magnolol	[mæg'nɔlɔl]	厚朴酚
mannitol	['mænɪtɔl]	甘露醇
matairesinol	[mæ'təaɪərezɪnɔl]	罗汉松树脂酚、罗汉松脂素
matairesinoside	[mætəaɪre'zi:nəusaɪd]	马太树脂酚苷、罗汉松脂苷
meta-position	['metə] [pə'zɪʃn]	间位
methylenedioxy	[meθɪleni'daɪɔksi]	亚甲二氧基
mild cold	[maɪld] [kəuld]	微寒的
monoepoxylignans	['mɔnəu:ɪ'pɔksi] ['lɪgnænz]	单环氧木脂素
myrcene	['mju:si:n]	月桂烯
myrcenol	['maɪrsenɔl]	香叶烯醇，月桂烯醇
Myristica otoba		奥托肉豆蔻
N		
nodakenin	[nə'deɪkənɪn]	紫花前胡苷
nodakenetin	[nə'deɪkɪntɪn]	紫花前胡苷元
O		
Oleaceae		木犀科
oleanolic acid	['əulɪə'nɔ:lɪk] ['æsɪd]	齐墩果酸
Orchidaceae		兰科
ortho-position	['ɔ:θəu] [pə'zɪʃn]	邻位
osthole	['ɔsθəul]	蛇床子素
otoboene	[əu'tɔbɔ:nə]	奥托肉豆蔻烯脂素
oxygen heterocyclic	['ɔksɪdʒən] [ˌhetərə'saɪklɪk]	氧杂环
P		
para-position	['pærə] [pə'zɪʃn]	对位
Peucedani decursivi Radix		紫花前胡
Peucedanum pareruptorum		白花前胡
phellandrene	['feləndri:n]	水芹烯

(continued)

4-phenyl-2, 3-naphthyl lactone		4– 苯代 –2, 3– 萘内酯
4-phenylnaphthalene	[ˈfiːnaɪl] [ˈnæfθəliːn]	4– 苯基萘类化合物
phenylpropanoids	[fenɪlˈprɔpənɔɪdz]	苯丙素
phenylpropene	[fenɪlˈprəupiːn]	苯丙烯
phenylpropionic acid	[fenɪlˈprɔpɪəunɪk][ˈæsɪd]	苯丙酸
phenylpropyl alcohol	[ˈfenɪlprɔpɪl][ˈælkəhɔl]	苯丙醇
phenylpropyl aldehyde	[ˈfenɪlprɔpɪl][ˈældɪhaɪd]	苯丙醛
phillygenin	[ˈfɪlɪdʒnɪn]	连翘脂素
phillygenol	[ˈfɪlɪdʒenɔl]	连翘脂素
phillyrin	[ˈfɪlɪrɪn]	连翘苷
phosphomolybdic acid	[fəusfəuˈməulɪbdɪk][ˈæsɪd]	磷钼酸
p-hydroxycinnamic acids	[haɪˈdrɔksi] [səˈnæmɪk] [ˈæsɪdz]	对羟基桂皮酸
phyllanthin	[ˈfɪlənθɪn]	叶下珠脂素
Phyllanthusnirui		珠子草
picropodophyllin	[ˈpɪkrɔːpuˈdɔːfɪliːn]	鬼臼苦素
pimpinellin	[ˈpɪmpaiːnəliːn]	虎耳草素
pinene	[ˈpaɪniːn]	蒎烯
pinocarveol	[ˌpaɪnəˈkaːvɪəul]	松香芹醇
pinoresinol	[ˌpaɪnəˈrezɪnɔl]	右旋松脂酚
Piper cubeba	[ˈpaɪpə][ˈkjuːbə]	毕澄茄
piperitol	[pɪˈperɪtɔl]	薄荷醇
podophyllotoxin	[ˌpɔdəˌfɪləˈtɔksɪn]	鬼臼毒脂素
Podophyllum genus		鬼臼
polyamide chromatography	[ˌpɔlɪˈeɪmaɪd] [ˌkrəuməˈtɔgrəfi]	聚酰胺色谱
Polygalae Radix		远志
potassium ferricyanide	[pəˈtæsɪəm] [ˌferɪˈsaɪənaɪd]	铁氰化钾
potassium hydroxide	[pəˈtæsɪəm] [haɪˈdrɔksaɪd]	氢氧化钾
praeroside Ⅱ	[ˈpraɪərɔːsɪd]	白花前胡苷 Ⅱ
pracrutorin A	[ˈpraɪkrəutɔːrɪn]	白花前胡丙素
preparative TLC	[prɪˈpærətɪv]	制备薄层色谱
propenyl benzene	[prəˈpenɪl] [ˈbenziːn]	丙烯苯
pteryxin	[ˈpteriːksɪn]	北美芹素
pseudo-γ-schisandrin		伪 γ– 五味子素
Psoraleae Fructus		补骨脂
psoralen	[ˈpsəurəlɪn]	补骨脂素
pyranone	[ˈpɪrənəun]	吡喃酮
pyranocoumarin	[paɪərənəuˈkəmərɪn]	吡喃香豆素

(continued)

Q		
quercetin	[ˈkwəːsɪtɪn]	槲皮素
R		
recrystallize	[riːˈkrɪstəlaɪz]	重结晶
rengyol	[ˈreɪndʒiːɔl]	连翘环己醇
rengyoside	[ˈreŋjɔːsɪd]	连翘环己醇苷
S		
Salviae miltiorrhizae Radix et Rhizoma		丹参
schisandrol	[ˈskiːsæˈdrɔːl]	五味子醇
Schisandra henryi		翼梗五味子
Schisandrae chinensis Fructus		五味子，北五味子
Schisandra chinensis (Turca) Baill		五味子
schisandrin (schisandrol A)		五味子素、五味子醇甲
schisanhenol	[ˈskiːsənˈhenɔːl]	五味子酚
schisantherin A、B、C、D	[ˈskiːsənθeiːrɪn]	五味子酯甲、乙、丙和丁
scoparone	[ˈskɔːpærɔːn]	滨蒿内酯
scopoletin	[ˈskəupəletɪn]	东莨菪亭
sesamin	[ˈsezəmɪn]	芝麻脂素
shashenoside		沙参苷
Silybi Fructus		水飞蓟
silymarin	[ˈsɪlɪmərɪn]	水飞蓟素
simple coumarin	[ˈsɪmpl] [ˈkuːmərɪn]	简单香豆素
simple lignans	[ˈsɪmpl] [ˈlɪgnænz]	简单木脂素
simple phenylpropanoids	[ˈsɪmpl] [fenilˈprɔpənɔɪdz]	简单苯丙素
sinapaldehyde	[ˌsɪnəˈpældəhaɪd]	芥子醛
sitosterol	[saɪˈtəstərɔl]	谷甾醇
small intestine	[smɔːl] [ɪnˈtestɪn]	小肠
sour	[ˈsauə]	酸的
stereoisomer	[ˌsterɪəuˈaɪsəmə]	立体异构体
sterols	[ˈsterɔlz]	甾醇类
stylosin	[staɪˈləuzɪn]	宿柱白蜡苷
sublimability	[ˈsʌblɪməˈbɪlɪti]	升华性
substituent	[səbˈstɪtjuənt]	取代基
sulfuric acid-ethanol solution	[sʌlˈfjuərɪk] [ˈæsɪd] [ˈeθənɔl][səˈluːʃn]	硫酸乙醇溶液
symmetrical	[sɪˈmetrɪkl]	对称的
syringaldehyde	[sɪˈrɪŋgəldɪhaɪd]	丁香醛
syringaresinol	[sɪrɪgəˈrezɪnɔl]	丁香脂素

(continued)

syringin	[sɪˈrɪŋɪn]	丁香苷
syringinoside	[sɪˈrɪŋɪnəusaɪd]	紫丁香酚苷
T		
taiwanin		台湾脂素
tannin	[ˈtænɪn]	鞣质
tanshinol	[ˈtenʃɪnɔːl]	丹参素
Taraxaciherba		蒲公英
Taxus cuspidata		中国紫杉
terpinene	[ˈtəːpɪniːn]	松油烯
tetrahydronaphthalene	[ˈtetrəˌhaɪdrəuˈnæfθəliːn]	四氢化萘
Thymelaeaceae		瑞香科
tigloylgomisin H	[ˈtaɪglɔːɪl] [ˈgɒmisiːn]	巴豆酰五味子脂素 H
trans-adjacent hydroxycinnamic acid	[trænz] [əˈdʒeɪsnt] [haɪˈdrɒksi] [səˈnæmɪk] [ˈæsɪd]	反邻羟基桂皮酸
trans-configuration	[trænz] [kənˌfɪgəˈreɪʃn]	反式构型
triacontanoic acid	[ˌtraɪəkɒnˈtemɔɪk] [ˈæsɪd]	三十烷酸
triterpenes	[traɪˈtəːpiːns]	三萜类
U		
umbelliferone	[ˌʌmbəˈlɪfərəun]	伞形花内酯
unsaturated	[ʌnˈsætʃəˌreɪtɪd]	不饱和
unsaturated side chain	[ʌnˈsætʃəˌreɪtɪd] [saɪd] [tʃeɪn]	不饱和侧链
unsubstituted	[ʌnsəbstɪˈtjuːtɪd]	未被取代的
ursolic acid	[əːˈsɔlɪk][ˈæsɪd]	熊果酸，乌索酸
W		
wogonin-7-*O*-glucoside	[ˈwɒgənɪn] [ˈgluːkəsaɪd]	黄芩素 –7–*O*– 葡萄糖苷
woody tissues	[ˈwudi] [ˈtisjuːz]	木质组织
Y		
yellow and brown	[ˈjeləu] [ənd] [ˈbraun]	黄棕色

重 点 小 结

　　苯丙素类是指基本母核具有一个或几个 C₆–C₃ 结构单元的天然有机化合物，均由桂皮酸途径合成而来。主要包括简单苯丙素、香豆素、木脂素、木质素、黄酮等。

　　简单苯丙素类可分为苯丙烯、苯丙醇、苯丙醛、苯丙酸等。苯丙烯、苯丙醛及苯丙酸的简单酯类衍生物多具有挥发性，是挥发油中芳香族化合物的主要组成部分。

　　香豆素是一类具有苯骈 α – 吡喃酮母核的天然产物的总称，在结构上可以看成是顺式邻羟基桂皮酸脱水而形成的内酯类化合物。依据在 α – 吡喃酮环上有无取代，以及 C₇ 位羟基是否与

C_6 或 C_8 位的异戊烯基缩合形成呋喃环、吡喃环，将香豆素分为四类：简单香豆素，呋喃香豆素（线型、角型），吡喃香豆素（线型、角型），其他香豆素（二聚体、三聚体、异香豆素等）。

　　游离香豆素多为结晶型固体，但也有一些呈液态。分子量小的游离香豆素多具有芳香气味、升华性与挥发性，能随水蒸气蒸馏。香豆素苷类一般呈粉末或晶体状，不具有挥发性和升华性。游离香豆素易溶于乙醚、三氯甲烷、丙酮、乙醇、甲醇等有机溶剂，能部分溶于沸水，不溶于冷水；香豆素苷类易溶于甲醇、乙醇，可溶于水，难溶于乙醚、三氯甲烷等低极性有机溶剂。

　　香豆素类成分结构中具有内酯环，碱性条件下可水解开环，生成顺式邻羟基桂皮酸的盐而溶解于水，经酸化后又可闭环恢复为内酯结构而沉淀析出，因此可用碱溶酸沉法提取游离香豆素。但需要注意：①如果与碱液长时间加热，开环产物顺式则会异构化为反式，酸化后不能再环合为内酯，因此需要注意控制条件，避免异构化；②当结构中含有其他酯基时，其他酯基也会水解；③结构中若在酚羟基的邻位有异戊烯基等不饱和侧链，酸化时能环合形成呋喃环或吡喃环等含氧杂环。

　　分离香豆素类成分常用硅胶柱色谱、制备薄层色谱和高效液相色谱等，葡聚糖凝胶 Sephadex LH-20 柱色谱等也可用于不同分子量的香豆素苷类成分的分离。

　　香豆素类化合物的检识可利用其荧光特性、化学检识和色谱检识。香豆素类化合物与异羟肟酸铁反应显红色，检识内酯环的存在；与三氯化铁生成绿色至墨绿色沉淀，检识酚羟基的存在；酚羟基的邻、对位无取代的，可与重氮化试剂反应显红色至紫红色；C_6 位无取代基的香豆素，可与 2,6- 二氯苯醌氯亚胺（Gibb's 试剂）反应而显蓝色，或与 Emerson 试剂（4- 氨基安替比林和铁氰化钾）反应显红色。

　　在 ^{1}H-NMR 中，3、4 位无取代的香豆素类成分 H-3、H-4 构成 AB 系统，δ_{H-4} 7.50~8.20 (d, $J = 9.5$ Hz)，在芳氢的最低场，δ_{H-3} 6.10~6.50 (d, $J = 9.5$ Hz)，在芳氢的最高场。香豆素类化合物在 EI-MS 中大多具有强的分子离子峰，简单香豆素类和呋喃香豆素类的分子离子峰经常是基峰，常出现一系列连续失去 CO、OH 或 H_2O、甲基或甲氧基的碎片离子峰。

　　木脂素是一类由两个或两个以上 C_6-C_3 结构单元聚合而成的天然化合物，主要存在于植物的木质部和树脂中，多呈游离态，少数与糖结合成苷。组成木脂素的单体有四种：桂皮酸（偶有桂皮醛）、桂皮醇、丙烯苯和烯丙苯。多数木脂素类化合物是无色结晶，一般无挥发性，少数有升华性（如二氢愈创木脂酸）。木脂素大部分具有光学活性，遇酸易异构化，且其光学活性往往与生物活性密切相关。因此在提取分离过程中应注意操作条件，尽量避免与酸、碱接触，以防止其构型的改变。

　　游离木脂素多具有亲脂性，易溶于乙醚、三氯甲烷及乙醇等溶剂，木脂素苷类极性较大，可溶于甲醇、乙醇等。木脂素的分离主要依靠色谱法，常用吸附剂为硅胶和中性氧化铝，洗脱剂可根据被分离物质的极性进行选择。木脂素没有特征性的理化检识反应，但可对其常有的官能团进行检识。如用三氯化铁反应检识酚羟基的有无；Labat 反应或 Ecgrine 反应检识亚甲二氧基的有无；异羟肟酸铁反应检识内酯环的有无等。

　　在环木脂内酯中，可用 ^{1}H-NMR 谱区别内酯环向上和向下两种类型；在双环氧木脂素的异构体中，根据 ^{1}H-NMR 谱中 H-7 和 H-8 的 J 值，可判断两个苯环是位于同侧还是异侧。

题库

目 标 检 测

一、单选题

1. 判断香豆素 C-6 位是否有取代基可用的反应是（　　）
   A. 异羟肟酸铁反应　　　　　　B. Gibb's 反应　　　　　　C. 三氯化铁反应
   D. 盐酸 – 镁粉反应　　　　　　E. 三氯化锑反应

2. 鉴别香豆素类化合物时，一般首选的显色反应是（　　）
   A. Molish 反应　　　　　　　　B. 浓硫酸反应　　　　　　C. Gibb's 反应
   D. 异羟肟酸铁反应　　　　　　E. Labat 反应

3. 下列化合物中可能具有挥发性的是（　　）
   A. 木质素　　　　　　　　　　B. 强心苷　　　　　　　　C. 游离香豆素
   D. 香豆素苷　　　　　　　　　E. 多糖

4. 以下叙述不正确的是（　　）
   A. 线型呋喃香豆素是由 C_7 位羟基与 C_6 位异戊烯基缩合形成
   B. 7- 羟基香豆素可视为香豆素的母核
   C. 简单香豆素一般在 C_3 和 C_4 位没有取代
   D. 角型吡喃香豆素是由 C_7 位羟基与 C_6 位异戊烯基缩合形成
   E. 香豆素还有二聚体、三聚体等

5. 欲从某药材中提取游离香豆素类化合物，下列方法一般不可用的是（　　）
   A. 水浸出法　　　　　　　　　B. 有机溶剂提取法　　　　C. 碱溶酸沉法
   D. 水蒸气蒸馏　　　　　　　　E. 乙醇回流提取

6. Labat 反应是以下哪个官能团的特征反应（　　）
   A. 酚羟基　　　　　　　　　　B. 亚甲二氧基　　　　　　C. 内酯环
   D. 甲氧基　　　　　　　　　　E. 异戊烯基

7. 组成木脂素类化合物的的基本结构骨架是（　　）
   A. C_5-C_3　　　　　　　　　　B. C_5-C_4　　　　　　　　C. C_6-C_3
   D. C_6-C_4　　　　　　　　　　E. C_6-C_6

8. 关于呋喃香豆素下列叙述中不正确的是（　　）
   A. 分为线型和角型
   B. 可以游离态或成苷形式存在
   C. 在 ^{1}H-NMR 中，6,7- 二取代香豆素的 H-5、H-8 分别呈现为单峰信号
   D. 由 C_8 位异戊烯基与 C_7 位羟基形成的为角型
   E. 由 C_6 位异戊烯基与 C_7 位羟基形成的为角型

9. 在香豆素类化合物的 IR 光谱中 1750~1700cm^{-1} 显示一个强吸收，是由以下哪个结构引起的（　　）
   A. 芳环　　　　　　　　　　　B. 内酯结构　　　　　　　C. 羟基
   D. 呋喃环　　　　　　　　　　E. 甲氧基

10. 厚朴酚与和厚朴酚属于以下哪一类木脂素（   ）

    A. 联苯型木脂素　　　　　　B. 联苯环辛烯型木脂素　　　C. 单环氧木脂素

    D. 环木脂素　　　　　　　　E. 简单木脂素

二、多选题

1. 检识含羟基取代的香豆素苷类化合物时，以下哪些反应显阳性（   ）

    A. Molish 反应　　　　　　　B. 碘化铋钾试剂　　　　　　C. 盐酸 – 镁粉反应

    D. 三氯化铁反应　　　　　　E. 异羟肟酸铁反应

2. 区别 6，7– 呋喃香豆素和 7，8– 呋喃香豆素时，可采用（   ）

    A. 异羟肟酸铁反应　　　　　B. Gibb's 反应　　　　　　　C. 醋酐 – 浓硫酸反应

    D. Emerson 反应　　　　　　E. 氨性氯化锶反应

3. 组成木脂素的单体有（   ）

    A. 桂皮酸　　　　　　　　　B. 桂皮醛　　　　　　　　　C. 桂皮醇

    D. 丙烯苯　　　　　　　　　E. 烯丙苯

4. 以下关于香豆素苷类化合物的叙述不正确的是（   ）

    A. 易溶于甲醇、乙醇　　　　B. 多具有芳香味　　　　　　C. 多具有升华性

    D. 一般呈粉末或晶体状　　　E. 可以用水蒸气蒸馏法提取

5. 在双环氧木脂素的异构体中，根据 ^{1}H-NMR 谱中的 J 值，可以判断 2 个苯环位于同侧还是位于异侧的质子是（   ）

    A. H-2　　　　　　　　　　B. H-7　　　　　　　　　　C. H-4

    D. H-3　　　　　　　　　　E. H-8

6. 以下属于苯丙素类化合物的是（   ）

    A. 木脂素　　　　　　　　　B. 甾体　　　　　　　　　　C. 香豆素

    D. 黄酮　　　　　　　　　　E. 木质素

7. 以下关于香豆素类化合物荧光性质叙述正确的是（   ）

    A. 一般显蓝色或紫色的荧光

    B. 7– 羟基香豆素类加碱后其荧光更强

    C. 香豆素类化合物都具有荧光

    D. 可作为薄层色谱的检视用

    E. 导入非羟基取代基往往使荧光强度减弱

8. 以下关于 7 位取代香豆素的核磁共振氢谱叙述正确的是（   ）

    A. H-5、H-8 分别呈现为单峰信号

    B. H-5 呈现为 d 峰（和 H-6 偶合）

    C. H-6 呈现为 d 峰（和 H-5 偶合）

    D. H-6 呈现为 dd 峰（和 H-5、H-8 均偶合）

    E. H-8 呈现为 d 峰（和 H-6 偶合）

9. 以下属于联苯环辛烯型木脂素的是（   ）

    A. 五味子素　　　　　　　　B. 厚朴酚　　　　　　　　　C. 五味子醇

    D. 和厚朴酚　　　　　　　　E. 连翘苷

10. 以下关于游离香豆素提取方法叙述正确的是（   ）

    A. 小分子游离香豆素可用水蒸气蒸馏法

B. 可用有机溶剂法提取

C. 可用冷水提取

D. 可用碱溶酸沉法

E. 有些可用升华法

三、思考题

1. 如何判断某药材中是否可能含有香豆素类化合物?

2. 香豆素类化合物为什么可以用碱溶酸沉法进行提取?需要注意什么问题?

3. 选择适当的试剂用化学反应鉴别下列三个化合物。

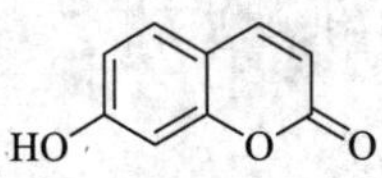

(A) 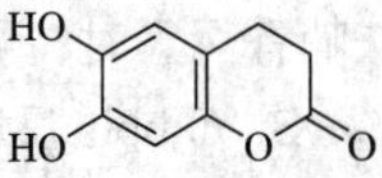　　　　　　　(B) 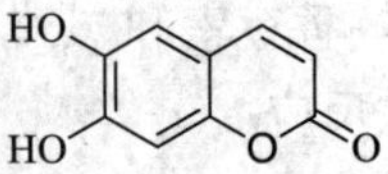　　　　　　　(C)

（邵　晶）

Chapter 6　Flavonoids

学习目标

知识要求：

1. 掌握　黄酮类化合物的主要理化性质、提取分离及检识方法。

2. 熟悉　黄酮的定义、分类、能熟练运用理化反应、紫外光谱及核磁共振氢谱等信息综合解析黄酮类化合物的结构。

3. 了解　黄芩、银杏叶、槐花和葛根中黄酮类主要活性成分的结构特征及其饮片的质量控制标准。

能力要求：

学会应用盐酸－镁粉反应检识黄酮类化合物，应用金属盐络合反应判断黄酮类化合物结构中邻二羟基、3－羟基取代特征；学会应用黄酮类化合物的理化性质选择适合的提取分离方法，解决黄酮类化合物在提取分离过程中存在的技术问题；学会运用理化反应、紫外光谱及核磁共振氢谱等信息综合解析黄酮类化合物的结构。

1　Introduction

Flavonoids (黄酮类) are a group of naturally occurring phenolic compounds that exit in various parts of plants both in aglycone and glycoside form. The term flavonoid is derived from the Latin word *flavus* meaning yellow, because most of flavonoids are yellow in color. They are also known as plant pigments (色素) or co-pigments (辅色素). Some flavonoids have various biological activities.

1.1　Definition

The classic definition of flavonoids was described as the derivatives of 2-phenylchromone (2-苯基色原酮). Nowadays, flavonoids are also described as the natural products with skeleton of C_6-C_3-C_6 system.

Chromone　　　　2-phenylchromone　　　　$C_6-C_3-C_6$

1.2　Distribution

Flavonoids are widely distributed in nature and especially common in higher plants belonging to families (科) Gesneriaceae (苦苣苔科), Labiatae, Scrophulariaceae (玄参科), Ericaceae (杜鹃花科), Rosaceae (蔷薇科), Faboideae (蝶形花亚科), Leguminosae, Zingiberaceae (姜科), Rutaceae, Primulaceae (报春花科), Polygonaceae, Salicaceae (杨柳科), Pinaceae (松科), Asteraceae, Lamiaceae, Moraceae (桑科), Betulaceae (桦木科), Rubiaceae, Bignoniaceae (紫葳科), and Myrtaceae (桃金娘科). Flavonoids also exist in some lower plants, e.g. algae (藻类). Flavonoids occur as glycosides and aglycones, and exist in different parts of plants such as root, bark, heartwood, leaf, flower, fruit and seed.

1.3　Pharmacological Activities

Flavonoids have various biological activities, such as antioxidant, antimicrobial, antiulcer, antiarthritic, anti-angiogenic, anticancer, antivirus, anti-inflammatory activities, neuroprotector, estrogenic, estrogen (雌性激素) receptor binding, and so on (Table 6-1).

Table 6-1　Some biological active flavonoids

Compounds	Main sources	Biological activities
Baicalin (黄芩苷)	*Scutellaria baicalensis*	Anticancer, anti-HIV, anti-inflammation, antioxidant, etc.
Daidzein (大豆素)	*Trifolium pratense*	Estrogen receptor, anticancer, neuroprotector, etc.
Ginkgetin (银杏黄酮)	*Ginkgo biloba*	Anti-inflammation, neuroprotector, antiherpesvirus, etc.
Luteolin (木犀草素)	*Arachis hypogaes*	Anticancer, antimicrobial, anti-inflammation, etc.
Puerarin (葛根素)	*Pueraria lobata*	Estrogen receptor, antihyperglycemic agent, etc.
Rutin (芦丁)	*Sophora japonica*	Antioxidant, cardioprotector, etc.
Silymarin (水飞蓟素)	*Silybum marianum*	Anticancer, liver protector, antioxidant, etc.
Hesperidin (橘皮苷)	*Citrus reticulata*	Neuroprotector, anti-inflammation, antihypolipidemic, etc.

1.4　Biosynthesis

The frame of flavonoids are divided into two parts, one part is ring A, the other part is phenylpropanoids moiety (C_6-C_3). The biogenesis (生物起源) of ring A is via acetate-malonate pathway (乙酸–丙二酸途径), while that of ring B is via shikimate pathway (莽草酸途径).

It has been found that chalcones (查尔酮) are the intermediate (中间体) for flavonoids and isoflavonoids (异黄酮类). The condensation of *p*-coumaoyl coenzyme (辅酶) -A with three molecules of malonyl (丙二酰基) coenzyme A (acetate units) catalyzed by chalcone synthase (合成酶) result in the formation of chalcones.

Dihydroflavonols (二氢黄酮) are formed by the action of chalcone isomerase (异构化酶) and flavanone-3-hydroxylase. The anthocyanins (花色素) are further formed from dihydroflavonols. Chalcones are converted to isoflavones *via* oxidation (氧化), rearrangement (重排) and cyclization reactions (环合反应). The biosynthesis (生物合成) of flavonoids are summarized as follows (Figure 6-1).

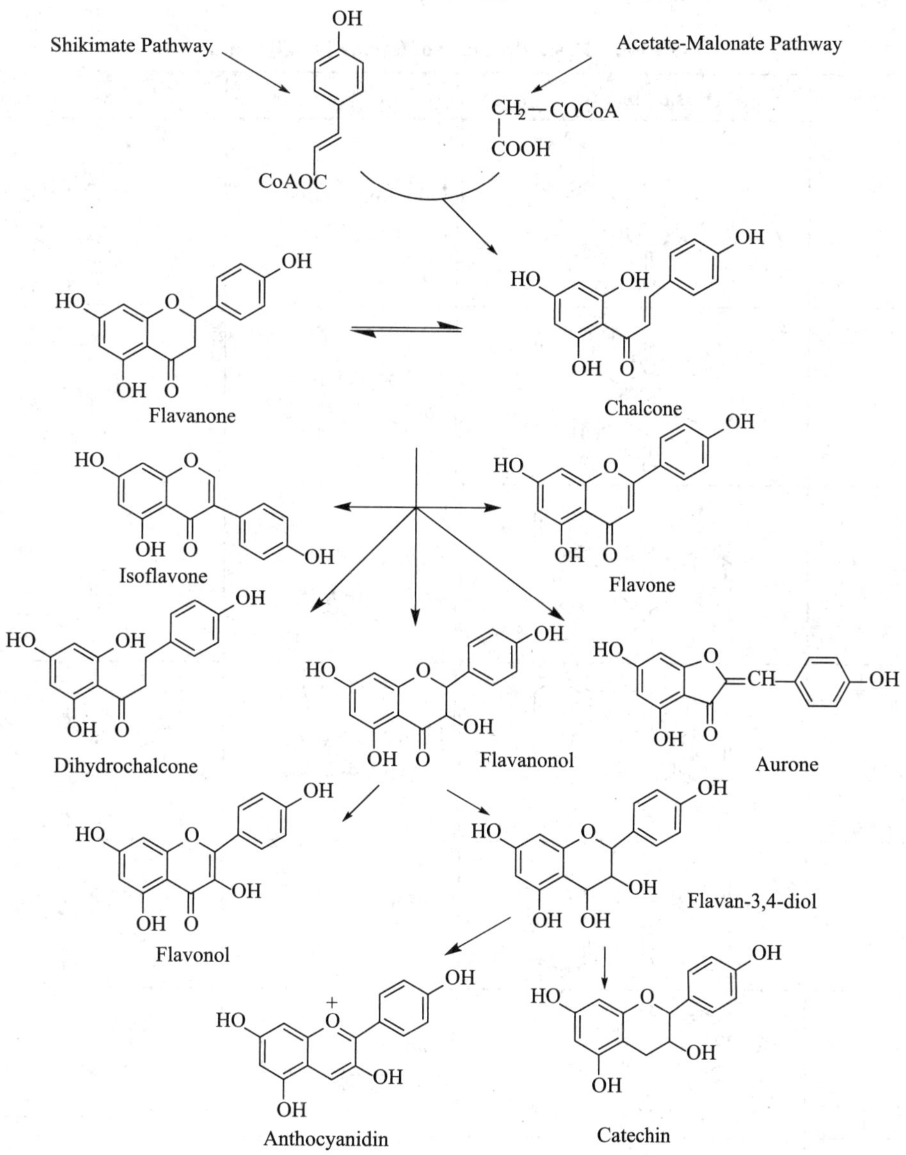

Shikimate Pathway

Acetate-Malonate Pathway

Flavanone

Chalcone

Isoflavone

Flavone

Dihydrochalcone

Flavanonol

Aurone

Flavonol

Flavan-3,4-diol

Anthocyanidin

Catechin

Figure 6-1　Biosynthesis of flavonoids

2　Structure and Classification

　　Flavonoids are classified into various types according to four factors: ① whether the three carbon bridge is open or close; ② the level of oxidation of the C-ring; ③ the position of attachment of the B-ring;

④ whether the compound is monomer (单体), dimer (二聚体), or a higher oligomer (寡聚体).

2.1 Flavonoid Aglycones

The basic types of flavonoids are listed in Table 6-2.

Table 6-2   Basic structure of flavonoid aglycones

Types	Basic Structure	Types	Basic Structure
Flavone (黄酮)		Dihydrochalcone (二氢查尔酮)	
Flavonol (黄酮醇)		Anthocyanidin (花色素)	
Flavanone (二氢黄酮)		Flavan-3-ol (黄烷-3-醇)	
Flavanonol (二氢黄酮醇)		Flavan-3, 4-diol (黄烷-3, 4-二醇)	
Isoflavone (异黄酮)		Aurone (橙酮)	
Isoflavanone (二氢异黄酮)		Xanthone (双苯吡酮)	
Chalcone (查尔酮)		Homoisoflavone (高异黄酮)	

2.1.1   Flavones (黄酮)

Flavones contain a chromone (色原酮) ring with phenyl (苯基) substitution at position C-2 of the pyrone (吡喃酮) ring. Most natural flavones are bonded hydroxyl groups at C-5 and C-7 position of ring A. The oxygenated (氧化的) groups, such as hydroxyl and methoxyl (甲氧基) often appear at C-4′ and C-3′ of ring B. The representative flavones include luteolin, baicalin, apigenin (芹菜素), etc.

Luteolin　　　　　　Baicalin　　　　　　Apigenin

2.1.2　Flavonols (黄酮醇)

Flavonols are characterized with their B-ring attached to C-2, and possess a hydroxyl group at C-3. The typical flavonols include quercetin (槲皮素), kaempferol (山奈酚), myricetin (杨梅素), etc.

Kaempferol　　　　Quercetin R=H　　　　Myricetin
　　　　　　　　　Rutin　　R= rhaα 1 ⟶ 6glc

2.1.3　Flavanones (二氢黄酮)

2, 3-Dihydroderivatives of flavone are called flavanones, which look like flavones except that they don't have the C-2/C-3 double bond. Hesperetin (橙皮素) and its glycosides from *Citrus aurantiun* (酸橙), liquintigenin (甘草素) and liquiritin (甘草苷) from Glycyrrhizae Radix et Rhizoma (甘草) are flavanones type.

Liguirtigenin　R = H　　　　Hesperitin　　　　　　R = H
Liquiritin　　　R = glc　　　　Hesperitin glcoside　R = rhaα1 ⟶ 6glc

2.1.4　Flavanonols (二氢黄酮醇)

Flavanonols are characterized as possessing a hydroxyl group at C-3 of flavanones. The structure of dihydroquercetin (二氢槲皮素) from the leaf of *Rhododendron dahuricum* (满山红), phellamurin (黄柏素–7–*O*–葡萄糖苷), an anti-cancer active ingredient from *Phellodendron chinense* (黄柏), and dihydromorin (二氢桑色素) from the branch of mulberry (桑树) are typical flavanonols.

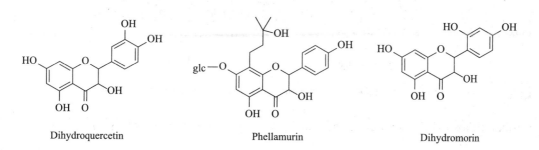

Dihydroquercetin　　　　　　Phellamurin　　　　　　Dihydromorin

2.1.5　Isoflavones (异黄酮) and Isoflavanones (二氢异黄酮)

Isoflavones contain chromone ring with a phenyl substitutent at C-3 of the pyrone ring and isoflavanones are dihydro-derivatives of isoflavones. Daidzein, daidzein-7, 4′-diglucoside, puerain and puerain-xyloside (葛根素木糖苷) are typical isoflavones. Pterocarpin (紫檀素), trifolirhizin (三叶豆紫檀苷), maackiain (马卡因) isolated from *Sophora subprostrata* (广豆根) and rotenone (鱼藤酮) came from *Derris elliptica* (毛鱼藤) are isoflavanone derivatives.

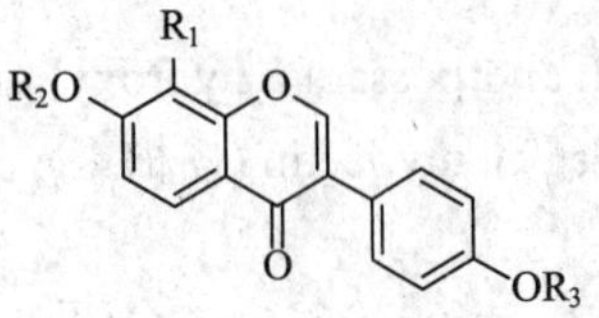

Daidzien	$R_1=R_2=R_3=H$	
Daidzin	$R_1=R_3=H$	$R_2=glc$
Puerarin	$R_2=R_3=H$	$R_1=glc$
Daidzien-7,4'-diglucoside	$R_1=H$	$R_2=R_3=glc$
Puerarin-xyloside	$R_1=glc$　$R_2=xyl$　$R_3=H$	

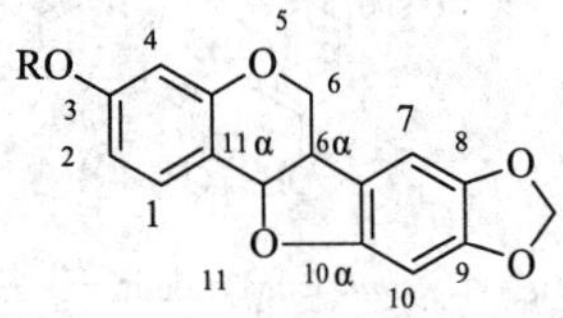

Pterocarpin	$R=CH_3$
Trifolirhizin	$R=glc$
Maackiain	$R=H$

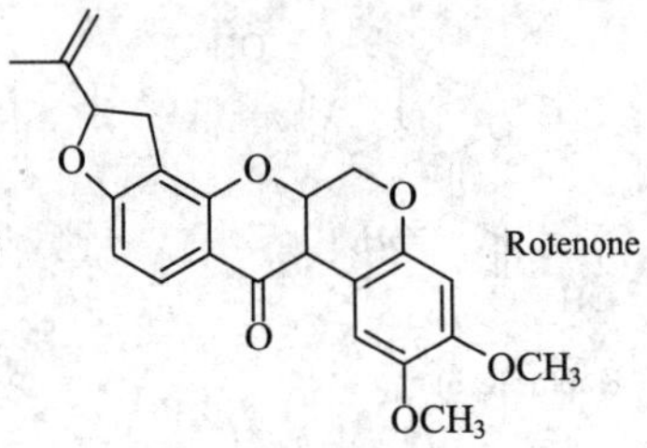

Rotenone

2.1.6　Anthocyanins

Anthocyanins possessing a flavylium (花色基元) salt structure are the glycosides of anthocyanidins. They are responsible for the color, such as color red, mauve (淡紫色), violet (蓝紫色), and blue in the flower of most plants. In general, the sugar moieties are linked with a hydroxyl group at C-3, C-5 or C-7.

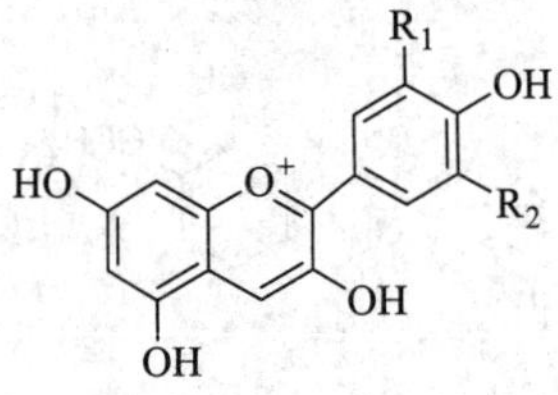

Cyanidin	$R_1=OH$	$R_2=H$
Delphinidin	$R_1=R_2=OH$	
Pelargonidin	$R_1=R_2=H$	

2.1.7　Chalcones and Dihydrochalcones (二氢查耳酮)

Chalcones are open chain flavonoids in which two aromatic rings (芳香环) are joined by a three carbon chain (3-unsaturated carbonyl system). The corresponding dihydro-derivatives are called dihydrochalcone. 2′-Hydroxychalcone is a isomer (异构体) of flavanone, and they are convertible each other. 2′-Hydroxychalcone can be converted to colorless flavanone in acid medium, and the latter can convert to brown yellow 2′-hydroxychalcone in base medium (Figure 6-2).

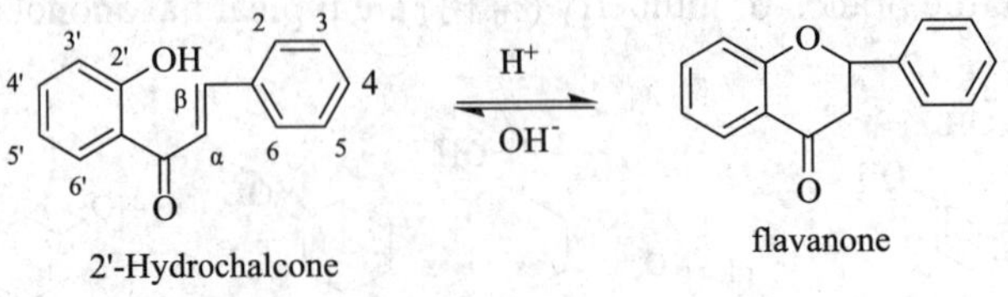

2′-Hydrochalcone　　　　　flavanone

Figure 6-2　Scheme of conversion of 2′-hydroxychalcone to flavanone

Carthami Flos (红花) contains carthamin (红花苷), neocarthamin (新红花苷) and carthamone (醌

式红花苷). At the beginning of blooming, it is light yellow because of possessing colorless neocarthamin and trace carthamin. It turns brown yellow in the middle stage due to carthamin as the main component. At last, it turns red due to forming carthamone *via* oxidation of carthamin (Figure 6-3).

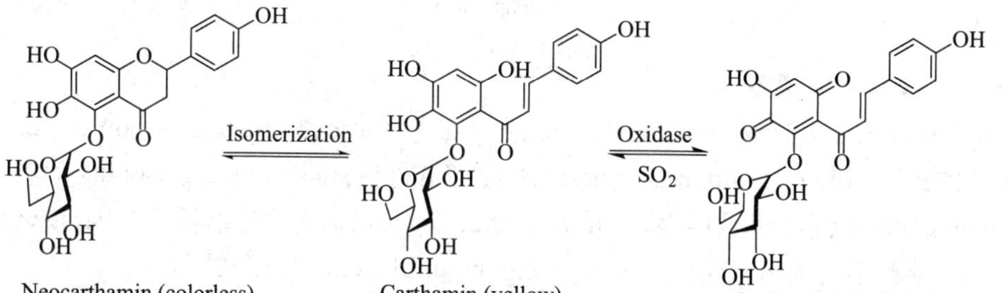

Neocarthamin (colorless)　　Carthamin (yellow)　　Carthamone (red)

Figure 6-3　Main constituents of Carthami Flos

Dihydrochalcones rarely occur in plants. The structure of phloridzin (梨根苷) belongs to dihydrochalcones type, which is a chemical component of the seed of apple.

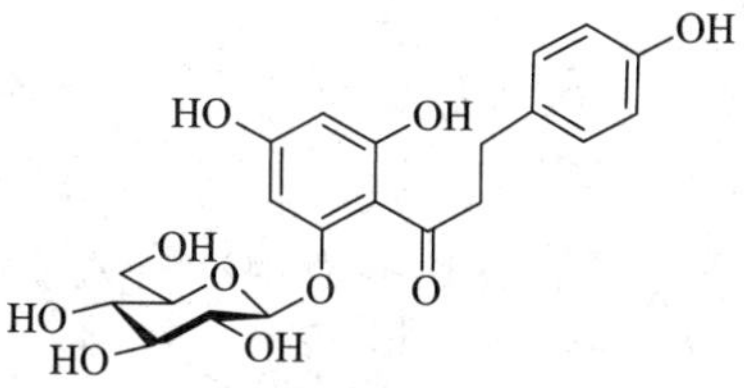

Phloridzin

2.1.8　Flavanols（黄烷醇）

Flavans (黄烷类) refer to a group of flavonoids lacking the C-4 carbonyl (羰基) on the C-ring. Flavan-3-ol (黄烷–3–醇) and flavan-3, 4-diols (黄烷–3, 4–二醇) are widely distributed in the plants containing tannins. The typical flavans are (+)-catechin (儿茶素) and (-)-epicatechin (表儿茶素) from *Acacia catechu* (儿茶), and leucosyanidin (无色矢车菊素), leucodelphinidin (无色飞燕草素) and leuco-pelargonidin (无色天竺葵素) from *Delphinium grandiflorum* (翠雀).

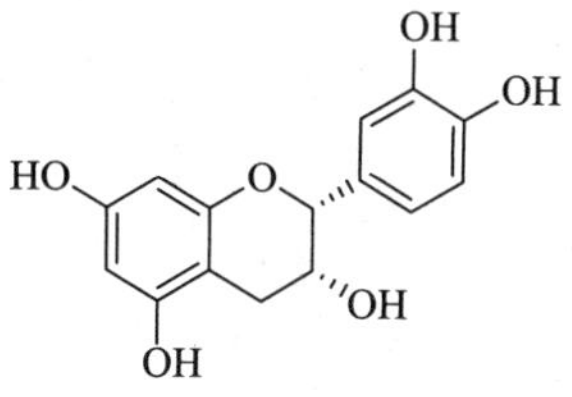

l-Epicatechin 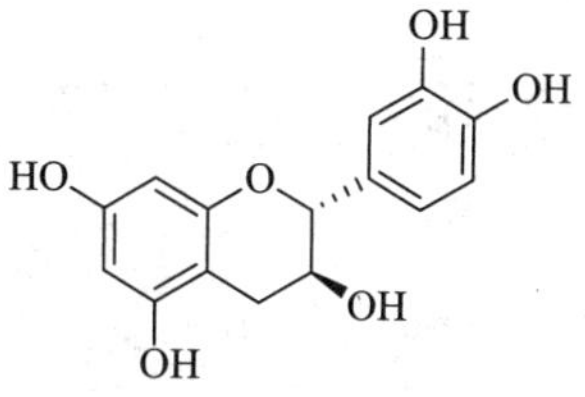　　　　　*d*-Catechin

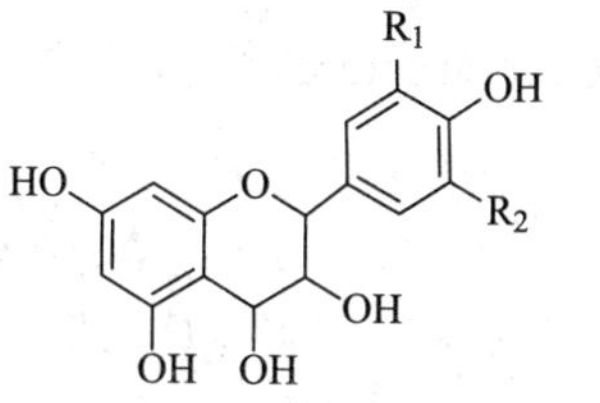

Leucocyanidin　　R_1= OH　R_2= H
Leucodelphinidin　R_1= R_2= OH
Leucopelargonidin　R_1= R_2= H

2.1.9　Aurones (橙酮)

Aurones are characterized by possessing a five-membered ring C rather than a six-membered ring C. Aurones are rare in nature and mainly distributed in Asteraceae (菊科), Scrophulariaceae, Cyperaceae (莎草科), Gesneriaceae (苦苣苔科). The structure of sulphuretin (硫磺菊素) belongs to aurones type.

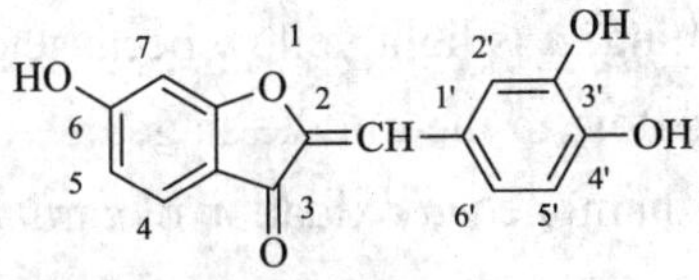

Sulphuretin

2.1.10 Biflavonoids (双黄酮)

Biflavonoids consist of two flavonoid skeletons linked through either a carbon-oxygen or carbon-carbon bond. They are divided into three types: ① 3', 8″-diapigenins type, e.g. isoginkgetin (异银杏素), ginkgetin (银杏素) and bilobetin (白果素) from ginkgo leaves (银杏叶); ② 8, 8″-diapigenins type, e.g. cupresuflavone (柏黄酮); ③ bibenzyl ether type, e.g. hinokiflavone (扁柏黄酮).

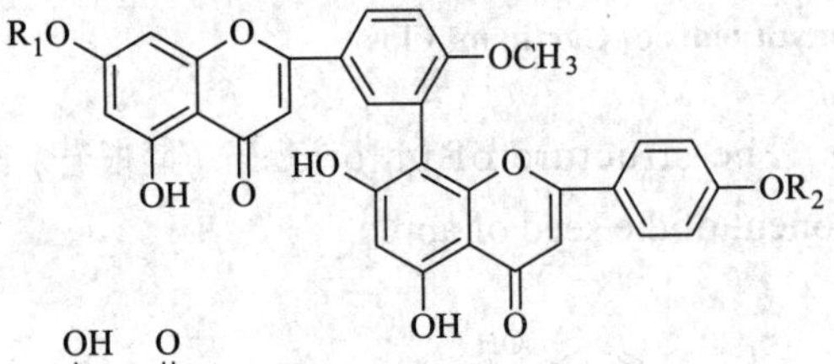

Isoginkgetin	R_1= H	R_2= CH$_3$
Ginkgetin	R_1= CH$_3$	R_2= H
Bilobetin	R_1= H	R_2= H

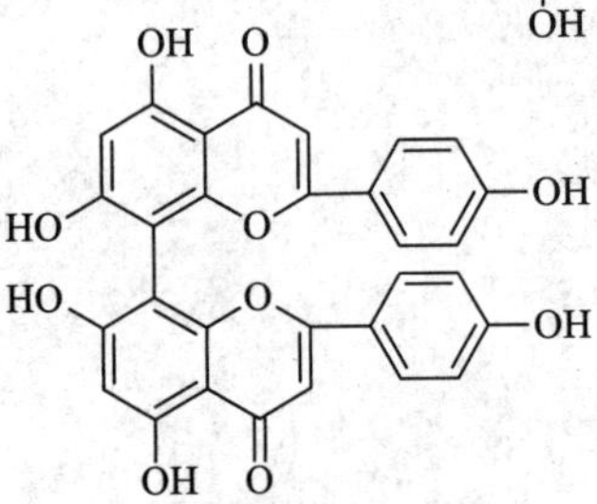

Cupresuflavone

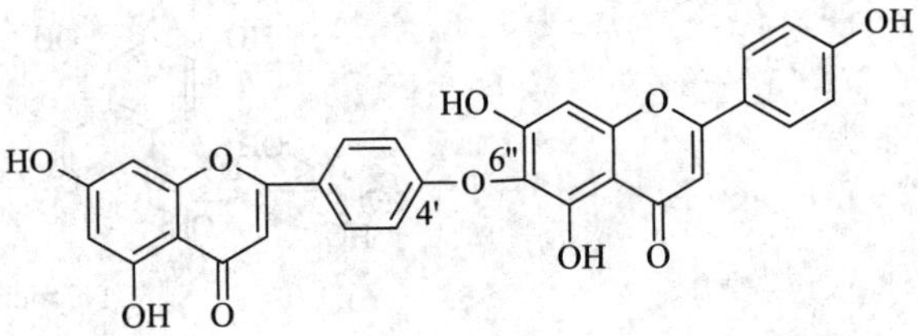

Hinokiflavone

2.1.11 Other Flavonoids

Xanthones (双苯吡酮, 氧杂蒽酮), named biphenylpyrone (双苯吡酮), consist of phenyl and chromone at C-2 and C-3. They are commonly distributed in Gentianaceae (龙胆科), Guttiferae (藤黄科), and Liliaceae (唇形科) plants. Isomerngiferin (异芒果素) is a component of Pyrrosiae Folium (石韦) and Anemarrhenae Rhizoma (知母). Its structure belongs to xanthones type.

Silymarin is flavonolignan (黄酮木脂素) consisting of a dihydroflavanol and a phenylpropanoid unit. While the structure of ficine (榕碱) and isoficine (异榕碱) are alkaloid flavonoids type.

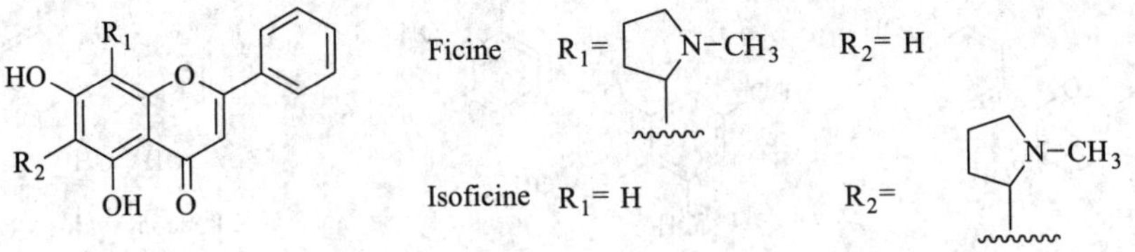

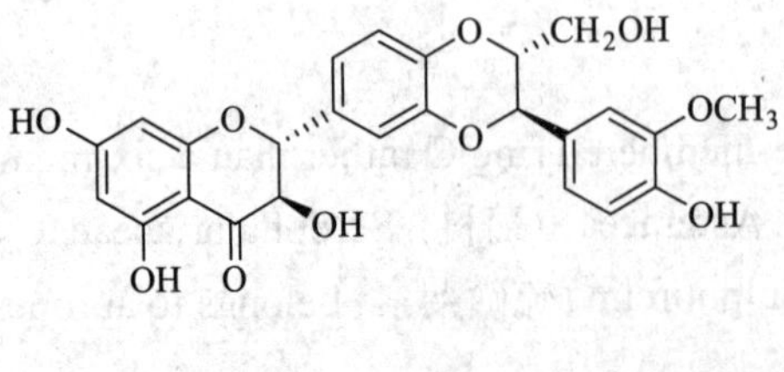

Ficine R_1= [pyrrolidine N-CH$_3$ group] R_2= H

Isoficine R_1= H R_2= [pyrrolidine N-CH$_3$ group]

Silymarin

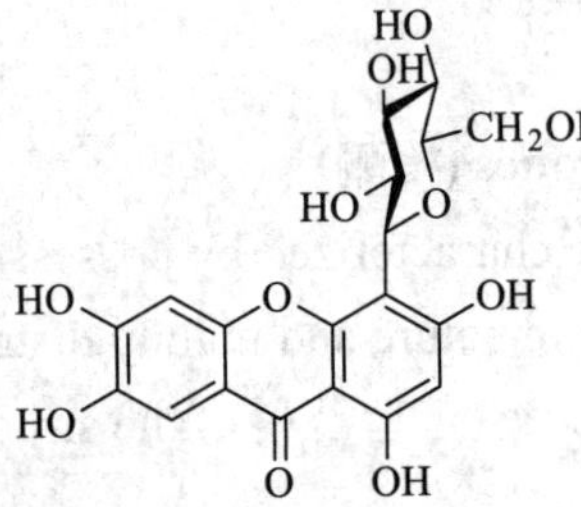

Isomergiferin

2.2 Flavonoid Glycosides

Most flavonoids present in nature as glycosides. The common saccharides in flavonoid glycosides are listed in Table 6-3.

Table 6-3 Common saccharides in flavonoid glycosides

Types	Common saccharides
monosaccharides	D-glucose, D-xylose, L-rhamnose, D-galactose, L-arabinose, D-glucuronic acid
disaccharides	Neohesperdose (rhaα1 $\rightarrow$ 2 glc), robinobiose (rhaα1 $\rightarrow$ 6 gal)
trisaccharides	Gentianose (glcβ1 $\rightarrow$ 6glcβ1 $\rightarrow$ 2fru), sophorotriose (glcβ1 $\rightarrow$ 2glcβ1 $\rightarrow$ 2glc)
acetyl saccharides	2-acetylglucose, caffeoylglucose

2.2.1 *O*-glycosides

O-glycosides are the most common type in flavonoid glycosides. Glycosylation (苷化) occur at any hydroxyl group but some are favored. For example, most flavonols occur as 3-*O*-glycosides and 7-*O*-glycosides. Flavones mostly occur as 7-*O*-glycosides.

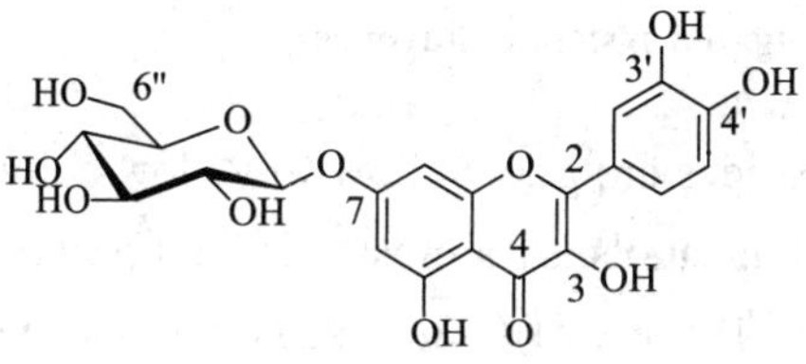

Quercetin7-O-β-D-glucopyanoside 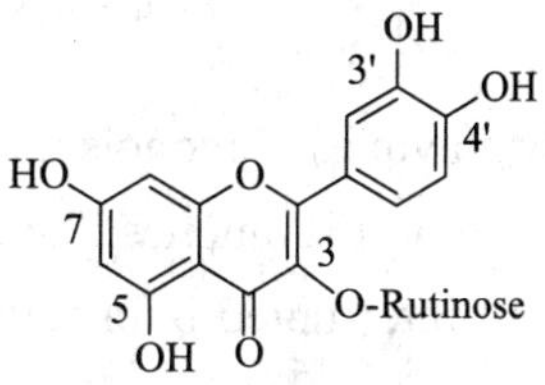   Rutin

2.2.2 *C*-glycosides

C-glycosyl flavonoids are also presented in Chinese herbs. C-6 or C-8, or C-6 and C-8 are the common positions of flavonoid aglycones attached to the sugar moieties. Vitexin and puerarin are the typical *C*-glycosides.

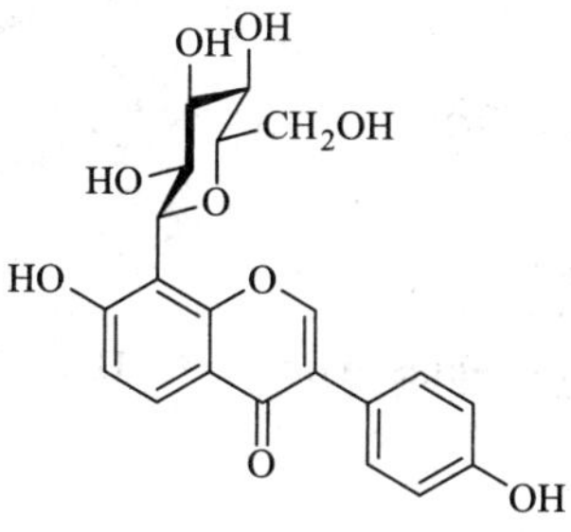

Puerarin 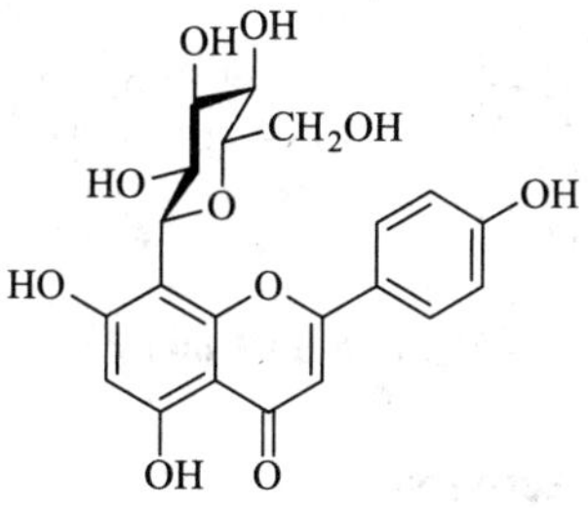   Vitexin

3   Physicochemical Properties

3.1   Physical Properties

3.1.1   Characteristics

Most flavonoids are yellow crystal. However, their color depends on whether the cross-conjugated (交叉共轭) system exist or not, also depends on the types, numbers and locations of substituents (取代基) bonding to flavonoid frame. For flavone and flavonol types, the groups (e.g. hydroxyl and methoxyl) attached to C-7 or C-4′ will bring intensive effects (Figure 6-4).

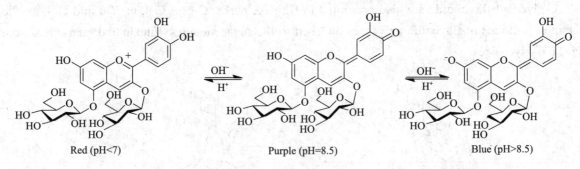

Figure 6-4   Cross-conjugated system of flavones

In generally, flavones, flavonols and their glycosides are gray yellow to yellow color. Chalcones are yellow to orange color. Flavanones, flavanonols and flavanols are almost colorless because of their cross-conjugated system interrupted by a saturated (饱和的) bond of C-2/ C-3. Isoflavones are slight yellow due to the phenyl group attached to C-3 position, in which the incompletely conjugated system is formed.

Anthocyanins can reversibly (可逆的) change color with pH value. For example, cyanin (花色素苷) presents as color red, purple and blue with the value of pH< 7, pH=8.5 and pH>8.5, respectively (Figure 6-5).

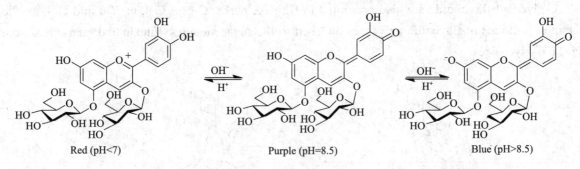

Red (pH<7)   Purple (pH=8.5)   Blue (pH>8.5)

Figure 6-5   Color conversion of anthocyanins in different pH

3.1.2   Optical Activity

Flavanones, flavanonols, flavanols aglycones and their derivatives are optically active due to the chiral (手性的) carbons presented. The rotation value is related to their absolute stereochemistry (立体化学). In general, flavonoid glycosides always are optically active.

3.1.3   Solubility (溶解性)

The solubility of flavonoids differs from each other due to their structure types and forms (e.g. glycoside or aglycone, monosaccharides, disaccharides or trisaccharides, etc.).

(1) Solubility of Flavonoid aglycones

Flavonoid aglycones are generally low soluble or insoluble in water, but soluble in organic solvents, e.g. methanol, ethanol, ethyl acetate, chloroform, ethyl ether, and dilute alkali aqueous (稀碱液).

The structure skeletons of flavonoids affect their solubility in water. For example, flavones, flavonols, chalcones are difficult to dissolve in water due to their planar structure (平面结构). However, flavanones and flavanonols are easier soluble in water than that of flavones owing to their non-planar structure [e.g. similar to a semi-chair structure (半椅式结构）]. Isoflavones are also non-planar structure because of the interaction of ring B and the carbonyl group at C-4, and they are more hydrophilic (亲水的) than that of flavonoids with planar structures. Although anthocyanins are of planar structures, they are soluble in water because of their ionic (离子的) structure possessing salt properties.

Dihydroflavones　　R=H
Dihydroflavonols　　R=OH

The more hydroxyl groups bonding up to flavonoids, the higher hydrophilic they are. The methoxylation (甲氧基化) of hydroxyl groups increase their liposolubility (亲脂性). For example, most polyhydroxyl (多羟基) flavonoids are insoluble in petroleum ether, but polymethoxylated flavonoids, e.g. nobiletin (川陈皮素） (5, 6, 7, 8, 3′, 4′-hexamethoxylflavone) are soluble in petroleum ether.

(2) Solubility of Flavonoid Glycosides

Flavonoid glycosides are generally soluble in water, ethanol, methanol, acetone, n-butanol, etc., but they are uneasily soluble or insoluble in benzene, chloroform, ethyl ether and so on.

The numbers of monosaccharide and their location attached to flavonoid aglycones affect their solubility. In general, polysaccharide glycosides are more soluble in water than that of monoscharide glycosides. Owing to the stereochemistry exclusion (排斥) between the 3-O-glucosyl and the carbonyl group at C-4, the quercetin-3-O-glucoside is more soluble in water than that of quercetin-7-O-glucoside.

3.2　Chemical Properties

3.2.1　Acidity (酸性)

Flavonoids are generally acidic due to possessing phenolic hydroxyl groups. The number and substituted location of phenolic hydroxyl group in flavonoids affect their acidic intensity. The sequence of acidic intensity of phenolic hydroxyl in flavonoids is as below.

7, 4′-di-OH>7-or 4′-OH>general phenolic OH > 5-OH

Flavonoids which consist of 7, 4′-di-OH, 7-or 4′-OH, general phenolic-OH or 5-OH are soluble in 5% $NaHCO_3$, 5%Na_2CO_3, 1%NaOH and 5%NaOH, respectively. These chemical properties can be used for extraction, isolation and structure determination of flavonoids.

3.2.2　Basicity (碱性)

Flavonoids are slightly basicity because of a pair of non-bonded (未成键的) electrons of oxygen at γ-pyranone ring. They may dissolve in a concentrate inorganic acid (e.g. concentrate sulphuric acid, concentrate hydrochloric acid) via formation of oxonium salt (锌盐) (Figure 6-6). But the oxonium salt is unstable, and can be easily decomposed after diluting.

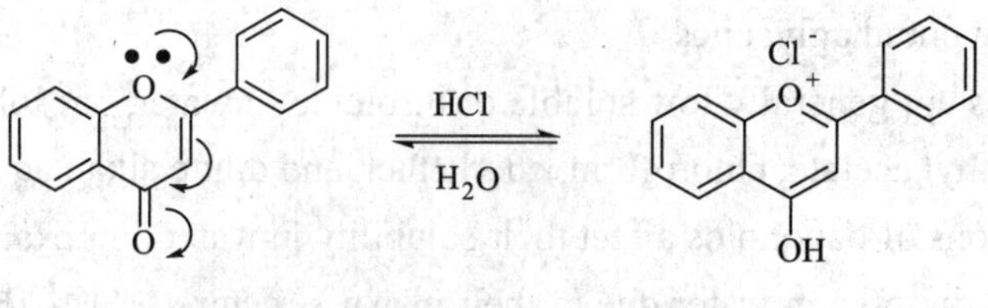

Figure 6-6   Oxonium salt of flavonoid

3.2.3   Color Reactions

Flavonoids can react with different chemical reagents due to the properties of phenolic hydroxyl and γ-pyranone structure. The common chemical reagents include reduction reagents, mental salts, bronic acid (硼酸), base, Lewis acid (路易斯酸) (e.g. $SbCl_5$), etc.

(1) HCl-Mg

Most of flavones, flavonols, flavanones and flavanonols have positive (阳性的) reaction with HCl-Mg and generally produce red color, and less are blue or green color. However, chalcones, aurones, catechin and most isoflavones have negative (阴性的) reaction with HCl-Mg.

It is worth noting that chalcones, anthocyanins and some aurones may change their color in concentrate hydrochloride acid. Therefore, the blank test is needed (without Mg powder added) to make sure the color change caused by HCl-Mg or just con. HCl.

(2) $NaBH_4$

$NaBH_4$ is a specific reductant (还原剂) to flavanones and flavanonols. Color red or purple-red indicates flavanones or flavanonols are presented. The reaction with $NaBH_4$ is negative in other flavonoid types.

(3) Complex Reaction with Metal Salt

Owing to consisting of the special group pairs, such as 3-OH/4-C=O, or 5-OH/4-C=O, or *ortho*- （邻位) di-OH, flavonoids can react with some metal salts, e.g. aluminum (铝) (Al), zirconium (锆)(Zr) and strontium (锶) (Sr) salt, to form colorful complexes (络合物) or precipitates (沉淀). Some complex salts have colorful fluorescence (荧光) under UV light.

① $AlCl_3$

This reaction can be carried out in a tube, on a TLC plate or a piece of filter paper. Most flavonoids complexes with aluminum salt (e.g. 1% $AlCl_3$) can present yellow color, and present bright yellow fluorescence under UV light. However, the complexes of 4′-hydroxyflavonols and 7, 4′-dihydroxyflavonols present blue fluorescence under UV light.

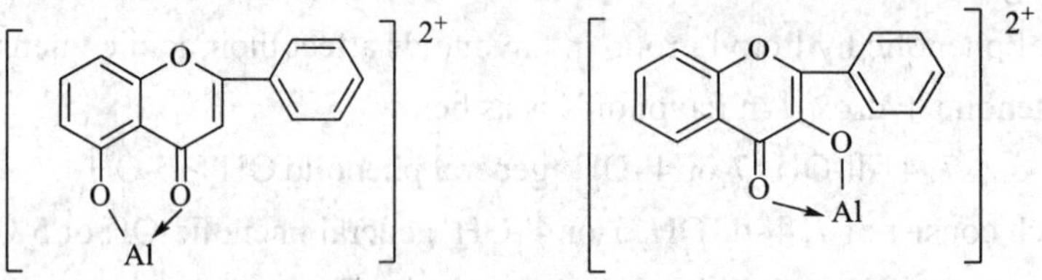

② $ZrOCl_2$-Citric Acid (枸橼酸)

This reaction is used to determine whether the 3- or 5- OH exists or not. Presence of color yellow in the test indicates that the complexes of 3- or 5-OH with $ZrOCl_2$ are formed. Then, 2% citric acid is added. If no color fading occurs, it indicates the existence of 3-OH or 3, 5-di-OH in flavonoids; otherwise, none 3-OH attached. This test may also be performed on a filter paper, and yellowish green fluorescence appears under UV light.

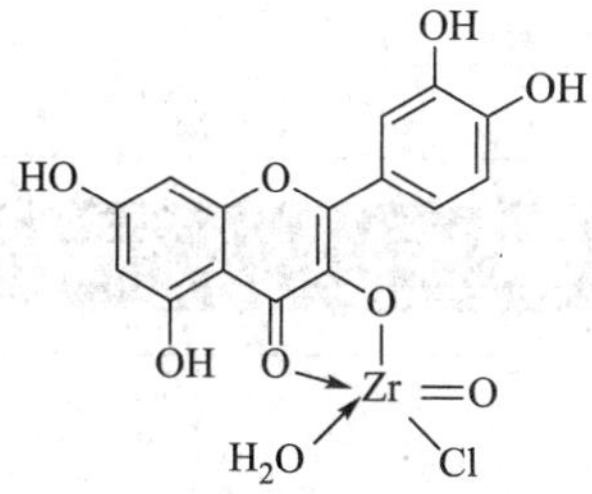

③ $SrCl_2$-$NH_3 \cdot H_2O$

Flavonoids with *ortho*-diphenolic hydroxyl groups reacting with $SrCl_2$-$NH_3 \cdot H_2O$ can present green, brown or black precipitates. This reaction can identify the *ortho*-diphenolic hydroxyl groups in flavonoids (Figure 6-7).

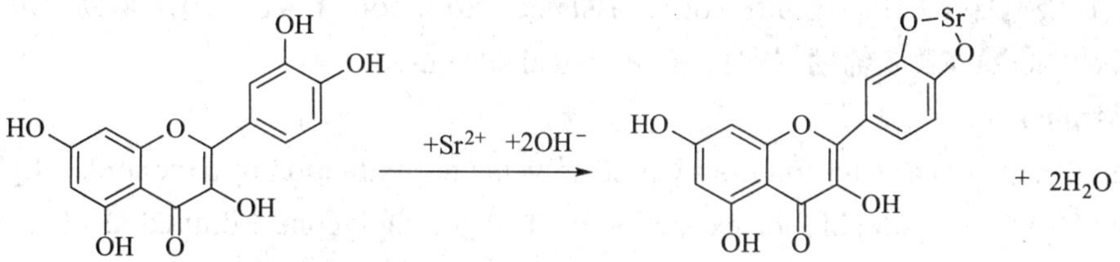

Figure 6-7 $SrCl_2$-$NH_3 \cdot H_2O$ reaction of flavonoids

④ $FeCl_3$

Flavonoids with phenolic hydroxyl groups can react with $FeCl_3$ in aqueous or methanol solution. The different color (e.g. color purple, green or blue) of this reaction can indicate the number and location of hydroxyl groups in flavonoids.

(4) Bronic Acid

5-Hydroxyflavone and 6′-hydroxychalcone can react with bronic acid to form a yellow complex in acidic solution. In general, the complex has yellowish green fluorescence in oxalic acid (草酸) solution, but no fluorescence in citric acid/acetone solution. Therefore, this reaction may be used to identify 5-hydroxyflavone and 6′-hydroxychalcone from other flavonoids.

(5) Base

Different flavonoid types present different color when they encounter base (Table 6-4).

Table 6-4   Color characters of reaction of flavonoids and base

Flavonoid type	Reaction condition	Color
flavones	cool or hot NaOH aqueous	red–orange
chalcones, aurones	NaOH aqueous	red–purple
flavanones	cool NaOH aqueous	red–orange
	hot NaOH aqueous	deep red–purplish red
flavonols	NaOH aqueous	yellow, then change to brown
flavonoids (*ortho*-tri-OH)	dilute NaOH aqueous	dark-green or blue-green precipitate

(6) $SbCl_5$

Chalcones reacting with 2% $SbCl_5$ in CCl_4 solution present red or purplish red precipitate, but flavones, flavanones and flavonols give color yellow or orange under the same condition. Therefore, this reaction can be used to identify chalcones.

4　Extraction and Isolation

4.1　Extraction

A frequently used method is solvent extraction. A suitable solvent should be chosen based on target compounds and co-existed (共存) impurities in the Chinese herb. In addition to solvent extraction method, other methods include supercritical fluid extraction (超临界提取) (SFE), pressurized liquid extraction (加压液相提取) (PLE), ultrasound-assisted extraction (UAE) (超声辅助提取) and micro-wave-assisted extraction (微波辅助提取) (MAE) can also be used.

4.1.1　Alcohol

Ethanol and methanol are the commonly used solvents for extraction of flavonoids. High concentrate alcohol (e.g. 90%–95%) is suitable for extraction of flavonoid aglycones, diluted alcohol (60%) is used to extract flavonoid glycosides. Maceration, reflux or percolation is generally used. For example, the total flavonoids of Ginkgo Folium is extracted by refluxing with 70% ethanol.

4.1.2　Hot Water

Hot water may be used for extraction of flavonoid glycosides. It is worth noting that hot water must be added to the Chinese herb materials to avoid the flavonoid glycosides hydrolyzed by enzyme and the boiling time and volume of hot water should also be considered in the process.

4.1.3　Alkali Aqueous Solution

Most of flavonoids are phenols, so they can dissolve in alkali aqueous or dilute alkali alcohol solution (e.g. 50% ethanol). The commonly used alkali includes NaOH, Na_2CO_3 or $Ca(OH)_2$. The alkali extract solution is further acidified, and then the flavonoid aglycones can be obtained as the precipitate form or by partitioning with organic solvent.

It is worth noting that a suitable intensity of alkali and acid should be considered. The strong alkali can destroy the skeleton when it is heated, and strong acid may make flavonoids to become a water-soluble oxonium salt. In general, bronic acid is used in order to avoid demage of ortho-dihydroxyl groups on flavonoids in this extraction process.

4.2　Isolation

Suitable isolation methods are chosen based on the polarity, acidity (酸度), molecular weight and the functional groups of flavonoids.

4.2.1　Solvent Partition (溶剂萃取)

The solvent partition method is generally used to isolate the crude extract. The procedure is that the crude extract is suspended in water, followed by ethyl ether, ethyl acetate or *n*-butanol to obtain flavonoid aglycones and flavonoid glycosides, respectively.

Petroleum ether is used to remove lipo-pigments (脂溶性色素), e.g. chlorophyll (叶绿素）and carotenes before partitioning with ethyl acetate. Water soluble impurities, e.g. protein and polysccacharides, can be removed by adding ethanol into the crude water solution.

4.2.2 Gradient pH Extraction

This method is used to separate flavonoid aglycones with different acidities. The procedure is similar to the separation of anthraquinones with different acidities. Dissolve the mixture of flavonoid aglycones in a lipophilic organic solvent, e.g. ethyl ether, followed by partitioning with 5%NaHCO$_3$, 5%Na$_2$CO$_3$, 0.2%NaOH, 4%NaOH aqueous to obtain 7, 4′-dihydroxyflavonoids, 7- or 4′-hydroxylflavonoids, general phenolic hydroxylflavonoids, and 5-hydroxylflavonoids, successively.

4.2.3 Chromatography

Conventional column chromatography (CC) is still widely used to isolate flavonoids. General support materials include silica gel, polyamide, Sephadex LH-20, macroporous resin and RP-C$_{18}$.

(1) Silica Gel CC

Silica gel is the most popular absorbent for separation of less polar flavonoids. The organic solvent system (e.g. chloroform-methanol with various ratio) is chosen for separation of flavonoids aglycones, but water containing solvent systems [e.g. chloroform-methanol-water (v/v, 80 : 20 : 1 or 80 : 18 : 2) and ethyl acetate-acetone-water (25 : 5 : 1)] are suitable for the isolation of flavonoid glycosides.

(2) Polyamide CC

Polyamide is suitable for separation of all flavonoids types. It should be thoroughly prewashed (预洗) with methanol and water before use. Moreover, it may require sieving to obtain adequately uniform particles in size.

The isolation mechanism of polyamide chromatography is the formation of hydrogen bond between the carbonyl group of the polyamide and phenolic hydroxyl of flavonoids. The adsorption intensity depends on the structure of flavonoids and the elution solvent system.

① In general, flavonoids with more hydroxyl groups have stronger adsorption intensity. For example, the adsorbability of morin with five hydroxyls is higher than that of kaempferol with four hydroxyls.

Morin   >   Kaempferol

② The position of hydroxyls on flavonoids also affects their adsorbability. The intramolecular hydrogen bond formation in flavonoids can decrease the adsorbability. For example, the adsorbability of daidzein is stronger than that of calycosin (卡米可新).

Daidzein   >   Calycosin

③ Flavonoids with more aromatic and conjugated double bonds will increase the adsorbability. For example, the adsorbability of hesperetin chalcone is stronger than that of hesperetin.

187

Hesperetin chalcone   Hesperetin

④The adsorbability of different types of flavonoids is ranked as: Flavonols > flavones > flavanonols > isoflavones.

⑤ Flavonoid glycosides are easily eluted than flavonoid aglycones in the water containing solvent system. In general, the eluted sequence is as below: Trisaccharide glycosides > disaccharide glycosides > monosaccharide glycosides > aglycones. However, the sequence is opposite in organic solvent system (e.g. chloroform-methanol). For example, the flavonoid aglycones will be eluted out of column first in organic solvent system.

⑥ The intensity of hydrogen bond formed between polyamide and flavonoids is the strongest in water, weaker in organic solvents and weakest in alkali aqueous solution. Therefore, the elute abilities of different solvents are ranked as: water < methanol or ethanol < acetone < dilute NaOH aqueous or ammonium (氨水) < formamide (甲酰胺) < DMF < urea (尿素) aqueous solution.

Chloroform-methanol-butanone-acetone (v/v, 40 : 20 : 5 : 1) or benzene-petroleum ether -butanone-methanol (v/v, 60 : 26 : 3.5 : 3.5) is generally used to isolate aglycones. The methanol-water or ethanol-water system is generally used to isolate flavonoid glycosides.

(3) Sephadex LH-20 CC

Sephadex LH-20 is ideally suitable for final clean-up of flavonoid aglycone and flavonoid glycoside which have been separated by using silica gel or polyamide. Methanol or ethanol or methanol-water or ethanol-water are generally used solvent systems in Sephadex LH-20 CC. Solution of 0.1M ammonia water (氨水), 0.5M NaCl, t-butanol-methanol (3 : 1) may also be used as solvent systems.

The flavonoid aglycones with more free hydroxyl groups will have stronger adsorbability on gel, and eluted out later from column; The flavonoid glycosides with larger molecular size will be eluted out earlier from column.

In Table 6-5, V_e and V_o represent the total eluted volume and volume retained (保留体积), respectively. The less V_e/V_o value indicates that the compound is easily eluted out from the column.

Table 6-5 V_e/V_o values of flavonoids on Sephadex LH-20 (methanol)

Flavonoids*	Substituted groups	V_e/V_o
kaempferol-3-O-galactosyl-rhamnosyl-7-O-rhamnoside	trisaccharide glycoside	3.3
quercetin-3-O-rutinoside	disaccharide glycoside	4.0
quercetin-3-O-rhanmoside	monosaccharide glycoside	4.9
apigenin	5, 7, 4′-tri-OH	5.3
luteolin	5, 7, 3′, 4′-tetra-OH	6.3
quercetin	3, 5, 7, 3′, 4′-penta-OH	8.3
myricetin	3, 5, 7, 3′, 4′, 5′,-hexa-OH	9.2

*Sample：2.5mg/0.5ml, flow rate 3–5ml/min.

(4) Macroporous Resin CC

Macroporous resin CC is generally used to purify a crude extract and obtain the total flavonoids. The types of resin, concentration of sample solution, elute solvent system, pH value of eluent and flow rate will affect the separation efficiency. The most commonly used solvent systems are methanol-water and ethanol-water.

(5) HPLC

Preparative HPLC is widely used for the isolation of flavonoids. In general, reversed-phase column, e.g. ODS is the first choice. The commonly used eluent systems are water-methanol or water-acetonitrile containing formic acid or acetic acid.

(6) Al_2O_3 CC

Al_2O_3 is less used for the separation of flavonoids due to the intensive interaction between flavonoids and aluminum. Just polymethoxylated flavonoids may use Al_2O_3 CC to do separation.

5　Identification

5.1　Physicochemical Identification

The types of flavonoids can be determined by color reactions. The reactions for flavonoids identification are listed in Table 6-6.

Table 6-6　Color reactions for flavonoids identification

Reaction	Color	Types of flavonoids
HCl-Mg	red	flavone(ol), flavanone(ol)
$NaBH_4$	red–purple	flavanone(ol)
$ZrOCl_2$-citric acid	yellow	3-OH or 5-OH flavone
$SrCl_2$-$NH_3 \cdot H_2O$	green–brown–black	vicinal hydroxyl groups
$SbCl_5/CCl_4$	red–purple	chalcone
Alkaline	red–purple	chalcone, aurone

5.2　TLC Identification

Silica gel and polyamide TLC are preferred to identify flavonoids.

5.2.1　Silica Gel

Silica gel TLC is mainly used to separate the less polar flavonoids. Commonly used development solvent systems are listed in Table 6-7.

Table 6-7　Commonly used development solvent systems for silica gel TLC

Flavonoids	Commonly used development solvent system (v/v)
flavonoid aglycones	toluene-methyl formate (甲酸甲酯) -formic acid (5 : 4 : 1), benzene-methanol (95 : 5)
	chloroform-methanol (8.5 : 1.5, 7 : 0.5), benzene-methanol-acetic acid (35 : 5 : 5)
flavonoid glycosides	n-butanol-acetic acid-water (3 : 1 : 1), formic acid-ethyl acetate-water (9 : 1 : 1),
	chloroform-ethyl acetate-acetone (5 : 1 : 4), chloroform-methanol-water (65 : 45 : 12)

5.2.2 Polyamide

Polyamide TLC is suitable to separate flavonoid aglycones and glycosides with free phenolic hydroxyl groups. The commonly used development solvent systems are listed in Table 6-8.

Table 6-8 Commonly used development solvent systems for polyamide TLC

Flavonoids	Commonly used development solvent system (v/v)
flavonoid aglycones	chloroform-methanol (94 : 6, 96 : 4), chloroform-methanol-butanone (12 : 2 : 1)
flavonoid glycosides	methanol-acetic acid-water (90 : 5 : 5), methanol-water (1 : 1), acetone-water (1 : 1)

6 Structure Elucidation

6.1 UV

UV spectroscopy is used to identify the flavonoid type and determine the location of substituted phenolic hydroxyl groups by adding diagnostic reagents (诊断试剂) into the test sample solution.

6.1.1 UV Spectrum in Methanol

The UV spectra of flavonoids are usually determined in methanol solution. However, 0.4M methanolic HCl is required for anthocyanins. The spectrum typically consists of two absorption bands: 240-280nm (Band II) and 300–400 (Band I). Band I is generated by ring B conjugated system, and Band II is produced by ring A conjugated system (Figure 6-8).

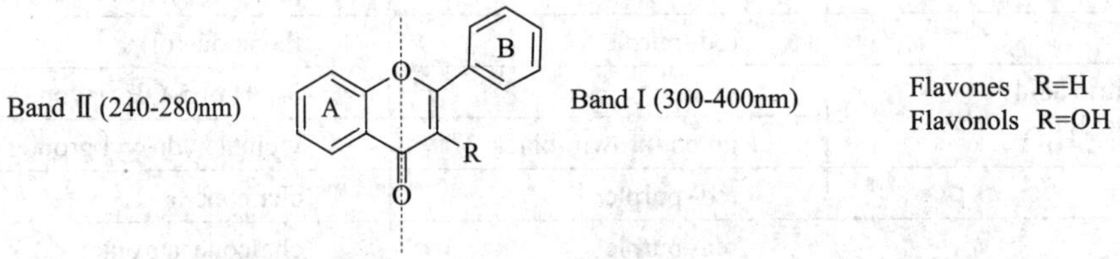

Band II (240-280nm) Band I (300-400nm) Flavones R=H
Flavonols R=OH

Figure 6-8 Basic UV absorption Band I and II of flavonoids

Different flavonoid types have different UV spectra (Table 6-9 and Figure 6-9).

Table 6-9 UV absorption bands of different flavonoid types

Flavonoid Types	λ_{nm} of Band II	λ_{nm} of Band I
flavones	250-280 (strong)	<350 (strong)
flavonols(3-OH free)	250-280 (strong)	>350 (strong)
isoflavones	<270 (strong)	310-330 (shoulder)
flavanones or flavanonols	>270 (strong)	300-330 (shoulder)
chalcones	220-270 (weak)	<390 (strong)
aurones	230-270 (weak)	>370 (strong)

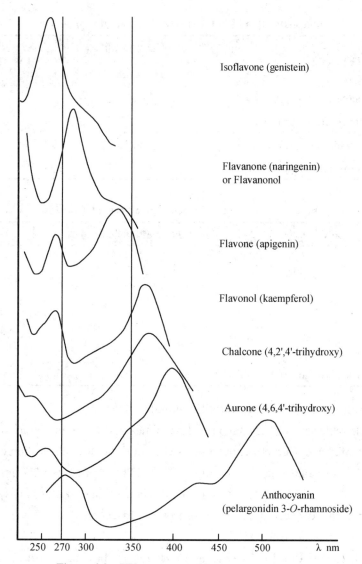

Figure 6-9　UV spectra of different flavonoid types

(1) UV Spectra of Flavones and Flavonols

The UV spectra of flavones and flavonols are similar to each other. The same characteristics are they both have two main bands in their UV spectra and Band Ⅱ is both located in 250-280nm. However, Band Ⅰ is different, Band Ⅰ of flavones locate at 304–350nm (less than 350nm), but Band Ⅰ of flavonols locate at 358-385nm (larger than 350nm). Therefore, it is easy to identify flavones and flavonols according to the location of Band Ⅰ.

Band Ⅰ and Ⅱ of flavones and flavonols are affected by the substituted oxygenated groups on ring B and A. In general, the more oxygenated groups substituted on ring B, the redder shift values of Band Ⅰ occur, but Band Ⅱ has no change (Table 6-10). The location of Band Ⅱ is mainly affected by the oxygenated level of ring A (Table 6-11).

Table 6-10   Band Ⅰ in UV spectra of different flavonoids

Flavonoids	Position of -OH		Band Ⅰ (nm)
	ring A and C	ring B	
3, 5, 7-trihydroxylflavone(galangin) (高良姜素)	3, 5, 7	—	359
3, 5, 7, 4′- tetrahydroxylflavone(kaempferol)	3, 5, 7	4′	367
3, 5, 7, 3′, 4′- pentahydroxylflavone(quercetin)	3, 5, 7	3′, 4′	370
3, 5, 7, 3′, 4′, 5′- hexahydroxylflavone(myricetin)	3, 5, 7	3′, 4′, 5′	374

Table 6-11   Band Ⅱ in UV spectra of different flavonoids

Flavonoids	Position of -OH on ring A	Band Ⅱ (nm)
flavones	—	250
5-hydroxylflavones	5	268
7-hydroxylflavones	7	252
5, 7-dihydroxylflavones	5, 7	268
5, 6, 7-trihydroxylflavones (baicalein)	5, 6, 7	274
5, 7, 8-trihydroxylflavones (norwogonin)	5, 7, 8	281

(2) Spectra of Isoflavones, Flavanones and Flavanonols

The same UV characteristics of isoflavones, flavanones and flavanonols are having strong Band Ⅱ absorption because of benzoyl structure, but a very weak or a shoulder-absorption of Band Ⅰ.

In general, Band Ⅱ of isoflavones is the range of 245–270nm (less than 270nm), while flavanones and flavanonols is the range of 270–295nm (larger than 270nm). Therefore, it is easy to tell isoflavones from flavanones and flavanonols according to the absorption of Band Ⅱ.

(3) Spectra of Chalcones and Aurones

The same UV characteristic of chalcones and aurones are having a strong Band Ⅰ and a weak Band Ⅱ absorption. Band Ⅰ absorption of chalcones is at the range of 340-390nm, but Band Ⅰ of aurones is at the range of 370–430nm.

6.1.2   UV Spectrum with Diagnostic Reagents

The common diagnostic reagents include NaOMe, NaOAc, NaOAc/H_3BO_3, $AlCl_3$ and $AlCl_3$/HCl. After measurement of the spectrum of the sample in methanol (the "MeOH" spectrum), the diagnostic reagents mentioned above are added and after mixing, the "diagnostic reagent" spectra are recorded. Comparing the "diagnostic reagent" spectrum with that of the "MeOH" spectrum, the detailed structure information will be acquired. The interpretation of these spectra is summarized in Table 6-12.

Table 6-12   Interpretation of "diagnostic reagents" spectra of flavonoids

Diagnostic reagents	Band Ⅰ	Band Ⅱ	Interpretation
NaOMe	+ 40–65nm, no decrease in intensity + 50–60nm, decrease in intensity		4'-OH 3-OH, no free 4'-OH
NaOAc		+ 5–20nm	7-OH
NaOAc/H_3BO_3	+ 12–30nm		B ring *ortho*-di-OH
		+ 5–10nm	A ring *ortho*-di-OH(6, 7,or 7, 8)

(continued)

Diagnostic reagents	Band Ⅰ	Band Ⅱ	Interpretation
AlCl₃ and AlCl₃/HCl	AlCl₃/HCl spectrum = AlCl₃ spectrum		no *ortho*-di-OH
	AlCl₃/HCl spectrum ≠ AlCl₃ spectrum		*ortho*-di-OH
	− 30–40nm		B ring *ortho*-di-OH
	− 50–60nm		A, B ring *ortho*-di-OH
	AlCl₃ spectrum = MeOH spectrum		no free 3-and (or)5-OH
	AlCl₃ spectrum ≠ MeOH spectrum		3-and (or)5-OH
	+ 35–55nm		5-OH
	+ 60nm		3-OH
	+ 50–60nm		3- and 5-OH
	+ 17–20nm		5-OH and 6-oxygenated

The UV spectra of rutin added with different diagnostic reagents are listed as below.

UV data (λ_{max} nm)

MeOH	259, 266sh, 299sh, 359
NaOMe	272, 327, 410
AlCl₃	275, 303sh, 433
AlCl₃/HCl	271, 300, 364sh, 402
NaOAc	271, 325, 393
NaOAc/H₃BO₃	262, 298, 387

6.2   NMR

NMR is a well-established and the most commonly used method for structure determination. The chemical shifts, coupling constants, multiplicity and intensity of resonances in 1D- and 2D-NMR allow for easy identification of the aglycone structure, the pattern of glycosylation and the sugar moiety.

6.2.1   ¹H-NMR

¹H-NMR is an important diagnostic tool to determine ① flavonoids type, e.g. isoflavones, flavanones and flavanonols; ② the oxygenation pattern (all three rings); ③ the information of substituted groups; ④ the number of monosaccharide.

The frequently used NMR solvents for flavonoids analyses include $(CD_3)_2CO$, CD_3OD and DMSO-d_6. Anthocyanins require the addition of an acid to ensure conversion to the flavylium form. CD_3OD has high solubility for both flavonoid aglycones and glycosides. In addition, CD_3OD combined with various proportions (2%–20%) of deuterotrifluoroacetic acid (CF_3COOD) is the most common NMR solvent used for anthocyanins.

The chemical shifts of TMS- ether derivatives of flavonoids in CCl_4 are listed in Table 6-13.

Table 6-13   Approximate chemical shift values (δ) for various flavonoid proton types

Chemical shifts (δ)	Proton types
0	tetramethylsilane(reference)
0–0.5	trimethylsilyl ether groups
c. 1.0	rhamnose C-CH₃ (broad doublet)

(continued)

Chemical shifts (δ)	Proton types
c. 1.7	prenyl $[\,—CH_2—CH = C(CH_3)_2\,]$ methyl groups
c. 2.0	acetate ($—OCOCH_3$) and aromatic C-CH$_3$
2–3	H-3 of flavanones (two proton-multiplet)
3.5–4.0	most sugar C-H
4.2–6.0	H-l of sugars
c. 6.0	methylenedioxy (O-CH$_2$-O), singlet
6.0–8.0	A- and B-ring protons
7.5–8.0	H-2 of isoflavones (singlet)
12–14	5-OH

(1) Protons on Ring C

The information of protons on ring C is useful for identification of the flavonoid types. The proton resonances of ring C are listed in Table 6-14.

Table 6-14 Proton resonances of ring C in flavonoids

Flavonoid type	H-2	H-3
flavones	no	6.30s
flavonols	no	no
isoflavones	7.60–7.80 s	no
flavanones	5.00–5.50 dd, J=11.0, 5.0Hz	about 2.80 dd, J=11.0, 5.0Hz
flavanonols	4.80–5.00 d, J=11.0Hz	4.10–4.30 d, J=11.0Hz
flavanonol-3-O-glycoside	5.00–5.60 d, J=11.0Hz	4.30–4.60 d, J=11.0Hz
chalcones	6.70–7.40 d, J=14~17.0Hz (H-α)	7.00–7.70 d, J=14–17.0Hz (H-β)
aurone	6.50–6.70 s (=CH—)	no

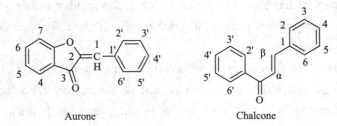

Aurone   Chalcone

(2) Protons on Ring A

① 5, 7-Dihydroxylflavonoids

The H-6 & H-8 resonances appear as a doublet (双重峰) (J=2.5Hz) at δ 5.70–6.90. The chemical shift of H-6 is up-field (高场) than that of H-8. The H-6 and H-8 will move to down-field (低场) after glycosidation of 7-hydroxyl group (Table 6-15).

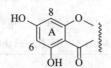

Table 6-15 Chemical shift values (δ) of H-6 & H-8 in 5, 7-dihydroxylflavonoids

5, 7-Dihydroxylflavonoids	δ_{H-6}	δ_{H-8}
flavones, flavonols, isoflavones	6.00–6.20 d	6.30–6.50 d
(flavones, flavonols, isoflavones) 7-O-glucoside	6.20–6.40 d	6.50–6.90 d
flavanones, flavanonols	5.75–5.95 d	5.90–6.10 d
(flavanones, flavanonols) 7-O-glucoside	5.90–6.10 d	6.10–6.40 d

② 7-Hydroxylflavonoids

The H-5 resonance locates at the deshielding (去屏蔽) zone of 4-C=O as doublet at δ 8.0 (J=ca. 8.0Hz). H-6 resonance appears as a dd signal due to coupling with H-5 and H-8. The H-8 signal appears as a doublet (J=ca. 2.0Hz) because of coupling with H-6 (Table 6-16).

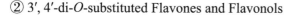

Table 6-16 Chemical shift values (δ) of H-5, H-6 & H-8 in 7-hydroxylflavonoids

7-Hydroxylflavonoids	δ_{H-5}	δ_{H-6}	δ_{H-8}
flavones, flavonols, isoflavones	7.90–8.20 d	6.70–7.10 dd	6.70–7.00 d
flavanones, flavanonols	7.70–7.90 d	6.40–6.50 dd	6.30–6.40 d

(3) Protons on Ring B

① 4′-O-substituted Flavonoids

The H-2′/H-6′ pair occurs in identical environments and is centered at ca. δ 7.7, while the H-3′ and H-5′ pair also occurs in identical environments, with a signal centered at ca. δ 6.8 (Table 6-17).

Table 6-17 Chemical shift values (δ) of H-2′, H-6′ and H-3′, H-5′ in 4′-O-substituted flavonoids

4′-O-Substituted flavonoids	$\delta_{H-2',6'}$	$\delta_{H-3',5'}$
flavanones	7.10–7.30 d	6.50–7.10 d
flavanonols	7.20–7.40 d	6.50–7.10 d
isoflavones	7.20–7.50 d	6.50–7.10 d
chalcones(H-2, 6 & H-3, 5)	7.40–7.60 d	6.50–7.10 d
aurones	7.60–7.80 d	6.50–7.10 d
flavones	7.70–7.90 d	6.50–7.10 d
flavonols	7.90–8.10 d	6.50–7.10 d

② 3′, 4′-di-O-substituted Flavones and Flavonols

H-5′ couple with H-6′ and its resonance appears as a doublet at δ 6.70–7.10 (J=ca. 8.0Hz). H-2′ signal appears as doublet at δ 7.2 (J=ca. 2.0Hz) due to the *meta*-coupling (间位偶合) with H-6′. The dd signal at δ 7.90 (J=ca. 8.0 and 2.0Hz) is assigned to H-6′, which is *meta*-coupling with H-2′ and *ortho*-coupling (邻位偶合) with H-5′ (Table 6-18).

Table 6-18　Chemical shift values (δ) of H-2′ and H-6′ in 3′, 4′-di-O-substituted flavonoids

3′, 4′-Di-*O*-substituted flavonoids	$\delta_{H-2'}$	$\delta_{H-6'}$
flavones(3′, 4′-OH & 3′-OH, 4′-OCH$_3$)	7.20–7.30 d	7.30–7.50 dd
flavonols(3′, 4′-OH & 3′-OH, 4′-OCH$_3$)	7.50–7.70 d	7.60–7.90 dd
flavonols(3′-OCH$_3$, 4′-OH)	7.60–7.80 d	7.40–7.60 dd
flavonols(3′, 4′-OH, 3-*O*-glycoside)	7.20–7.50 d	7.30–7.70 dd

③ 3′, 4′, 5′-tri-*O*-substituted Flavonoids

In 3′, 4′, 5′-trihydroxylflavonoids, H-2′, 6′ signals appear as a singlet at δ 6.5–7.50. When 3′ or 5′-OH is substituted with methyl or sugar moiety, the H-2′, 6′ signals appear as a doublet (J=ca. 2.0Hz).

(4) Protons of Saccharide Moiety

① Monosaccharide glycosides

The anomeric proton (端基质子) (H-1″) is observed as a doublet at downfield compared to those of other protons in the saccharide. The chemical shift of anomeric proton (H-1″) is related to the attached position and type of the saccharide. The detailed anomeric proton resonances for various flavonoid monosaccharide glycosides are listed in Table 6-19.

Table 6-19　Chemical shifts values (δ) of H-1″ in flavonoid monosaccharide glycosides

Flavonoid monosaccharide glycosides	$\delta_{H-1''}$
flavones 7-*O*-glucoside	4.80–5.20 d
flavones 4′-*O*-glucoside	4.80–5.20 d
flavones 5-*O*-glucoside	4.80–5.20 d
flavones 6-and 8-*C*-glycoside	4.80–5.20 d
flavonols 3-*O*-glucoside	5.70–6.00 d
flavonols 3-*O*-rhamnoside	5.00–5.10 d
flavonols 7-*O*-rhamnoside	5.10–5.30 d
flavanonols 3-*O*-glucoside	4.10–4.30 d
flavanonols 3-*O*-rhamnoside	4.00–4.20 d

② Di-*O*-glycosides

The common flavonoid di-*O*-glycosides consisting of glucose and rhamnose have two types: aglycone-rutinosyl, e.g. [aglycone-*O*-β-D-glucosyl(6 → 1)-α-L-rhamnose]; aglycone-neohesperidosyl, e.g.[aglycone-*O*-β-D-glucosyl(2 → 1)-α-L-rhamnose].

The anomeric proton (H-1‴) of terminal sugar moieties appear at up-field compared to that of anomeric proton (H-1″) because of a long distance from the flavonoid skeleton. The linked position of the rhamnose can be determined according to the chemical shift values of anomeric proton (H-1‴) and rha-CH_3 (H-6‴) (Table 6-20).

Table 6-20   Chemical shift values (δ) of H-1‴and H-6‴ of rhamnose in di-*O*-glycosides

Sugar moiety	H-1‴	H-6‴
rutinosyl	4.20–4.40 (d, *J*=2.0Hz)	0.70–1.00 (d)
neohesperidosyl	4.90–5.00 (d, *J*=2.0Hz)	1.10–1.30 (d)

(5) Other Protons on Flavonoids

① Phenolic Hydroxyl Protons

The phenolic -OH proton signals of flavonoids can be detected in DMSO-d_6 solvent, which appear at δ12.99(5-OH), δ10.01(4′-OH) and δ9.42(3′-OH), respectively, and disappear after adding of D_2O.

② Protons of Methyl attached to C-6 and C-8

The chemical shifts of CH_3-6 appear at up-field than that of CH_3-8 (about 0.2). For example, the CH_3-6 of isoflavones appears at δ2.04–2.27 and the CH_3-8 appears at δ2.14–2.45.

③ Methoxyl Protons

Methoxyl protons appear as a singlet at the range of δ3.50–4.10, which is easily identified with the saccharide protons.

④ Protons of Acetyl Group

The protons of acetyl group on saccharide moiety appear as a singlet at δ1.65–2.10. However, the protons of phenolic acetyl group on the flavonoid skeleton appear as a singlet at δ2.30–2.50.

6.2.2 ^{13}C-NMR

^{13}C-NMR is a very powerful technique for structure determination. The typical applications include ① establishment of the total number of carbon atoms, the number of oxygenated carbons on the flavonoid skeleton and the number of carbons in the saccharide moiety; ② determination of the glycosidic linkage position; ③ identification of *C*-(and *O*-) linked glycosides; ④ identification of substituents and the position of substituted.

(1) Determination of Flavonoid Types

The resonances of the three-carbon between ring A and B are good guide to the flavonoid types. The detailed ^{13}C NMR data of various flavonoid types are listed in Table 6-21.

Table 6-21   Detailed ^{13}C-NMR data of the three-carbon between ring A and B

Flavonoid type	C=O	C-2	C-3
flavones	176.3–184.0 (s)	160.0–165.0 (s)	103.0–111.8 (d)
flavonols	172.0–177.0 (s)	145.0–150.0 (s)	136.0–139.0 (s)
isoflavones	174.5–181.0 (s)	149.8–155.4 (d)	122.3–125.9 (s)

(continued)

Flavonoid type	C=O	C-2	C-3
flavanones	189.5–195.5 (s)	75.0–80.3 (d)	42.8–44.6 (t)
flavanonols	188.0–197.0 (s)	82.7 (d)	71.2 (d)
chalcones*	188.6–194.6 (s)	136.9–145.4 (d)*	116.6–128.1 (d)*
aurones	182.5–182.7 (s)	146.1–147.7 (s)	111.6–111.9 (d) (=CH—)

* In chalcones, the C-2 as C-β, C-3 as C-α.

(2) Determination of Substituted Pattern

The detailed ^{13}C-NMR data of unsubstituted flavone are completely assigned as below.

① Effects of Substituents

When the substituted group (X) is bonding up to ring B, the effect of chemical shift is similar to that of the benzene derivatives (Table 6-22).

Table 6-22　Chemical shifts of carbons on ring B after substituted by X

X	Z_i	Z_o	Z_m	Z_p
—OH	+26.0	−12.8	+1.6	−7.1
—OCH$_3$	+31.4	−14.4	+1.0	−7.8

The 5-hydroxyl group substituted on ring A not only affects on the chemical shift values of ring A, but also increases the chemical shift value of C-4 and C-2 with 4.5 and 0.87, respectively, and decreases the chemical shift value of C-3 (about 1.99).

② C-6 and C-8 Characteristics of 5, 7-Dihydroxylflavones

The C-6 and C-8 signals of most 5, 7-dihydroxylflavones appear in the range of δ 90–100 , and the shift value of C-6 is larger than that of C-8. The shift value difference between C-6 and C-8 is about 0.9 in flavanones, but is about 4.8 in flavones and flavonols.

The chemical shift values of C-6, C-8 can be used to determine whether the alkyl or aromatic groups substituted on C-6 and C-8 or not. For example, the δ values of the C-6 and C-8 which have attached to a methyl group will move down-field 6.0–10.0, while the δ value of unsubstituted C-6 and C-8 will have a small change in comparing with that of the skeleton.

③ Position of Saccharide Moiety in O-flavonoid Glycosides

When flavonoids are bonded with saccharides, all the signals of related carbons both on the flavonoids and the saccharide moieties will be shifted. The changes are related to the kinds of saccharide and their attached positions.

In O-glucosides, the anomeric carbon of saccharide is shifted to down-field 4–6. The anomeric carbon signals of 7- or 2′ - or 3′- or 4′-O-glucosides are in the range of δ 100.0–102.5. However, the anomeric carbon signals of 5-*O*-glucoside and 7-*O*-rhamnoside are in the range of δ98.0–109.0.

The glycosylation shifts of aglycones are used to determine the position of saccharide in flavonoid glycosides. In *O*-glucosides, δ value of the carbons attached to saccharide are shifted to up-field as much as 2, while the δ values of the adjacent (邻近的) carbons (the *ortho*-carbons) are shifted to down-field about 1–4. In 3-*O*-glycoside, the glycosidation shift value of C-2 is larger than that of the *ortho*-carbons. The glycosidation of 5-OH will destroy the hydrogen-bond between 4-C=O and 5-OH, and bring large effect on the carbons of ring C. In this case, δC-2 and C-4 are shifted to up-field obviously, but δC-3 is shifted to down-field (Table 6-23).

Table 6-23　^{13}C-NMR glycosidation shift values (δ) of flavonoides

Positions	The mean glycosidation shift values of flavonoid														
	2	3	4	5	6	7	8	9	10	1'	2'	3'	4'	5'	6'
7-*O*-glucose					+0.8	−1.4	+1.1		+1.7						
7-*O*-rhamnose					+0.8	−2.4	+1.0		+1.7						
3-*O*-glucose	+9.2	−2.1	+1.5	+0.4					+1.0	−0.8	+1.1	−0.3	+0.7		+1.5
3-*O*-rhamnose	+10.3	−1.1	+2.0	+0.6					+1.1						
5-*O*-glucose	−2.8	+2.2	−6.0	−2.7	+4.4	−3.0	+3.2	+1.4	+4.3	−1.3	−1.2	−0.4	−0.8	−1.0	−1.2
3'-*O*-glucose	−0.5	+0.4									+1.6	0	+1.4	+0.4	+3.2
4'-*O*-glucose	+0.1		+1.0							+3.7	+0.4	+2.0	−1.2	+1.4	0

C-glycosylations cause the aromatic ring carbon down-field shift about 10, but only a little change to the adjacent carbons on saccharide.

6.3　MS

MS is a very sensitive analytical method used to identify flavonoids or to perform partial structural characterization by using microgram amounts of sample. In addition to giving accurate molecular masses, fragmentation patterns may provide:① structural information about the nature of the aglycones and substituents (saccharides, acyl groups, etc.); ② glycosidic linkages and aglycone substitution positions; ③ even some stereochemical information.

The highest energy transfer occurs during EI-MS of flavonoid aglycones, and the molecular ion ([M]$^+$) is normally observed as a base peak (基峰). But most of flavonoid glycosides are polar, nonvolatile and often thermally labile (热不稳定的). Therefore, conventional EI-MS and CI-MS are not suitable because they require flavonoids to be in the gas phase for ionization. At present, ESI-MS, FAB-MS and FD-MS (场致裂解质谱) techniques are commonly used to analyze flavonoid glycosides.

6.3.1　Interpretation EI-MS of Flavonoid aglycone

Commonly encountered fragments in flavonoid aglycones are shown in Figure 6-10.

The molecular ion of a flavonoid aglycone can undergo fission (裂解) in different ways, one by the reverse Diels-Alder (RDA) route to yield A$_1$ and B$_1$ fragments, the second route to yield B$_2$ fragment from B-ring and fragments arising from A- and C-ring. Other fragments that may be appear include [A$_1$+H]$^+$, the ethylenic analogue of B$_1$, [M-l]$^+$, [M-15]$^+$(-CH$_3$), [M-17]$^+$(-OH), [M-18]$^+$(-H$_2$O), [M-28]$^+$(CO),

$[M-43]^+(- CH_3CO)$ and $[M-55]^+ [- CH_2-CH=C(CH_3)_2]$(see Figure 6-11).

The dominant route of decomposition depends on the nature of the flavonoid: flavones and isoflavones tend to give $(A_1+H)^+$ and B_1^+ fragments, flavonols give A_1^+ and B_2^+ fragments, flavanones give A_1 and $(B_1+2H)^+$ fragments, and flavanonols give A_1^+ and $(B_1+H_2O)^+$ fragments.

Molecular ion (M^+) normally appears as a major peak in the EI-MS of flavonoid aglycone. M^+ must be an even mass number and it must represent a reasonable molecular weight (the molecular weight of the basic flavonoid nucleus, i.e. flavones, isoflavones and aurones, 222; Flavanones and chalcones, 224; Flavonols, 238; Flavanonols, 240; and the 16 mass units must be added for each —OH, the 30 mass units for each —OCH₃).

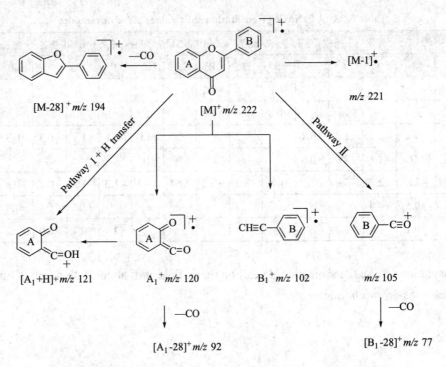

Figure 6-10   Common fragments of flavonoid aglycone in EI-MS

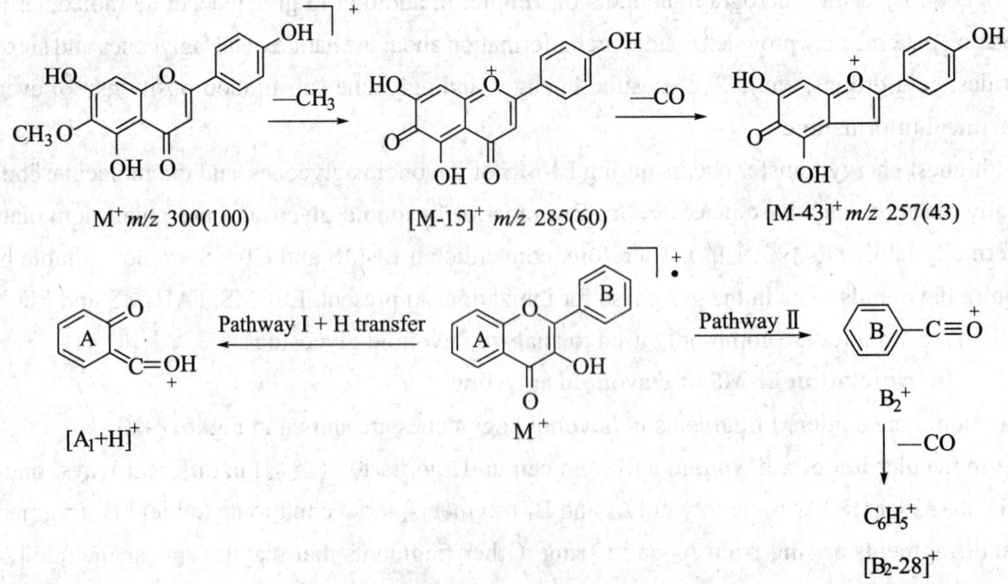

Figure 6-11   Common fragments of flavones and flavonols

6.3.2　Interpretation of Flavonoid Glycosides MS

In the past, EI-MS was used to analyze the permethyl (PM) or perdeuteromethyl (PDM) ethers of flavonoid glycosides to acquire the structure information. At present, the flavonoid glycosides can be directly analyzed by the ESI-MS, FAB-MS, FD-MS methods.

FAB-MS has been widely used for the characterization of flavonoid glycosides dissolved in a variety of matrices and normally involve the use of xenon or argon atoms for bombardment. The quasi-molecular ion (准分子离子) $[M+H]^+$, $[M+Na]^+$, $[M+K]^+$ signals are commonly observed. HR-FAB-MS can provide exact masses and for determining the molecule formula of flavonoid glycosides.

ESI is the most popular technique used to analyze polar and nonvolatile flavonoid glycosides. This technique permits the detection of the molecular ion, either as a protonated ion, $[M+H]^+$ or and adduct, $[M+Na]^+$ in positive model (正离子模式), or as a deprotonated ion, $[M-H]^-$ in negative model (负离子模式), and causes only moderate fragmentation of the molecule which occurs in other higher energy types of ionization techniques. It is commonly used to analyze large molecular weight flavonoid glycosides.

FD-MS is the first technique employed for the direct analysis of polar flavonoid glycosides. It can provide molecular mass data and little structural fragment information.

6.4　An Example for Structural Determination of Flavonoids

Compound X, a slight yellow crystal, mp. 260–262°C, was obtained from *Chryanthemum morifolium* (杭白菊). The $[M]^+$ peak of X at m/z 446.4056 in the HR-EIMS corresponds to the molecular formula of $C_{22}H_{22}O_{10}$. The molecular formula shows twelve degrees of unsaturation (不饱和度). The reaction with HCl/Mg is red. So it indicates that X is a flavone, flavonol, flavanone or flavanonol type. Molish reaction of X is positive, and a glucose unit is detected in its hydrolyzed product. $ZrOCl_2$-citric acid reaction indicates that the 5-OH but none 3-OH included in X.

All the information above suggests compound X is a flavone monoglucoside with 5-OH.

The UV spectrum (in methanol) of X shows the typical UV characteristics of flavone with λ_{max} at 267nm (Band Ⅱ) and 324nm (Band Ⅰ). The main EI-MS fragments of X are listed in Figure 6-12. The ions of aglycone at *m/z* 284 (100), 152 $[A_1]^+$, and 132 $[B_1]^+$ indicate that two hydroxyl groups on ring A of X and one methoxyl on ring B of X. The IR (KBr) signals at 3248, 3102, 1657, 1616, 1584, 1469, 975, 832, 770cm^{-1} suggest that hydroxyl group, unsaturated C=O, and phenyl group are presented in X.

The NMR data are listed in Table 6-24. The proton signal at δ 12.92 (1H, s) is presented from 5-OH, which appears at down-field due to the hydrogen bond formed with 4-C=O, and disappears after addition of D_2O. The proton signal at δ 6.95(1H,s) is assigned to H-3. A pair of symmetric *ortho*-coupled protons δ 8.05 (2H, d,*J*=8.9Hz) and δ 7.14(2H, d,*J*=8.9Hz) is characteristics of a C-4′ substituted B-ring. The evidences of signal δ 3.87(3H, s) and the fragment ions 132 $[B_1]^+$ in EI-MS prove a methoxyl group substituted at C-4′ position. H-8 and H-6 signals are observed as doublet at δ 6.86 (1H,d,*J*=1.8Hz) and 6.64 (1H,d,*J*=1.8Hz), respectively. Therefore, di-*O*-substituted groups are at C-5, 7 positions of ring A.

The 5-OH occurrence indicates 7-*O*-glucosyl group attached in X. The signal at δ 5.08 (1H, d, *J*=7.4Hz) is assigned to the anomeric proton of glucose. The configuration of glucose is determined as β type due to the coupling constant of anomeric proton $J_{H1''-2''}$ is 7.4Hz.

^{13}C-NMR signals of δ 182.17(C=O), 163.97(C-2) and 103.94(C-3) correspond to a flavone skeleton. A group of carbon signals of δ 100.12, 77.34, 76.57, 73.27, 69.66 and 60.81 are assigned to the glucose

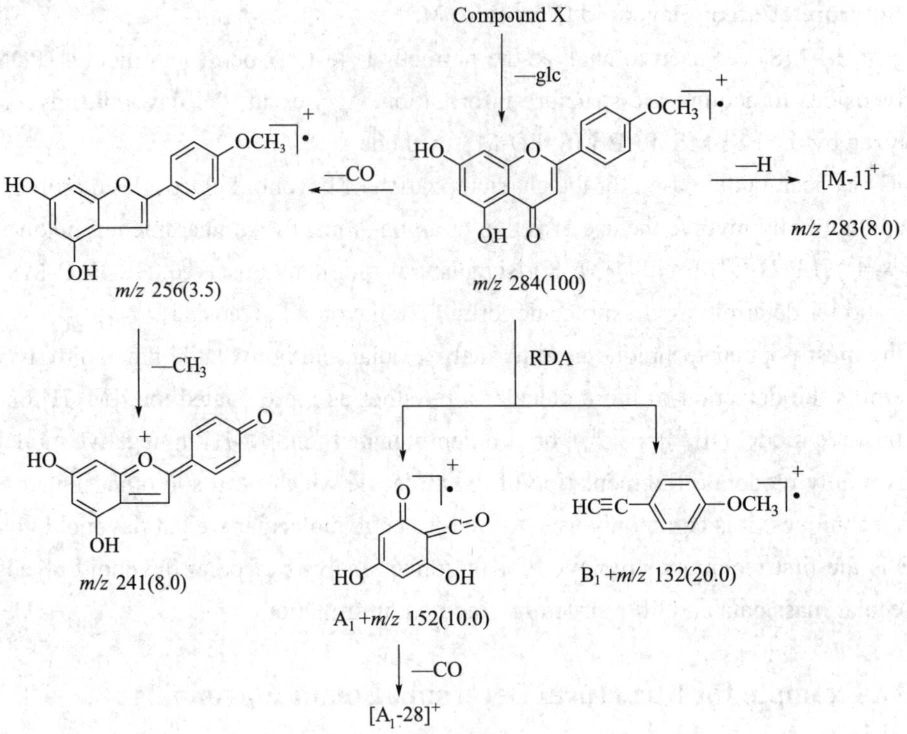

Figure 6-12   Fragment pathway of compound F₁

unit. The other ¹³C-NMR data are listed in Table 6-24.

All information mentioned above indicates that X is acacetin-7-*O-β*-D-glucoside.

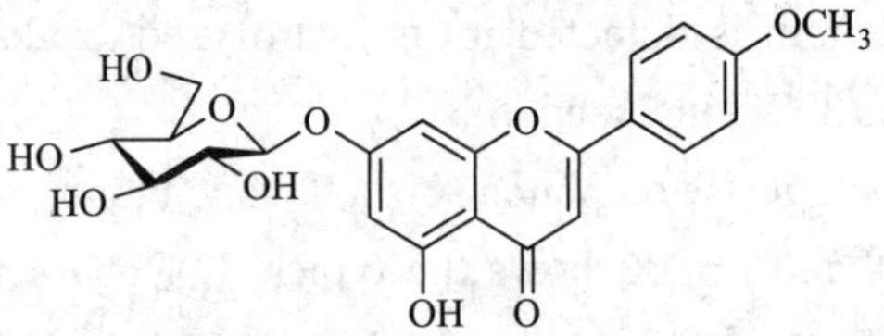

Table 6-24   Detailed NMR data for compound X (DMSO-*d₆*)

Position	δ_C	δ_H	Position	δ_C	δ_H
2	163.97		1′	122.83	
3	103.94	6.95(1H, s)	2′	128.56	8.05 (2H，d, J=8.9Hz, 2′, 6′-H)
4	182.17		3′	114.76	7.14 (2H，d，J=8.9Hz, 3′, 5′-H)
5	162.62		4′	161.27	
6	99.74	6.46(1H,d,J=1.8Hz)	5′	114.76	7.14 (2H，d，J=8.9Hz, 3′, 5′-H)
7	163.18		6′	128.56	8.05 (2H，d,J=8.9Hz, 2′, 6′-H)
8	95.11	6.86(1H,d,J=1.8Hz)	1″	100.12	5.08 (1H，d，J=7.4Hz)
9	157.12		2″	73.27	3.18–3.73 (6H, m, protons on glucose); 4.60–5.41 (4H, m, —OH protons on glucose, disappear after adding D₂O)
10	105.55		3″	76.57	
OCH₃	55.73	3.87(3H, s)	4″	69.66	
C₅-OH		12.92 (1H, s, disappear after adding D₂O)	5″	77.34	
			6″	60.81	

7　Examples of Chinese Herbs Containing Flavonoids

7.1　Scutellariae Radix（黄芩）

7.1.1　Introduction

(1) Biological Source

Scutellariae Radix is the dried root of *Scutellaria baicalensis* Georgi.(Fam. Labiatae)

(2) Property, Flavor and Channels Entered

Property and Flavor: cold, bitter.

Channels Entered: lung, gallbladder, spleen, large intestine, small intestine.

(3) Actions& Indications

To clear heat and dry dampness, purge fire to remove toxin, stop bleeding, prevent miscarriage. For dampness-warmth, summer heat-dampness, vomiting and nausea, oppression in the chest, dampness-heat stuffiness and fullness, diarrhea and dysentery, jaundice, cough caused by lung-heat, high fever with vexation and thirst, swelling abscess, blood heat with hematemesis, sore and toxin, threatened abortion.

(4) Pharmacological Activities

The pharmacological activities associated with Scutellariae Radix include Central Nervous System (CNS) actions, hepatoprotective actions, antiviral, antimicrobial, anti-inflammatory, anti-oxidation effects, etc.

7.1.2　Main Chemical Constituents

The main chemical constituents of Scutellariae Radix include flavonoids (flavones and flavone glycosides, flavanones, chalcones), volatile oils and others. Some representative compounds are listed in Table 6-25.

Table 6-25　Chemical constituents of Scutellariae Radix

Type	Compounds
flavones	baicalein, wogonin, norwogonin, 7-methoxynorwogonin, chrysin, oroxylin A
favanones	7, 2′, 6′-trihydroxy-5-methoxy-flavanone, 5, 7, 4′-trihydroxy-6-methoxyflavanone
flavonoid glycosides	baicalin, dihydrobaicalin, scutellarin, wogonoside, chrysin-7-*O*-glucuronide, norwogonin-7-*O*-glucuronide, wogonin-5-*O*-β-D-glucoside
chalcones	2, 6, 2′, 4′-tetrahydroxy-6-methoxychalcone, 7, 2′, 6′-trihydroxy-5-methoxychalcone
others	phenylethanol glycosides, volatile oils, amino acids, steroids

The main flavonoids in Scutellariae Radix include baicalein (黄芩素), baicalin ,wogonin (汉黄芩素), wogonoside (汉黄芩苷), etc. Baicalin as the main active component has various pharmacological activities, including anti-HIV, anti-inflammatory, anti-oxidant, anti-bacterial, antifibrogenic and anti-cancer effects.

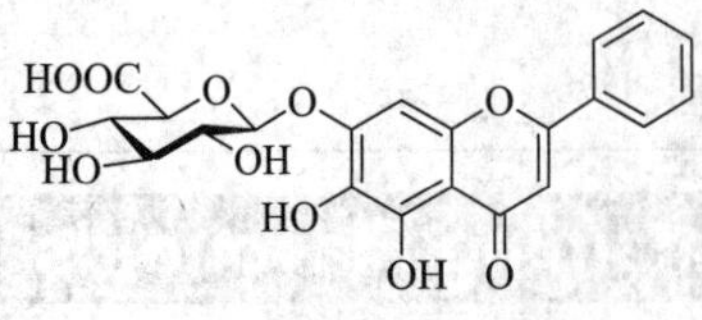

Baicalin

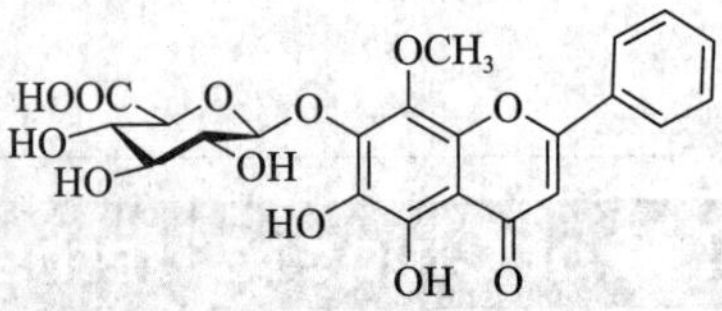

Wogonoside

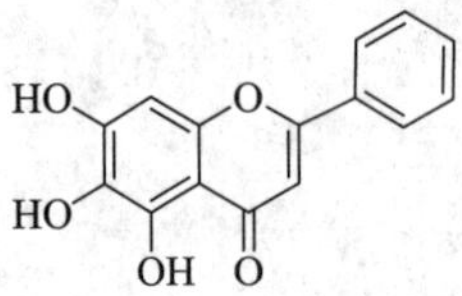

Baicalein

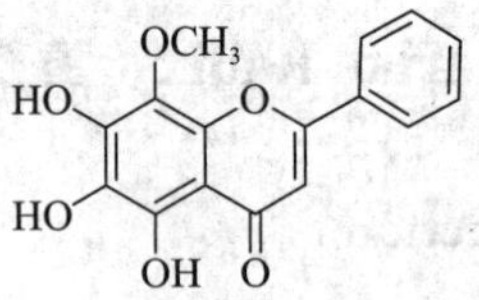

Wogonin

Baicalin is a slight yellow crystal, soluble in water, diluted ethanol, hot acetic acid. Owing to the *ortho*-trihydroxyl attached to ring A of baicalein, the aglycone of baicalin, is unstable and can be oxidized to a green quinone derivative (Figure 6-13). Therefore, it is needed to protect Scutellariae Radix from the degradation of enzyme during preparation and storage.

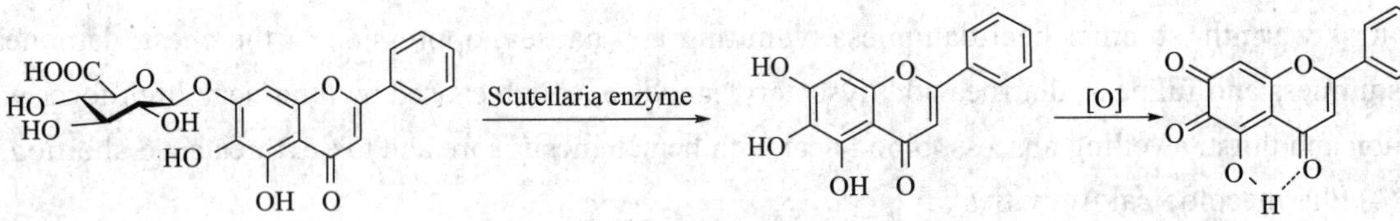

Baicalin   Scutellaria enzyme   Baicalein (yellow)   [O]   green

Figure 6-13   Enzymolysis (酶解) of baicalin

The extraction and purification procedure for baicalin is shown in Figure 6-14.

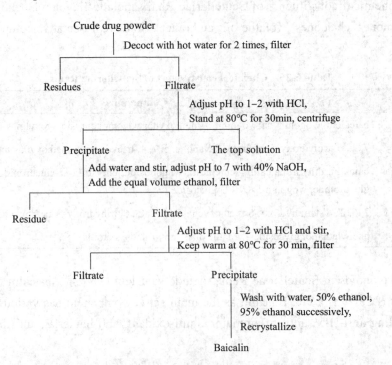

Crude drug powder

Decoct with hot water for 2 times, filter

Residues   Filtrate

Adjust pH to 1–2 with HCl,
Stand at 80°C for 30min, centrifuge

Precipitate   The top solution

Add water and stir, adjust pH to 7 with 40% NaOH,
Add the equal volume ethanol, filter

Residue   Filtrate

Adjust pH to 1–2 with HCl and stir,
Keep warm at 80°C for 30 min, filter

Filtrate   Precipitate

Wash with water, 50% ethanol,
95% ethanol successively,
Recrystallize

Baicalin

Figure 6-14   Extraction and purification procedure for baicalin

7.1.3 Quality Control Standards

(1) TLC Identification

Stationary Phase: polyamide plate.

Standard: authentic crude drug.

Development System: toluene-ethyl acetate-methanol-formic acid (10 : 3 : 1 : 2, v/v), pre-saturated for 30min.

Visualization: 365nm UV light.

(2) Tests

Water: not more than 12.0%.

Total Ash: not more than 6.0%.

Heavy Metals and Other Harmful Elements: Pb $\leqslant$ 5 ppm; Cd $\leqslant$ 0.3 ppm; As $\leqslant$ 2 ppm; Hg $\leqslant$ 0.2 ppm; Cu $\leqslant$ 20 ppm.

Extract (diluted ethanol): not less than 40.0%.

(3) Assay

Baicalin: not less than 9.0% (HPLC).

7.2 Puerariae Lobatae Radix (葛根)

7.2.1 Introduciton

(1) Biological Source

Puerariae Lobatae Radix is the dried root of *Pueraria lobata* (Willd.)Ohwi.(Fam. Leguminosae)

(2) Property, Flavor and Channels Entered

Property and Flavor: cool; sweet, pungent.

Channels Entered: spleen, stomach, lung.

(3) Actions& Indications

To release the flesh and reduce fever, increase body fluid to quench thirst, promote eruption, upraise the middle qi to quench diarrhea, unblock the meridian, activate collaterals, remove wine toxin. For external contraction with fever and headache, the stiff and pain nape and neck, wasting-thirst, unerupted measles, diarrhea, heat dysentery, dizziness and headache, hemiplegia caused by wind-stroke, chest impediment and heart pain, wine toxin damaging the middle.

(4) Pharmacological Activities

The pharmacological activities associated with Puerariae Lobatae Radix include anti-hypertension, cardioprotective effect, improving cerebral vessels and peripheral circulation, effecting on smooth muscle, anti-inflammatory, anti-cancer, etc.

7.2.2 Main Chemical Constituents

The chemical constituents of Puerariae Lobatae Radix include flavonoids, triterpenoids, coumarins, organic acids, etc. The examples are listed in Table 6-26.

Table 6-26 Main chemical constitutes of Puerariae Lobatae Radix

Types	Main chemical constitutes
flavonoids	daidzein, daidzin, puerarin, 4′-methoxypuerarin, diadzein-7-(6-O-malony)-glucoside, daidzein-4′, 7-diglucoside, 4′, 7-dihydroxyisoflavone, genistein, puerarin-7-xyloside, 4′-methoxypuerarin, 3′-hydroxypuerarin, 3′-methoxypuerarin

(continued)

Types	Main chemical constitutes
triterpenoids	sophoradiol, cantoniensistriol, soyasapogenol A, B, kudzusapogenol A, C
coumarins	6, 7-dimethoxycoumarin , puerarol
organic acids	succinic acid, behenic acid, carnaubic acid, arachidic acid, docosanoic acid
others	allantoin, 5-methylhydantion, tuberosin, cholin chloride, glycerol-1-monotetrecosanoate, β-sitosterol

The main constituents of Puerariae Lobatae Radix are isoflavones, such as daidzien, daidzin and puerarin, etc.

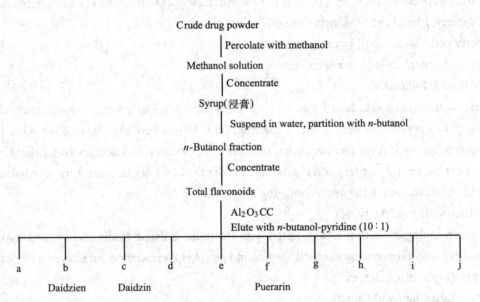

Daidzien $R_1=R_2=R_3=H$
Daidzin $R_1=R_3=H$ $R_2=glc$
Puerarin $R_2=R_3=H$ $R_1=glc$

Daidzein, daidzin and puerarin as phytoestrogen（植物雌激素）can protect primary neurons from β-amyloid toxicity and also have anti-inflammation, anti-breast cancer and anti-apoptosis effects, etc. Their isolation scheme is shown in Figure 6-15.

Crude drug powder
Percolate with methanol
Methanol solution
Concentrate
Syrup(浸膏)
Suspend in water, partition with n-butanol
n-Butanol fraction
Concentrate
Total flavonoids
Al$_2$O$_3$CC
Elute with n-butanol-pyridine (10 : 1)

a   b   c   d   e   f   g   h   i   j

Daidzien   Daidzin   Puerarin

Figure 6-15   Isolation of daidzein, daidzin and puerarin from Puerariae Lobatae Radix

Puerariae Lobatae Radix also contains triterpenoids, e.g. sophoradiol (槐花二醇), cantoniensistriol (广东相思子三醇), soyasapogenol (大豆皂醇) A, B, kudzusapogenol (葛根皂醇) A, C, etc. Sophoradiol and soyasapogenol A, B have anti-herpes virus activity.

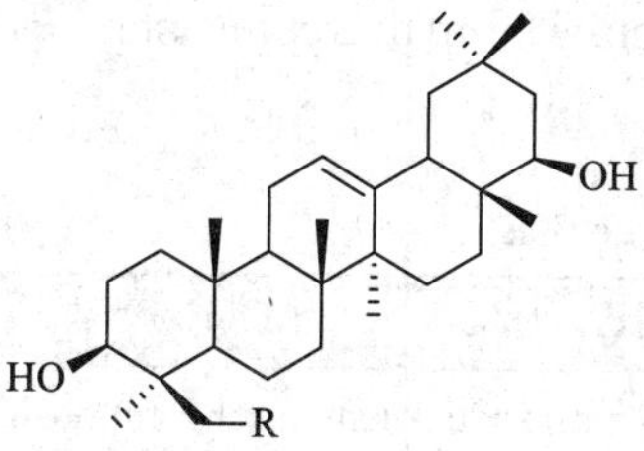

Sophoradiol　　　　R=H
Soyasapogenol B　R=OH

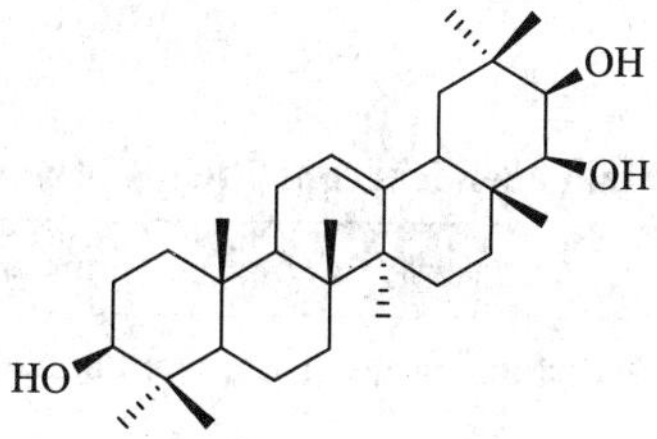

Cantoniensistriol

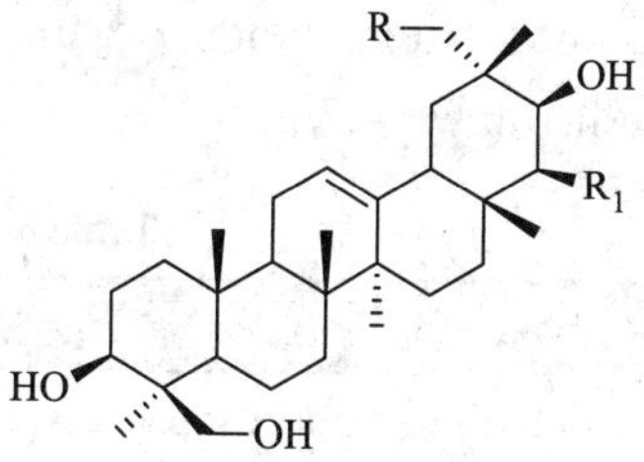

Soyasapogenol　A　R=H,　　R₁=OH
Kudzusapogenol　A　R=OH,　R₁=OH
Kudzusapogenol　C　R=H,　　R₁=H

7.2.3　Quality Control Standards

(1) TLC Identification

Stationary Phase: silica gel plate.

Standard: authentic crude drug.

Development System: chloroform-methanol -water (7 : 2.5 : 0.25, *v/v*).

Visualization: 365nm UV light.

(2) Tests

Water: not more than 14.0%.

Total Ash: not more than 7.0%.

Heavy Metals and Other Harmful Elements: Pb ⩽ 5 ppm;　Cd ⩽ 0.3 ppm; As ⩽ 2 ppm; Hg ⩽ 0.2 ppm; Cu ⩽ 20 ppm.

Extract (diluted ethanol): not less than 24.0%.

(3) Assay

Puerarin: not less than 2.4% (HPLC).

7.3　Sophorae Flos (槐花)

7.3.1　Introduction

(1) Biological Source

Sophorae Flos is the dried flower or bud of *Sophora japonica* L. The former is known as "*Huaihua*", and the later "*Huaimi*".(Fam. Leguminosae)

(2) Property, Flavor and Channels Entered

Property and Flavor: mild cold; bitter.

Channels Entered: liver, large intestine.

(3) Actions& Indications

To cool the blood to stanch bleeding, clear the liver and purge fire. For bloody stool, hemorrhoid bleeding, blood dysentery, flooding and spotting, epistaxis, hematemesis, red eyes caused by liver-heat, headache and dizziness.

(4) Pharmacological Activities

The pharmacological activities associated with Sophorae Flos include anti-inflammatory, anti-tumor, anti-obesity, anti-platelet and anti-hemorrhagic activities.

7.3.2　Main Chemical Constituents

The chemical constituents of flower, root, seed, and pericarp (果皮) of *S. japonica* include flavonoids, triterpenoids, organic acids, coumaronochromone and so on. The main representatives are listed in Table 6-27.

Table 6-27　Main chemical constituents of Sophorae Flos

Type	Main chemical constituents
flavonoids	rutin, sophora A, B, C, quercetin, isorhamnetin, isorhamnetin-3-rutinoside, kaempferol-3-rutinoside
triterpenoids	azukisasponin Ⅰ, Ⅱ, Ⅴ, soyasaponin Ⅰ, Ⅲ, kaikasaponin Ⅰ, Ⅱ, Ⅲ
organic acids	lauric acid, dodecenoic acid, myristic acid, tetradecenoic acid, tetradecadienoic acid
others	betulin, sophoradiol, β-sitosterol

The main flavonoids in Sophorae Flos include rutin, quercetin, isorhamnetin (异鼠李素), isorhamnetin-3-rutinoside, etc.

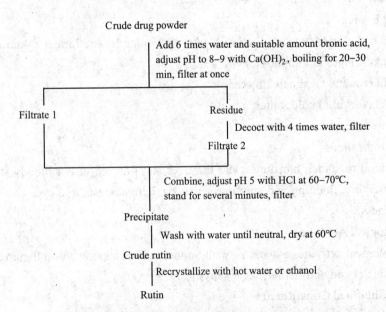

Rutin	R = rutinosyl, R_1 = H
Isorhamnetin	R = H, R_1 = Me
Quercetin	R = R_1 = H
Isorhamnetin-3-rutinoside	R = rutinosyl, R_1 = H

Rutin is an important nutritional supplement because of its many pharmacological activities. For example, it has anti-carcinogenic, cytoprotective, anti-platelet, anti-thrombic, vasoprotective and cardioprotective activities. In addition, rutin is a powerful antioxidant and anti-inflammatory polyphenol. Rutin and its analogues are efficient radical inhibitors and can rescue spatial memory impairment in rats with cerebral ischemia. Moreover, they are promising agents for the treatment of Alzheimer disease (AD).

Rutin is water soluble, and can be extracted from Sophorae Flos with boiling water. The industrial production procedure is shown in Figure 6-16.

Crude drug powder

Add 6 times water and suitable amount bronic acid,
adjust pH to 8–9 with Ca(OH)$_2$, boiling for 20–30
min, filter at once

Filtrate 1 ｜ Residue

Decoct with 4 times water, filter

Filtrate 2

Combine, adjust pH 5 with HCl at 60–70℃,
stand for several minutes, filter

Precipitate

Wash with water until neutral, dry at 60℃

Crude rutin

Recrystallize with hot water or ethanol

Rutin

Figure 6-16　Preparation of rutin from Sophorae Flos

Sophorae Flos also contains triterpenoids, such as azukisasponin I, II, V, soyasaponin (大豆皂苷) I, III, kaikasaponin (槐花皂苷) I, II, III, etc. They have anti-herpes virus activity.

Soyasaponin I:　　$R_1 = S_1, R_2 = OH$
Kaikasaponin I:　　$R_1 = S_2, R_2 = H$
Kaikasaponin III:　　$R_1 = S_1, R_2 = H$

$S_1 = GlcA \overset{2}{-\!-} Gal \overset{2}{-\!-} Rha$

$S_2 = GlcA \overset{2}{-\!-} Ara \overset{2}{-\!-} Rha$

7.3.3　Quality Control Standards

(1) TLC Identification

Stationary Phase: silica gel plate.

Standard: authentic crude drug.

Development System: ethyl acetate-formic acid-water (8 : 1 : 1, v/v).

Visualization: $AlCl_3$, 365nm UV light.

(2) Tests

Water: not more than 11.0%.

Total ash: not more than 9.0% (flower), not more than 14.0% (bud).

Acid-insoluble Ash: not more than 8.0% (flower), not more than 3.0% (bud).

Heavy Metals and Other Harmful Elements: Pb ≤ 5 ppm, Cd ≤ 0.3 ppm, As ≤ 2 ppm, Hg ≤ 0.2 ppm, Cu ≤ 20 ppm.

Extract (30% methanol): not less than 43.0% (bud), not less than 37.0% (flower).

(3) Assay

Total Flavonoids (rutin): not less than 8.0% (flower), not less than 20.0% (bud) (UV-VIS).

Rutin: not less than 6.0% (flower), not less than 15.0% (bud) (HPLC).

7.4　Ginkgo Folium（银杏叶）

7.4.1　Introduction

(1) Biological Source

Ginkgo Folium is the dried leaves of *Ginkgo biloba* L. (Fam. Ginkgoaceae).

(2) Property, Flavor and Channels Entered

Property and Flavor: neutral; sweet, bitter, astringent.

Channels Entered: heart, lung.

(3) Actions & Indications

To activate blood and resolve stasis, unblock the collaterals and relieve pain, constrain the lung to relieve panting, resolve turbidity and lower lipid. For obstruction of collaterals by blood stasis, chest impediment and heart pain, cough and panting caused by lung deficiency, hemiplegia caused by wind-stroke, hyperlipemia.

(4) Pharmacological Activities

The pharmacological activities associated with Ginkgo Folium include free radical scavenging, anti-inflammatory, anti-anxiety/stress, anti-tumor, neuroprotective, cardioprotective, delay-aging effects, etc.

7.4.2 Main Chemical Constituents

Ginkgo Folium contains various compounds, such as flavonoids, diterpenoids, steroids, polyphenols, organic acids, carbohydrates, straight chain hydrocarbons, alcohol, ketones and hexenol (己烯醇), etc.

One main type of chemical constituents in Ginkgo Folium is flavonoids. The common flavonoids are proanthocyanidins (原花青素类) [e.g. catechins (儿茶素), dehydrocatechins (脱氢儿茶素), etc.], flavones (e.g. quercetin, kaempferol, isorhamnetin, etc.) and biflavones [e.g. ginkgetin, bilobetin (去甲银杏双黄酮), sciadopitysin (金松双黄酮), etc.].

Amentoflavone	$R_1 = R_2 = R_3 = R_4 = H$
Bilobetin	$R_1 = CH_3$ $R_2 = R_3 = R_4 = H$
Isoginkgetin	$R_1 = R_3 = CH_3$ $R_2 = R_4 = H$
Ginkgetin	$R_1 = R_2 = CH_3$ $R_3 = R_4 = H$
Sclareol	$R_1 = R_2 = R_3 = CH_3$ $R_4 = H$
1-5′-methoxylbilobetin	$R_1 = CH_3$ $R_2 = R_3 = H$ $R_4 = OCH_3$

The flavonoids of Ginkgo Folium have various pharmaceutical activities. For example, ginkgetin exhibits anti-inflammatory, antifungal, antiherpes virus, cytotoxicity, neuroprotective and anti-influenza virus activities.

The other main type of chemical constituents in Ginkgo Folium is diterpenoids, including bilobalide (白果内酯), and ginkgolides (银杏内酯) A, B, C, J and M. Bilobalide and ginkgolides are rare natural products possessing a *tert*-butyl group.

Ginkgolides are potent and selective antagonists of platelet activating factor (PAF). They also exert antagonistic effect on glycine receptors and an anxiolytic effect. Bilobalide lacks PAF antagonistic activity but has neuroprotective effect.

Bilobalide

| Ginkgolide A: $R_1 = R_2 = H$, $R_3 = OH$ |
| Ginkgolide B: $R_1 = R_3 = OH$, $R_2 = H$ |
| Ginkgolide C: $R_1 = R_2 = R_3 = OH$ |
| Ginkgolide J: $R_1 = H$, $R_2 = R_3 = OH$ |
| Ginkgolide M: $R_1 = R_2 = OH$, $R_3 = H$ |

Several techniques for total extraction of Ginkgo Folium have been studied so far. The major one is shown in Figure 6-17.

7.4.3 Quality Control Standards

(1) TLC Identification

Method Ⅰ:

Stationary Phase: silica gel plate.

Standard: authentic crude drug.

Development System: toluene-ethyl acetate-acetone-methanol (10:5:5:0.6, *v/v*) below 15℃.

Visualization: stand in acetic anhydride for 15min, 140-150℃ 30 min, 365nm UV light.

Method Ⅱ:

Stationary Phase: silica gel plate.

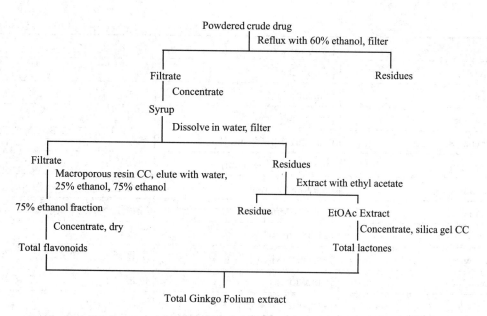

Figure 6-17 Preparation of total Ginkgo Folium extract by macroporous resin

Standard: authentic crude drug

Development System: ethyl acetate-butanone（丁酮）-formic acid-water (5 : 3 : 1 : 1, v/v).

Visualization: 3% $AlCl_3$, 365nm UV light.

(2) Tests

Impurities: not more than 2%.

Water: not more than 12.0%.

Total Ash: not more than 10.0%.

Acid-insoluble Ash: not more than 2.0%.

Heavy Metals and Other Harmful Elements: Pb ≤ 5 ppm, Cd ≤ 0.3 ppm, As ≤ 2 ppm, Hg ≤ 0.2 ppm, Cu ≤ 20 ppm.

Extract (diluted ethanol): not less than 25.0%

(3) Assay

Total flavonoid glycosides [content of (quercetin，kaempferol，isorhamnetin) × 2.51]: not less than 0.40% (HPLC).

Total terpernoid lactones (ginkgolide A, B, C and bilobalide): not less than 0.25% (HPLC).

词 汇 表
An Alphabetical List of Words and Phrases

A		
Acacia catechu (L.f.)Willd.		儿茶
acetate-malonate pathway	[ˈæsɪteɪt][mæləʊˈneɪt][pɑːθweɪ]	乙酸－丙二酸途径
acidity	[əˈsɪdəti]	酸性，酸度
adjacent	[əˈdʒeɪsənt]	毗邻的

(continued)

algae	[ˈældʒiː]	藻类植物
aluminum (Al)	[əˈluːmənəm]	铝
ammonium	[əˈməunɪəm]	氨水
ammonia water	[əˈməunɪə][ˈwɔːtə]	氨水
Anemarrhenae Rhizoma	[ˈənmærɪniː][raɪˈzəmə]	知母
anomeric proton	[æˈnəumerɪk][ˈprəutɔn]	端基质子
anthocyanidin	[ˌænθəsaɪˈænɪdɪn]	花青素
anthocyanin	[ˌænθəˈsaɪənɪn]	花色素，花色苷
apigenin	[ˈæpaɪdʒnɪn]	芹菜素
aromatic ring	[ˌærəˈmætɪk][rɪŋ]	芳香环
aurantiun	[ɔːrɔnˈtiːjuːn]	酸橙
aurones	[auˈrəunz]	橙酮
B		
baicalein	[ˈbeɪkəleɪn]	黄芩素
base peak	[beɪs][piːk]	基峰
Basicity	[beˈsɪsəti]	碱性
Betulaceae		桦木科
biflavonoids	[baɪˈflævənəuɪdz]	双黄酮类
biphenylpyrone		双苯吡酮
bilobalide	[baɪˈləubælaɪd]	白果内酯，银杏内酯
bilobetin	[ˈbiːləbɪtɪn]	白果素
biogenesis	[ˌbaɪəuˈdʒenɪsɪs]	生物起源
Bignoniaceae		紫葳科
biosynthesis	[ˌbaɪəuˈsɪnθɪsɪs]	生物合成
boric acid	[ˌbɔːrɪkˈæsɪd]	硼酸
butanone	[ˈbjuːtənəun]	丁酮
C		
calycosin	[ˈkælɪkəusiːn]	毛蕊异黄酮
cantoniensistriol	[kæntəunɪənˈsɪstriːəul]	广东相思子三醇
carbonyl	[ˈkɑːbənɪl]	羰基
Carthami Flos		红花
carthamin	[kɑːˈθeɪmiːn]	红花苷
carthamone	[kɑːθæmˈwʌn]	醌式红花苷
catechin/catechol/catechuic acid	[ˈkætɪtʃɪn]/[ˈkɪtɪʃəul][ˈæsɪd]	儿茶素，儿茶酸，儿茶酚，邻苯二酚
chalcone	[ˈkælkəun]	查耳酮
chiral	[ˈtʃɪrən]	手性的
chlorophyll	[ˈklɔrəfɪl]	叶绿素

(continued)

chromone	[ˈkrəuməun]	色原酮
Chryanthemum morifolium		杭白菊
Citrus aurantiun		酸橙
coenzyme	[kəuˈenzaɪm]	辅酶
co-existed	[kəuɪɡˈzɪstɪd]	共存
complexes	[ˈkɔmpleksɪz]	络合物
co-pigments	[kəuˈpɪɡmənts]	辅色素
cross-conjugated	[krɔsˈkɔndʒəˌɡeɪtɪd]	交叉共轭的
cupresuflavone	[kʌprɪzʌˈfleɪvn]	柏黄酮
cyanin	[ˈsaɪənɪn]	花色素苷
cyclization reactions	[saɪklɪˈzeɪʃən][riˈækʃənz]	环合反应
Cyperaceae		莎草科
D		
daidzein	[deɪdˈzeən]	大豆苷元
dehydrocatechins	[diːˌhaɪdrəuˈkætəkɪnz]	脱氢儿茶素
Delphinium grandiflorum		翠雀
Derris elliptica		毛鱼藤
deshielding	[dɪˈʃiːldɪŋ]	去屏蔽
diagnostic reagent	[ˌdaɪəɡˈnɔstɪk][rɪˈeɪdʒənt]	诊断试剂
dihydrochalcones	[diːhaɪdrəukælˈkəunz]	二氢查耳酮类
dihydroflavonol	[daɪˌhaɪdrəˈflævənɔl]	二氢黄酮醇
dihydromorin	[daɪˌhaɪdrəˈmɔːrɪn]	二氢桑色素
dihydroquercetin	[diːhaɪdrəukəˈsetɪn]	二氢槲皮素
dilute alkali aqueous	[daɪˈluːt][ˈælkəlaɪ][ˈeɪkwɪəs]	稀碱液
dimer	[ˈdaɪmə]	二聚体
doublet	[ˈdʌblət]	双重峰
down-field	[daun][fiːld]	低场
E		
enzymolysis	[ˌenzaɪˈmɔlɪsɪs]	酶解
epicatechin	[ˌepɪˈkætɪtʃɪn]	表儿茶素
Ericaceae		杜鹃花科
ESI-MS		电喷雾电离质谱
estrogen	[ˈestrədʒən]	雌性激素
exclusion	[ɪkˈskluːʒn]	排斥
F		
Faboideae		蝶形花亚科
fam. (family)	[ˈfæməli]	科

(continued)

fast atom bombardment (FAB)	[fɑ:st]['ætəm][bɔm'bɑ:dmənt]	快原子轰击
FD-MS		场致裂解质谱
ficine	['fɪsɪn]	黄酮榕碱
fission	['fɪʃn]	裂解
flavan-3,4-diol	['fleɪvən]['daɪəul]	黄烷 –3,4– 二醇
flavan-3-ol	['fleɪvən]	黄烷 –3– 醇
flavanol	['fleɪvənɔl]	黄烷醇
flavanones	['fleɪvənəunz]	二氢黄酮类
flavanonols	[fleɪ'vænənɔlz]	二氢黄酮醇类
flavans	['fleɪvənz]	黄烷
flavones	['fleɪvəunz]	黄酮类（狭义的黄酮）
flavonoids	['fleɪvənəuɪdz]	黄酮类
flavonols	[fleɪvə'nɔlz]	黄酮醇类
flavonolignan	[fleɪvə'nɔlɪgnæn]	黄酮木脂素
flavylium	[flæ'vaɪlɪəm]	花色基元
fluorescence	[flu:ə'resəns]	荧光
formamide	[fɔ:'mæmɪd]	甲酰胺
G		
galangin	[gə'læŋgɪn]	高良姜精，三羟基黄酮
Gentianaceae		龙胆科
Gesneriaceae		苦苣苔科
ginkgetin	[ˌgɪŋ'getɪn]	银杏素
ginkgo leaves	['gɪŋkgəu][li:vz]	银杏叶
ginkgolide	['gɪŋkgɔlɪd]	银杏内酯
Ginkgo biloba L.		银杏
glycosylation	[ˌglaɪkəsɪ'leɪʃən]	糖基化
Glycyrrhizae Radix et Rhizoma		甘草
Guttiferae		藤黄科
H		
hesperetin	['hespərɪtɪn]	橙皮素
hesperidin	[he'sperɪdɪn]	橙皮苷
hexenol	['heksɪnɔl]	己烯醇
hinokiflavone	[ɪnəukɪf'leɪvn]	扁柏黄酮
hydrophilic	[ˌhaɪdrɔ'fɪlɪk]	亲水的
I		
intermediate	['ɪntə'mi:djət]	中间体
ionic	[aɪ'ɔnɪk]	离子的

(continued)

isoficine	[ˌaɪsɔˈfɪsɪn]	黄酮异榕碱
isoflavanones	[ˌaɪsɔːfleɪˈvænənz]	二氢异黄酮类
isoflavones	[ˌaɪsəuˈfleɪvəunz]	异黄酮
isoginkgetin	[aɪˈsɔdʒɪnkdʒɪtɪn]	异银杏素
isomer	[ˈaɪsəmə]	异构体
isomerase	[aɪˈsɔməreɪs]	异构酶
isomerngiferin	[ˌaɪsəumənˈdʒɪfərɪn]	异芒果素
isorhamnetin	[aɪsəˈhæmnɪtɪn]	异鼠李素
K		
kaempferol	[ˈkiːmpfərɔl]	山萘酚
kaikasaponin	[kaɪkæsæˈpɔnɪn]	槐花皂苷
kudzusapogenol		葛根皂醇
L		
leucocyanidin	[ˌljuːkəˌsaɪˈænɪdɪn]	白矢车菊素
leucodelphinidin	[ljuːkədelfɪˈnaɪdɪn]	无色飞燕草素
leucopelargonidin	[ljuːkəpiːləgəˈnaɪdɪn]	无色天竺葵素
Lewis acid	[ˈluɪs][ˈæsɪd]	路易斯酸
liquintigenin		甘草素
liquiritin	[ˈlɪkwɪərɪtɪn]	甘草苷
lipo-pigments	[ˈlɪpəu][ˈpɪgmənts]	脂溶性色素
liposolubility	[lɪpəsɔljuˈbɪlɪtɪ]	脂溶性
Luteolin	[ˈluːtɪəlɪn]	木犀草素
M		
maackiain	[məkˈɪeɪɪn]	马卡因
malonyl	[ˈmælənɪl]	丙二酰基
mauve	[məuv]	淡紫色，苯胺紫
meta-coupling	[ˈmetə][ˈkʌplɪŋ]	间位偶合
methoxyl	[ˈmetɔksɪl]	甲氧基
methyl formate	[ˈmeθɪl][ˈfɔːmeɪt]	甲酸甲酯
microwave-assisted extraction (MAE)	[ˈmaɪkrəweɪv][əˈsɪstɪd][ɪkˈstrækʃn]	微波辅助提取
monomer	[ˈmɔnəmə]	单体
Moraceae		桑科
mulberry	[ˈmʌlbəri]	桑树
myricetin	[mɪˈrɪsətɪn]	杨梅素
Myrtaceae		桃金娘科
N		
negative	[ˈnegətɪv]	阴性的

(continued)

negative model	['negətɪv]['mɒdl]	负离子模式
neocarthamin	[ni:əukɑ:'θeɪmi:n]	新红花苷
nobiletin	[nəuaɪ'letɪn]	川陈皮素
non-bonded	[nʌn'bɒndɪd]	未成键的
O		
oligomer	['ɒlɪgəumə]	寡聚体
ortho-	['ɔ:θəu]	邻位
ortho-coupling	['ɔ:θəu]['kʌplɪŋ]	邻位偶合
oxalic acid	[ɒk'sælɪk]['æsɪd]	草酸
oxidation	[ˌɒksɪ'deɪʃn]	氧化
oxonium salt	[ɒk'səunjəm] [sɔ:lt]	盐
oxygenated	['ɒksɪdʒɪneɪtɪd]	氧化的
P		
pericarp	['perɪkɑ:p]	果皮
phellamurin	[feləm'juərɪn]	黄柏素 –7–*O*– 葡萄糖苷
Phellodendron chinense	[felə'dendrən]	黄柏
phenyl	['fenəl]	苯基
phenylchromone	[fenɪl'krəuməun]	苯基色原酮
phloridzin	[flə'rɪdzɪn]	根皮苷
phytoestrogen	[ˌfaɪtəu'estrədʒən]	植物雌激素
pigment	['pɪgmənt]	色素
Pinaceae		松科
planar structure	['pleɪnə]['strʌktʃə]	平面结构
polyhydroxyl	[pɒlɪhaɪ'drɒksɪl]	多羟基
positive	['pɒzətɪv]	阳性的
positive model	['pɒzətɪv]['mɒdl]	正离子模式
precipitate	[prɪ'sɪpɪteɪt]	沉淀
pressurized liquid extraction	['preʃəraɪzd]['lɪkwɪd][ɪk'strækʃn]	加压液相提取
prewashed	['prewɒʃt]	预洗
Primulaceae		报春花科
proanthocyanidins	[prəuntəsaɪə'naɪdɪnz]	原花青素类
pterocarpin	[tərəu'kɑ:pɪn]	紫檀素
Puerariae Lobatae Radix		葛根
puerain-xyloside		葛根素木糖苷
pyrone	['paɪrəun]	吡喃酮
Pyrrosiae Folium		石韦
2-phenylchromone	[fenɪl'krəuməun]	2– 苯基色原酮

(continued)

Q		
quasi-molecular ion	['kweɪsaɪ][mə'lekjələ]['aɪən]	准分子离子
quercetin	['kwə:sɪtɪn]	槲皮素
R		
Rosaceae		蔷薇科
rearrangement	[ˌri:ə'reɪndʒmənt]	重排
reductant	[rɪ'dʌktənt]	还原剂
reversibly	[rɪ'və:səbl]	可逆的
Rhododendron dahuricum		兴安杜鹃
rotenone	['rəutnəun]	鱼藤酮
S		
saturate	['sæʃəreɪt]	饱和的
Salicaceae		杨柳科
sciadopitysin	[ʃɪædəpɪ'taɪzɪn]	金松双黄酮
Scrophulariaceae		玄参科
semi-chair structure	['semɪ][tʃeə]['strʌktʃə]	半椅式结构
shikimate pathway		莽草酸途径
silymarin	['sɪlɪmərɪn]	水飞蓟素
solubility	[ˌsɔlju'bɪlɪti]	溶解性
Solvent Partition	['sɔlvənt][pɑ:'tɪʃn]	溶剂萃取
Sophorae Flos		槐花
sophoradiol	[səufəreɪd'ɪəul]	槐花二醇
Sophora subprostrata		广豆根
soyasapogenol	[sɔɪeɪzæ'pɔdʒɪnɔl]	大豆皂醇
soyasaponin	[sɔɪeɪzæ'pɔnɪn]	大豆皂苷
stereochemistry	[ˌstɪərɪə'kemɪstrɪ]	立体化学
strontium (Sr)	['strɔnʃɪəm]	锶
substituent	[sʌb'stɪtjuənt]	取代基
supercritical fluid extraction	[ˌsju:pə'krɪtɪkəl]['flu:ɪd][ɪk'strækʃn]	超临界提取
sulphuretin	[sʌlfju'ri:tɪn]	硫磺菊素
T		
thermally labile	['θə:məli]['leɪbaɪl]	热不稳定的
trifolirhizin	[traɪfə'lə:haɪzɪn]	三叶豆紫檀苷
U		
ultrasound-assisted extraction	[ˌʌltrə'saund][ə'sɪstɪd][ɪk'strækʃn]	超声提取技术
up-field	[ʌp][fi:ld]	高场
urea	[ju'ri:ə]	尿素

(continued)

V		
violet	['vaɪəlɪt]	紫色的
volume retained	['vɒlju:m][rɪ'teɪnd]	保留体积
W		
wogonin	['wɒgənɪn]	汉黄芩素
wogonoside	[wɒgə'nəusaɪd]	汉黄芩苷
X		
xanthone	['zænθæn]	双苯吡酮，氧杂蒽酮
Z		
zirconium (Zr)	[zə'kəunɪəm]	锆
citric acid		枸橼酸
Zingiberaceae		姜科

重 点 小 结

　　狭义的黄酮是指一类以 2- 苯基色原酮为母核的天然产物及其衍生物；广义的黄酮是指具有 $C_6-C_3-C_6$ 结构母核的天然产物及其衍生物的总称。黄酮依据其苷元结构中央 C 部分的氧化程度、成环与否、B- 环取代位置及聚合度的不同分类，主要分为黄酮（醇）、二氢黄酮（醇）、异黄酮、黄烷醇、花色素、橙酮、查尔酮、双黄酮等类型；黄酮苷主要有氧苷（常见 3, 7 位成苷）、碳苷（常见 8 位成苷）。

　　黄酮类化合物一般为黄色固体，黄酮苷元多呈晶型，黄酮苷多为粉末状。黄酮颜色的深浅与助色团（如，酚羟基）多少与位置有关，助色团越多，颜色越深，7, 4′- 羟基对颜色影响较大。溶解性方面，游离黄酮（苷元）一般易溶于甲醇、乙醇、乙酸乙酯、三氯甲烷、乙醚等有机溶剂，不溶于水，但因酚羟基的酸性，可溶于碱水；黄酮苷一般易溶于水、甲醇、乙醇，不溶于三氯甲烷、乙醚等亲脂性有机溶剂。黄酮类化合物在水中溶解性，还与其结构有关，二氢黄酮（醇）、黄烷醇类、异黄酮类属于非平面结构，其水溶性大于黄酮（醇）、查耳酮等平面性分子，花色素类属于离子型，易溶于水；酚羟基甲醚化后水溶性降低；取代位置也影响水溶性，如，黄酮 -3-O- 苷水溶性大于黄酮 -7-O- 苷。黄酮类化合物的苷元有无旋光性取决于其母核结构中有无手性碳原子，在黄酮的各游离苷元中，二氢黄酮、二氢黄酮醇、黄烷醇类具有旋光性，其余类型黄酮苷元无旋光性。黄酮苷则因糖基的存在都有旋光性，且多为左旋。

　　黄酮类化合物因含酚羟基显酸性，其酸性大小与酚羟基的数目与位置有关。一般规律为：7, 4′-OH>7 或 4′-OH> 一般酚羟基 >5-OH，分别可溶于 5%NaHCO₃、5%Na₂CO₃、1%NaOH、4%NaOH 溶液中，这一性质常用于黄酮化合物的 pH 梯度萃取分离。

　　黄酮类化合物的显色反应：HCl-Mg 反应中，黄酮（醇）、二氢黄酮（醇）显示红色，并有气泡产生，可用于检识；硼氢化钠反应是二氢黄酮的专属反应，显红色；含有 3-OH 或 5-OH 的黄酮在滴加 ZrOCl₂ 后显黄色，如再加入枸橼酸不褪色，预示有 3-OH，若褪色，则无 3-OH；含有邻二酚羟基结构的黄酮滴加 SrCl₂-NH₃ · H₂O 后显示墨绿色；三氯化铁是酚羟基的常用显色剂，一般呈墨绿色，对酚羟基类型无选择性；含酚羟基的黄酮，在碱液中呈现不同颜色。

　　黄酮类化合物的常用提取方法有醇提法、热水提取法、碱提酸沉法：黄酮苷及游离黄酮苷元均能溶于甲醇或乙醇；含糖基多的黄酮苷在热水中有比较好的溶解度。分离方法包括色谱法和pH 梯度萃取分离，色谱法常用硅胶、聚酰胺、大孔树脂和葡聚糖凝胶。硅胶色谱法常用于分离极性较小的黄酮苷元和黄酮苷的粗分离；聚酰胺利用氢键原理分离，对黄酮有较理想的分离效果，一般来说酚羟基越多、共轭程度越高、芳香性越强，吸附越强，R_f 越小，难于洗脱。大孔树脂主要用于黄酮苷的富集分离；葡聚糖凝胶色谱分离黄酮苷元时，化合物极性小的黄酮苷元容易洗脱，分离黄酮苷时，分子量大的苷易被洗脱；pH 梯度萃取分离黄酮时，7,4′- 二羟基者溶于 5% $NaHCO_3$，7或 4′- 羟基者溶于 5% Na_2CO_3，一般羟基者溶于 0.2% NaOH，5-OH 者溶于 4%NaOH。

　　黄酮类化合物紫外光谱（UV）特征：B 环桂皮酰基系统产生Ⅰ带（300~400nm），A 环苯甲酰基系统产生Ⅱ带（240~280nm）。根据紫外光谱的峰型可以判断黄酮母核类型：Ⅰ，Ⅱ带都强者，为黄酮（醇）类（再根据Ⅰ带的最大吸收峰位置判断是黄酮还是黄酮醇，350nm 为界）；Ⅰ带强Ⅱ带弱者，为橙酮和查耳酮类；Ⅰ带弱Ⅱ带强者，为异黄酮、二氢黄酮（醇）类（再根据Ⅱ带的最大吸收峰位置判断是异黄酮还是二氢黄酮或二氢黄酮醇，270nm 为界）。诊断试剂主要根据加入试剂前后谱图变化情况分析推测 −OH 取代位置。如，NaOMe 加入后Ⅰ带明显红移时则表明有4′-OH；NaOAC 加入后Ⅱ带明显红移时则表明有 7-OH；$AlCl_3$/HCl 图谱与 $AlCl_3$ 图谱相同时，表明无邻二酚羟基；$AlCl_3$/HCl 图谱与 $AlCl_3$ 图谱不同时，表明有邻二酚羟基；$AlCl_3$/HCl 图谱与MeOH 图谱相同者，表明无 3- 及（或）5-OH；$AlCl_3$/HCl 图谱与 MeOH 图谱不同者，表明可能有 3- 及（或）5-OH。

　　^{1}H−NMR 是黄酮类化合物结构测定的重要方法。A 环常见 5, 7 取代和 7 位取代，5, 7- 取代 A 环时，只有 6, 8 两组信号（1H,d,J=2.5Hz），H-8 较 H-6 在低场；7- 取代则有三组氢信号，H-5（1H,d,J=8.5Hz）处于低场，H-6（1H,dd,J=2.5, 8.5Hz），H-8（1H,d,J=2.5Hz）；B 环取代模式有 4′- 取代、3′, 4′- 取代、3′, 4′, 5′- 取代三种模式：4′- 取代时，有 2′, 6′（2H,d,J=8.5Hz），3′, 5′（2H,d,J=8.5Hz）两组氢信号；3′, 4′- 取代时，有三组氢信号，H-2′（1H,d,J=2.5Hz），H-6′（1H,dd,J=2.5,8.5Hz），H-5′（1H,d,J=8.5Hz）；3′, 4′, 5′-取代时有两种情况，如 3′, 5′-取代基相同时，只有一组氢信号，H-2′，H-6′ 对称（2H,s），3′, 5′ 取代基不同时，有两组氢信号 H-2′，H-6′（1H,d,J=2.5Hz）。二氢黄酮有三组氢信号 Ha-3 δ 2.80（1H,dd, J=11.0, 5.0Hz），Hb-3 δ 2.80（1H,dd, J=11.0, 5.0Hz），H-2 ~ δ 5.6ppm（1H,dd, J=11.0, 5.0Hz）。黄酮苷上糖基的端基氢约 5~6ppm（1H,d），端基氢的个数可判断糖的数目，其偶合常数则常用于苷键构型的判断，当 J=2~4Hz 时，苷键为 α 构型，J 值为 6~8Hz 时苷键 β- 构型。黄酮类化合物结构中还存在羟基、甲氧基、甲基等取代基团，如鼠李糖甲基化学位移 ~1ppm 左右（3H,d），苯环上甲基 2.0ppm 左右，苯环上甲氧基则 ~3.8ppm 左右（3H,s）；酚羟基氢是活泼氢，其化学位移一般 8ppm 以上，5-OH 因与 4- 羰基形成分子内氢键，其化学位移大于 12ppm。

　　^{13}C−NMR 谱在鉴定结构中发挥重要的作用。根据中央三个碳信号的位置可以推测黄酮的母核类型。依据苷元的苷化位移规律，可知糖连接在苷元结构上的位置。苷化位移：苷元成苷后与糖相连的碳原子向高场位移，其邻、对位碳原子向低场位移，且对位移动尺度较大。

　　高分辨质谱 HRMS 可以获知化合物分子量、分子式和结构碎片。黄酮苷元可由 EI 方式电离，其分子离子峰（M$^+$）常为基峰。黄酮苷一般用 ESI、FAB、FD 等方式电离，正离子模式下常见 [M+H]$^+$、[M−H]$^−$、[M+Na]$^+$、[M+K]$^+$，负离子模式下常见 [M−H]$^−$、[M−Cl]$^−$ 等准分子离子峰，以及丢失糖基的碎片峰。

　　黄芩主要有效成分为黄芩苷、黄芩素、汉黄芩素、汉黄芩苷等。葛根主要有效成分有大豆素、大豆苷、葛根素等。槐花主要有效成分有槲皮素、芦丁等。银杏叶主要黄酮类有效成分有儿茶素、去氢儿茶素、槲皮素、山奈酚、异鼠李素、银杏双黄酮、金松双黄酮等。

目 标 检 测

一、单选题

1. 黄酮类化合物的颜色主要与下列哪项因素有关（   ）
    A. 结构中有酚羟基   B. 结构中有邻二酚羟基
    C. A+D 项   D. 分子中存在交叉共轭体系
    E. 结构中有色原酮

2. 黄酮类化合物的基本骨架是（   ）
    A. C_3-C_6-C_3 B. C_6-C_6-C_6 C. C_6-C_3
    D. C_6-C_3-C_6 E. C_6-C_6-C_3

3. 黄酮类化合物加 2%$ZrOCl_2$ 甲醇液呈黄色，再加入 2% 枸橼酸甲醇溶液，黄色显著消退，该黄酮类化合物是（   ）
    A. C_3–OH 黄酮   B. 异黄酮   C. C_5–OH 黄酮
    D. 二氢黄酮   E. 4′, 7– 二羟基黄酮

4. 二氢黄酮、二氢黄酮醇类苷元在水中溶解度稍大于黄酮（醇）类是因为（   ）
    A. 羟基多   B. 有羧基   C. 离子型
    D. C 环为平面型   E. C 环为非平面型

5. 黄酮苷类化合物不能采用的提取方法是（   ）
    A. 酸提碱沉法   B. 碱提酸沉法   C. 沸水提取法
    D. 乙醇提取法   E. 甲醇提取法

6. 下列黄酮都为黄或橙黄色，除了（   ）
    A. 黄酮   B. 黄酮醇   C. 异黄酮
    D. 查耳酮   E. 橙酮

7. 四氢硼钠反应用于鉴别（   ）
    A. 黄酮、黄酮醇   B. 异黄酮
    C. 查耳酮   D. 二氢黄酮、二氢黄酮醇
    E. 花色素

8. pH 梯度萃取法分离黄酮苷元类，加碱液萃取的顺序应是（   ）
    A. $NaHCO_3 \rightarrow NaOH \rightarrow Na_2CO_3$ B. $NaHCO_3 \rightarrow Na_2CO_3 \rightarrow NaOH$
    C. $NaOH \rightarrow NaHCO_3 \rightarrow Na_2CO_3$ D. $NaOH \rightarrow Na_2CO_3 \rightarrow NaHCO_3$
    E. $Na_2CO_3 \rightarrow NaHCO_3 \rightarrow NaOH$

9. 测定某黄酮类化合物的紫外光谱，$AlCl_3$+HCl 谱与 $AlCl_3$ 谱比较，带 I 向紫移 30~40nm，说明该化合物（   ）
    A. B 环上有邻二酚羟基   B. 有 5–OH
    C. 有 3–OH   D. A 环上有邻二酚羟基
    E. A、B 环上有邻二酚羟基

10. 下列化合物的醇溶液中加入少许镁粉，再添加几滴浓盐酸，出现微红色或红色，除了（   ）

A. 异黄酮   B. 黄酮   C. 二氢黄酮

D. 黄酮醇   E. 二氢黄酮醇

二、多选题

1. 下列哪几类黄酮类化合物具有旋光性（   ）

     A. 黄酮醇   B. 二氢黄酮   C. 黄烷醇

     D. 查耳酮   E. 二氢黄酮醇

2. 黄酮类化合物常用的提取方法有（   ）

     A. 碱溶酸沉法   B. 酸溶碱沉法   C. 醇提取法

     D. 金属配合物沉淀法   E. 水蒸气蒸馏法

3. 用于总黄酮纯化、分离的方法有（   ）

     A. pH 梯度萃取法   B. 活性炭吸附法   C. 聚酰胺柱层析分离法

     D. 金属配合物沉淀法   E. 醇沉淀法

4. 黄酮苷元按结构分类，主要是依据（   ）

     A. 三碳链的氧化程度   B. 是否连接糖链   C. B 环连接位置

     D. 来自何种植物   E. 三碳链是否成环

5. 中药槐米中的主要有效成分（   ）

     A. 是槲皮素   B. 在冷水和热水中溶解度相差悬殊

     C. 能与四氢硼钠反应   D. 能与硼酸发生络合反应

     E. 可用碱溶酸沉法提取

6. 与二氢黄酮化合物成阳性的反应是（   ）

     A. 盐酸－镁粉反应   B. 四氢硼钠反应   C. 锆－枸橼酸反应

     D. 醋酸铅反应   E. 醋酸镁反应

7. pH 梯度萃取法分离黄酮类化合物（   ）

     A. 将总黄酮溶解在亲脂性有机溶剂中

     B. 以碱液为萃取剂

     C. 适用于分离苷类和苷元类

     D. 适用于分离酸性强弱不同的苷元类

     E. 酸性弱的黄酮类先被萃取出来

8. 黄酮类化合物的紫外光谱中（   ）

     A. 黄酮和黄酮醇有带 I 和带 II 两个强峰

     B. 异黄酮带 I 为主峰，带 II 则较弱

     C. 二氢黄酮带 II 为主峰，带 I 则较弱

     D. 查耳酮带 II 为主峰，带 I 则较弱

     E. 黄酮和黄酮醇谱形相似，但带 I 位置不同

9. 在芦丁的 ^{1}HNMR 谱中（   ）

     A. H–3 为一个尖锐的单峰信号

     B. H–6 和 H–8 都是二重峰

     C. H–6 信号比 H–8 信号位于较低磁场区

     D. H–2′ 为二重峰

     E. H–5′ 和 H–6′ 为双二重峰

10.芦丁经酸水解后，可得到的单糖有（　　　）

A. 葡萄糖 B. 半乳糖 C. 鼠李糖

D. 果糖 E. 阿拉伯糖

三、思考题

1. 从某中药中得一黄色结晶 I，分子式 $C_{21}H_{21}O_{11}$，HCl-Mg 反应呈淡粉红色，$FeCl_3$ 反应及 α- 萘酚 - 浓 H_2SO_4 反应均为阳性，氨性氯化锶反应阴性，二氯氧锆反应呈黄色，加枸橼酸后黄色消褪，可被苦杏仁酶水解，水解产物经鉴定为葡萄糖及黄色结晶 II，分子式 $C_{15}H_{10}O_6$，HCl-Mg 反应及 $FeCl_3$ 反应均为阳性，α- 萘酚 - 浓 H_2SO_4 反应阴性，二氯氧锆反应呈黄色，加枸橼酸后黄色不褪。晶 I 的光谱数据如下：

UV（λ_{max} nm）：

MeOH: 267,348; NaOMe: 275,326,398 (强度不降); $AlCl_3$: 274,301,352;

$AlCl_3$/HCl: 276,303,352; NaOAc: 275,305(sh), 372; NaOAc/H_3BO_3: 266,300,353。

^{1}H-NMR (DMSD-d_6,TMS) δ:

3.2~3.9(6H, m), 3.9~5.1(4H, 加 D_2O 后消失); 5.68(1H, d, J=8.0Hz), 6.12(1H, d, J=2.0Hz), 6.42(1H, d, J=2.0Hz), 6.86(2H, d, J=9.0Hz), 8.08(2H, d, J=9.0Hz)。

请根据以上提供的信息解析结晶 I 的结构，并指出苷键的构型。

2. 黄芩在贮存过程中为什么变绿？化学成分有何变化（请用化学式表达）?

（何细新）

Chapter 7　Tannins

PPT

学习目标

知识要求：

1. **掌握** 鞣质的定义、分类及主要理化性质。
2. **熟悉** 鞣质的提取分离及检识方法。
3. **了解** 鞣质的波谱特征及五倍子和肉桂的主要有效成分。

能力要求：

学会应用蛋白质沉淀反应检识鞣质；学会应用鞣质与蛋白质沉淀的性质，解决鞣质在提取分离过程中存在的技术问题。

1　Introduction

Tannins (鞣质) are defined as polyphenols (多酚) (molecular weights usually ranging from 500 to 3000) that can precipitate proteins from aqueous solutions. Deriving the name from the technical word 'tanning (鞣制)' that means converting animal hides to leather through chemical processes. They are composed of a very diverse group of oligomers (低聚物) and polymers (多聚物).

One of popular definition of tannins given by Karamali Khanbabaee and Teunis van Ree is: "Tannins are polyphenolic (多聚酚) secondary metabolites of higher plants, and are either galloyl esters (没食子酸酯) and their derivatives (衍生物), in which galloyl moieties or their derivatives are attached to a variety of polyol-, catechin- and triterpenoid cores [gallotannins (没食子鞣质), ellagitannins (逆没食子鞣质) and complex tannins(复合鞣质)], or they are oligomeric and polymeric proanthocyanidins that can possess different inter flavanyl coupling and substitution patterns (condensed tannins) (缩合鞣质)".

In nature, tannins are found world-wide in many families of higher plants such as Rhei Radix et Rhizoma from Polygonaceae, Chinese sumac (盐肤木) from Anacardiaceae (漆树科), Chebulae Fructus (诃子) from Combretaceae (使君子科) or plant galls (植物虫瘿), etc. Tannins can be found in nearly every part of the plant, such as the bark, wood, leaves, fruit, roots, and seeds. Frequently an increased tannin production can be associated with some sickness of the plant. Therefore, it is assumed that the biological role of tannins in plants is related to protection against infection, insects, or animal herbivory (食草性).

Tannins are used in medicines as astringents (收敛剂), diuretics (利尿药), anti-inflammatory, antiseptics (防腐剂) and haemostatic pharmaceuticals (止血药). Tannins are most definitely antioxidants, which mean that they can reduce the risk of developing coronary artery disease and a number of other health problems. In commercial, tannins are used chiefly in tanning leather, dyeing fabric, making ink, clarifying wine and beer, reducing viscosity of oil-well drilling mud, preventing scale (水垢) in boiler water. Their extracts are widely used in food and feed additives (添加剂), photography (摄影), metallurgy (冶金), etc.

The search for new leading compounds for the development of novel pharmaceuticals (药物) has become increasingly important, especially as the biological action of tannin-containing plant extracts has been well documented. During the last twenty years, many representatives of this class of compounds have been isolated and characterized. Currently known tannins with unambiguously (明白地) determined structures already number far more than 1000.

Biosynthetically, hydrolysable tannins (可水解鞣质) are derived from the shikimate pathway and condensed tannins are derived from acetate and shikimate pathways.

2　Structure and Classification

Tannins have a great structural diversity (多样性), but they are usually divided into three groups based on their chemical structures, i.e. hydrolysable tannins, condensed tannins, and complex tannins.

2.1　Hydrolysable Tannins

As the name indicated, they can be hydrolysed by acid, base or enzyme quickly. Members of this class consist of several molecules of phenolic acids united by ester linkage to a central polyol (多元醇) moiety. Hydrolysable tannins can be subdivided into two categories: gallotannins and ellagitannins.

gallic acid　　　　pyrogallol　　　hexahydroxydiphenic acid　　　　ellagic acid

2.1.1　Gallotannins

On hydrolysis, they give gallic acid and glucose or other polyols. The basic building block is β-glucogallin (葡萄糖没食子鞣苷). Typical form of the complex gallotannins is the addition of further gallic acid moieties and the formation of depsidic meta-bonds between suitably positioned galloyl moieties in the molecule. Variations in structures come from the degree of esterification (酯化反应) of the glucose centre and the degree of depside (缩酚酸) esterification.

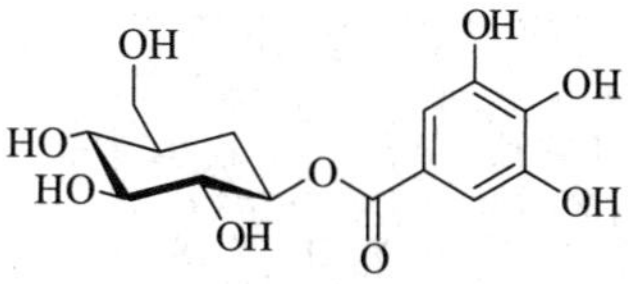

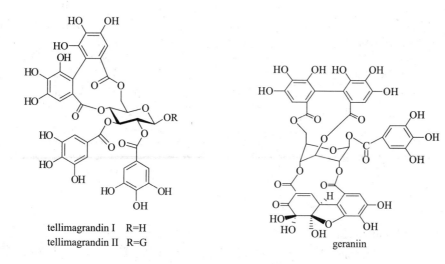

β-glucogallin

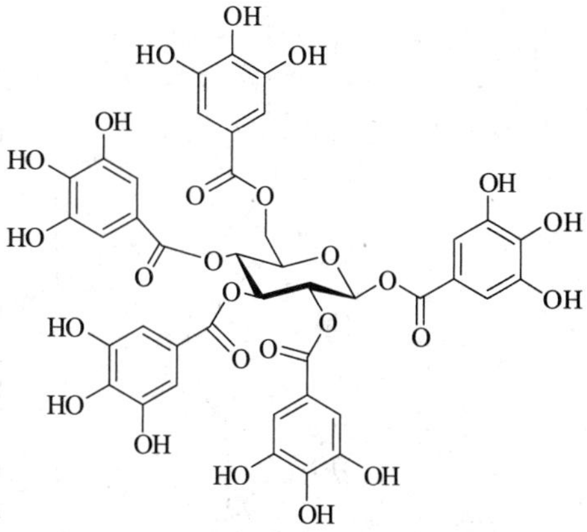

pentagalloylglucose

2.1.2 Ellagitannins

Ellagitannins are characterized by the presence of one or more hexahydroxydiphenoyl（HHDP,六羟基联苯二甲酰基) unit(s) on a glucopyranose core. The HHDP group is biosynthetically formed through intramolecular (分子内的) oxidative C-C bond formation between neighboring galloyl groups in galloyl-glucoses(GGs)（没食子酰基葡萄糖).They are easily hydrolysed, either enzymatically or with acid, to produce a stable dilactone (双内酯) form of hexahydroxydiphenic acid (六羟二酚酸), ellagic acid (逆没食子酸).

In addition to the HHDP group, other constituent acyl units in ellagitannins include a galloyl group and HHDP derivatives such as valoneoyl (Val) (橡腕酰基), sanguisorboyl (Sang) (地榆酰基), dehydro-hexahydroxydiphenoyl (DHHDP)（脱氢六羟基联苯二甲酰基）and chebuloyl (Che) (诃子酰基) groups. Their oxidative coupling of ellagitannin monomers leads proposedly to the formation of more complex oligomeric structures. The relationship between HHDP and derivatives is shown in Figure 7-1.

Ellagitannins can be further subdivided into monomeric ellagitannins (简单逆没食子鞣质), oligo-meric ellagitannins (逆没食子鞣质低聚体),*C*-glycosidic ellagitannins（*C*–苷鞣质),and caffeetannins (咖啡鞣质) according to the products of hydrolysis and chemical structure characters.

(1) Monomeric Ellagitannins

Monomeric ellagitannins refer to those ellagitannins containing only one glucose core, for example, tellimagrandin (特马里素) Ⅰ、Ⅱ, and geraniin (老鹳草素).

tellimagrandin I   R=H
tellimagrandin II   R=G

geraniin

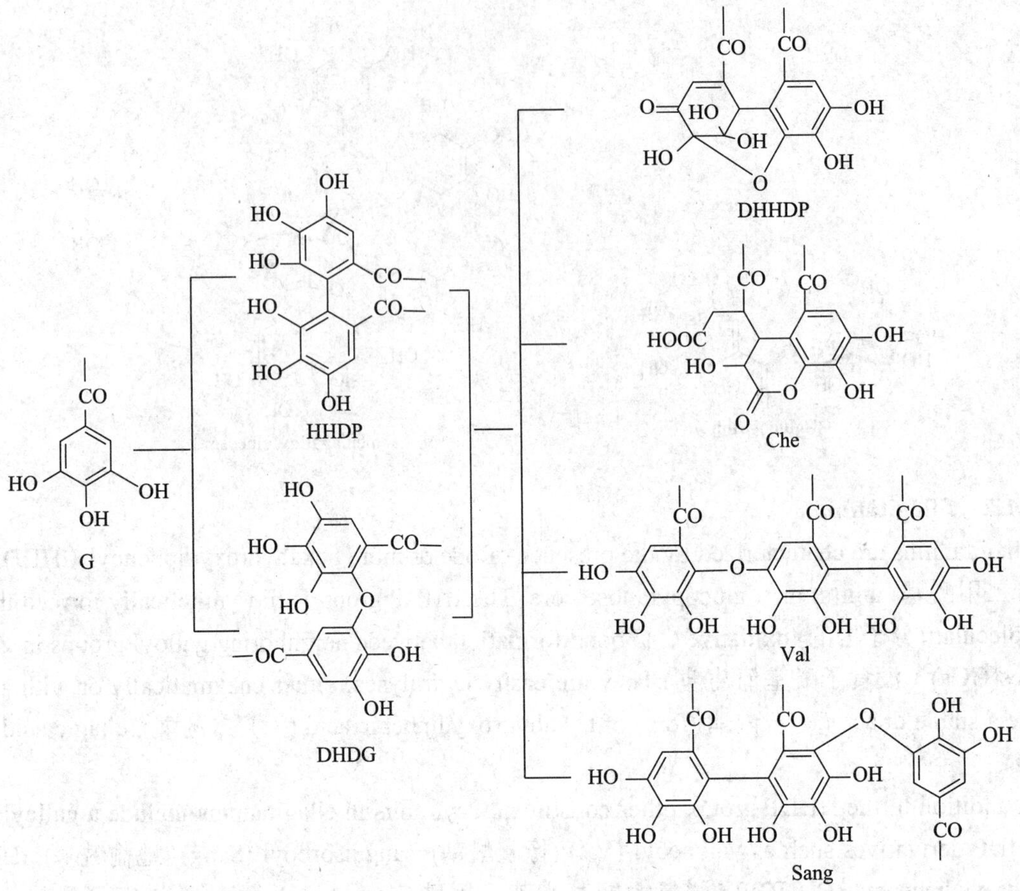

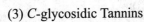

Figure 7-1   HHDP's lineage

(2) Oligomeric Ellagitannins

Hydrolysable tannin oligomers are produced through intermolecular C-O or C-C bonds between monomeric ellagitannins. They can be divided into dimers, trimers (三聚体), tetramers (四聚体) up to pentamers (五聚体) according to the number of glucopyranose cores which are susceptible to bond formation, positions and their condensation degree of HHDP and other groups of monomers. For exemple, agrimoniin (仙鹤草素) is composed of two different monomers.

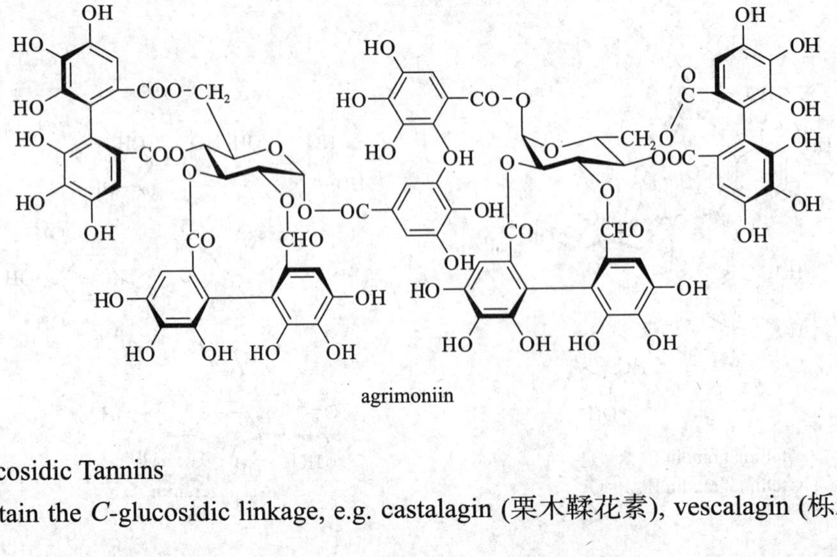

agrimoniin

(3) C-glycosidic Tannins

They contain the C-glucosidic linkage, e.g. castalagin (栗木鞣花素), vescalagin (栎木鞣花素), casuarinin (木麻黄鞣宁) and stachyurin (旌节花素).

castalagin: R=OH, R'=H
vescalagin: R=H, R'=OH

casuarinin: R=OH, R'=H
stachyurin: R=H, R'=OH

(4) Caffeetannins

Caffeetannins are formed by esterification of quinic acid (奎宁酸) with several molecules of caffeic acid (咖啡酸) or by mutual esterification between caffeic acids. However, the latter was rarely found. The tannin activities of east-Asian medicinal plants of Artemisia (蒿属) species were found to be mainly attributable to that of 3, 5-di-*O*-caffeoylquinic acid (3, 5- 二 -*O*- 咖啡酰奎宁酸) and its isomers.

3,5-dicaffeoylquini cacid

2.2   Condensed Tannins

Condensed tannins are related to flavonoid pigments, because they are formed via derivatives of flavones, such as catechin or flavan-3-ol or flavan-3, 4-diols. Unlike hydrolysable tannins, condensed tannins can not be hydrolyzed to simpler molecules and they do not contain a saccharide moiety, but can convert into red water-insoluble compounds known as tannin reds or phlobaphenes (鞣红). So they are also called non-hydrolysable tannins, phlobatannins (鞣红鞣质) or proanthocyanidins.

Phlobaphenes are flushed precipitates found in some plants that have reddish tints (淡红色) and this is an indication that these plants are abundant of condensed tannins. Phlobaphenes give the characteristic red color to many herbs such as Cinnamomi Cortex (肉桂).

Condensed tannins are much more resistant to decomposition and merely yield polymers or precipitates when acidified (酸化). The basic monomer of condensed tannins is epicatechin and catechin (儿茶素); These are then extended by the successive addition of similar phenol units to produce polymers. They are polymers of 2 to 50 (or more) flavonoid units linked together by C-C bonds, most often 4-8 or 4-6, which result from coupling between the electrophilic C-4 of a flavanyl unit of a flavan-3-ol (catechin) or flavan-3, 4-diol (leucocyanidin) and a nucleophilic position (C-8, less commonly C-6) of another unit, generally a flavan-3-ol, which are not easy to being cleaved (裂解) by hydrolysis.

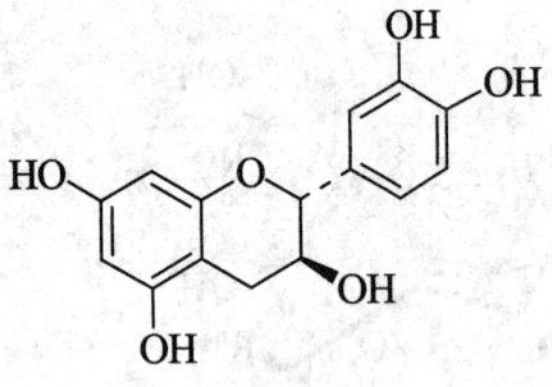

(*l*) catechin 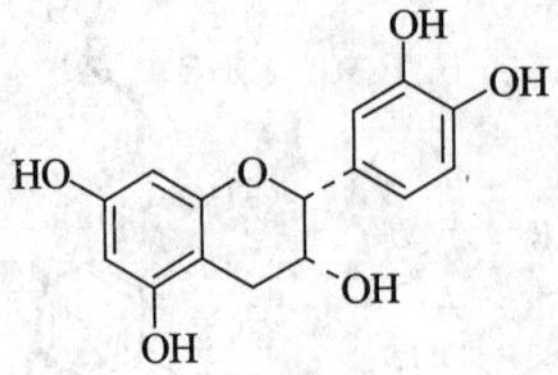 (*d*) epicatechin 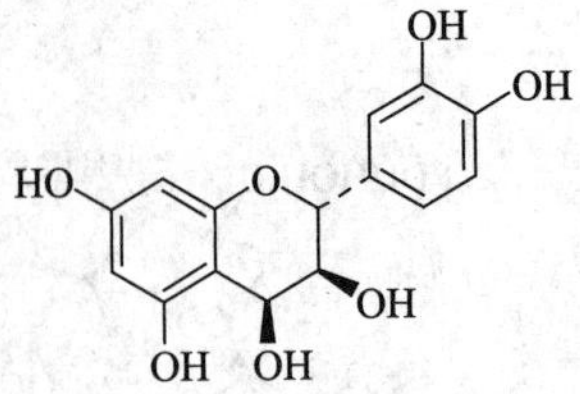 leucocyanidin

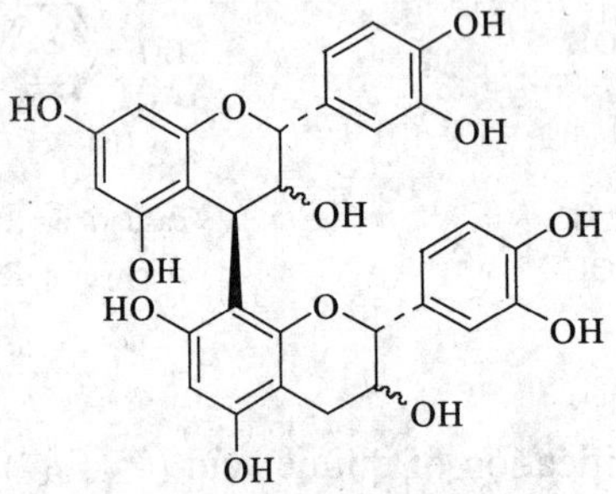

catechin dimer

Condensed tannins are more widely distributed in plants than hydrolysable tannins. For example, cinchona (金鸡纳树皮), Cinnamomi Cortex and wild cherry bark, Dryopteridis crassirhizomatis rhizoma (绵马贯众), cocoa (可可树), cola (可乐树) and Arecae semen (槟榔), Rhei radix et rhizoma. Some Chinese herbs contain both hydrolysable and condensed tannins.

2.3 Complex Tannins

Complex tannins include both hydrolysable tannin moiety and condensed tannin moiety, in which a hydrolysable gallotannin or ellagitannin moiety is bound glycosidically to a condensed tannin moiety.

Complex tannins are a series of compounds first isolated from a Fagaceous (壳斗科) plant and now found to occur widely in plants. For example, acutissimin (野牡丹鞣质) A and B, camelliatannin (山茶鞣质) A-H, mongolicin (蒙古栎素) A and B, guavin (番石榴素) A, etc.

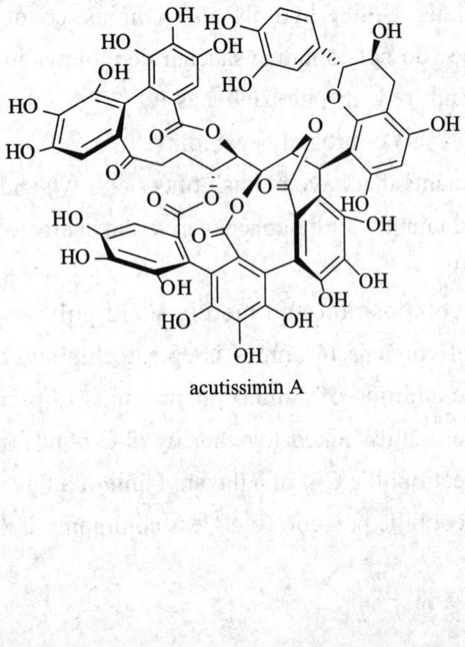

acutissimin A 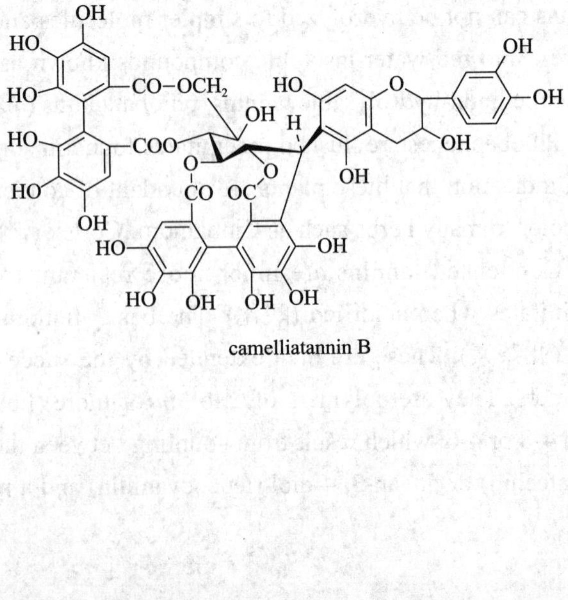 camelliatannin B

3 General Physicochemical Properties

3.1 Physical Properties

Tannins generally are slight yellow or white amorphous powder or shiny and with a characteristic strange smell and astringent taste. They are soluble in water, alcohol, and acetone, insoluble in ethyl ether, chloroform, benzene and other low polar organic solvents.

3.2 Chemical Properties

Tannins have many phenolic hydroxyl groups, so they have strong reduction property. They are easy to be oxidized by agents such as Fehling's reagent.

When encountered with proteins, some alkaloids, heavy metal salts [copper, tin (锡), and lead (铅)], tannins can form precipitates. These reactions can be used in isolation/purification of tannins.

Tannins show color reaction with iron salts. Ferric chloride gives bluish-black or greenish-black color. Tannins react with potassium ferricyanide (铁氰化钾) and ammonia (氨) to give deep red color.

4 Extraction and Isolation Methods

4.1 Extraction Methods

The plant material should be fresh for the best extraction result. The fresh material should be immediately extracted or stored in acetone or cut into small pieces and freeze with liquid nitrogen. At any stage of extracting, care should be taken of the sample temperature, moisture and oxygen, to avoid destroying the tannins structure.

The general extraction solvent is 50% to 70% aqueous acetone. The ratio depends on the moisture presented in the fresh material. Aqueous acetone is a more effective solvent than alcohol and it can inhibit tannin-protein interaction. The extraction procedures are shown in Figure 7-2.

The traditional extraction method usually requires much time. Recently, ultrasound is applied effectively and rapidly to extract tannins from the plant material.

4.2 Isolation Methods

Owing to the large number of structurally similar tannins in plants, isolation of individual tannins is comparatively difficult and complicated. Isolation of tannins is almost invariably achieved by a

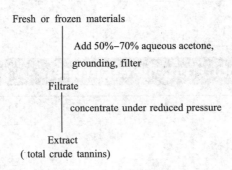

Figure 7-2   General extraction procedure for total crude tannins

combination of methods, such as solvent, precipitation and chromatography methods.

4.2.1   Solvent Method

Tannins are natural water-soluble products. Usually, the aqueous solution containing tannins are defatted with low polar solvent, such as ethyl ether, to remove the low polar impurities(杂质); then extracted with ethyl acetate to obtain tannins. Another procedure is dissolving total crude tannins in small amount of alcohol or ethyl acetate, then adding ethyl ether gradually to obtain tannins as precipitate.

4.2.2   Precipitation Method

Precipitation with gelatin is commonly used to separate tannins. The procedure is described in Figure 7-3.

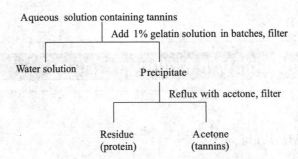

Figure 7-3   Isolation procedure for tannins by the precipitation method

4.2.3   Chromatography Method

Chromatography is the main method for isolation and purification of tannins from plant materials. The universal stationary phases include Diaion HP-20, Toyopearl HW-40, Sephadex LH-20, MCI Gel CHP-20 and polyamides. The commonly used solvent systems are the water solution of ethanol, methanol, or acetone.

Diaion HP-20 is commonly used first in separating tannins from non-tannin impurities, the procedures are shown in Figure 7-4.

Tannins can be fractionated (分离) by HPLC to provide both qualitative information on the homogeneity of a particular preparation, estimation of molecular weight and quantitative information on specific compounds. Either normal phase or reversed phase HPLC can be used.

The molecular sizes of hydrolysable tannins can be estimated by normal phase HPLC and as retention time extends. The ranking is in the order of monomers, dimmers, trimers, tetramers as seen in Figure 7-5.

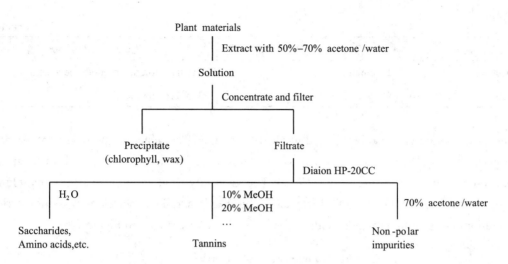

Figure 7-4 Isolation procedure for tannins using Diaion HP-20

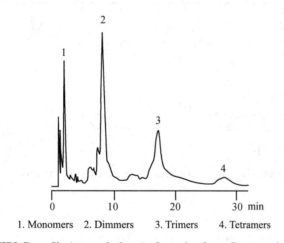

1. Monomers 2. Dimmers 3. Trimers 4. Tetramers

Figure 7-5 HPLC profile (normal phase) of tannins from *Reaumuria hirtella* (硬毛红砂)

5 Identification

The gelatin test is commonly used to identify the existence of tannins. The method is adding 1% solution of gelatin containing 10% sodium chloride to the solution of tannins (0.5%–1%). If the solution becomes turbid, it indicates that the solution may contain tannins.

Hydrolysable tannins and condensed tannins can be distinguished preliminarily by chemical reactions (Table 7-1).

Table 7-1 Chemical reactions of hydrolysable tannins and condensed tannins

Reagent	Hydrolysable tannins	Condensed tannins
Dilute acid (boil)	No precipitate	Dark-red precipitate
Bromine water	No precipitate	Yellow or brown precipitate
Ferric chloride	Bluish black precipitate	Dark-green precipitate

(continued)

Reagent	Hydrolysable tannins	Condensed tannins
Lead acetate	Precipitate	Precipitate (soluble in dilute acetic acid)
Lime-water	Gray or blue precipitate	Pink or brown precipitate

The TLC method can also be applied to identify tannins. The generally used TLC plates are silica gel G plates; the developing solvent system is chloroform-acetone-water-formic acid (different portion) or benzene-ethyl formate-formic acid (2 : 7 : 1); The generally used spraying reagents include ethanol solution of ferric chloride ($FeCl_3$), anisaldehyde-sulphuric acid and ferric chloride-potassium ferricyanide (1 : 1) solution. The preliminary judgments of compound types are shown in Figure 7-6.

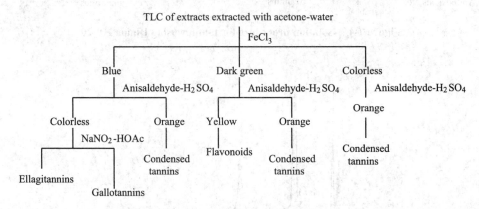

Figure 7-6　TLC identification procedure for tannins

6　Structure Determination

The structures of tannins are elucidated by using all kinds of spectral methods.

6.1　^{1}H-NMR

^{1}H-NMR spectroscopy is one of the powerful methods used in determination of tannins structures. The number of phenolic hydroxyl groups in tannins is frequently determined by ^{1}H-NMR spectroscopy of their methylated derivatives. The number of saccharides can be inferred from the NMR based on the numbers of signals from the anomeric protons of the saccharides. Coupling constants can be used to evaluate the protons of the saccharides. The replacement of aromatic rings can be judged from the number of the proton of aromatic ring and their chemical shifts. In addition, the ^{1}H-^{1}H COSY is used to detect the relationship between protons.

For hydrolysable tannins, the application of ^{1}H-NMR is listed in Table 7-2.

Table 7-2   Chemical shifts of protons on benzene rings

The aromatic moiety	Chemical shift (δ_H)
Gallic acid residues (G)	6.9–7.2 (2H,s)
Hexahydroxydiphenoyl (HHDP)	H_A, H_B 6.3–6.8 (2H,s)
Valoneoyl (Val)	H_A, H_B 6.3–6.8 (2H,s), H_C 6.9–7.2 (1H,s)
Sanguisorboyl (Sang)	H_A, H_B 6.8–7.4 (2H,d), H_C 7.0–7.2 (1H,s)

The glycosyl of tannins is mainly β-D-glucose. Its proton signals are all split and shifted to lower field.

6.2 ^{13}C-NMR

^{13}C-NMR spectroscopy is used to identify the number of gallic acid residues and HHDP, the position of acylation (酰化) and the configuration of glycosidic linkages.

6.3   MS

FAB-MS makes it possible to obtain molecular ion of tannins that are high polar, non-volatile and thermally unstable. It has become the most commonly used method for determination of tannins without derivatization.

MS^n spectra are useful in identification of compounds in complex samples and permit more complete fingerprinting of plant materials.

6.4   CD

As a conventional technique, CD spectrum is mainly used to determine the absolute configuration of ellagitannins (Table 7-3 and Figure 7-7).

Table 7-3   Characters of CD spectra for different structures of ellagitannins

Structures of ellagitannins	Characters of CD spectra	Configuration
Mono-HHDP	235nm, 265nm (+ Cotton effect)	S
	235nm, 265nm (– Cotton effect)	R
Double-HHDP	235nm, 265nm (+ Cotton effect double)	S
	235nm, 265nm (– Cotton effect double)	R
One or two HHDP and galloyl groups	235nm, 265nm and 285nm	

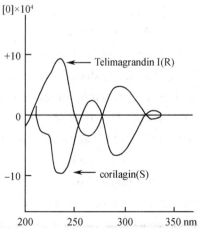

Figure 7-7   CD spectra of monomeric hydrolysable tannins in MeOH

tellimagrandin I
(R)

corilagin
(S)

7 Examples of Chinese Herbs Containing Tannins

7.1 Galla Chinensis (五倍子)

7.1.1 Introduction

(1) Biological Source

Galla Chinensis is the gall (虫瘿) produced mainly by parastic (寄生的) aphids (蚜虫) of *Melaphis chinensis* (Bell) Baker (五倍子蚜) on the leaf of *Rhus chinensis* Mill. (盐肤木), *Rhus potaninii* Maxim. (青麸杨) or *Rhus punjabensis* Stew.var. sinica (Diels) Rehd. et Wils (红麸杨). (Fam. Anacardiaceae).

(2) Property, Flavor, and Channels Entered

Property and Flavor: Cold; Sour, astringent.

Channels Entered: Lung, Large Intestine, Kidney.

(3) Actions & Indications

To constrain the lung and downbear fire, astringe the intestines to check diarrhea, stanch bleeding, check sweating, drain dampness and promote wound healing. For chronic cough caused by lung deficiency, expectoration of phlegm and cough caused by lung-heat, chronic dysentery and diarrhea, spontaneous sweating and night sweating, wasting-thirst, swelling abscess, bloody stool caused by hemorrhoid bleeding, traumatic bleeding, sore and toxin, damp ulceration of skin.

(4) Pharmacological Activities

The pharmacological activities associated with Galla Chinensis include antiviral, antibacterial, anticancer, antidiarrhea, antioxidant, hepatoprotective, suppressing HIV-1, inhibiting enamel demineralization, enhancing remineralization of dental enamel with fluoride, etc.

Gallic acid (3, 4, 5-trihydroxybenzoic acid) isolated from *Rhus chinensis* induces apoptosis in human monocytic lymphoma cell line U937 and may be a potential chemotherapeutic agent against lymphoma.

7.1.2 Main Chemical Constituents

Galla Chinensis is a native product of China, but it is also produced in small quantity in Turkey, India, Japan and Korea. The main chemical constituents of Galla Chinensis are tannins, and it also contains a few fatty acids, resins, starch, wax, protein, fiber, etc.

(1) Tannins

The main bioactive compounds of Galla Chinensis are gallotannins (50%–70%), a type of hydrolysable tannins, which have strong antioxidant and antimicrobial activities. Gallotannins is comprised of 5–12 molecules of gallic acid attached to a central glucose.

Chinensis gallotannins

(2) Other Constituents

2-hydroxy-6-pentadecyl benzoic acid, 4-(pentadec-8-enyl) phenol, palmitic acid-1, 3-dipropyl ester, β-sitosterol, pentacosane (二十五烷), 4-hydroxy-3-methoxy-benzoic acid, palmitic acid, lauric acid (月桂酸), myristic acid (豆蔻酸) are also isolated from Galla Chinensis.

7.1.3   Quality Control Standards

(1) TLC Identification

Stationary Phase: Silica gel GF_{254} plate

Standard: Authentic crude drug; gallic acid (Chemical Reference Substance, CRS).

Development System: Chloroform-ethyl formate-formic acid (5∶5∶1).

Visualization: 254nm UV light.

(2) Tests

Water: Not more than 12.0%.

Total Ash: Not more than 3.5%.

(3) Assay

Tannins: Not less than 50.0% (Spectrophotometric method).

Gallic Acid: Not less than 50.0% (HPLC).

7.2   Cinnamomi Cortex(肉桂)

7.2.1   Introduction

(1) Biological Source

Cinnamomi Cortex is the dried stem bark of *Cinnamomum cassia* Presl (肉桂). (Fam. Lauraceae)(樟科)

(2) Property, Flavor and Channels Entered

Propert and Flavor: Highly hot; Pungent, sweet.

Channels Entered: Kidney, Spleen, Heart, Liver.

(3) Actions & Indications

To tonify fire and assist yang, conduct fire back to its origin, dissipate cold and relieve pain, warm and unblock the meridian. For impotence and uterine coldness, cold pain in the lower back and knees, panting caused by kidney deficiency, dizziness and red eyes, upfloating of deficiency yang, cold pain in the heart and abdomen, deficiency cold vomiting and diarrhea, abdominal pain caused by cold abdominal colic, dysmenorrhea and amenorrhea.

(4) Pharmacological Activities

The pharmacological activities associated with Cinnamomi Cortex include anti-inflammatory, anti-bacterial, antioxidant, antidiabetic, anti-platelet aggregation, anticancer effects, sedative, improving blood circulation, etc. In addition, it is also used as stomachic, carminative, mildly astringent.

7.2.2 Main Chemical Constituents

Cinnamomi Cortex grows in Guangdong, Guangxi and Hainan provinces of China, Indonesia, Laos, and Viet Nam. It contains essential oils, phenols, organic acids, polysaccharides, glycosides, coumarins, tannins and mucilage.

(1) Volatile Oils

It contains up to 4% of volatile oils consisting primarily of cinnamaldehyde (60%–80%), others include 2-methoxycinnamaldehyde (邻甲氧基肉桂醛), phellandrene, eugenol, methyleugenol (丁香酚甲醚), cinnamyl acetate (乙酸肉桂酯), β-caryophyllene (β-石竹烯), δ-cadinene (δ-荜澄茄烯), linalool and cineole.

(2) Tannins

It chiefly contains condensed tannins, namely, *d*-catechin, *l*-epicatechin, procyanidin B-1, procyanidin B-2, arecatannin A1 (槟榔鞣质 A1), cinnamtannin (肉桂鞣质) B2 and C2.

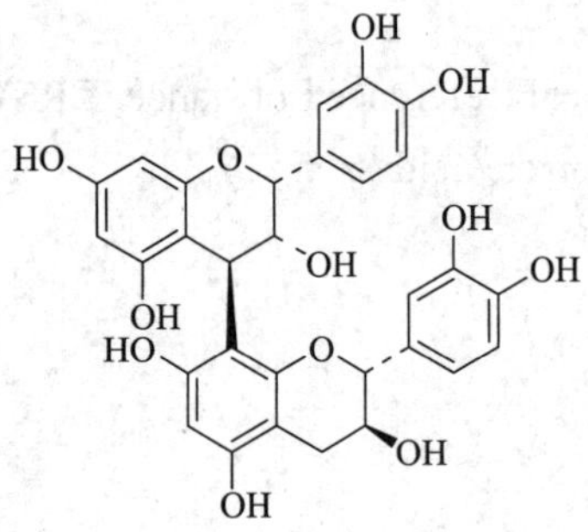

procyanidin B-1

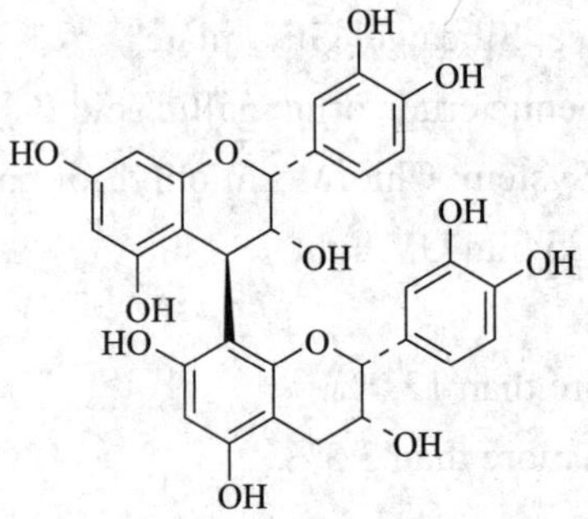

procyanidin B-2

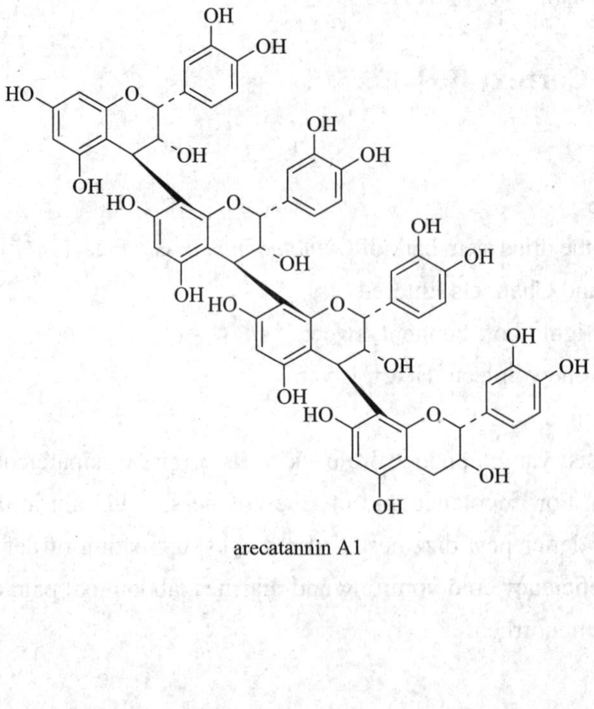

arecatannin A1

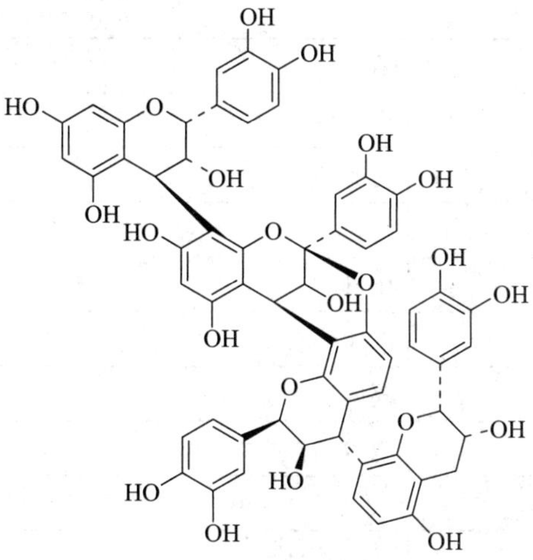

cinnamtannin B2

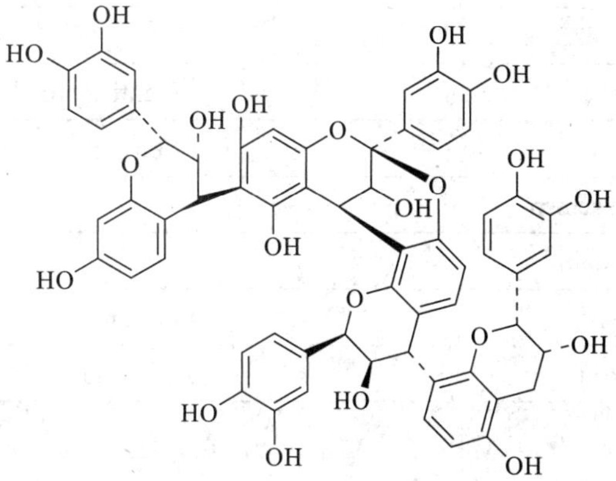

cinnamtannin C2

(3) Other Constituents

Cinnamomi Cortex also contains pentacyclic diterpenes such as cinnzeylanol (桂二萜醇) and its acetyl derivative cinnzeylanine (乙酰桂二萜醇), which have insecticidal effect, and other diterpene derivatives like cinncassiol (肉桂萜醇) A-E, which are present as both glycosides and free aglycones. In addition, Cinnamomi Cortex contains cinnamic acid, phenolic acids and saccharides like mannitol, L-arabino-D-xylanase, L-arabinose, D-xylose, α-D-glucane as well as mucilage, etc.

7.2.3　Quality Control Standards

(1) TLC Identification

Stationary Phase: silica gel plate.

Standard: Cinnamaldehyde (Chemical Reference Substance, CRS).

Development System: Petroleum ether (60–90℃)-ethyl acetate (17∶3).

Visualization: Spray the solution of dinitrophenylhydrazine (二硝基苯肼) in ethanol.

(2) Tests

Water: Not more than 15.0%.

Total Ash: Not more than 5.0%.

(3) Assay

Volatile Oils: Not less than 1.2% (determination method for volatile oils).

Cinnamaldehyde: Not less than 1.5% (HPLC).

词　汇　表

An Alphabetical List of Words and Phrases

A		
acidified	[əˈsɪdɪfaɪ]	酸化
acutissimin		野牡丹鞣质
acylation	[ˈæsəleɪʃən]	酰化
additives	[ˈædɪtɪvz]	添加剂
agrimoniin		仙鹤草素

(continued)

ammonia	[ə'məunjə]	氨
Anacardiaceae		漆树科
antiseptics	[ˌæntɪ'septɪks]	防腐剂
aphids	['eɪfɪdz]	蚜虫
Arecae semen		槟榔
arecatannin		槟榔鞣质
artemisia	[ˌɑːtɪ'mɪzɪə]	蒿属
astringent	[ə'strɪndʒənt]	收敛剂，涩
C		
δ-cadinene	[keɪdaɪ'niːn]	δ– 荜澄茄烯
caffeetannin		咖啡鞣质
caffeic acid	[ke'fiːɪk]['æsɪd]	咖啡酸
camelliatannin		山茶鞣质
β-caryophyllene	[keəriːəfɪ'liːn]	β– 石竹烯
castalagin	[kæs'təlɪdʒɪn]	栗木鞣花素
casuarinin	['kæʒuərɪnɪn]	木麻黄鞣宁
catechin / catechol / catechuic acid	['kætɪtʃɪn] / ['ktɪtɪʃəul]['æsɪd]	儿茶素，儿茶酸，儿茶酚，邻苯二酚
Chebulae Fructus		诃子
chebuloyl (Che)		诃子酰基
Chinese sumac	[ˌtʃai'niːz]['suːmæk]	盐肤木
cinchona	[sɪŋ'kəunə]	金鸡纳树皮
Cinnamomi Cortex		肉桂
cinnamtannin	[sɪ'næmtænɪn]	肉桂鞣质
cinnamyl acetate	[sɪ'næmɪl]['æsɪteɪt]	乙酸肉桂酯
cinncassiol	[sɪn'kæsiːəul]	肉桂萜醇
cinnzeylanine		乙酰桂二萜醇
cinnzeylanol		桂二萜醇
cleave	[kliːv]	裂解
cocoa	['kəukəu]	可可树
cola	['kəulə]	可乐树
Combretaceae		使君子科
complex tannins	['kɔmpleks]['tænɪnz]	复合鞣质
condensed tannins	[kən'denst]['tænɪnz]	缩合鞣质
Cinnamomum cassia Presl		肉桂
D		
dehydrohexahydroxydiphenoyl (DHHDP)		脱氢六羟基联苯二甲酰基
depside	['depsaɪd]	缩酚酸

(continued)

derivative	[dɪˈrɪvətɪv]	衍生物，派生物
dilactone	[daɪˈlæktəun]	双内酯
dinitrophenylhydrazine	[daɪnaɪtrəufenɪlhaɪdreɪˈzɪ]	二硝基苯肼
3,5-di-*O*-caffeoylquinic acid		3,5- 二 –*O*- 咖啡酰奎宁酸
diuretics	[daɪˈjuəreɪtɪks]	利尿药
diversity	[daɪˈvə:səti]	多样性
Dryopteridis crassirhizomatis rhizoma		绵马贯众
E		
ellagic acid	[ɪˈlædʒɪk][ˈæsɪd]	逆没食子酸
ellagitannins	[ˈelɪdʒɪtənɪnz]	逆没食子鞣质，鞣花酸鞣质
esterification	[eˌsterɪfɪˈkeɪʃən]	酯化反应
F		
Fagaceous plant		壳斗科植物
fractionate	[ˈfrækʃəneɪt]	分离
G		
galloyl ester	[ˈgælɔɪl][ˈestə]	没食子酸酯
gall	[gɔ:l]	虫瘿
gallotannins	[ˈgæləutænɪnz]	没食子鞣质
galloylglucoses (GGs)	[ˌgælɔɪlˈglu:kəus]	没食子酰基葡萄糖
geraniin	[dʒeˈræni:n]	老鹳草素
glucogallin	[glu:ˈkɔgælɪn]	葡萄糖没食子鞣苷
C-glycosidic ellagitannins	[glaɪkəuˈsɪdɪk] [ˈelɪdʒɪtənɪnz]	*C*– 苷逆没食子鞣质
guavin		番石榴素
Galla chinensis		五倍子
H		
haemostatic pharmaceuticals	[hɪˌməuˈstætɪk] [ˌfɑ:məˈsju:tɪklz]	止血药
herbivory	[ˈhə:bɪvərɪ]	食草性
hexahydroxydiphenic acid		六羟二酚酸
hexahydroxydiphenoyl (HHDP)		六羟基联苯二甲酰基
hydrolysable tannins	[haɪˈdrɔlaɪzəbl][ˈtænɪnz]	可水解鞣质
I		
lead	[li:d]	铅
impurities	[ɪmˈpjuərɪtɪs]	杂质
intramolecular	[ˌɪntrəməˈlekjulə]	分子内的
L		
Lauraceae		樟科
lauric acid	[ˈlɔ:rɪk][ˈæsɪd]	月桂酸

(continued)

M		
metallurgy	[məˈtælədʒiː]	冶金
2-methoxycinnamaldehyde		邻甲氧基肉桂醛
methyleugenol	[ˈmetɪljuːdʒenɔl]	丁香酚甲醚
mongolicin		蒙古栎素
monomeric ellagitannins	[ˌmɔnəˈmerɪk][ˈelɪdʒɪtənɪnz]	简单逆没食子鞣质
myristic acid	[mɪˈrɪstɪk][ˈæsɪd]	豆蔻酸
Melaphis chinensis (Bell) Baker	[tʃaɪˈnensɪs]	五倍子蚜
O		
oligomer	[ˈɔlɪɡəʊmə]	低聚物，低聚体
oligomeric ellagitannins	[ɔlɪɡəʊˈmerɪk] [ˈelɪdʒɪtənɪnz]	逆没食子鞣质低聚体
P		
parastic	[ˌpærəˈstɪk]	寄生的
pentacosane	[pentəˈkəʊseɪn]	二十五烷
pentamers	[ˈpentəməz]	五聚体
pharmaceuticals	[ˌfɑːmeˈsjuːtɪklz]	药物
phlobaphene	[fləʊˈbæfiːn]	鞣红，鞣酐
phlobatannins	[ˈfləʊbətənɪnz]	鞣红鞣质
photography	[fəˈtɔɡrəfi]	摄影
plant galls	[plɑːnt][ɡɔːlz]	植物虫瘿
polymers	[ˈpɔləməz]	高聚物，高聚体
polyols	[ˈpɔlɪɔlz]	多元醇
polyphenol	[ˌpɔlɪˈfiːnɔl]	多酚
polyphenolic	[ˌpɔlɪfɪˈnɔlɪk]	多聚酚
potassium ferricyanide	[pəˈtæsɪəm][ˌferɪˈsaɪənaɪd]	铁氰化钾
Q		
quinic acid	[ˈkwɪnɪk][ˈæsɪd]	奎宁酸，金鸡纳酸
R		
reddish tints	[ˈredɪʃ][tɪnts]	淡红色
Reaumuria hirtella		硬毛红砂
Rhus chinensis Mill.		盐肤木
Rhus potaninii Maxim.		青麸杨
Rhus punjabensis Stew.var. sinica (Diels) Rehd. et Wils		红麸杨
S		
sanguisorboyl (Sang)	[ˌsæŋgwɪˈsɔːbɔɪl]	地榆酰基
scale	[skeɪl]	水垢

(continued)

stachyurin		旌节花素
T		
tannin	['tænɪn]	鞣质
tannin reds	['tænɪn][redz]	鞣红
tanning	['tænɪŋ]	鞣制，鞣革
tellimagrandin		特里马素
tetramers	['tetrəməz]	四聚体
tin	[tɪn]	锡
trimer	['traɪmə]	三聚体
U		
unambiguously	[ˌʌnæm'bɪgjuəsli]	含糊地，不明白地
V		
valoneoyl (Val)		橡腕酰基
vescalagin	[ves'kɑːlɪdʒɪn]	栎木鞣花素

重 点 小 结

　　鞣质是由没食子酸（或其聚合物）的葡萄糖（及其他多元醇）酯、黄烷醇及其衍生物的聚合物以及两者混合共同组成的植物多元酚。鞣质分为可水解鞣质、缩合鞣质和复合鞣质三大类。

　　鞣质大多为灰白色无定性粉末，多具引湿性。极性较强，溶于水、亲水性有机溶剂、乙酸乙酯，难溶或不溶于亲脂性有机溶剂。

　　鞣质为强还原剂，能还原斐林试剂；可与蛋白质结合产生沉淀，可据此性质用明胶提纯、鉴别鞣质；鞣质的水溶液可与生物碱生成沉淀，可作为生物碱沉淀试剂；与三氯化铁产生蓝黑色或绿黑色反应或产生沉淀，故可作为工业原料制造蓝黑墨水；鞣质与铁氰化钾氨溶液反应呈现深红色，进一步变为棕色。

　　鞣质可使明胶溶液变混浊或生成沉淀，可用于检识鞣质。

　　鞣质因其具有强还原性，故提取时多采用新鲜原料且宜立即浸提，原料的干燥尽可能在短时间内完成，以避免鞣质在水分、日光、氧气和酶作用下变质。多采用组织破碎法，以50%~70%含水丙酮作为提取溶剂进行提取。分离方法有溶剂法、沉淀法、柱色谱法、高效液相法等。

目 标 检 测

题库

一、单选题

1. 提取鞣质类成分最常用的方法是（　　　　）

　　A. 煎煮法　　　　　　　　　B. 渗漉法　　　　　　　　　C. 回流提取法

　　D. 组织破碎提取法　　　　　E. 超临界流体萃取法

2. 以下不能溶解鞣质的溶剂是（　　）
    A. 水　　　　　　　　　　　　B. 甲醇　　　　　　　　　　C. 乙醇
    D. 丙酮　　　　　　　　　　　E. 石油醚

3. 制造蓝黑墨水利用的是鞣质与（　　）作用产生蓝黑色
    A. 蛋白质　　　　　　　　　　B. 生物碱　　　　　　　　　C. 铁氰化钾
    D. 石灰水　　　　　　　　　　E. 三氯化铁

4. 从中药水提液中分离或者除去鞣质可采用的方法是（　　）
    A. 硅胶柱层析法　　　　　　　B. 明胶沉淀法
    C. 雷氏盐沉淀法　　　　　　　D. 碱溶酸沉淀法
    E. 水提醇沉法

5. 以下不能与鞣质形成沉淀的是（　　）
    A. 明胶　　　　　　　　　　　B. 生物碱　　　　　　　　　C. FeCl₃
    D. 乙酸铅　　　　　　　　　　E. 乙酸乙酯

二、多选题

1. 根据鞣质的化学结构特征，鞣质的类型包括（　　）
    A. 可水解鞣质　　　　　　　　B. 缩合鞣质　　　　　　　　C. 复合鞣质
    D. 混合鞣质　　　　　　　　　E. 聚合鞣质

2. 可水解鞣质在酸、碱、酶作用下，可水解成（　　）
    A. 小分子酚酸类　　　　　　　B. 糖　　　　　　　　　　　C. 苷元
    D. 鞣红　　　　　　　　　　　E. 多元醇

3. 分离鞣质类成分常用的方法有（　　）
    A. 溶剂法　　　　　　　　　　B. 沉淀法　　　　　　　　　C. 色谱法
    D. 透析法　　　　　　　　　　E. 盐析法

4. 缩合鞣质的基本结构有（　　）
    A. 黄酮醇　　　　　　　　　　　　　　　　B. 黄烷 -3- 醇类
    C. 黄烷 -3, 4- 二醇类　　　　　　　　　　D. 查耳酮
    E. 花色素

5. 关于鞣质表述正确的有（　　）
    A. 多为灰白色无定型粉末
    B. 多为红色无定型粉末
    C. 多具有吸湿性
    D. 极性较小
    E. 能沉淀生物碱

三、思考题

1. 简述鞣质的常用提取方法及注意事项。
2. 简述沉淀法分离鞣质的原理及操作方法。
3. 对鞣质类成分进行薄层鉴别时，为什么需在展开剂中加入少量酸？

（王　薇）

Chapter 8　Alkaloids

PPT-2

知识要求：

1．掌握　生物碱的定义、主要理化性质及其提取分离，以及检识方法。掌握麻黄、黄连、洋金花、防己中主要生物碱成分的结构特点、主要理化性质、提取分离与检识方法。

2．熟悉　生物碱的结构与分类；熟悉延胡索、苦参中主要生物碱成分的结构特点、主要理化性质及提取分离方法；熟悉脂溶性和水溶性生物碱的提取分离方法。

3．了解　生物碱的分布、生物活性及结构研究的一般方法。

能力要求：

学会应用生物碱专属性反应检识生物碱类化合物；学会应用 pH 梯度萃取法分离不同碱性的生物碱；学会应用雷氏铵盐沉淀法分离纯化季铵碱；学会应用生物碱的碱性和溶解性的不同，针对不同生物碱选择适合的提取分离方法，解决生物碱类化合物在提取分离过程中存在的技术问题。

1　Introduction

1.1　Definition of Alkaloids

Alkaloids are a naturally occurring large group of physiologically active nitrogen-containing organic compounds from organisms (mainly are plants). In general, the naturally occurring nitrogen-containing organic compounds are all considered as alkaloids except for the organism need, for example amino acids, amino sugars, peptides, proteins, nucleic acids (核酸), nucleotide acids (核苷酸), nitrogen-containing vitamines, and so on. In most alkaloids, there is a complex heterocyclic ring system, and the nitrogen atom is part of the rings. They show alkaline and form salts with acid.

1.2　Distribution of Alkaloids

Alkaloids exist in about 15% of all terrestrial plants and in more than 150 different plant families. Most of them present in dicotyledon (双子叶植物) of higher plants. They are also detected in microorganisms, marine organisms, insects, animals and some of the lower plants. Among the angiosperms (被子植物), the Apocynaceae (夹竹桃科), Papaveraceae (罂粟科), Ranunculaceae (毛茛科), Rubiaceae, Solanaceae, and Berberidaceae (小檗科) are outstanding for alkaloid-yielding plants. Some common alkaloids sources are listed in Table 8-1.

In plants, alkaloids may be found in the whole plant, but most of them gather in one organ, such as bark, rhizome, marrow, etc., for example quinine (奎宁) mainly exists in the bark of quina. One plant generally contains one class of alkaloids with the same parent nucleus due to their similar biosynthetic path way. Moreover, the same family and genus plants generally contain the same class of alkaloids.

Table 8-1　Some common alkaloids sources

Family	Chinese Herb	Main alkaloids	Chemical type
Ranunculaceae	Coptidis rhizoma Aconiti lateralis radix praeparata, （北乌头） Aconiti radix	Coptisine (黄连碱) Aconitine	Diterpene
Papaveraceae	Papaveris pericarpium (罂粟壳) Corydalis rhizoma	Morphine (吗啡) Palmatine (巴马丁) Tetrahydropulmatine （延胡索乙素）	Morphine
Solanaceae	Daturae flos (洋金花) Belladonnae herba (颠茄) Hyoscyami semen (天仙子)	Scopolamine (东莨菪碱) Atropine (阿托品)	Tropane (莨菪烷) Pyridine
Leguminosae Fabaceae （蝶形花科）	Cassia obtusifolia (草决明) Sophorae flavescentis radix (苦参)	Cytisine (胞苷) Matrine (苦参碱)	Quinolizidine (喹诺里西啶)
Menispermaceae （防己科）	Stephania tetrandrae radix (防己) Menipermi rhizome (北豆根)	Tetrandrine (汉防己碱)	Dibenzyltetrahydroiso-quinolin (二苄基四氢异喹啉)
Berberidaceae	Berberidis radix (三颗针)	Berberine	Isoquinoline (异喹啉)

1.3　Pharmacological Activities of Alkaloids

Alkaloids have distinguished bioactivities. Some of alkaloids and their pharmacological activities are listed in Table 8-2.

Table 8-2　Pharmacological activities of some alkaloids

Alkaloids	Pharmacological activities
Morphine, tetrahydropulmatine	Narcotic analgesic, Relieve pain
Ephedrine	Relieving cough and asthma
Atropine	Spasmolysis
Matrine, oxymatrine (氧化苦参碱)	Anti-arrhythmia
Colchicine (秋水仙碱), camptothecine (喜树碱), vincristine (长春新碱), cephalotaxin (三尖杉碱), taxol (紫杉醇)	Anticancer
Quinine	Antimalaria

(continued)

Alkaloids	Pharmacological activities
Berberine, dauricine (蝙蝠葛碱)	Antisepsis, eliminate and inflammation
Quinidine (奎尼丁)	Cardiac depressant

2   Structure and Classification

There are many categories of alkaloids. Various methods proposed for classification of alkaloids are as follows:

The term alkaloid covers proto-alkaloids (原生物碱), true-alkaloids, and pseudo-alkaloids (伪生物碱). Proto-alkaloids are simple amines in which the nitrogen is not in a heterocyclic ring. Generally they are basic in property and come from amino acids. True-alkaloids are heterocyclic nitrogen-containing compounds which are derived from amino acids and always basic in property. They are normally presented in plants as salts of organic acids. Pseudo-alkaloids mainly include steroidal and terpenoid alkaloids and purines (嘌呤). They are not derived from amino acids, and they do not show many of the typical characteristics of alkaloids, but show positive reactions to precipitation reagents for alkaloids.

Depending on the physiological response, the alkaloids are classified under various pharmacological categories, like central nervous system stimulants or depressants, analgesics, purgatives, etc. This method does not take into account the chemical nature of alkaloids.

The third one is taxonomic classification. This method classifies alkaloids based on their distribution in various plant families, like solanaceous (茄科的) or papillionaceous (蝶形科的) alkaloids. From this classification, the chemotaxonomic classification has been further derived.

The chemical classification is the type of fundamental (normally heterocyclic) ring structure present in alkaloids. The new classification is biosynthetic classification combining with chemical classification. This method gives significance to the precursor from which the alkaloids are biosynthesized in the organisms. Hence, the variety of alkaloids with different taxonomic distributions and physiological activities can be brought under the same group, if they are derived from the same precursor. For example, all indole alkaloids (吲哚生物碱类) from tryptophan (色氨酸) are grouped together. Alkaloids are categorized on the fact whether they are derived from amino acid precursor such as ornithine (鸟氨酸), lysine (赖氨酸), tyrosine (酪氨酸), phenylalanine (苯丙氨酸), tryptophan, etc.

The types of alkaloids and their occurrence in various plants along with basic chemical ring are listed in Table 8-3.

Table 8-3   Main true-alkaloids and pseudo-alkaloids

Categories	N-containing structure	Biosynthetic precursor	Example
Pyrrole (吡咯) and Pyrrolidine (吡咯烷)		Aspartic acid (天冬氨酸)	Nicotine (烟碱), hygrine (古柯碱)
Pyridine and Piperidine (哌啶)		Lysine	Piperine (胡椒碱), arecolidine (槟榔碱), coniine (毒芹碱), pelletierine (石榴皮碱), anabasin (八角枫碱), trigonelline (胡芦巴碱)
Quinolizidine		Lysine	Lupinine (羽扇豆碱)
Indolizidine (吲哚里西啶)		Lysine	Securinine (一叶萩碱)
Pyrrolizidine		Ornithine	Senecionine (千里光宁碱)
Tropane		Ornithine	Atropine, hyoscine (东莨菪碱), cocaine (可卡因)
Quinoline (喹啉)		Tyrosine	Quinine, quinidine
Isoquinoline		Tyrosine	Berberine, emetine (吐根碱), codeine (可待因), morphine, dl-tetrahydropalmatine
Indole (吲哚)		Tryptophan	Reserpine (利血平) strychnine (士的宁), evodiamine (吴茱萸碱), camptothecine
Imidazole (咪唑)		Histidine (组氨酸)	Pilocarpine (毛果芸香碱)
Terpenes		Monoterpenes, Sesquiterpene, Diterpenes	Gentianine (龙胆碱), Dendrobine (石斛碱), Aconitine
Steroidal			Veratramine (藜芦胺)
Alkylamine (有机胺类)	CHOH CHCH₃ NHCH₃		Ephedrine

3　Physical and Chemical Properties

3.1　Physical Properties

3.1.1　Characteristics

Most of alkaloids are colorless, crystalline solids with a sharp melting point or decomposition range. Some alkaloids are amorphous gums. Some small alkaloids such as nicotine, coniine, sparteine, etc., are liquid and can volatile. Some alkaloids have color. For example, berberine and serpentine are yellow, betanidin is red, and salts of sanguinarine (血根碱) are copper red. Some alkaloids, such as ephedrine, nicotine, etc., are volatile. Some free form alkaloid, such as caffeine, can sublimate.

3.1.2　Optical Activity

Alkaloids generally have optical activity due to the chiral carbon atom in their structures. The solvent and pH value, and the concentration of alkaloids can affect the optical activity of alkaloids. For example, hydrastine (白毛茛碱) shows laevorotation in 95% ethanol and dextrorotation in low concentrated ethanol. Ephedrine shows dextrorotation in water but laevorotation in chloroform.

The pharmacological activities of alkaloids are related to their optical activity. The pharmacological activities of levorotary alkaloids generally are much stronger than those of dexiotropic alkaloids. For example, the mydriasis effect of *l*-hyoscyamine is 100 times stronger than *d*-hyoscyamine.

3.1.3　Solubility

Alkaloids present in organisms either in free form as amine, or as salt with acid, or alkaloid *N*-oxides.

In general, the free form alkaloids are soluble in non-polar organic solvents and insoluble in water. For example, most of tertiary amines (叔胺) and secondary amine (仲胺) are lipophilic (亲脂性的) when they present in free form. They are easy to dissolve in chloroform. While quaternary alkaloids (季铵碱) and *N*-oxides are more polar and can dissolve in water, methanol and ethanol. Some alkaloids, e.g. ephedrine, matrine, oxymatrine, scopolamine, nicotine can dissolve either in water and ethanol or in non-polar organic solvents, which is because they are small molecules, or with ether bond (醚键), or with coordinate bond (配位键), or liquid. The amphoteric alkaloids (两性生物碱) with phenolic hydroxyl or carboxyl group are soluble either in acid water or in alkaline water, but easy to be precipitated when pH value is 8–9, e.g. morphine, berbamine, arecaidine etc.

The salts of alkaloids generally are soluble in water and insoluble in organic solvents. Their solubility in water is related to acid. For example, quinine hydrochloride (盐酸盐) is highly soluble in water (1 part of quinine hydrochloride is soluble in less than 1 part of water), while 1 part of quinine sulphate (硫酸盐) is only soluble in 1000 parts of water.

The solubility of alkaloids and their salts does not always follow the above rule. For example, free form morphine is soluble in alkaline water, but difficult to dissolve in chloroform or ether. Free form lycorine (石蒜碱) is soluble in water and insoluble in organic solvents. Free form camptothecine is insoluble in organic solvents but soluble in acidic chloroform. Some salts of alkaloids are soluble in non-polar organic solvents. For example, homolycorine (高石蒜碱) hydrochloride is soluble in chloroform and difficult to dissolve in water. Some salts of alkaloids are insoluble in water, e.g. berberine hydrochloride, ephedrine oxalate.

3.2 Chemical Properties

3.2.1 Basicity

The basicity of alkaloids is the most important chemical property and can be used for its extraction, isolation and identification. Most alkaloids are basic due to the availability of a pair of non-bonded electrons on nitrogen. In the Lewis sense, an acid is defined as an electron pair acceptor and a base as an electron pair donor. The strength of a base is expressed by the equilibrium constant K_b (basicity constant):

$$B + H_2O \rightleftharpoons BH^+ + OH^- \qquad K_b = [BH^+][OH^-] / [B]$$

The pK_b is defined as the negative logarithm of K_b. The pK_a is the negative logarithm of K_a.

$$pK_b = -\log K_b \qquad pK_a + pK_b = 14\ (pK_W) \qquad pK_a = 14 - pK_b$$

The larger the K_b and pK_a of an alkaloid, the stronger the basicity of the alkaloid, and vice versa.

The degree of basicity is greatly depending on the structure of the alkaloid. The relationship among the basicity, pK_a, and structures of alkaloids is shown in Table 8-4.

Table 8-4　Basicity, pK_a, and structures of alkaloids

Structure	Basicity	pK_a
Carbamidine (胍), quaternary ammonium	Strong	>11
Alkyl heterocyclic (烷基杂环), aliphatic amines (脂肪胺)	Medium strong	7~11
Aromatic heterocyclic-N (芳香杂环), aromatic amines (芳香族胺)	Weak	2~7
Amides, pyrrole	Nearly neutral	<2

3.2.2 Relationship between Basicity and Structure

The basicity of alkaloids is depended on the hybridization (杂化) of the nitrogenin in alkaloids and it is affected by inductive effect (诱导效应), inductive-field effect (诱导–场效应), conjugative effect (共轭效应), space effect (空间效应) and hydrogen bonding effect (氢键效应) etc.

(1) Hybridization of Nitrogen

In the hybrid orbital (杂化轨道), p electron is easy to supply electron due to its activity. When the ratio of p electron becomes higher, its basicity will be stronger, i.e. $sp^3 > sp^2 > sp$. Examples are listed in Table 8-5.

Table 8-5　Basicity of alkaloids and the hybridization of nitrogen

Alkaloids	Structure	Hybridization	pK_a
Tetrahydroisowuinolin (四氢异喹啉)		sp^3	9.5
Pyridine		sp^2	5.17
Isoquinoline		sp^2	5.4
Cyanide ion (氰离子)	CN^-	sp	Neutral

(2) Inductive Effect

The electron atmosphere density (电子云密度) on nitrogen of the alkaloids is affected by the electron donors (alkyl groups) and electron acceptor (—OCH₃, —OH, —Ar, —C=O) near the nitrogen. Electron donors can increase the electron atmosphere density of the nitrogen and increase its basicity. The electron acceptor can decrease the electron atmosphere density of the nitrogen and decrease its basicity. For example, the basicity of ephedrine (pK_a 9.58) is stronger than that of demethyl-ephedrine (去甲基麻黄碱）(pK_a 9.00) due to the electron donor's inductive effect of methyl group in ephedrine. But the basicity of them is all weaker than that of amphetamine (pK_a 9.80), because the electron acceptor's inductive effect of hydroxyl group connects with C-1 in ephedrine and demethyl-ephedrine.

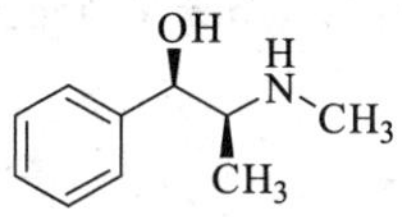

l-ephedrine (1*R*, 2*S*)
pK_a = 9.58

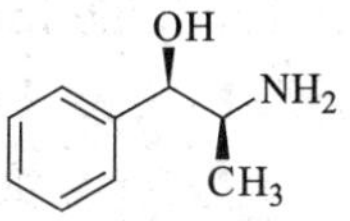

l-demethyl-ephedrine (1*R*, 2*S*)
pK_a = 9.00

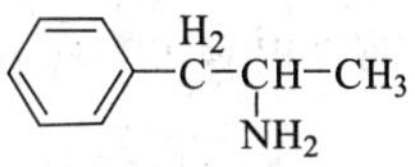

amphetamine
pK_a = 9.80

There is an exception when a double bond or hydroxyl group is presented next to the nitrogen atom of an alkaloid. Its basicity can become much strong, e.g. berberine (Figure 8-1).

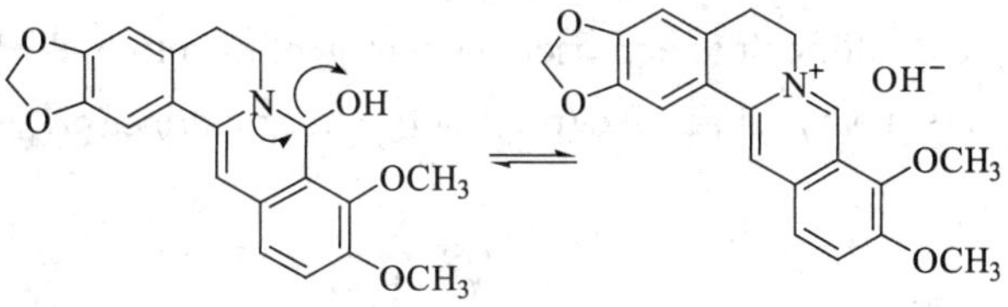

Figure 8-1 Basicity of berberine in different types

(3) Inductive-Field Effect

The basicity of every nitrogen atom is different when there are more than one nitrogen atoms in an alkaloid even though the hybridization and chemical environment of each nitrogen atom are same. After one of the nitrogen atoms hybridize, an electron acceptor (—N⁺HR₂) will be created, which can produce two kinds of effects to decrease the basicity of other nitrogen atoms in the alkaloid. These effects include inductive effect and static electricity field effect. For example the basicities of two nitrogen atoms in sparteine (无叶豆碱) are different (ΔpK_a is 8.1) because they are close in the space and exist inductive-field effect.

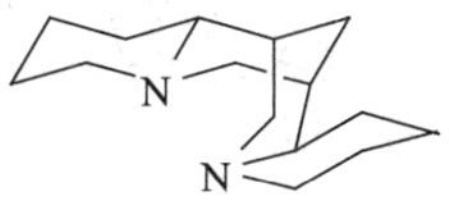

sparteine

(4) Conjugative Effect

When the pair of non-bonded electrons on nitrogen of alkaloids conjugate with π-electrons, the basicity of the alkaloid will decrease due to the decreasing of electron density of nitrogen. Phenylamines (苯胺) and amides alkaloids are common. For example, the basicities of two nitrogen atoms of physostigmine (毒扁豆碱) are different due to the conjugation effect. The pair of non-bonded electrons on nitrogen of amide conjugate with carbonyl to create the p-π conjugated system, which makes its basicity very weak. For example, piperine (pK_a 1.42), colchicines (pK_a 1.84), and caffeine (pK_a 1.22) are all amides with very weak basicity.

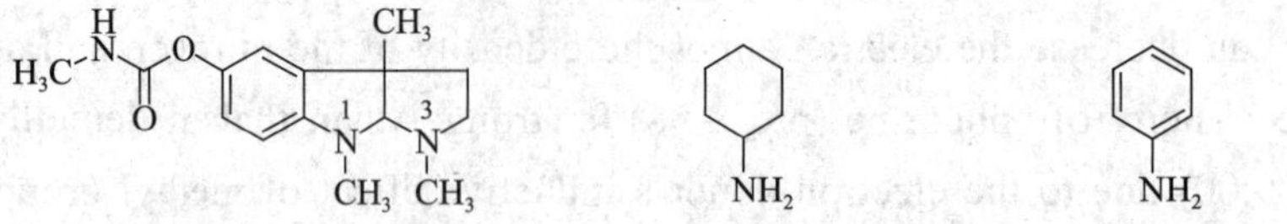

physostigmine　　　　　　　　　cyclohexylamines　　　　phenylamines

pK_a　　1.76 (N$_1$)　　7.88(N$_3$)　　　　　10.64　　　　　　4.58

An exception is that the basicity of carbamidine increases greatly when it accepts a proton and becomes quaternary amine ion (季铵离子) (pK_a 13.6, see Figure 8-2).

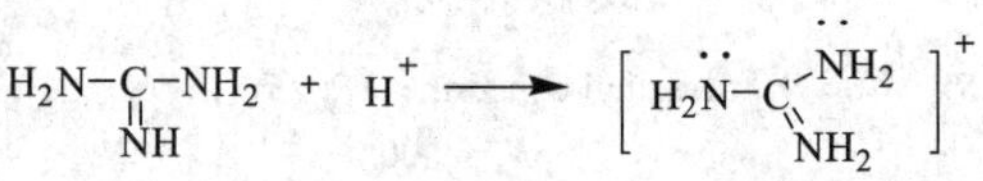

Figure 8-2　Conjugative effect of carbamidine

(5) Space Effect

The factors of the steric hindrance (空间位阻) and molecular conformation (构象) of the substituent near the nitrogen make the proton difficult to approach the nitrogen, therefore, the basicity of the alkaloid will decrease: scopolamine (pK_a 7.5), methyl-ephedrine (pK_a 9.30), and ephedrine (pK_a 9.58), etc.

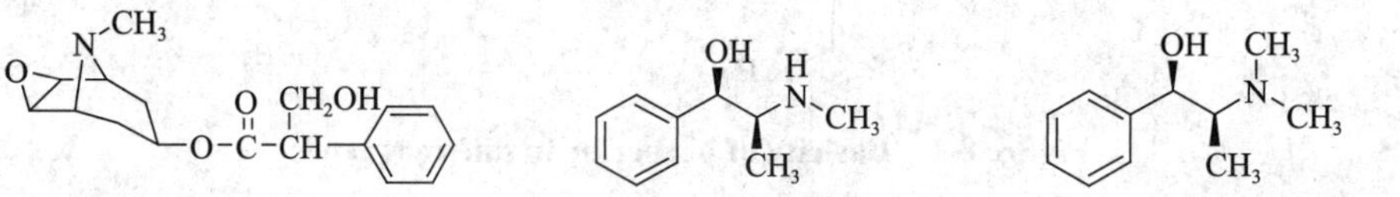

scopolamine　　　　　　l-ephedrine (1R, 2S)　　　　l-methyl-ephedrine (1R, 2S)

pK_a 7.5　　　　　　　　　pK_a 9.58　　　　　　　　　pK_a 9.30

(6) Hydrogen Bonding Effect

When alkaloids accept a proton, there is hydroxyl or carbonyl (-OH, -C=O) near the nitrogen atom, and if it is beneficial to form an intramolecular hydrogen bond, the basicity of the alkaloid will increase because the proton on nitrogen is not easy to leave. For example, the basicity of ephedrine (pK_a 9.58, see Figure 8-3) is weaker than that of pseudoephedrine (伪麻黄碱) (pK_a 9.74, see Figure 8-4).

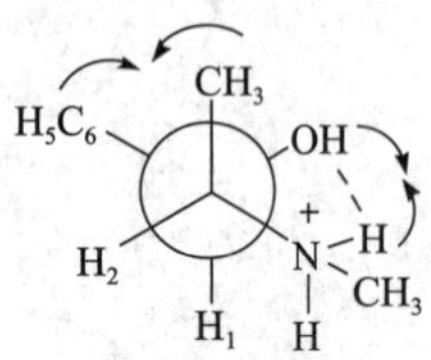

Figure 8-3　Conjugate acid of ephedrine 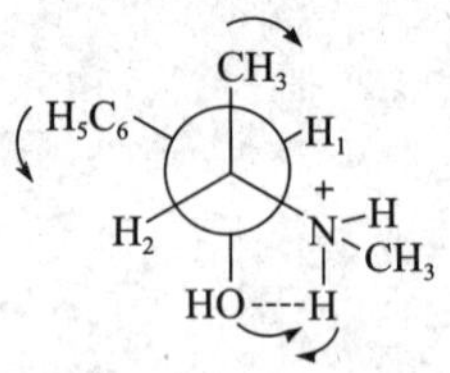　　　　**Figure 8-4　Conjugate acid of pseudoephedrine**

For some alkaloids, there are more than one factor affecting their basicity. The co-existing factors need to be discussed. In general, when the space effect and inductive effect co-exist in one alkaloid molecule, the former factor is predominant, when the inductive effect and conjugative effect co-exist, the latter will be predominant.

3.2.3　Precipitation Reactions

The general chemical tests used for identification of alkaloids are precipitation reactions. Most alkaloids can give positive precipitation reactions with large organic acids or salts of heavy metals, such as mercury (汞), platinum (铂), gold, etc.

(1) Condition

Precipitation reactions of alkaloids generally accomplish in acidic water or acidic dilute alcohol.

(2) Reagents

The commonly used precipitation reagents are listed in Table 8-6.

Table 8-6　Commonly used reagents of precipitation reactions

Reagent	Composition	Result
Dragendorff's reagent	$KBiI_4$	Reddish brown amorphism precipitate (无定形沉淀)
Mayer's reagent	K_2HgI_4	Off-white color precipitate
Wagner's reagent	$KI-I_2$	Reddish brown precipitate
Hager's reagent	2, 4, 6-trinitrophenol (2, 4, 6– 三硝基苯酚)	Yellow precipitate
Reinecke's salt (雷氏铵盐)	$NH_4[Cr(NH_3)_2(SCN)_4]$	Red precipitate

(3) Application and Cautions

① Precipitation reactions of alkaloids should accomplish in acidic water or acidic dilute alcohol. But the reaction of Hager's reagent can carry out in neutral water.

② Pay attention to the false negative or positive reactions. In general, secondary amine, such as ephedrine, is not easy to react with the precipitation reagents of alkaloids. Protein, peptides and tannins in water solution can also react with these reagents to produce false positive reaction. Therefore, these constituents should be removed from the test solution first. The following procedure is used to avoid false positive reactions (Figure 8-5).

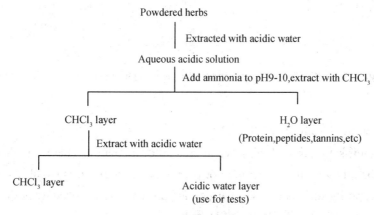

Figure 8-5　Preparation of test solution for identification of alkaloids

4　Extraction and Isolation

The extraction of alkaloids is based on their basicity and solubility. Seeds and leaves of Chinese herbs are generally defatted first with petroleum ether. Then different methods of isolation are followed.

4.1　Extraction

4.1.1　Extract with Water or Acidic Water

Most alkaloids present as salts in plants, so they can be extracted with water or acidic water. Inorganic acids are commonly used. For example, 0.1%–1% sulfuric acid (硫酸) or hydrochloric acid. Acetic acid and tartaric acid (酒石酸) can also be used. In general, maceration and percolation methods are used to extract alkaloids. Followed the acidic water extraction of alkaloids, the extracted aqueous solution can be treated to get total alkaloids by partition or cation exchange resin chromatography. The processes are showed in Figure 8-6.

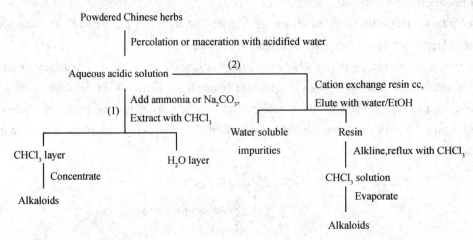

Figure 8-6　Purification procedure for aqueous acidic extraction of alkaloids

4.1.2　Extract with Methanol or Ethanol

Alkaloids and their salts can both dissolve in ethanol or methanol. Therefore, they can be extracted with methanol or ethanol by reflux, maceration or percolation method. It is suitable for various alkaloids with water-soluble impurity such as polysaccharides and proteins. The procedure is shown in Figure 8-7.

4.1.3　Extract with Lipophilic Organic Solvents

Moisten the herb with alkali to free the alkaloids first, then to extract the free form alkaloids with lipophilic organic solvents. This method is not applicable to quaternary alkaloids because they can not dissolve in lipophilic solvents.

The process of extraction with lipophilic organic solvent is as follows (Figure 8-8).

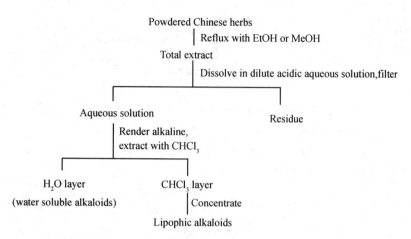

Figure 8-7　Purification procedure for alcohol extract of alkaloids

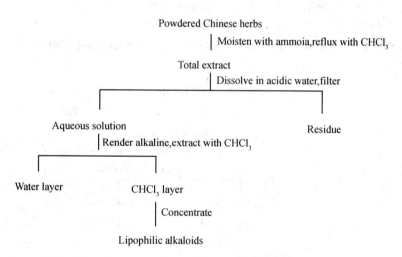

Figure 8-8　Extraction procedure with non-polar organic solvent for alkaloids

4.2　Isolation

Further purification of crude alkaloids can be done by the following methods, which may vary for individual alkaloid.

4.2.1　According to the Types of Alkaloids

Total alkaloids are divided into five types according to the basicity, the water-solubility, and with or without phenolic character. The scheme for isolation of five types of alkaloids is as follows (Figure 8-9).

4.2.2　According to the Basicity (Gradient pH Technique)

There are variations in the extent of basicity of various alkaloids from the same plant. Depending on this character, the crude alkaloidal mixture can be dissolved in dilute hydrochloric acid solution and extracted with chloroform so that the first fraction contains neutral and/or very weakly basic alkaloids. Adjust the pH of the aqueous solution gradually upto pH 11 and the organic solvent extraction is followed at each pH level. By this way, alkaloids with different basicity are extracted. Strongly basic alkaloids are extracted at the end. The scheme of gradient pH extraction for isolation of alkaloids is as follows (Figure 8-10).

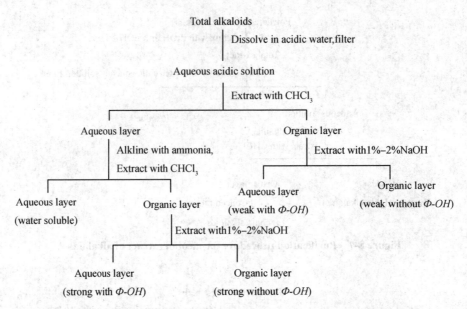

Figure 8-9   Isolation procedure of alkaloids based on the types of alkaloids

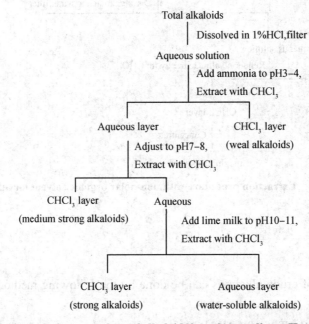

Figure 8-10   Isolation procedure of alkaloids by using gradient pH technique (1)

The other method is that the crude alkaloids is dissolved in chloroform and extracted with different acidic buffer solution so that the first fraction contains strong basicity alkaloids. The scheme for isolation of alkaloids is shown in Figure 8-11.

4.2.3   According to the Solubility

Each costituent of total alkaloids has different solubility in one organic solvent due to their different polarities. Based on this character, a specific alkaloid compound can be isolated from the others. For example, total alkaloids from Sophorae flavescentis Radix are dissolved in chloroform, then add ethyl ether over 10 times in volume, and oxymatrine can be precipitated because it is polar than others. It is difficult to dissolve in ethyl ether, while matrine and others still dissolve in the solution.

Total alkaloids
| Dissolve in CHCl₃,filter

CHCl₃ solution
| Extract with pH5–6 buffer

CHCl₃ layer 　　　　Aqueous layer
| Extract with pH3–4 buffer　(string alkaloids)

Aqueous layer 　　CHCl₃ layer
(medium strong alkaloids)　| Extract with pH1–2 buffer

Aqueous layer　　　CHCl₃ layer
(weak alkaloids)　(lipophilic impyrities)

Figure 8-11　Isolation procedure of alkaloids by using gradient pH technique (2)

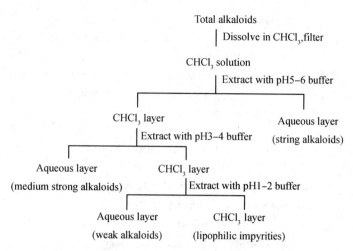

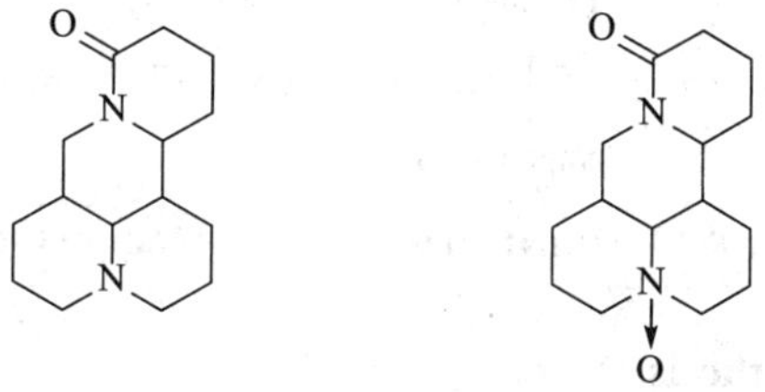

matrine　　　　　　oxymatrine

The solubility of different alkaloidal salts may be different. Based on this character, some alkaloidal salts can be isolated. For example, ephedrine and pseudoephedrine can be separated according to the different water-solubility of their oxalates (草酸盐). Ephedrine oxalate can be crystallized by extracting with oxalic acid solution because of its poor water-solubility, while pseudoephedrine oxalate is still dissolved in the mother liquor.

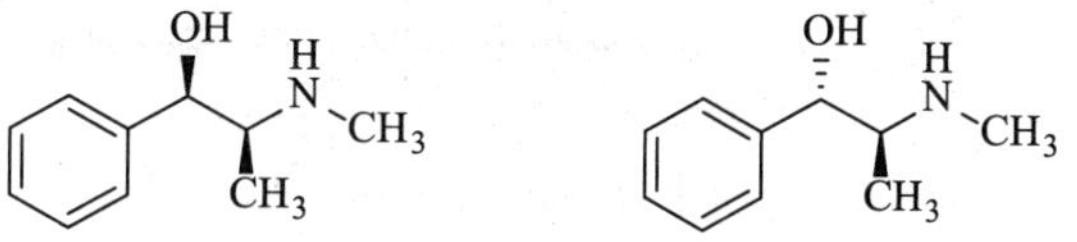

l-ephedrine (1*R*, 2*S*)　　　*d*-pseudoephedrine (1*S*, 2*S*)

4.2.4　According to the Functional Groups

Alkaloids with special functional groups including the phenolic hydroxyl group (酚羟基), carboxyl group, lactone (内酯), lactam (内酰胺), etc., can be separated according to the reversible chemical reactions of these groups. For example, camptothecine can be separated by using the property of its lactone-ring from the root of *Camptotheca acuminata* (喜树) (Figure 8-12, 8-13).

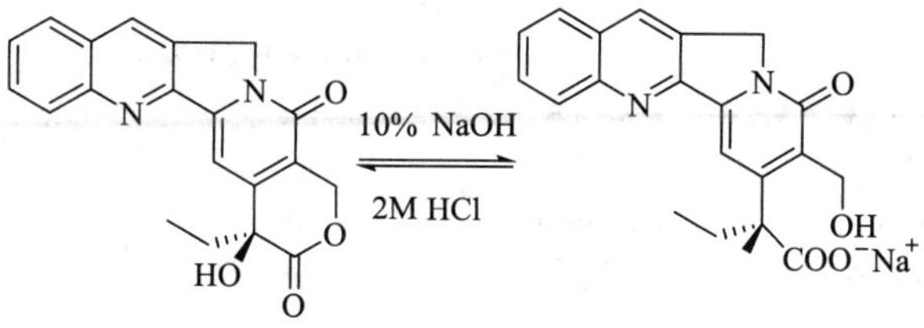

10% NaOH
2M HCl

Camptothecine

Figure 8-12　Reaction of lactone ring in camptothecine

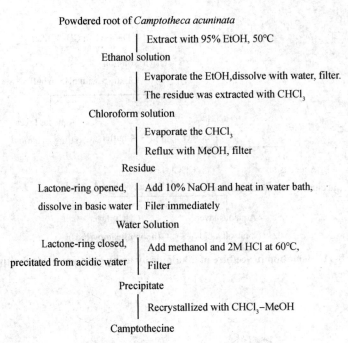

Figure 8-13　Isolation procedure of camptothecine

4.2.5　Chromatography Methods

Chromatography method has been proved to be ideal for isolation of alkaloids. Different types of chromatography (absorption, partition, ion exchange chromatography, etc.) methods are used for isolation of individual alkaloids from complex mixtures. For example, four steroidal alkaloids are isolated from *Fritillaria thunbergii* var. *chekiangensis* (东贝母) by the silica gel column chromatography method. The isolation scheme is as follows (Figure 8-14).

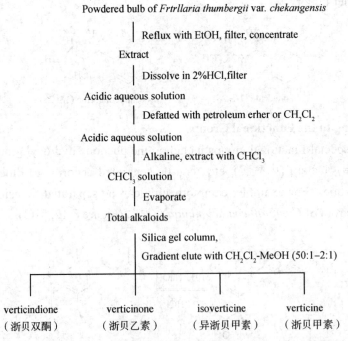

Figure 8-14　Isolation procedure of steroidal alkaloids from *Fritillaria thunbergii* var. *chekiangensis*

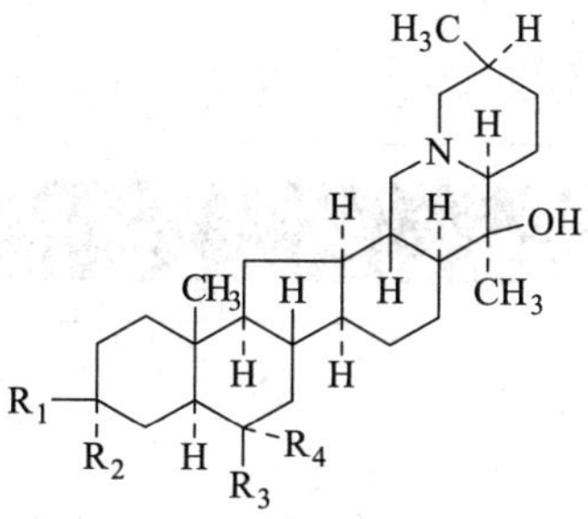

	R₁	R₂	R₃	R₄
verticine	OH	H	H	OH
isoverticine	OH	H	OH	H
verticinone	OH	H	=O	
verticindione	=O		=O	

4.2.6　Isolation of Water-soluble Alkaloids

Water-souble alkaloids can be precipitated from the water by adding the precipitation reagent and separated from the impurities in the aqueous solution. Reinecke's salt is a popular precipitation reagent for this purpose. The procedure is shown in Figure 8-15.

Aqueous solution contains quaternary alkaloids

　　　│ Add HCl to pH 2-3,filter

Filtrate

　　　│ Add Reineckes's salt and filter

Precipitate

　　　│ Al₂O₃CC,elute with acetone

Acetone solution

　　　│ Add Ag₂SO₄, filter

Filtrate(Alkaloid sulphate)

　　　│ Add BaCl₂, filter, recrystallize

Quatenary alkaloid chloride

Figure 8-15　Isolation procedure of water-soluble alkaloids

The chemical reactions in above procedure are as follows (Figure 8-16).

$$B^+ + NH_4[Cr(NH_3)_2(SCN)_4] \longrightarrow B[Cr(NH_3)_2(SCN)_4]\downarrow$$

$$2B[Cr(NH_3)_2(SCN)_4] + Ag_2SO_4 \longrightarrow B_2SO_4 + 2Ag[Cr(NH_3)_2(SCN)_4]\downarrow$$

$$Ag_2SO_4 + BaCl_2 \longrightarrow BaSO_4\downarrow + 2AgCl\downarrow$$

$$B_2SO_4 + BaCl_2 \longrightarrow 2BCl + BaSO_4\downarrow$$

Note: B represents quaternary alkaloids

Figure 8-16　Reactions in purification of water-soluble alkaloids

Water-soluble alkaloids can not only dissolve in water, but also in polar solvents such as water saturated *n*-butanol or isoamyl alcohol (异戊醇) etc. Therefore, the basic aqueous solution containing water-soluble alkaloids can also be directly extracted with these kinds of solvents. Then the water-soluble alkaloids will be isolated from the water-soluble impurities.

5 Identification

5.1 Chemical Tests

Precipitation reactions of alkaloids are commonly used to identify the presence of alkaloids in Chinese herbs. The commonly used reagents are listed in Table 8-6. It is worth noticing that Chinese herbs containing alkaloids usually also contain proteins, peptides and tannins that can cause false positive reactions with precipitation reagents of alkaloids. Therefore, these impurities need to be removed before testing.

Some individual alkaloids give color reactions with certain specific reagents. These color reactions can also be used to do identification (see Table 8-7).

Table 8-7   Color reactions of some alkaloids

Reagent	Alkaloid	Color
Mandelin [1% ammonium vanadate (钒酸铵) in concentrated sulfuric acid]	Hyoscyamine, Atropine	Red
	Quinine	Slight orange
	Morphine, Strychine	Blue-purple
	Codeine	Blue
Fröhde [1% sodium molybdate (钼酸钠) in concentrate sulfuric acid]	Aconitine	Yellow-brown
	Morphine	Purple turn to brown
	Berberine	Brown-green
	Reserpine	Yellow turn to blue
Marquis [0.2ml 30% formaldehyde (甲醛) mixed with 10ml sulfuric acid]	Morphine	Orange to purple
	Codeine	Red to yellow-brown

5.2   Chromatography Methods

Alkaloids can also be identified by TLC, PC, HPLC and GC methods.

The silica gel TLC method is the most commonly used for identification of alkaloids. However, small value of R_f and the tailing of colored patches of alkaloids may appear because silica gel is slightly acidic. These can be avoided by three methods: Using basic development solvent system; Saturating with concentrate ammonium hydroxide (氢氧化铵) before development; Preparing the silica gel plate with alkaline buffer solution.

Volatile alkaloids can be identified by GC method.

6 Structure Determination

The structure determination of alkaloids is very difficult due to their complicated structure. Chemical methods and spectroscopy methods are used to elucidate the structure of alkaloids.

6.1 Chemical Methods

Chemical degradation is the classic and traditional method, which is less used today.

In order to explore the structures of alkaloids, the C-N linkage in alkaloids can be broken by reactions such as the Hofmann degradation (霍夫曼降解), Emde degradation and Von Braun reaction. In the Hofmann degradation, primary (RNH_2) and secondary (R_2NH) amines are converted to quaternary ammonium (季铵) salts, which undergo β-H elimination, when heated with base to give alkenes (烯烃) and tertiary amines (Figure 8-17, 8-18, 8-19, 8-20). The primary structure of alkaloid is deduced according to the structure of small degradation products.

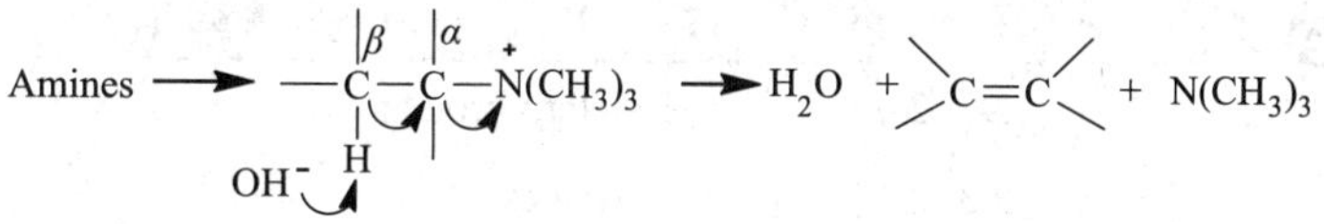

Figure 8-17 Principle of Hofmann degradation

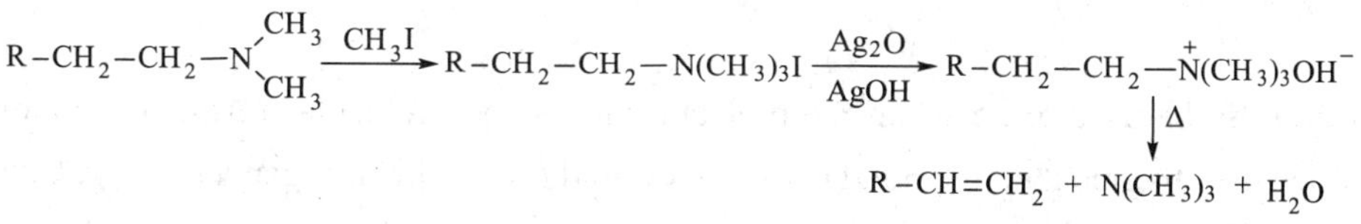

Figure 8-18 Hofmann degradation of alkaloids with straight chain

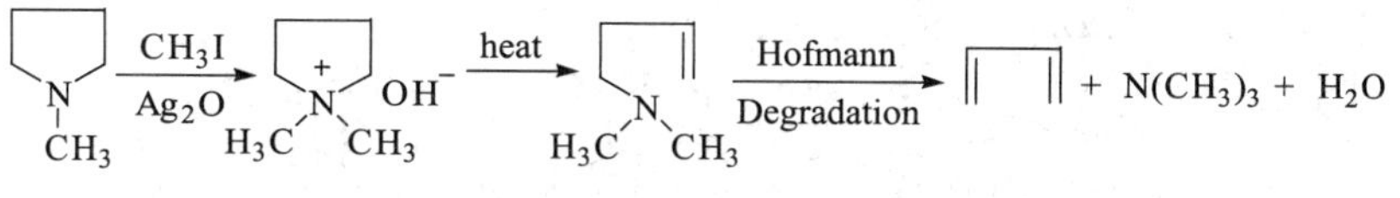

Figure 8-19 Hofmann degradation of alkaloids with divalent nitrogen atom in the ring

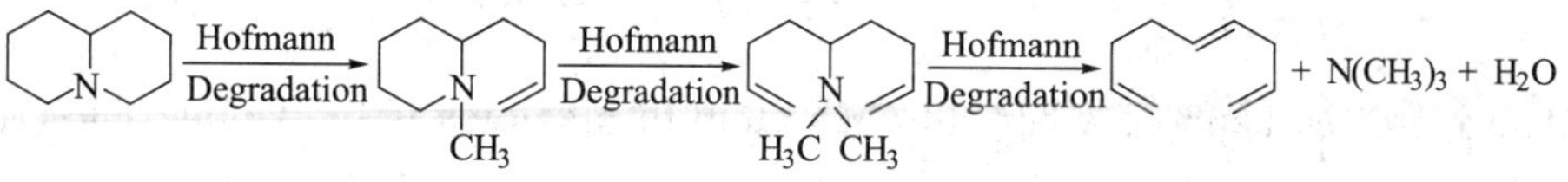

Figure 8-20 Hofmann degradation of alkaloids with trivalent nitrogen atom in the ring

6.2　Spectroscopy Methods

Spectroscopy methods are the main approachs to determine the structure of alkaloids.

UV spectra of alkaloids may help to identity the structure class of alkaloids based on the information from the conjugated system in molecules. IR spectra of alkaloids can be used to identify the functional groups in molecules. Moreover, IR spectra has been used to assign the relative stereochemistry and conformational preferences for indolizidines, quinolizidines, pyrrolizidines and other fused 6/5 and 5/5 ring systems, as well as their derivatives for many years.

NMR is the most useful technique in determining the structure and stereochemistry of alkaloids, especially 2D-NMR such as HSQC (HMQC), HMBC, NOESY.

The ^{1}H-NMR spectrum of a primary or secondary amine will show a broad signal for the N-H in the region 0.5–4.5, which will disappear from the spectrum if the sample is shaken with deuterated water (氘代水). For aromatic amines, the signal of N-H is typically in the range of 3–6. The chemical shifts of neighboring groups can also help to indicate the presence of an amine group indirectly. For example, an N-CH$_3$ gives a signal near 2.3 in the ^{1}H-NMR spectrum and a signal in the region of 30–45 in the ^{13}C-NMR spectrum (Table 8-8).

Table 8-8　Chemical shifts of different types of N-CH$_3$ in ^{1}H-NMR (CDCl$_3$)

Type of nitrogen atom	N-CH$_3$ (δ)	Type of nitrogen atom	N-CH$_3$ (δ)
Tertiary amines	1.97–2.56	Hetero-aromatic ring	2.7–4.0
Secondary amines	2.3–2.5	Amides	2.6–3.1
Aromatic tertiary or secondary amines	2.6–3.1	Quaternary ammonium	2.7–3.5*

* In DMSO-d$_6$, or C$_5$D$_5$N or CD$_3$OD

MS spectra can be used to determin the molecular mass and molecular formula. Alkaloids undergo α-cleavage when they fragment on the bond between α-C and β-C of the nitrogen atom, e.g. Cinchonine (辛可宁）(Figure 8-21).

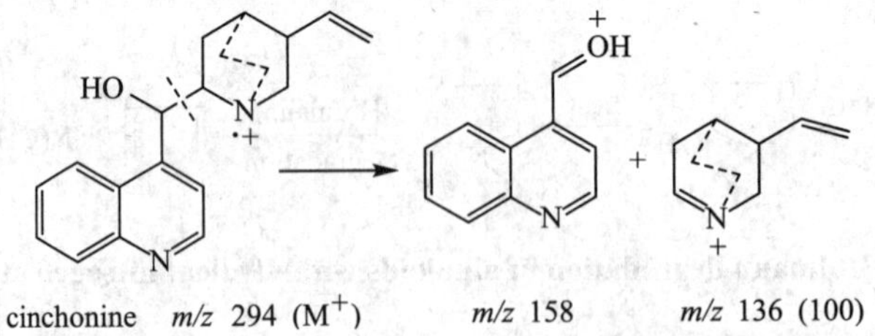

cinchonine　m/z 294 (M$^+$)　　m/z 158　　m/z 136 (100)

Figure 8-21　α-cleavage of cinchonine

RDA-cleavage often happens when nitrogen atom of alkaloids is in cyclohexene (环己烯). The RDA-cleavage of tetrahydroberberine (四氢小檗碱) is shown in Figure 8-22.

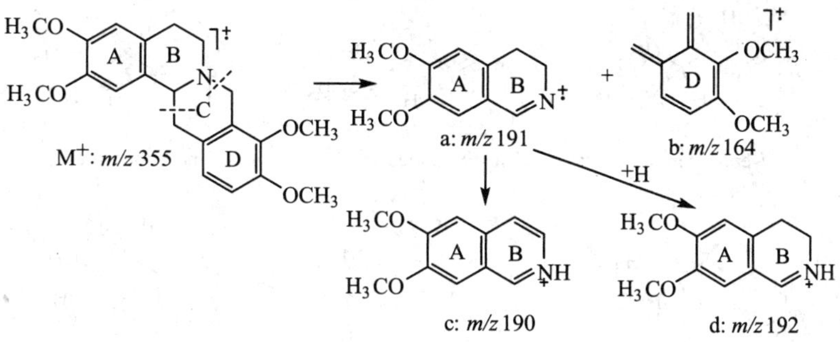

Figure 8-22 RDA-cleavage of tetrahydroberberine

7 Examples of Chinese Herbs Containing Alkaloids

7.1 Ephedrae Herba(麻黄)

7.1.1 Introduction

(1) Biological Source

Ephedrae Herba is the dried herbaceous stem of *Ephedra sinica* Stapf (草麻黄), *E. intermedia* Schrenk et C. A. Mey. (中麻黄) or *E. equisetina* Bge (木贼麻黄) (Fam. Ephedraceae) (麻黄科).

(2) Property, Flavor and Channels Entered

Property and Flavor: Warm; Pungent, mild bitter.

Channels Entered: Lung, Bladder.

(3) Actions & Indications

To promote sweating, dissipate cold, diffuse the lung to relieve panting, promote urination to alleviate edema. For common cold caused by wind-cold, edema caused by wind, panting and cough, oppression in the chest.

(4) Pharmacological Activities

The pharmacological activities associated with Ephedrae Herba include stimulating the central and peripheral nervous system, losing bronchial muscles, exciting breathing, contracting blood vessels, increasing blood pressure, etc. Ephedrine has a similar action as adrenaline, but it is less toxic and taken orally.

7.1.2 Main Chemical Constituents

Ephedrae Herba is mainly produced in Xinjiang, Inner Mongolia, Shanxi, Shanxi and Ningxia. It contains alkaloids such as *l*-ephedrine and *d*-pseudoephedrine, volatile oils, tannins, flavonoids, saponins, etc. As a common important Chinese herb, Ephedrae Herba must be prescribed carefully and its use is supervised because of its constituents, alkaloids.

(1) Alkaloids

Ephedrae Herba contains alkaloids 0.5%–2.0%, the major active principle is *l*-ephedrine taking part in 40%–90% concentrations in the total alkaloid fraction, accompanied by *d*-pseudoephedrine. Other trace alkaloids include *l*-norephedrine, *d*-norpseudoephedrine, *l*-*N*-methylephedrine, *d*-*N*-methylpseudoephedrine, ephedroxane (麻黄噁唑酮), etc.

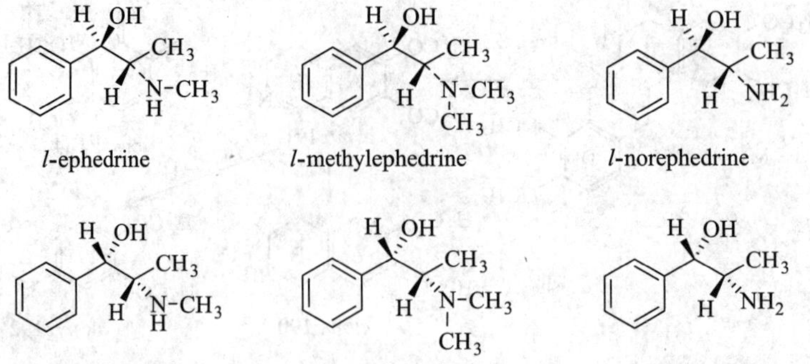

l-ephedrine   *l*-methylephedrine   *l*-norephedrine

d-pseudoephedrine   *d*-methylpseudoephedrine   *d*-norpseudoephedrine

① Properties of Main Alkaloids

a. Characteristics   Ephedrine and pseudoephedrine are colorless rhombic crystals, the melting point (m.p.) of free base (anhydrous) of ephedrine is at 38.1℃; the hemihydrate of ephedrine is at 40℃; The m.p. of pseudoephedrine is at 118℃. Ephedrine and pseudoephedrine both can volatile.

b. Basicity   Ephedrine and pseudoephedrine as the secondary amines are medium strong in basicity. Because the stability of intramolecular hydrogen bond forms in pseudoephedrine, its basicity ($pK_a = 9.74$) is stronger than that of ephedrine ($pK_a = 9.58$).

c. Solubility   Ephedrine and pseudoephedrine as small molecules, both can dissolve in water, but pseudoephedrine is much less soluble in water than ephedrine. They also dissolve in ethanol, chloroform, and ethyl ether. The ephedrine oxalate is much less soluble in cold water than the pseudoephedrine oxalate. Ephedrine hydrochloride is not soluble in chloroform, but pseudoephedrine hydrochloride can dissolve in it.

② Identification

Ephedrine and pseudoephedrine are the secondary amines. They do not give positive reaction to precipitation reagents of alkaloids, but they can be identified by the following reactions.

a. CS₂-CuSO₄ Reaction   The reaction mechanism is shown in Figure 8-23.

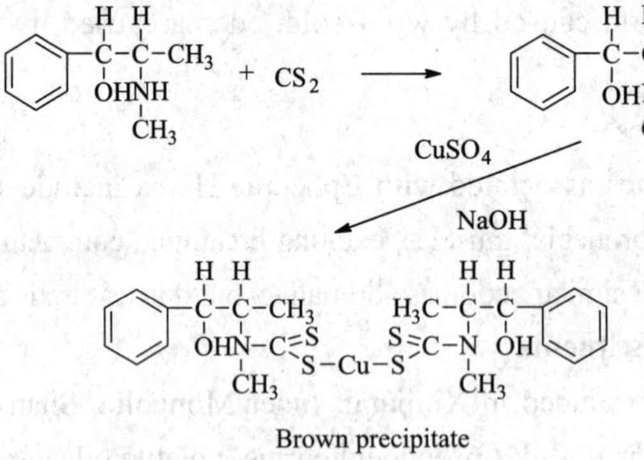

Brown precipitate

Figure 8-23   Mechanism of CS₂-CuSO₄ reaction

b. Chen's Test (Copper Sulphate Test)   Dissolve ephedrine (or pseudoephedrine) in water, add 5% CuSO₄ and NaOH reagent, the solution will show violet color. Then add ethyl ether and mix, the ethyl ether layer shows purple-red and the water layer shows blue. The reaction mechanism is shown in Figure 8-24.

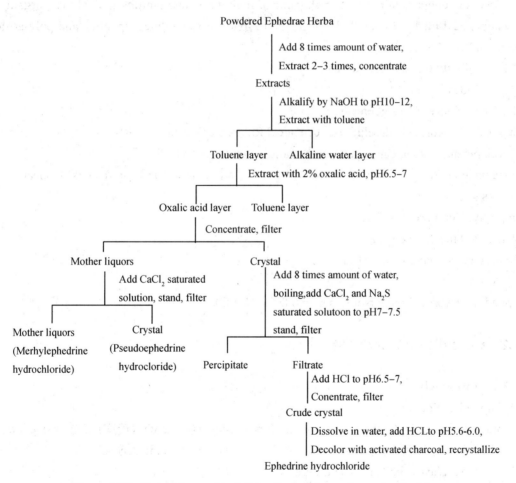

Figure 8-24　Chen-kao complex formation between ephedrine and copper sulfate

③ Extraction and Isolation of Ephedrine and Pseudoephedrine

Ephedrine and pseudoephedrine may be extracted from the plant material by the following methods.

a. Solvent Method　Ephedrine and pseudoephedrine can dissolve in both water and organic solvents, so they can be extracted with water and organic solvents. Ephedrine oxalate can be separated from pseudoephedrine oxalate because ephedrine oxalate is much less soluble than pseudoephedrine oxalate in cold water. The process is illustrated in Figure 8-25.

Powdered Ephedrae Herba

Add 8 times amount of water,
Extract 2–3 times, concentrate

Extracts

Alkalify by NaOH to pH10–12,
Extract with toluene

Toluene layer　　　　Alkaline water layer

Extract with 2% oxalic acid, pH6.5–7

Oxalic acid layer　　　Toluene layer

Concentrate, filter

Mother liquors　　　　　　　Crystal

Add CaCl₂ saturated
solution, stand, filter

Add 8 times amount of water,
boiling, add CaCl₂ and Na₂S
saturated solutoon to pH7–7.5
stand, filter

Mother liquors　　　Crystal
(Merhylephedrine　　(Pseudoephedrine
hydrochloride)　　　hydrocloride)

Percipitate　　　　Filtrate

Add HCl to pH6.5–7,
Conentrate, filter

Crude crystal

Dissolve in water, add HCLto pH5.6–6.0,
Decolor with activated charcoal, recrystallize

Ephedrine hydrochloride

Figure 8-25　Extraction and isolation of ephedrine and pseudoephedrine

b. Steam Distillation Method　The free form of ephedrine and pseudoephedrine can volatile with steam, so they can be extracted by the steam distillation method. This method does not use any organic solvent, but it is time consuming and under high temperature, decomposition of ephedrine may happen. The yielding will be decreased.

c. Ion-exchange Resin Method　Ephedrine and pseudoephedrine can be separated by using strong acid cation resin column chromatography. Because the basicity of ephedrine is weaker than pseudoephedrine, it is eluted out of the column first.

(2) Volatile Oils

Volatile oils account for 0.25% in Ephedrae Herba, including terpinen-4-ol (松油烯–4–醇), *l*-α-terpineol (松油醇), linalool, benzoic acid, 2, 3, 5, 6-tetramethylpyrazine (苄基甲胺2, 3, 5, 6– 四甲基吡嗪), *p*-meth-2-en-7-ol, *p*-hydroxybenzoic acid, *p*-coumaric acid, cinnamic acid, vanillic acid (香草酸), protocatechuic acid (原儿茶酸), *p*-cymene (对伞花烃), *d*-limonene (柠檬烯), etc.

(3) Flavonoids

Flavonoids isolated from Ephedrae Herba include leucodelphinidin, apigenin (芹菜素), tricin (小麦黄素), 3-*O*-*β*-D-glucopyranoyl-5, 9, 4′-trihydroxy-8-methoxyflavone, kaempferol (山奈酚), kaempferol rhamnoside, herbacetin (草质素), 3-methoxyherbacetin, etc.

(4) Others

Diterpenes (ephedrannin A and mahuannin), monoterpenes, tannins (catechins), organic acids (octadecanoic acid methyl ester), 2, 3, 4-trimethyl-5-phenyloxazolidine, saponins, and polysaccharides also found in Ephedrae Herba.

7.1.3　Quality Control Standards

(1) TLC Identification

Stationary Phase: Silica gel plate.

Standard: Ephedrine hydrochloride (Chemical Reference Substance, CRS).

Development System: Chloroform-methanol-ammonia (20∶5∶0.5).

Visualization: Spray the solution of ninhydrin (茚三酮), heat to 105℃ until spots are clear.

(2) Tests

Impurity: Not more than 5%.

Water: Not more than 9.0%.

Total Ash: Not more than 10.0%.

(3) Assay

Ephedrine Hydrochloride: Not less than 0.80% (HPLC).

7.2　Coptidis Rhizoma(黄连)

7.2.1　Introduction

(1) Biological Source

Coptidis Rhizoma is the dried rhizome of *Coptis chinensis* Franch. (黄连), *Coptis deltoidea* C. Y. Cheng et Hsiao (三角叶黄连) or *Coptis teeta* Wall. (云连) (Fam. Ranunculaceae).

(2) Property, Flavor and Channels Entered

Property and Flavor: Cold; Bitter.

Channels Entered: Heart, Spleen, Stomach, Liver, Gallbladder, Large Intestine.

(3) Actions & Indications

To clear heat and dry dampness, purge fire and remove toxin. For dampness-heat stuffiness and fullness, eczema, dampness sore, purulent discharge from the ear, acid regurgitation, vomiting, diarrhea and dysentery, jaundice, high fever with loss of consciousness, intense heart fire, palpitation and unrest, insomnia caused by vexation, blood heat with hematemesis, toothache, red eyes, wasting-thirst, swelling abscess, deep-rooted boil and sore.

(4) Pharmacological Activities

The pharmacological activities associated with Coptidis Rhizoma include broad spectrum antibiotic properties, hypoglycemia activity, anti-inflammatory, antioxygen and free radical's (自由基) scavenging and anticancer effects etc. The major component of this herb, berberine also has many pharmacological effects including inhibition of adipocyte differentiation, anti-cancer, anti-microbial, anti-inflammatory, and Low Density Lipoprotein (LDL)-lowering effects.

7.2.2   Main Chemical Constituents

Coptis deltoidea C. Y. Cheng et Hsiao is mainly from Hongya, Emei of Sichuan province. *C. chinensis* Franch mainly grows in Sichuan, Hubei provinces. *C. teeta* Wall is mainly from Yunnan province. Alkaloids are their main constituents. It also contains lignans and other phenolic compounds such as ferulic acid (阿魏酸), etc.

(1) Alkaloids

Isoquinoline alkaloids: Berberine, coptisine, epiberberine (表小檗碱),berberrubine (小檗红碱), palmatine, hydrastine, jatrorrhizine (药根碱), worenine (甲基黄连碱), columbamine (非洲防己碱), magnoflorine (木兰碱), berberastine（5-羟基小檗碱）, groenlandicine (四去氢碎叶紫堇碱).

The major constituents are berberine and related protoberberine alkaloids. Berberine occurs in the range of 4%–8% (*C. chinensis*: 5%–7%, *C. deltoides*: 4%–8%, *C. japonica*: 7%–9%), followed by palmatine (*C. chinensis*: 1%–4%, *C. deltoides*: 1%–3%, *C. japonica*: 0.4%–0.6%), coptisine (*C. chinensis*: 0.8%–2%, *C. deltoides*: 0.8%–1%, *C. japonica*: 0.4%–0.6%) among others.

Compound	R_1	R_2	R_3	R_4	R_5
berberine	—CH₂—		CH₃	CH₃	H
palmatine	CH₃	CH₃	CH₃	CH₃	H
coptisine	—CH₂—		—CH₂—		H
worenine	—CH₂—		—CH₂—		CH₃
jatrorrhizine	H	CH₃	CH₃	CH₃	H
epiberberine	CH₃	CH₃	—CH₂—		H

① Properties of Berberine

a. Characteristics   The free berberine crystallizes from water or preferably dilute alcohol as a hydrate in brilliant yellow needle. If dried at 100℃ ,the crystals lose three molecules of water and their luster, at 110℃ they turn yellow-brown and at 160℃ decomposition sets in. Berberine hydrochloride is yellow to orange crystalline powder.

b. Basicity   Berberine is a quarternary alkaloid, pK_a 11.5.

c. Solubility   Berberine can dissolve in water, hardly dissolve in benzene, chloroform and acetone. The water-solubility of its hydrochloride is 1 in 500, its sulphate and phosphate are 1∶30 and 1∶15, respectively. The salts of large organic acids are always hardly dissolved in water. That is why Coptidis Rhizoma should not decoct with *Gancao*, *Huangqin* or *Dahuang* together. Berberine in Coptidis Rhizoma can form salts with glycyrrhizic acid (甘草酸), baiclin, rhein (大黄酸) and precipitate result in decreasing of the content of these active components in the decoction.

d. Stability   Berberine is stable in acidic and neutral solutions, but it converts to a number of products in basic solution. It manifests as quaternary ammonium, carbinol and amino-aldehyde tautomers, of which the most stable form is quaternary ammonium type. The tautomerization (互变异构) is shown in Figure 8-26.

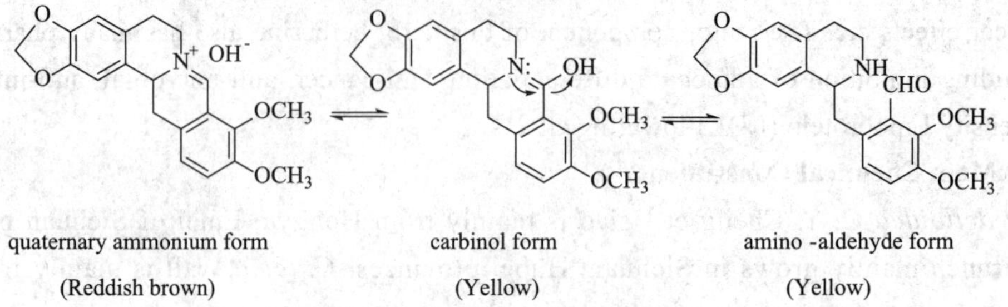

| quaternary ammonium form | carbinol form | amino -aldehyde form |
| (Reddish brown) | (Yellow) | (Yellow) |

Figure 8-26   Tautomerization of berberine

② Identification

a. Berberrubine Reaction   When heated to 220℃, berberine hydrochloride breaks down into reddish brown berberrubine.

b. Labat Reation or Ecgrine Reation   Berberine contains methylenedioxy group (亚甲二氧基), so it has positive Labat reation or Ecgrine reation (Table 8-9).

Table 8-9   Labat reation or Ecgrine reation of berberine

Reation	Reagent	Result
Labat	Gallic acid-con. H_2SO_4	Blue-green
Ecgrine	Chromotropic acid-con. H_2SO_4	Blue-purple

c. Addition Reaction with Acetone   Berberine hydrochloride can form a yellow crystal compound with acetone in the basic water solution. The product is called berberine acetone adduct. This reaction can be used to do identification or purification of berberine (Figure 8-27).

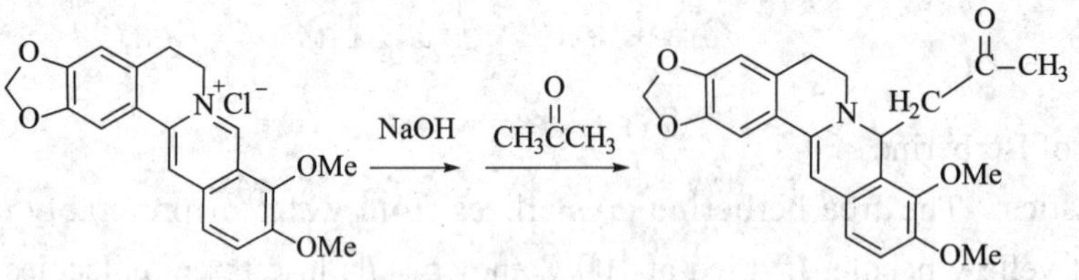

Figure 8-27   Addition reaction of berberine hydrochloride with acetone

d. Reaction with Bleaching Powder (漂白粉)   When bleaching powder or calcium hypochlorite (次氯酸钙) is added into the acidic water solution of berberine, the yellow color solution will turn into cherry red color.

③ Extraction and Isolation

The powder of Coptidis Rhizoma is extracted with methanol or ethanol. They are good solvents for both free bases and their salts. Further isolation and purification process is illustrated in Figure 8-28.

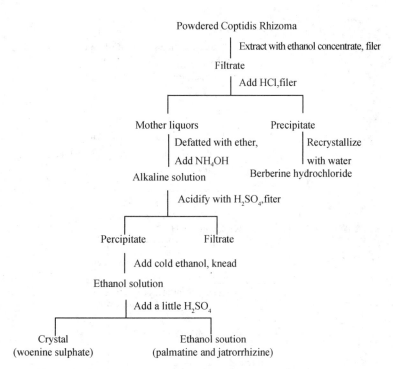

Figure 8-28　Extraction and isolation of berberine and worenine

The preparation of total alkaloids from Coptidis Rhizoma is shown in Figure 8-29.

(2) Phenolic Acids and Their Derivatives

Coptis chinensis Franch contains ferulic acid, 3, 4-dihydroxyphenylethylalcoholglucoside, 5-*O*-feruloyl-D-quinic acid, 3-methoxy-4-hydroxybenzoic acid, 4-*O*-feruloyl-D-quinic acid, vanillic acid-4-*O*-*β*-D-glucopyranoside, 3-(3', 4'-dihydroxyphenyl)-(2*R*)-lactic acid-4'-*O*-*β*-D-glucopyranoside, 3-(4'-hydroxyphenyl)-(2*R*)-lactic acid, 3-(3', 4'-dihydroxyphenyl)-(2*R*)-lactic acid methyl ester, 3-(3', 4'-dihydroxyphenyl)-(2*R*)-lactic acid, etc.

(3) Lignans

Isolarisiresinol-9-*O*-*β*-D-glucopyranoside, 7*S*, 8*R*, 8'*R*-*d*-larisiresnol-4, 4'-*O*-*β*-D-diglucopyranoside, *d*-pinoresinol-4, 4'-*O*-*β*-D-diglucopyranoside, and 7*S*, 8*R*, 8'*R*-*d*-larisiresinol-4-*O*-*β*-D-glucopyranoside are isolated from the decoction of *Coptis chinensis* Franch.

7.2.3　Quality Control Standards

(1) TLC Identification

Stationary Phase: Silica gel plate.

Standard: Authentic crude drug; Berberine hydrochloride.

Development System: Cyclohexane-acetyl acetate-isopropanol-methanol-water-triethylamine (3 : 3.5 : 1 : 1.5 : 0.5 : 1) (lower layer, saturated the developing tank with concentrated ammonia solution for 20 minutes in advance).

Visualization: 365nm UV light.

(2) Tests

Water: Not more than 14.0%.

Total Ash: Not more than 5.0%.

Extract (alcohol): Not less than 15.0%.

(3) Assay

Berberine: Not less than 5.5% (HPLC).

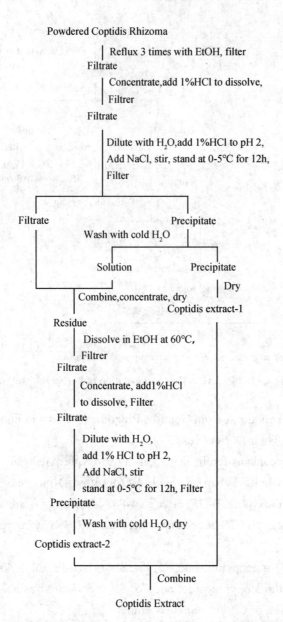

Figure 8-29   Preparation of total alkaloids of Coptidis Rhizoma

Epiberberine: Not less than 0.8% (HPLC).

Coptisine: Not less than 1.6% (HPLC).

Palmatine: Not less than 1.5% (HPLC).

7.3   Daturae Flos(洋金花)

7.3.1   Introduction

(1) Biological Source

Daturae Flos is the dried flower of *Datura metel* L. (白花曼陀罗) (Fam. Solanaceae).

(2) Property, Flavor and Channels Entered

Property and Flavor: Warm; Pungent; Toxic.

Channels Entered: Lung, Liver.

(3) Actions & Indications

To relieve panting, suppress cough and relieve pain. For asthma, cough, cold pain in the epigastrium and abdomen, chronic infantile convulsion, painful impediment caused by wind-dampness, anaesthesia in surgery.

(4) Pharmacological Activities

The pharmacological activities associated with Daturae Flos include depressing of the central nervous system, reducing bronchial mucus secretion, relieving pain, antishock, etc. The extracts of Daturae Flos have significant effect on psoriasis.

7.3.2   Main Chemical Constituents

Daturae Flos widely grows in China, India, England and other tropical and subtropical regions. It is a potent toxic herb, containing tropane alkaloids which can cause anti-cholinergic poisoning, and hence is classified in Schedule 1 of the Chinese Medicine Ordinance. Besides, a number of withanolides (醉茄内酯类), flavonoids, megastigmane sesquiterpenes (大柱香波龙烷型倍半萜烯), hydroxycoumarins, and other compounds have also been isolated from it.

(1) Alkaloids

Daturae Flos contains upto 0.5% total alkaloids, among which hyoscine (scopolamine) is the main component, it has an epoxide (环氧的) ring. While *l*-hyoscyamine (scopoline) is present in very less quantities. Atropine is the racemic form (外消旋体) of hyoscyamine. Others include anisodine (樟柳碱), *N*-demethylhyoscyamine, tigloidine (巴豆酰莨菪碱), valtropine (瓦托品), etc.

hyoscyamine (atropine)   R=H
anisodamine   R=OH

anisodine

scopolamine

N-demethylhyosodamine

① Properties of Main Tropane Alkaloids

a. Characteristics   Pure hyoscyamine crystallizes in tufts or stellate, silky needles, mp 108.5℃, and atropine is colorless long columnar crystals, mp 118–119℃. Scopolamine is semi-liquid. It can dissolve in water and recrystallizing from hot water. Natural Anisodamine is colorless needle crystals, mp 62–64℃ (from benzene). Anisodine is similar to scopolamine in structure, it is also semi-liquid, while its hydrobromide is white needle crystals, mp 162–165℃.

b. Optical Activity   These tropane alkaloids all are optical active (laevorotation) expect for atropine. The optical activity of hyoscyamine and scopolamine stems from the chiral center in the acid moiety, (*S*)-tropic acid, but the optical activity of anisodamine stems from all chiral carbons. In most cases, atropine is formed by racemization of hyoscyamine during extraction.

Hyoscyamine is readily converted into atropine (the *dl*-form) by melting or by the addition of small quantities of caustic alkali to its cold alcoholic solution. The same change is also brought about by sodium carbonate or ammonia.

c. Solubility   Hyoscyamine (atropine) is insoluble in water, easily soluble in alcohol, chloroform, soluble in ether and benzene. Scopolamine is soluble in water, easily soluble in alcohol, acetone, ether, and chloroform, and insoluble in benzene. Anisodamine is soluble in water and ethanol.

d. Basicity   The basicity of scopolamine and anisodine is weak (pK_a 7.5) due to space effect and inductive effect. Hyoscyamine is stronger alkaline (pK_a 9.65) and can form crystallizable salts with acids. The space effect of the 6-hydroxyl group of anisodamine is smaller to scopolamine, so the basicity of anisodamine is somewhere in between hyoscyamine and scopolamine.

e. Hydrolysis   In aqueous solution, hyoscyamine (atropine) is very unstable, can be decomposed by heat, especially in basic water, then yields tropine and tropic acid (Figure 8-30).

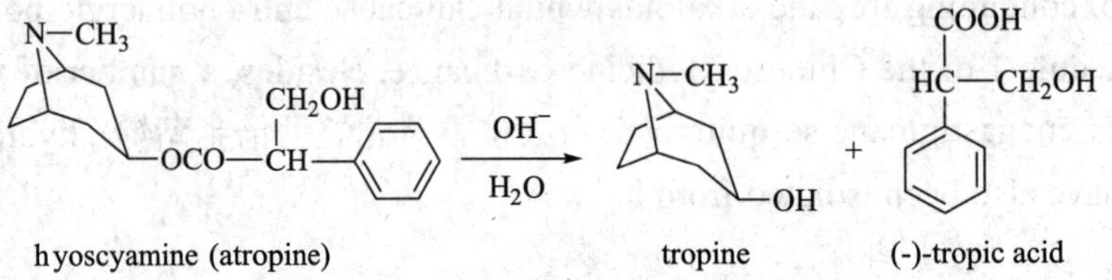

Figure 8-30　Hydrolysis reaction of hyoscyamine (atropine)

② Identification

They can be precipitated by alkaloidal reagents and tannic acid, like most of alkaloids. In addition to these precipitation reactions, they can also be identified by the following reactions.

a. Vitali-Morin Reaction   Alkaloids that are esters of tropic acid are easy to characterize by the Vitali-Morin reaction: The tropane alkaloid is treated with fuming nitric acid (发烟硝酸), followed by evaporation to dryness and addition of ethanolic potassium hydroxide solution to an acetone solution of nitrated residue. Violet coloration will appear because of forming of the quinonoid derivative (Figure 8-31).

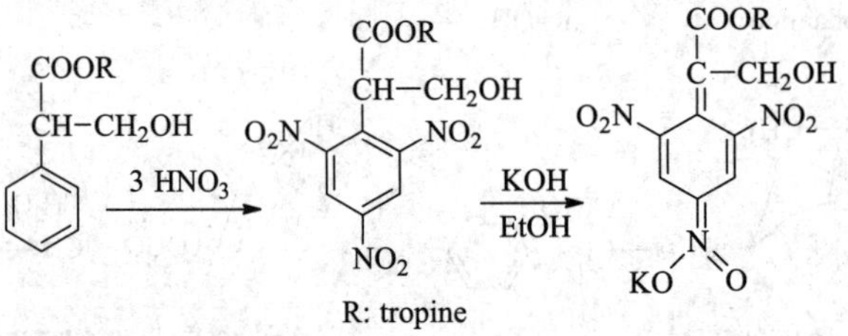

Figure 8-31　Vitali-Morin reaction of tropane alkaloids

b. Gerrard's Test   Tropane alkaloids can give positive results in Gerrard's test (Table 8-10).

Table 8-10　Gerrard's test of tropane alkaloids

Name of alkaloid	Reagent	Result
Hyoscyamine (Atropine)	2% $HgCl_2$ in 50% Ethanol	Red after warming
Scopolamine	2% $HgCl_2$ in 50% Ethanol	White precipitate
Anisodine	2% $HgCl_2$ in 50% Ethanol	White precipitate

c. Hantzsch Reaction   Due to the vicinal diol in the part of tropic acid, anisodine can be oxidized to formaldehyde by periodic acid (过碘酸). Then formaldehyde is condensed with acetylacetone (乙酰丙酮) in acetamide (乙酰胺) to produce diacetyldimethyldihydropyridine (二乙酰基二甲基二氢吡啶）(DDL), which gives a yellow color. This reaction is called Hantzsch reaction (Figure 8-32).

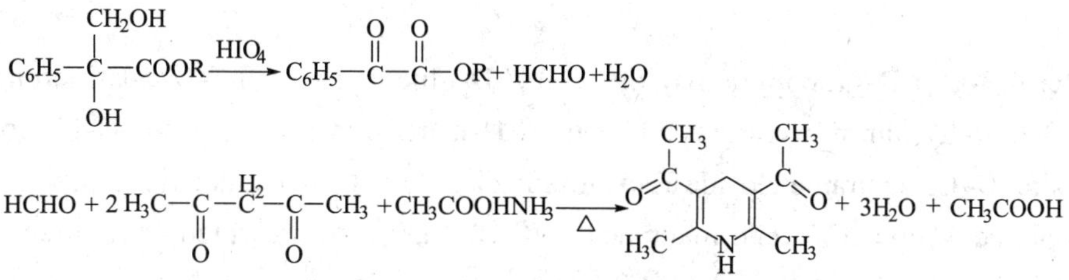

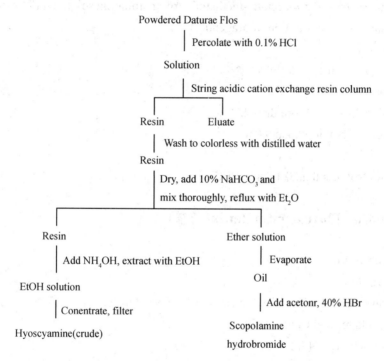

Figure 8-32   Hantzsch reaction of anisodine

③ Extraction and Isolation of Scopolamine and Hyoscyamine

Based on the difference of basicity between scopolamine and hyoscyamine, a common method for isolation of scopolamine and hyposcyamine is shown in Figure 8-33.

Powdered Daturae Flos
 | Percolate with 0.1% HCl
Solution
 | String acidic cation exchange resin column
Resin Eluate
 | Wash to colorless with distilled water
Resin
 | Dry, add 10% NaHCO₃ and
 | mix thoroughly, reflux with Et₂O

Resin   Ether solution
 | Add NH₄OH, extract with EtOH | Evaporate
EtOH solution   Oil
 | Conentrate, filter | Add acetonr, 40% HBr
Hyoscyamine(crude)   Scopolamine
          hydrobromide

Figure 8-33   Extraction and isolation of scopolamine and hyoscyamine

(2) Withanolide Lactones

1, 10-seco-withanolide (1, 10-裂环醉茄内酯), baimantuoluoline G, and baimantuoluoside H have been isolated from Daturae Flos.

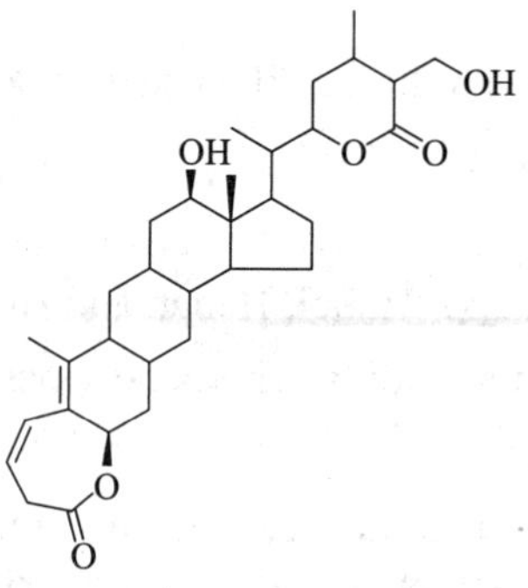

baimantuoluoline G 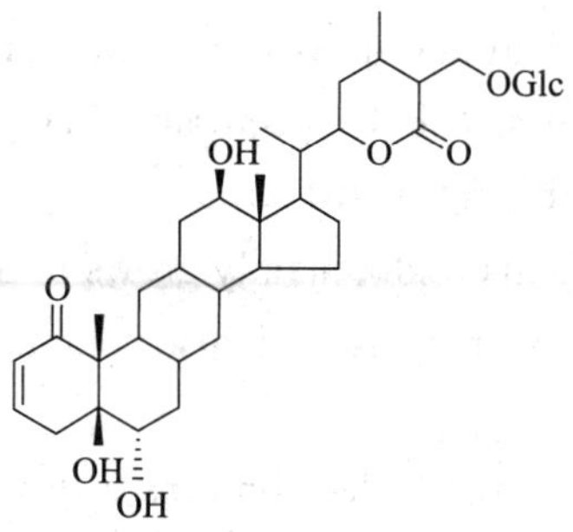   baimantuoluoside H

(3) Others

Kaempferol-3-*O*-*β*-D-gIucopyranosyl(1 → 2)-*β*-D-glucopyranosyl-7-*O*-*a*-L-rhamnopyranoside, kaempferol-3-*O*-*a*-L-rhamnopyranosyl(1 → 6)-*β*-D-glucopyranosyl-7-*O*-*β*-D-glucopyranoside, daturameteloside B–C, daturameteloside F, daturameteloside I–L, withametelin C, hydroxycoumarins, including scopoline, scopoletine, and malic acid (苹果酸) are also presented in Daturae Flos. Daturae Flos also contains a trace amount of volatile oils, gum, resin, starch and so on.

7.3.3 Quality Control Standards

(1) TLC Identification

Stationary Phase: Silica gel plate.

Standard: Atropine sulfate; Scopolamine hydrobromide.

Development System: Ethyl acetate -methanol-strong ammonia solution (17 : 2 : 1).

Visualization: Spray the solution of dragendorff.

(2) Tests

Water: Not more than 11.0%.

Total Ash: Not more than 11.0%.

Acid-insoluble Ash: Not more than 2.0%.

Extract (alcohol): Not less than 9.0%.

(3) Assay

Scopolamine: Not less than 0.15% (HPLC).

7.4 Sophorae Flavescentis Radix(苦参)

7.4.1 Introduction

(1) Biological Source

Sophorae Flavescentis Radix is the dried root of *Sophora flavescens* Ait. (苦参) (Fam. Leguminosae).

(2) Property, Flavor and Channels Entered

Property and Flavor: Cold; Bitter.

Channels Entered: Heart, Liver, Stomach, Large Intestine, Bladder.

(3) Actions & Indications

To clear heat and dry dampness, kill worms, disinhibit urine. For trichomonas vaginitis, heat dysentery, bloody stool, red or white vaginal discharge, jaundice with annuria, pudendal swelling and itch, eczema, dampness sore, itching of skin, scabies and tinea leprosy.

(4) Pharmacological Activities

The pharmacological activities associated with Sophorae Flavescentis Radix include inhibiting histamine release, antitussive and expectorant effect, etc.

7.4.2 Main Chemical Constituents

Sophorae Flavescentis Radix mainly grows in Shanxi, Hubei, Henan and Hebei provinces. The main constituents are alkaloids. In addition, it also contains flavonoids, triterpene saponins and so on.

(1) Alkaloids

Sophorae Flavescentis Radix contains a dozen of alkaloids, matrine and oxymatrine being the highest, together with hydroxymatrine, sophocarpine (槐果碱), sophoranol (槐花醇), sophoramine (槐胺碱), sophoridine (槐啶碱), allomatrine (别苦参碱), isomatrine (异苦参碱), *N*-oxysophocarpine,

N-methylcytisine（*N*– 甲基金雀花碱）, anagyrine (安那吉碱), baptifoline (野靛叶碱), and so on. Matrine and oxymatrine are unique tetracyclo-quinolizindine alkaloids found only in Sophora species so far.

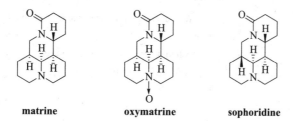

matrine   oxymatrine   sophoridine

① Properties of Matrine and Oxymatrine

a. Characteristics   Matrine exists in *α*-, *β*-, *γ*-, *δ*- four forms, *α*-form: flat prisms or needles, mp. 77℃, *β*-form: rhombs, mp. 87℃, *γ*-form: a liquid, bp. 223℃/6mmHg, *δ*-form: prisms, mp. 84℃, but the α-form is most common. Oxymatrine is colorless dice crystal (acetone), mp. 207–208℃ (decomposition), but its monohydrate has mp. of a 77–78℃ .

b. Basicity   Sophora alkaloids contain two nitrogen atoms. One is tertiary amine with middle strong basicity, the other is amide nitrogen, almost neutral.

c. Solubility   Matrine dissolves in water, but is also soluble in chloroform, ethyl ether and other lipophilic organic solvents. Oxymatrine, a nitrogen oxide, is more hydrophilic than matrine. It easily dissolves in water. It is soluble in chloroform, but insoluble in ethyl ether.

The polarity of sophora alkaloids are: Oxymatrine > hydroxymatrine > matrine.

d. Hydrolysis and Oxidative and Reductive Reactions   Matrine and oxymatrine have a lactam group which can be hydrolyzed in potassium hydroxide to potassium matrinate. Matrine and oxymatrine can be converted into each other (Figure 8-34).

Figure 8-34   Hydrolysis and oxidative and reductive reactions of matrine and oxymatrine

② Extraction and Isolation of Matrine and Oxymatrine

Matrine and oxymatrine can be separated according to the difference of solubility and basicity. The process is shown in Figure 8-35.

(2) Flavonoids

Sophorae Flavescentis Radix also contains many flavonoids, such as kushenol A–O, kuraridin (次苦参素), kushenin (苦参素), kuraridinol (苦参啶醇), kurarinol (苦参醇), neokurarinol (新苦参醇), norkurarinol (降苦参醇), isokurarinone (异苦参酮), kurarinone (苦参酮), norkurarinone (降苦参酮), formononetin (刺芒柄花素), methylkushenol C (甲基苦参新醇C）, *l*-maackiain, trifolirhizin (三叶豆紫檀苷), isoanhydroicaritin (异脱水淫羊藿素), noranhydroicaritin, xanthohumol (黄腐醇), isoxanthohumol (异黄腐酸), and luteolin-7-glucoside, etc.

Powdered Sophorae Flavescentis Radix
| Percolate with 0.1% HCl
Solution
| Strong acidic cation exchangge resin column
Resin
| Wash to colorless with distilled water;
| Dry the resin; Alkalify with $NH_3 \cdot H_2O$
Resin
| Rflux with $CHCl_3$
$CHCl_3$ solution
| Evaportate, dehydrate with
| anhydrous sodium sulfate
Synupy cnde product
| Recrystallize with acetone
Total alkaloids crysal
| Dissolve with a few $CHCl_3$
$CHCl_3$ solution
| Add Et_2O 10 times
Precipitate ─────────── Ether oslution
| Recrystallize with acetone Al_2O_3 CC
Oxymatrine   Elute with   Elute with benzene
            Et_2O—MeOH
                Matrine   Sophocarpine

Figure 8-35　Extraction and isolation procedure for matrine and oxymatrine

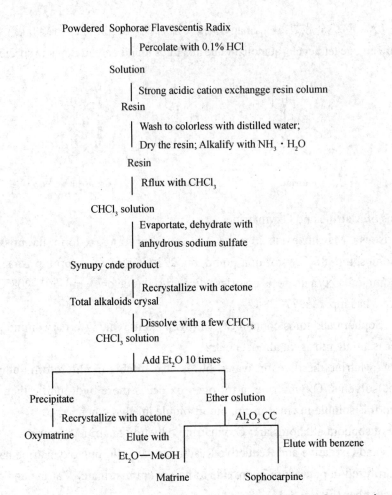

kuraridin　　　　　　　　　**norkurarinone**

(3) Triterpene Saponins

Sophoraflavoside Ⅰ–Ⅳ (苦参皂苷) and soyasaponin Ⅰ(大豆皂苷 Ⅰ) have been found in Sophorae Flavescentis Radix.

soyasaponin Ⅰ　　　　　R=H
sophoraflavoside Ⅰ　　　R=ara-glc

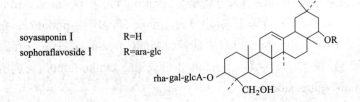

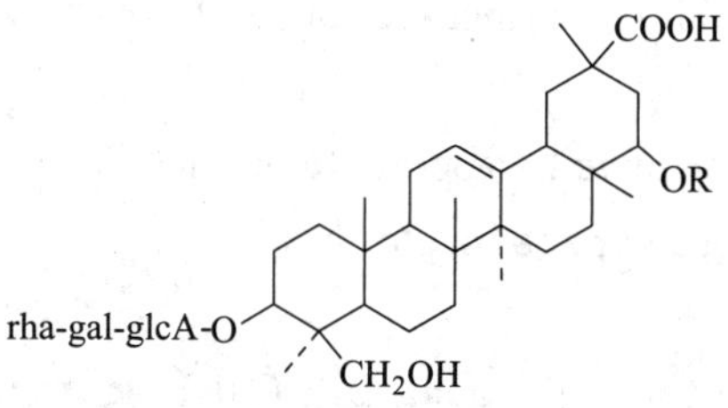

sophoraflavoside Ⅱ　　R = H
sophoraflavoside Ⅲ　　R = ara
sophoraflavoside Ⅳ　　R = ara-glc

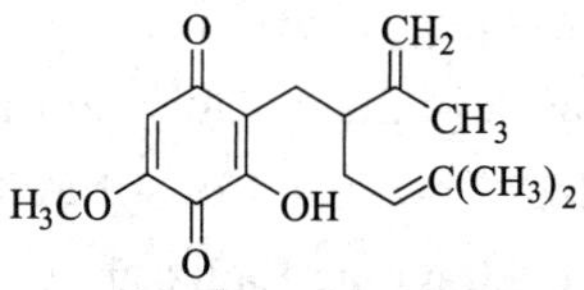

kushequinone A

(4) Others

Sophorae Flavescentis Radix also contains quinone compounds, such as kushequinone A.

7.4.3　Quality Control Standards

(1) TLC Identification

① Stationary Phase: Silica gel plate.

Standard: Matrine ; Sophoridine.

Development System: Methylbenzene-acetone-methanol (8∶3∶0.5); Methylbenzene-ethyl acetate-ethanol-water (2∶4∶2∶1) (Stand for at 10℃ below, upper layer).

Visualization: Spray the solution of bismuth potassium iodide (碘化铋钾) and sodium nitrite (亚硝酸钠) in ethanol successively.

② Stationary Phase: Silica gel plate prepared with sodium hydroxide solution.

Standard: Matrine ; Sophoridine.

Development System: Chloroform-methanol-concentrate ammonia (5∶0.6∶0.3) (Stand for at 10 ℃ below, lower layer).

Visualization: Spray the solution of bismuth potassium iodide and sodium nitrite in ethanol.

(2) Tests

Water: Not more than 11.0%.

Total Ash: Not more than 8.0%.

Extract (water): Not less than 20.0%.

(3) Assay

Matrine and Oxymatrine: Not less than 1.2% (HPLC).

7.5　Stephaniae Tetrandrae Radix(防己)

7.5.1　Introduction

(1) Biological Source

Stephaniae tetrandrae Radix is the dried root of *Stephania tetrandra* S. Moore. (粉防己) (Fam. Menispermaceae).

(2) Property, Flavor and Channels Entered

Property and Flavor: Cold; Bitter.

Channels Entered: Bladder, Lung.

(3) Actions & Indications

To dispel wind and relieve pain, promote urination to alleviate edema. For eczema, edema and tinea pedis, painful impediment caused by wind-dampness, inhibited urination, sore and toxin.

(4) Pharmacological Activities

The pharmacological activities associated with Stephaniae tetrandrae Radix include antihypertensive, anti-arrhythmic, anti-inflammatory, anti-tumor, cardiovascular action, etc.

7.5.2　Main Chemical Constituents

Stephaniae tetrandrae Radix grows in Shanxi, Yunnan and Guangxi of China. It contains alkaloids (2.3%–5%), flavones, phenols, volatile oils, etc.

(1) Alkaloids

The major chemical constituents of Stephaniae tetrandrae Radix are alkaloids, which can be classified into bisbenzylisoquinoline (双苄基异喹啉), protoberberine (原小檗碱), morphinane (吗啡烷) and phenanthrene (菲) types. The main components are tetrandrine and fangchinoline (防己诺林碱). Other constituents include bisbenzylisoquinoline type［berbamine (小檗胺), oxofanchirine, quaternary alkaloid of the protoberberine type cyclanoline (轮环藤酚碱）］, alkaloid with a phenanthrene skeleton and a tertiary armine side chain (stephenanthrine (防己菲碱), trilobine (木防己碱), etc.

Dimethyltetrandrine iodide generated from the reaction between tetrandrine or fangchinoline and methyl iodide (碘甲烷) in alkaline conditions has the effect of muscle relaxant.

fangchinoline　R=H
tetrandrine　R=CH₃

cyclanoline　　stephenanthrine

① Properties of Tetrandrine and Fangchinoline

a. Characteristics　Tetrandrine and fangchinoline are all white crystal. Tetrandrine has mp. 217–218 ℃ (acetone), $[\alpha]_D^{28}$ +268.7° (CHCl₃). Fangchinoline has mp. 237–238 ℃, $[\alpha]_D^{28}$ +255.1° (CHCl₃), which on –OH methylation yields tetrandrine, and is regarded as a demethyltetrandrine.

b. Basicity　They are tertiary bases, so the basicity is medium strong.

c. Solubility　Tetrandrine and fangchinoline are soluble in methanol, ethanol, ethyl ether, chloroform and benzene, insoluble in water. Fangchinoline has a phenolic hydroxyl group. It gives positive reaction to the ferric chloride color reaction and can be methylated with diazomethane, but it is not soluble in aqueous alkali.

② Extraction and Isolation of Tetrandrine, Fangchinoline and Cyclanoline

The process is illustrated in Figure 8-36.

(2) Others

Stephaniae tetrandrae Radix also contains flavonoids, phenols and volatile oils.

7.5.3　Quality Control Standards

(1) TLC Identification

Stationary Phase: Silica gel plate.

Standard: Tetrandrine; Fangchinoline.

Development System: Chloroform-acetone-methanol-strong ammonia solution (6∶1∶1∶0.1).

Visualization: Spray the solution of bismuth potassium iodide.

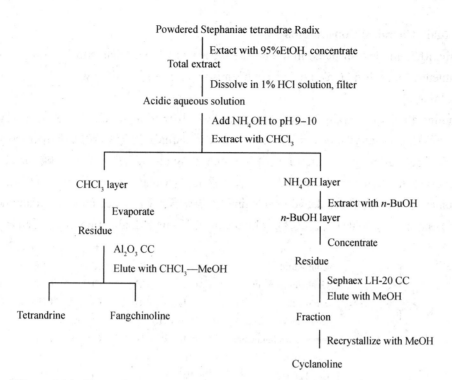

Figure 8-36 **Extraction and isolation of tetrandrine, fangchinoline and cyclanoline**

(2) Tests

Water: Not more than 12.0%.

Total Ash: Not more than 4.0%.

Extract (methanol): Not less than 5.0%.

(3) Assay

Fangchinoline and Tetrandrine: Not less than 1.6% (HPLC).

7.6 Corydalis Rhizoma (延胡索)

7.6.1 Introduction

(1) Biological Source

Corydalis Rhizoma is the dried tuber of *Corydalis yanhusuo* W. T. Wang (延胡索) (Fam. Papaveraceae).

(2) Property, Flavor and Channels Entered

Property and Flavor: Warm; Pungent, bitter.

Channels Entered: Liver, Spleen.

(3) Actions & Indications

To activate blood, move qi, relieve pain. For pain in the chest, the hypochondrium, epigastrium and abdomen, amenorrhea and dysmenorrhea, chest impediment and heart pain, postpartum stasis and obstruction, swelling and pain caused by injuries from falls.

(4) Pharmacological Activities

The pharmacological activities associated with Corydalis Rhizoma include increasing blood circulation, promoting stagnant blood, relieving heart arrhythmia, cardio tonic, killing pain, sedative, anti-cancer, antitussive, etc.

7.6.2 Main Chemical Constituents

Corydalis Rhizoma is distributed in the northern parts of China, Japan and Siberia. Alkaloids are its major constituents. More than 20 alkaloids have been isolated from it until now.

(1) Alkaloids

Isoquinoline alkaloids: tetrahydropalmatine, tetrahydroberberine, tetrahydrocoptisine (四氢黄连碱), corybulbine (紫堇球碱), corydaline (紫堇碱), dehydrocorydaline (去氢紫堇碱), dehydrocorybulbine (去氢紫堇鳞茎碱), palmatine, protopine (原阿片碱), dehydroglaucine (去氢海罂粟碱), α-allocryptopine (α- 别隐品碱), N-methyllaurotetanine (N- 甲基六驳碱), yuanhunine (延胡宁), leonticine (牡丹草碱), dihydrosanguinarine (二氢血根碱), dehydronantenine (去氢南天宁碱), bicuculline, corydalmine (紫堇单酚碱), bererine, coptisine, stylopine (人血草碱), columbamine, 13-methylpalmatine (去氢延胡索素), etc.

Compound	R_1	R_2	R_3	R_4	R_5
tetrahydropalmatine	CH_3	CH_3	CH_3	CH_3	H
corydaline	CH_3	CH_3	CH_3	CH_3	CH_3
tetrahydrocopetisine	—CH_2—		—CH_2—		H
tetrahydrocolumbanine	CH_3	H	CH_3	CH_3	H
d-corybulbine	H	CH_3	CH_3	CH_3	CH_3
corydalmine	CH_3	CH_3	CH_3	H	H

Compound	R_1	R_2	R_3	R_4	R_5
l-copetisine	—CH_2—		—CH_2—		H
dehydrocorydaline	CH_3	CH_3	CH_3	CH_3	CH_3
columbanine	CH_3	H	CH_3	CH_3	H

Compound	R_1	R_2
protopine	—CH_2—	
allocryptopine	CH_3	CH_3

The major alkaloids include tertiary alkaloids and quaternary alkaloids, and their structures are very similar. Tetrahydropalmatine is the known active compound as a pain killer. The extraction and isolation procedure is illustrated in Figure 8-37.

Other methods including microwave-assisted extraction (微波辅助萃取), supercritical fluid extraction (超临界流体萃取), HPLC, and high-speed countercurrent chromatography have been developed to extract and separate the alkaloids from Corydalis Rhizoma.

(2) Others

Corydalis Rhizoma also contains a large number of starch, small quantity of mucilage, β-glucoside, volatile oils besides alkaloids.

7.6.3 Quality Control Standards

(1) TLC Identification

Stationary Phase: Silica gel G plate (with 1% sodium hydroxide-impregnated).

Standard: Authentic crude drug; Tetrahydropalmatine.

Development System: Toluene-acetone (9 : 2).

Visualization: 365nm UV light.

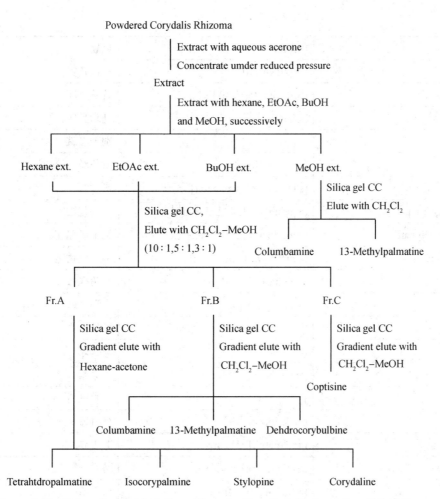

Figure 8-37   Extraction and isolation of isoquinoline alkaloids from Corydalis Rhizoma

(2) Tests

Water: Not more than 15.0%.

Total Ash: Not more than 4.0%.

Extract (dilute alcohol): Not less than 13.0%.

(3) Assay

Tetrahydropalmatine: Not less than 0.050% (HPLC).

词 汇 表

An Alphabetical List of Words and Phrases

A		
acetamide	[æsɪˈtæmaɪd]	乙酰胺
acetylacetone	[ˌæsɪtɪlˈæsɪtəun]	乙酰丙酮
Aconiti lateralis radix praeparata		北乌头
aliphatic amines	[ˌæləˈfætɪk] [əˈmiːns]	脂肪胺

(continued)

alkene	['ælki:n]	烯烃
alkylamine	[ˌælkɪlə'mi:n]	有机胺类
alkyl heterocyclic	['ælkɪl][hetərə'saɪklɪk]	烷基杂环
allocryptopine	[æləukrɪptə'paɪn]	别隐品碱
allomatrine		别苦参碱
aminophylline	[æmi:nəu'fɪlɪn]	氨茶碱
ammonium vanadate	[ə'məunjəm]['vænədeɪt]	钒酸铵
ammonium hydroxide	[ə'məunjəm][haɪ'drɒksaɪd]	氢氧化铵
amorphism precipitate	[ə'mɔ:fɪzəm][prɪ'sɪpɪteɪt]	无定形沉淀
amphoteric alkaloids	[æmfə'terɪk]['ælkələɪdz]	两性生物碱
anabasine	[ə'næbəsi:n]	八角枫碱
anagyrine	[æ'nædʒi:ri:n]	安那吉碱，臭豆碱
angiosperm	['ændʒɪə'spə:m]	被子植物
anisodine	[enɪ'səudɪn]	樟柳碱
apigenin	['æpaɪdʒnɪn]	芹菜素
Apocynaceae		夹竹桃科
arecolidine	[ərekə'lɪdɪn]	槟榔碱
aromatic amine	[ære'mætɪk][ə'mi:n]	芳香族胺
aromatic heterocyclic-N	[ære'mætɪk][hetərə'saɪklɪk]	芳香杂环
aspartic acid	[əs'pɑ:tɪk]['æsɪd]	天冬氨酸
atropine	['ætrɔpi:n]	阿托品
B		
baptifoline	[bæptɪ'fəulɪn]	野靛叶碱，膺靛叶碱
Belladonnae herba	[ˌbelə'dɒnə][hə:b]	颠茄
berbamine	['bə:bəmi:n]	小檗胺
berberastine	[bə:be'ræsti:n]	5–羟基小檗碱
Berberidaceae	[bə:bərɪ'deɪsi:i:]	小檗科
Berberidis radix		三颗针
berberrubine	[bə:bə'rʌbaɪn]	小檗红碱
bismuth potassium iodide	['bɪzməθ][pə'tæsɪəm]['aɪədaɪd]	碘化铋钾
bisbenzylisoquinoline	[bɪsbenzɪlɪsəkwaɪ'nəlɪn]	双苄基异喹啉
bleaching powder	['bli:tʃɪŋ]['paudə(r)]	漂白粉
C		
calcium hypochlorite	['kælsɪəm][ˌhaɪpəu'klɔ:raɪt]	次氯酸钙
camptothecine	[kæmptəu'θesɪn]	喜树碱
Camptotheca acuminata		喜树
Carbamidine	[kɑ:'bæmɪdi:n]	胍

(continued)

Cassia obtusifolia		草决明
cephalotaxin	[ˈsefələutæksɪn]	三尖杉碱
cinchonine	[ˈsɪnkəni:n]	辛可宁
cocaine	[kəuˈkeɪn]	可卡因
codeine	[ˈkəudi:ɪn]	可待因
colchicine	[ˈkɔltʃɪsi:n]	秋水仙碱
conformation	[ˌkɔnfɔ:ˈmeɪʃn]	构象
columbamine	[kɔləmˈbæmɪn]	非洲防己碱
coniine	[ˈkəunɪi:n]	毒芹碱
coordinate bond	[kəuˈɔ:dɪneɪt] [bɔnd]	配价键
Coptis chinensis Franch		黄连
Coptis deltoidea C.Y.Cheng et Hsiao		三角叶黄连
coptisine	[ˈkɔptɪsɪn]	黄连碱
Coptis teeta Wall.		云连
corybulbine	[kɔri:ˈbʌlbɪn]	紫堇球碱，紫堇鳞茎碱
corydaline	[kɔ:ˈraɪdəlaɪn]	紫堇碱
corydalmine	[kɔ:ˈraɪdɑ:lmaɪn]	紫堇单酚碱
cyanide ion	[ˈsaɪənaɪd] [ˈaɪən]	氰离子
cyclanoline	[sɪkˈlænəli:n]	轮环藤酚碱
cyclohexene	[ˈsaɪkləuhɪksi:n]	环己烯
cytidine	[ˈsaɪtədɪn]	胞苷
D		
Datura metel L.		白花曼陀罗
Daturae flos		洋金花
dauricine	[dɔ:ˈraɪsɪn]	蝙蝠葛碱
dehydrocorybulbine	[di:haɪdrəuˌkɔri:ˈbʌlbɪn]	去氢紫堇鳞茎碱
dehydrocorydaline	[di:haɪdrəukəˈraɪdəlaɪn]	去氢紫堇碱
dehydroglaucine	[di:haɪˈdrəglausɪn]	去氢海罂粟碱
dehydronantenine	[di:haɪdrəuˈnæntɪni:n]	去氢南天宁碱
demethylation ephedrine	[dɪmeθɪˈleɪʃn][eˈfedrɪn]	去甲基麻黄碱
dendrobine	[ˈdendrəubaɪn]	石斛碱
deuterated water	[ˈdju:təreɪtɪd][ˈwɔ:tə]	氘代水
diacetyldimethyldihydropyridine		二乙酰基二甲基二氢吡啶
dibenzyl-tetrahydroisoquinolin	[daɪˈbenzɪl][tetrəˌhaɪdrəuaisəˈkwɪnəlɪn]	二苄基四氢异喹啉
dicotyledon	[ˌdaɪkɔtɪˈli:dən]	双子叶植物
dihydrosanguinarine	[daɪˌhaɪdrəˌsæŋgwɪˈnæri:n]	二氢血根碱

(continued)

E		
electron atmosphere density	[ɪ'lektrɔn]['ætməsfɪə]['densəti]	电子云密度
emetine	['eməti:n]	吐根碱
Ephedra equisetina Bge.		木贼麻黄
Ephedra intermedia Schrenk et C.A.Mey.		中麻黄
Ephedra sinica Stapf.		草麻黄
Ephedraceae		麻黄科
ephedroxane	['efdrɔkseɪn]	麻黄恶唑酮
epiberberine	[e'paɪbəbərɪn]	表小檗碱
epoxide	[e'pɔksaɪd]	环氧的
ether bond	['i:θə][bɔnd]	醚键
evodiamine	[e,vəudɪ'æmɪn]	吴茱萸碱
F		
Fabaceae		蝶形花科
fangchinoline	['fæŋ'tʃɪnɔlɪn]	防己诺林碱，汉防己乙素
ferulic acid	[fə'ru:lɪk]['æsɪd]	阿魏酸
Formononetin	['fəmɔnəunɪtɪn]	刺芒柄花素
formaldehyde	[fɔ:'mældɪhaɪd]	甲醛
free radical	[fri:]['rædɪkəl]	自由基
Fritillaria thunbergii var. *chekiangensis*		东贝母
fuming nitric acid	[fjumɪŋ]['naɪtrɪk]['æsɪd]	发烟硝酸
G		
gentianine	['dʒeʃənɪn]	龙胆碱
glycyrrhizic acid	[,glɪsɪ'raɪzɪk]['æsɪd]	甘草酸
groenlandicine		四去氢碎叶紫堇碱
H		
herbacetin	[hə'beɪseɪn]	草质素
histidine	['hɪstɪdi:n]	组氨酸
homolycorine	[həu'mɔli:kəri:n]	高石蒜碱
Hofmann degradation		霍夫曼降解
hybridization	[,haɪbrɪdaɪ'zeɪʃn]	杂化
hydrastine	[haɪ'drɑsti:n]	白毛茛碱
hydrochloride	[haɪdrə'klauraɪd]	盐酸盐
hydrogen bonding effect	['haɪdrədʒən]['bɔndɪŋ][ɪ'fekt]	氢键效应
hygrine	['haɪgrɪn]	古柯碱
hyoscine	['haɪəsi:n]	东莨菪碱
hyoscyamine	[,haɪə'saɪəmi:n]	莨菪碱

(continued)

Hyoscyami semen		天仙子
I		
imidazole	[ɪmɪˈdɔzəul]	咪唑
indole	[ˈɪndəul]	吲哚
indole alkaloids	[ˈɪndəul][ˈælkələɪd]	吲哚生物碱类
indolizidine	[ˌɪndəuˈlɪzɪdaɪn]	吲哚里西啶
inductive effect	[ɪnˈdʌktɪv][ɪˈfekt]	诱导效应
inductive-field effect	[ɪnˈdʌktɪv][fiːld][ɪˈfekt]	诱导 – 场效应
isoanhydroicaritin	[aɪsəunˈhaɪdrɔɪkærɪtɪn]	异脱水淫羊藿素
isokurarinone	[aɪˈsəukjuərərɪnwʌn]	异苦参酮
isomatrine	[aɪsəmeɪtˈriːn]	异苦参碱
isoamyl alcohol	[aɪsəuˈæmɪl][ˈælkəhɔl]	异戊醇
isoquinoline	[ˌaɪsəuˈkwɪnəliːn]	异喹啉
isoxanthohumol	[aɪsəuˌzænθəˈhjuːmɔl]	异黄腐酸
isoverticine	[aɪsəuvəˈtɪsɪn]	异浙贝甲素
J		
jatrorrhizine	[dʒætˈrɔraɪzɪn]	药根碱
K		
kaempferol	[ˈkiːmpfərɔl]	山奈酚
kuraridin	[kjuəræˈraɪdɪn]	次苦参素，苦参查尔酮
kuraridinol	[kjuəræˈraɪdɪnɔl]	苦参啶醇，苦参查尔酮醇
kurarinol	[ˈkjuərərɪnl]	苦参醇
kurarinone	[ˈkjuərərɪnwʌn]	苦参酮，苦参黄素
kushenin	[ˈkʌʃenɪn]	苦参素
L		
lactone	[ˈlæktəun]	内酯
leonticine	[ˈlɪəuntiːsɪn]	牡丹草碱
Liliaceae		百合科
limonene	[ˈlɪməniːn]	柠檬烯
lipophilicp	[ˌlɪpəˈfɪlɪk]	亲脂性的
lupinine	[ˈluːpəniːn]	羽扇豆碱
lycorine	[ˈlɪkərɪn]	石蒜碱
lysine	[ˈlaɪsiːn]	赖氨酸
M		
maackiain	[məkˈɪeɪɪn]	山槐素，高丽槐素
magnoflorine	[mægˈnɔflɔriːn]	木兰碱
malic acid	[ˈmælɪk][ˈæsɪd]	苹果酸

(continued)

matrine	[meɪt'ri:n]	苦参碱
megastigmane sesquiterpenes		大柱香波龙烷型倍半萜烯
Menispermaceae		防己科
Menipermi rhizome		北豆根
mercury	['mə:kjuri]	汞
methylenedioxy group	[meθɪləni:da'ɪɔksɪ][gru:p]	亚甲二氧基
methyl iodide	['meθɪl]['aəɪdaɪd]	碘甲烷
methylkushenol C		甲基苦参新醇 C
13-methylpalmatine	['mɪɔɪlpælməti:n]	去氢延胡索素
methylpseudoephedrine	[ˌmeθɪlˌsu:dəʊɪ'fedrɪn]	甲基伪麻黄碱
microwave-assisted extraction (MAE)	['maɪkrəweɪv][ə'sɪstɪd][ɪk'strækʃn]	微波辅助萃取
morphinane	['mɔ:fɪnən]	吗啡烷
morphine	['mɔ:fi:n]	吗啡
N		
neokurarinol	[ni:əuk'juərərɪnl]	新苦参醇
nicotine	['nɪkəti:n]	烟碱，尼古丁
ninhydrin	[nɪn'haɪdrɪn]	茚三酮
N-methylcytisine	['meθɪl'sɪtaɪsɪn]	甲基金雀花碱
N-methylephedrine	[metɪ'lefedrɪn]	N– 甲基麻黄碱
N-methyllaurotetanine	[meθɪlɔ:rəʊ'tetənaɪn]	N– 甲基六驳碱
norkurarinol	['nɔ:rkjuərərɪnl]	降苦参醇
norkurarinone	['nɔ:rkjuərərɪnwʌn]	降苦参酮
nucleic acids	['nju:klɪɪk]['æsɪdz]	核酸
nucleotide acids	['nju:klɪətaɪd]['æsɪdz]	核苷酸
O		
ornithine	['ɔ:nɪθi:n]	鸟氨酸
oxalate	['ɔksəleɪt]	草酸盐
oxymatrine	[ɔk'sɪmətrɪn]	氧化苦参碱
P		
palmatine	['pælməti:n]	巴马丁
Papaveraceae		罂粟科
Papaveris pericarpium		罂粟壳
papillionaceous		蝶形科的
p-cymene	['saɪmi:n]	对伞花烃
pelletierine	[pelɪ'tɪəri:n]	石榴皮碱
periodic acid	[ˌpɪərɪ'ɔdɪk]['æsɪd]	过碘酸
phenanthrene	[fɪ'nænθri:n]	菲

(continued)

phenolic hydroxyl group	[fɪˈnɔlɪk][haɪˈdrɔksɪl][gru:p]	酚羟基
phenylalanine	[ˌfenəlˈæləni:n]	苯丙氨酸
phenylamine	[fenəlˈæmi:n]	苯胺
physostigmine	[faɪsəuˈstɪgmi:n]	毒扁豆碱
pilocarpine	[ˌpaɪləuˈkɑ:pɪn]	毛果芸香碱
piperine	[ˈpɪpərɪn]	胡椒碱
piperidine	[pɪˈperɪdi:n]	哌啶
platinum	[ˈplætɪnəm]	铂
proto-alkaloids	[ˈprəutə][ˈælkəlɔɪdz]	原生物碱
protoberberine	[ˌprəutəuˈbə:bəri:n]	原小檗碱
protocatechuic acid	[ˌprəutəukəˈtektʃuəɪk][ˈæsɪd]	原儿茶酸
protopine	[ˈprəutəpɪn]	原阿片碱，普托品
pseudo-alkaloids	[ˈsju:dəu][ˈælkəlɔɪdz]	伪生物碱
pseudoephedrine	[ˌsju:dəuˈfedrɪn]	伪麻黄碱
purine	[ˈpjuəri:n]	咖啡碱，嘌呤
Pyrrole	[ˈpaɪərəul]	吡咯
Pyrrolidine	[pɪˈrəulɪdi:n]	吡咯烷
Q		
quaternary amine ion	[kwəˈtə:nərɪ][ˈæmi:n][ˈaɪən]	季铵离子
quaternary ammonium	[kwəˈtə:nərɪ][əˈməunjəm]	季铵
quinidine	[kwɪˈnaɪdɪn]	奎尼丁
quinina	[kwɪˈni:nə]	金鸡纳碱
quinine	[ˈkwaɪˌnaɪn]	奎宁
quinoline	[ˈkwɪnəli:n]	喹啉
quinolizidine	[ˈkwɪnəlɪˈzaɪdɪn]	喹诺里西啶
R		
racemic form	[rəˈsi:mɪk][fɔ:m]	外消旋体
Ranunculaceae		毛茛科
reserpine	[rɪˈsə:pɪn]	利血平
Reinecke's salt		雷氏铵盐
rhein	[raɪn]	大黄酸
S		
sanguinarine	[sæŋgwɪˈneəri:n]	血根碱
scopolamine	[skəuˈpɔləmi:n]	东莨菪碱
secondary amine	[ˈsekəndrɪ][əˈmi:n]	仲胺
securinine	[sɪˈkju:rɪni:n]	一叶萩碱
senecionine	[sɪni:sɪˈəuni:n]	千里光宁碱

(continued)

sodium nitrite	[ˈsəudɪəm][ˈnaɪtraɪt]	亚硝酸钠
sodium molybdate	[ˈsəudɪəm][məˈlɪbdeɪt]	钼酸钠
solanaceous	[sɔləˈneɪʃəs]	茄科的
sophocarpine	[səufəˈkɑːpiːn]	槐果碱
Sophorae flavescentis radix		苦参
sophoraflavoside	[ˌsəufərəˈfleɪvəsaɪd]	苦参皂苷
sophoramine	[ˌsɔfəˈræmiːn]	槐胺碱
sophoranol	[sɔfəˈrænɔl]	槐花醇
sophoridine	[səuˈfɔːraɪdɪn]	槐定碱
soyasaponin	[sɔɪeɪzæˈpɔnɪn]	大豆皂苷
space effect	[speɪs][ɪˈfekt]	空间效应
sparteine	[ˈspɑːtɪiːn]	无叶豆碱
starch	[stɑːtʃ]	淀粉
Stephania tetrandra S. Moore.		粉防己
Stephania tetrandrae radix		防己
stephenanthrine		防己菲碱
steric hindrance	[ˈsterɪk][ˈhɪndrəns]	空间位阻
strychnine	[ˈstrɪkniːn]	士的宁，番木鳖碱
stylopine	[ˈstaɪləpɪn]	人血草碱
sulphate	[ˈsʌlfeɪt]	硫酸盐
sulfuric acid	[sʌlˈfjuːrɪk][ˈæsɪd]	硫酸
supercritical fluid extraction (SFE)	[ˌsjuːpəˈkrɪtɪkəl][ˈfluːɪd][[ɪkˈstrækʃn]	超临界萃取技术
T		
tartaric acid	[tɑːˈtærɪk][ˈæsɪd]	酒石酸
tautomerization	[ˈtɔːtɔmraɪˈzeɪʃən]	互变异构
taxol	[ˈtæksl]	紫杉醇
terpinen–4–ol		松油烯 –4– 醇
2,3,5,6–tetramethylpyrazine	[tetræmiːθɪlˈpaɪreɪzɪn]	苄基甲胺 2,3,5,6– 四甲基吡嗪
2,4,6–trinitrophenol	[traɪnaɪtrəuˈfiːnɔl]	2,4,6– 三硝基苯酚
terpinen	[ˈtəːpɪniːn]	松油烯
terpineol	[təˈpɪnɪəul]	松油醇
tertiary amines	[ˈtəːʃəri][əˈmiːns]	叔胺
tetrahydroberberine	[ˈtetrəaɪdrəubəːbərɪn]	四氢小檗碱
tetrahydrocoptisine	[tetrəaɪdrəukɔpˈtaɪsaɪn]	四氢黄连碱
tetrahydroisowuinolin	[tetrəaɪdrɔɪzaˈuuːnəlɪ]	四氢异喹啉
tetrahydropulmatine	[tetrəaɪdrəuˈpʌlmətiːn]	延胡索乙素
tetrandrine	[ˈtetrændraɪn]	汉防己碱，汉防己甲素

(continued)

tigloidine	[tɪˈglɔɪdɪn]	巴豆酰莨菪碱
tricin	[ˈtraɪsɪn]	小麦黄素
trifolirhizin	[traɪfəˈlə:haɪzɪn]	三叶豆紫檀苷，红车轴草根苷
trigonelline	[trɪˈgənelaɪn]	葫芦巴碱
trilobine	[traɪˈləbɪn]	木防己碱
tropane	[ˈtrəupeɪn]	莨菪烷
tryptophan	[ˈtrɪptəfæn]	色氨酸
tyrosine	[ˈtɪərəsi:n]	酪氨酸
V		
valtropine		瓦托品
vanillic acid	[vəˈnɪlɪk][ˈæsɪd]	香草酸
veratramine	[ˌverəˈtræmi:n]	藜芦胺
verticindione		浙贝双酮
verticinone	[vəˈtɪsɪnwʌn]	浙贝乙素
verticine	[vəˈtɪsɪn]	浙贝甲素
vincristine	[vɪŋˈkrɪsti:n]	长春新碱
W		
withanolides	[ˈwɪθənɔlɪdz]	醉茄内酯类
worenine	[ˈwɔ:rɪni:n]	甲基黄连碱
X		
xanthohumol	[ˌzænθəˈhju:mɔl]	黄腐醇
Y		
yuanhunine	[ju:ɑ:nhəˈnaɪn]	延胡宁

重 点 小 结

　　生物碱指主要来源于植物界的一类含氮有机化合物，多呈碱性，大多有较复杂的环状结构，氮原子常结合在环内。一般来说，生物界除生物体必需的含氮有机化合物（如氨基酸、蛋白质、肽类、核酸、核苷酸、氨基糖、含氮维生素等）外，其他含氮有机化合物均被视为生物碱，多具有显著而特殊的生物活性。

　　游离生物碱的溶解性：①亲脂性生物碱。大多数叔胺碱和仲胺碱为亲脂性，易溶于亲脂性有机溶剂，可溶于酸水，不溶或难溶于水和碱水。②亲水性生物碱。主要指季铵碱和某些含氮－氧化物的生物碱，可溶于水、甲醇、乙醇，难溶于亲脂性有机溶剂。③具特殊官能团的生物碱。具酚羟基或羧基的生物碱既可溶于酸水，也可溶于碱水，但在 pH 8~9 时易产生沉淀，这样的生物碱称为两性生物碱，其中具酚羟基者常称为酚性生物碱。具内酯或内酰胺结构的生物碱，在碱水溶液中，其内酯或内酰胺结构可开环形成羧酸盐而溶于水中，加酸又可环合析出。

　　生物碱盐一般易溶于水，可溶于醇类，难溶于亲脂性有机溶剂。一般生物碱的无机酸盐水溶性大于有机酸盐；含氧酸盐的水溶性大于卤代酸盐；在卤代酸盐中，盐酸盐水溶性最大，而氢碘酸盐的水溶度最小；小分子有机酸盐水溶性大于大分子有机酸盐；多元酸盐的水溶性大于一元酸盐的水溶性。但有些生物碱盐的溶解性比较特殊，如小檗碱盐酸盐、麻黄碱草酸盐等难溶于水，高石蒜碱（homolycorine）的盐酸盐难溶于水而易溶于三氯甲烷等。

生物碱的碱性大小与氮原子的杂化方式、诱导效应、诱导－场效应、共轭效应、空间效应及分子内氢键等因素有关。学习时应理解氮原子在生物碱碱性中所起的关键作用、pK_a的含义及其与碱性的关系，并能结合实例分析说明影响碱性强弱的因素。

沉淀反应在生物碱的提取分离、鉴别及含量测定等方面具有重要用途，应熟悉生物碱沉淀反应的条件、生物碱沉淀试剂的种类，重点掌握碘化铋钾试剂在生物碱检识中的应用。

生物碱的提取：①水或酸水提取法。酸水提取后可以采用阳离子树脂交换法和萃取法进行总生物碱的富集。②醇类溶剂提取法。可用醇回流或渗漉、浸渍，缺点是脂溶性杂质较多，可配合酸水－碱化－萃取法处理去除脂溶性杂质。③亲脂性有机溶剂提取法。大多数生物碱在游离状态下是亲脂性的，但在植物中多以盐的形式存在，因此在用三氯甲烷、乙醚及二氯甲烷等溶剂提取之前，必须先将药材粉末用氨水充分湿润，以使生物碱游离出来。

生物碱的分离：①不同类别生物碱的分离。采用萃取法将总生物碱按碱性强弱、酚性有无及是否水溶性初步分离。②利用生物碱的碱性差异进行分离。pH梯度萃取法分离总生物碱中碱性不同的各单体生物碱。③利用生物碱或生物碱盐溶解度的差异进行分离。④利用生物碱特殊官能团进行分离。例如用2%NaOH水溶液萃取酚性生物碱，使其与其他脂溶性生物碱分离。⑤利用色谱法进行分离。可采用氧化铝吸附柱色谱、分配柱色谱和高效液相色谱法（HPLC）进行分离和纯化。

中药麻黄中的生物碱40%～90%为麻黄碱，其次为伪麻黄碱及微量的$l-N-$甲基麻黄碱、$d-N-$甲基伪麻黄碱、$l-$去甲基麻黄碱、$d-$去甲基伪麻黄碱、麻黄次碱。麻黄碱和伪麻黄碱为仲胺衍生物，互为立体异构体，游离时具有挥发性。游离的麻黄生物碱可溶于水，能溶解于三氯甲烷、乙醚及醇类溶剂中。草酸麻黄碱较难溶于水，而草酸伪麻黄碱则易溶于水。麻黄碱和伪麻黄碱不能与生物碱沉淀试剂发生沉淀反应，可用二硫化碳－硫酸铜反应、铜络盐反应两种特征反应进行鉴别。麻黄碱和伪麻黄碱具有挥发性，还可用水蒸气蒸馏法提取。麻黄碱和伪麻黄碱的分离也可利用其碱性强弱不同，先将两者交换到强酸型阳离子树脂柱上进行分离。

中药黄连的有效成分主要有小檗碱、巴马丁、黄连碱、甲基黄连碱、药根碱等，均为季铵碱。游离小檗碱缓溶于水中，易溶于热水或热乙醇，在冷乙醇中溶解度不大，难溶于苯、三氯甲烷、丙酮等有机溶剂。盐酸小檗碱在水中溶解度仅为1∶500。小檗碱与大分子有机酸在水中加热会结合成难溶于水的大分子复合物，因此为了避免有效成分流失，含有小檗碱的中药黄连、黄柏等不能与大黄、甘草等中药一起煎煮。小檗碱除了能与一般生物碱沉淀试剂产生沉淀反应外，还具有以下特征性鉴别反应：小檗红碱反应、丙酮加成反应、漂白粉显色反应和变色酸反应。

中药洋金花中所含生物碱是由莨菪醇类和芳香族有机酸结合生成一元酯类化合物，习惯上称为莨菪烷类生物碱，主要有莨菪碱（阿托品）、山莨菪碱、东莨菪碱、樟柳碱和$N-$去甲莨菪碱。东莨菪碱和樟柳碱由于6、7位氧环立体效应和诱导效应的影响，碱性较弱（pK_a 7.5）；莨菪碱无立体效应障碍，碱性较强（pK_a 9.65）；山莨菪碱的6位羟基的立体效应影响较东莨菪碱小，故其碱性介于莨菪碱和东莨菪碱之间。莨菪烷类生物碱能与多种生物碱沉淀试剂产生沉淀反应，此外还可采用Vitali反应、氯化汞沉淀反应和过碘酸氧化乙酰丙酮缩合反应进行检识。

防己所含生物碱主要为粉防己碱（汉防己甲素）、防己诺林碱（汉防己乙素）、氧化防己碱和防己菲碱，还含有少量的轮环藤酚碱。粉防己碱和防己诺林碱均为双苄基异喹啉衍生物，为叔胺碱；轮环藤酚碱为季铵碱。利用防己生物碱都可溶于乙醇，用乙醇进行提取，再利用防己中粉防己碱、防己诺林碱和轮环藤酚碱的碱性和极性的差异，采用溶剂法和色谱法进行分离。

目 标 检 测

一、单选题

1. 分离季铵碱和水溶性杂质常用（　　　）
   A. 氧化铝层析法　　　　　　　　B. 葡聚糖凝胶层析法　　　　C. 铅盐沉淀法
   D. 明胶沉淀法　　　　　　　　　E. 雷氏铵盐沉淀法

2. 亲水性生物碱主要指（　　　）
   A. 酰胺生物碱　　　　　　　　　B. 叔胺生物碱　　　　　　　C. 仲胺生物碱
   D. 季铵生物碱　　　　　　　　　E. 两性生物碱

3. 下列化合物不能与生物碱沉淀试剂产生沉淀的是（　　　）
   A. 小檗碱　　　　　　　　　　　B. 麻黄碱　　　　　　　　　C. 苦参碱
   D. 莨菪碱　　　　　　　　　　　E. 马钱子碱

4. 具有隐性酚羟基的生物碱是（　　　）
   A. 小檗胺　　　　　　　　　　　B. 粉防己碱　　　　　　　　C. 防己诺林碱
   D. 烟碱　　　　　　　　　　　　E. 槟榔碱

5. 以下生物碱的碱性由强到弱的顺序是（　　　）
   A. A>C>D>B　　　　　　　　　　B. A>C>B>D　　　　　　　　C. B>C>D>A
   D. C>A>B>D　　　　　　　　　　E. D>C>A>B

6. 不属于常用生物碱检识试剂的是（　　　）
   A. 碘化铋钾试剂　　　　　　　　B. 硅钨酸试剂　　　　　　　C. 硼酸
   D. 苦味酸试剂　　　　　　　　　E. 碘－碘化钾试剂

7. 生物碱沉淀反应的介质是（　　　）
   A. 酸水　　　　　　　　　　　　B. 高浓度乙醇　　　　　　　C. 碱水
   D. 碱性醇　　　　　　　　　　　E. 三氯甲烷

8. 下列生物碱中碱性最弱的是（　　　）
   A. 季铵碱　　　　　　　　　　　　　　　　B. 胍类生物碱
   C. 脂胺类生物碱　　　　　　　　　　　　　D. 苯胺类生物碱
   E. 酰胺类生物碱

9. 毒扁豆碱中三个氮原子（N1、N2、N3）的碱性大小顺序是（　　　）

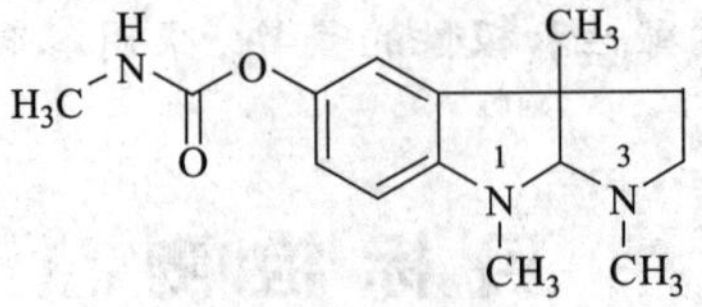

A. N1>N2>N3　　　　B. N1>N3>N2　　　　C. N3>N2>N1

D. N2>N1>N3　　　　E. N3>N1>N2

10. 下列生物碱具有挥发性的是（　　　）

    A. 小檗碱　　　　　　B. 咖啡因　　　　　　C. 黄连碱

    D. 甜菜碱　　　　　　E. 麻黄碱

11. 碱性不同生物碱混合物的分离可选用（　　　）

    A. 简单萃取法　　　　　　　　　　　B. 酸提取碱沉淀法

    C. pH 梯度萃取法　　　　　　　　　D. 有机溶剂回流法

    E. 分馏法

12. 溶解游离亲脂性生物碱的最好溶剂为（　　　）

    A. 水　　　　　　　　B. 甲醇　　　　　　C. 正丁醇

    D. 三氯甲烷　　　　　E. 苯

13. 从苦参总碱中分离苦参碱和氧化苦参碱是利用二者（　　　）

    A. 在水中溶解度不同　　　　　　　B. 在乙醇中溶解度不同

    C. 在三氯甲烷中溶解度不同　　　　D. 在苯中溶解度不同

    E. 在乙醚中溶解度不同

14. 若将中药中所含生物碱盐和游离生物碱都提取出来，应选用的溶剂是（　　　）

    A. 水　　　　　　　　B. 乙醇　　　　　　C. 三氯甲烷

    D. 石油醚　　　　　　E. 乙醚

15. 在除去脂溶性生物碱的碱水中，提取水溶性生物碱宜用（　　　）

    A. 酸化后乙醇提取　　　　　　　　B. 乙醇直接从碱水提取

    C. 丙酮直接从碱水提取　　　　　　D. 正丁醇直接从碱水提取

    E. 酸化后乙醇提取

二、多选题

1. 以下说法不正确的有（　　　）

    A. 吗啡和防己诺林碱均含有酚羟基

    B. 麻黄碱和伪麻黄碱互为立体异构体

    C. 苦参碱为喹诺里西啶类

    D. 黄连碱和延胡索乙素均为叔胺碱

    E. 苦参碱和氧化苦参碱均能溶于乙醚

2. 以下对小檗碱正确的描述有（　　　）

    A. 游离小檗碱易溶于热水或热乙醇

    B. 具有抗菌抗病毒作用

    C. 属于季铵型生物碱

    D. 其含氧酸盐在水中的溶解度小于卤代酸盐

E. 与大分子有机酸在水中加热会结合成难溶于水的大分子复合物

3. 对生物碱的分布描述正确的是（　　　）

 A. 主要分布于植物界，绝大多数存在于高等植物的双子叶植物中

 B. 裸子植物中不存在生物碱

 C. 多集中在植物的某一器官

 D. 多种生物碱共存

 E. 在植物不同器官中含量差别不大

4. 影响生物碱碱性的因素主要有（　　　）

 A. 氮原子的杂化方式   B. 分子内氢键   C. 空间效应

 D. 分子量大小   E. 诱导效应

5. 以下关于生物碱盐特殊溶解性的正确描述为（　　　）

 A. 麻黄碱草酸盐难溶于水

 B. 奎宁盐酸盐难溶于三氯甲烷

 C. 伪麻黄碱盐酸盐可溶于三氯甲烷

 D. 罂粟碱盐酸盐难溶于三氯甲烷

 E. 小檗碱盐酸盐难溶于水

6. 下列关于生物碱盐溶解性的正确描述为（　　　）

 A. 碱性极弱的生物碱易与酸成盐   B. 能溶于醇类有机溶剂

 C. 不溶或难溶于亲脂性有机溶剂   D. 一般易溶于水

 E. 一般生物碱无机酸盐的水溶性大于有机酸盐

7. 以下生物碱呈液态的是（　　　）

 A. 烟碱   B. 小檗碱   C. 槟榔碱

 D. 毒芹碱   E. 苦参碱

8. 对生物碱沉淀反应的正确描述为（　　　）

 A. 一般在酸水溶液中进行

 B. 可用于生物碱的分离纯化

 C. 有些沉淀反应可作为生物碱纸色谱或薄层色谱的显色剂

 D. 与一种生物碱沉淀试剂发生沉淀反应，即可判断有生物碱的存在

 E. 为了排除假阳性结果，中药的酸水提取液有必要进行酸碱处理

9. 常用的生物碱检识试剂有（　　　）

 A. 碘化铋钾试剂   B. 硼酸   C. 硅钨酸试剂

 D. 茚三酮试剂   E. 碘－碘化钾试剂

10. 采用硅胶薄层色谱分离生物碱时，可以采用的处理方法是（　　　）

 A. 展开剂中加入少量氨水   B. 以 $CHCl_3$ 为展开剂

 C. 展开剂中加入少量二乙胺   D. 制成碱性硅胶薄层板

 E. 展开前用氨蒸气饱和薄层板

11. 提取生物碱常用的方法有（　　　）

 A. 醇提取丙酮沉淀法   B. 酸水提取法

 C. 亲脂性有机溶剂提取法   D. 醇类溶剂提取法

 E. 碱提取酸沉淀法

12. 亲水性生物碱通常指（　　　）

 A. 两性生物碱   B. 游离生物碱

  C. 季铵生物碱
             D. 具有 N→O 配位键的生物碱

  E. 仲胺生物碱

13. 用亲脂性有机溶剂提取总生物碱时，一般（   ）

  A. 先用酸水湿润药材
          B. 先用碱水湿润药材

  C. 先用石油醚脱脂
          D. 用三氯甲烷等溶剂提取

  E. 用正丁醇、乙醇等溶剂提取

14. 以下对洋金花中生物碱描述正确的是（   ）

  A. 所含生物碱为莨菪烷衍生物

  B. 阿托品无旋光性，其他生物碱均具有左旋旋光性

  C. 莨菪碱亲脂性较强，东莨菪碱有较强的亲水性

  D. 山莨菪碱的碱性介于莨菪碱和东莨菪碱之间

  E. 莨菪烷类生物碱不易水解

15. 下列关于中药麻黄描述正确的是（   ）

  A. 具有发汗散寒、宣肺平喘、利水消肿等功效

  B. 麻黄中的主要生物碱为麻黄碱

  C. 麻黄碱和伪麻黄碱属仲胺衍生物

  D. 伪麻黄碱在水中的溶解度较麻黄碱大

  E. 麻黄碱和伪麻黄碱能与生物碱沉淀试剂发生沉淀反应

三、思考题

1. 什么是生物碱？指出小檗碱、莨菪碱、苦参碱、樟柳碱、麻黄碱、延胡索乙素、汉防己碱、轮环藤酚碱二级分类及存在的中药。

2. 简述生物碱的溶解性特点。

3. 影响生物碱碱性大小的因素有哪些？

4. 请举出 3 个常用的生物碱沉淀试剂，在沉淀反应中如何避免假阳性的产生？

5. 某中药含有季铵碱、叔胺碱、酚性叔胺碱，以及水溶性和脂溶性杂质，试设计提取分离三种生物碱的试验流程。

（吴　霞　张　薇）

Chapter 9　Steroids

PPT

 学习目标

知识要求:

1. **掌握**　强心苷的分类、主要理化性质及检识反应,强心苷类化合物的苷键裂解反应条件。

2. **熟悉**　甾类化合物的结构分类及颜色反应,强心苷的结构与活性的关系。

3. **了解**　胆汁酸、植物甾醇及 C_{21}- 甾苷的结构特征。

能力要求:

学会应用 Liebermann–Burchard 反应,Legal 反应,Keller–Kiliani 反应等检识强心苷类化合物;学会应用苷键裂解的原理,结合具体化合物的结构特征选择适合的苷键裂解方法,解决强心苷类化合物在提取分离过程中存在的技术问题。

1　Introduction

Steroids (甾体) are compounds that contain a cyclopentanoperhydrophenanthrene (环戊烷骈多氢菲) nucleus. They are widely distributed in nature. With cholesterol (胆甾醇) as the fundamental structure, steroids are further modified, especially to the side chain on C_{17} to create a wide range of natural products bearing bioactivities, e.g. cardiac glycosides (强心苷), bile acids (胆汁酸), C_{21}-steroids, Phytosterols (植物甾醇), and steroidal (甾体的) saponins. Cholesterol in all animal tissues is a constituent of cell membrane. Digoxin (地高辛), a cardiac glycoside from *Digitalis lanata* (毛花洋地黄), is used in congestive heart failure and atrial fibrillation. Chenodeoxycholic acid (鹅去氧胆酸) and ursodeoxycholic acid (熊去氧胆酸) are the main constituents of Bovis calculus belonging to the bile acids and are used to dissolve cholesterol gallstones as an alternative to surgery. Sterioid saponins are glycosides formed by the steroidal aglycone and sugar moiety. Due to the similar physicochemical properties, this type of steroid is included in the following chapter Saponins.

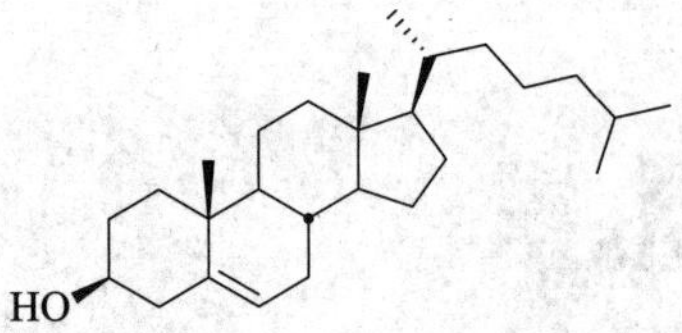

cholesterol
(sterols) (固醇)

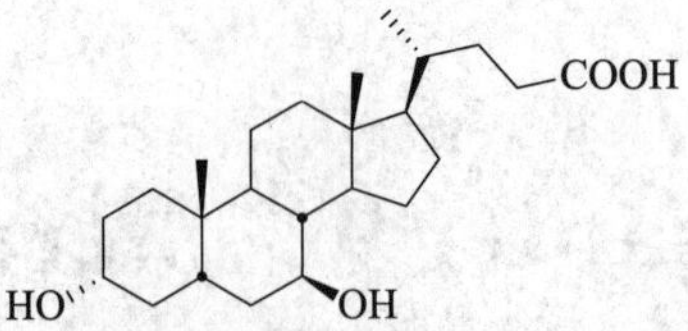

chenodeoxycholic acid
(bile acids)

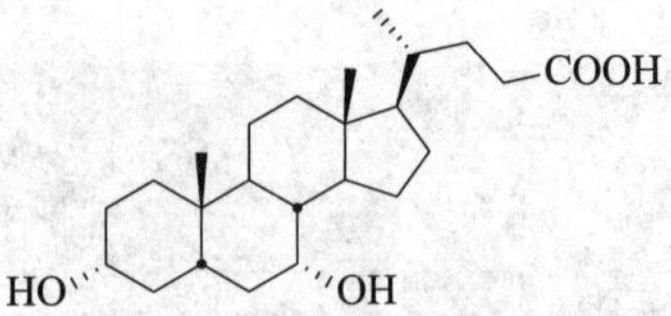

ursodeoxycholic acid
(bile acids)

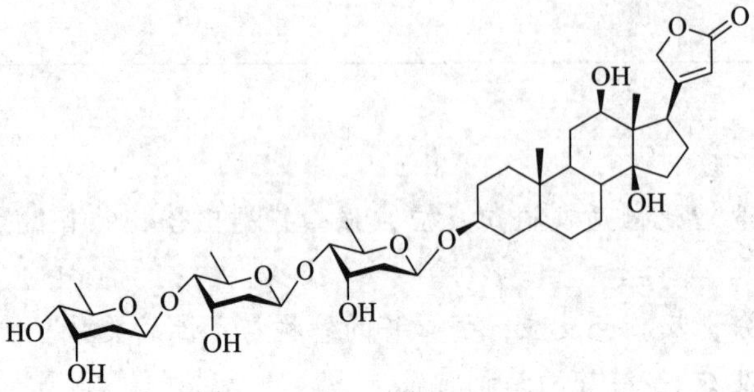

digoxin
(cardiac glycosides)

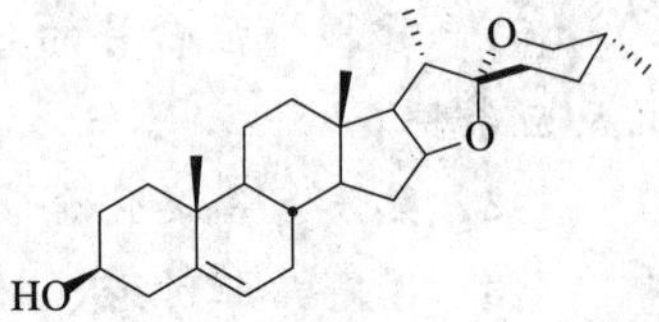

diosgenin (薯蓣皂苷元)
(aglycone of steroidal saponins)

Because of the profound biological activities encountered, many natural steroids together with a considerable number of synthetic and semi-synthetic steroidal compounds are routinely employed in medicine. The markedly different biological activities observed emanating from steroids are in part due to the functional groups attached to the steroid nucleus, and in part to the overall shape conferred on this nucleus by the stereochemistry of ring fusions.

1.1 Definition and Classification of Steroids

Steroids are compounds that contain a cyclopentanoperhydrophenanthrene nucleus. They are numbered and their rings are lettered as indicated in the structure of cholesterol. If one or more of carbon atoms in the structure is not present, the numbering of the remainder is undisturbed.

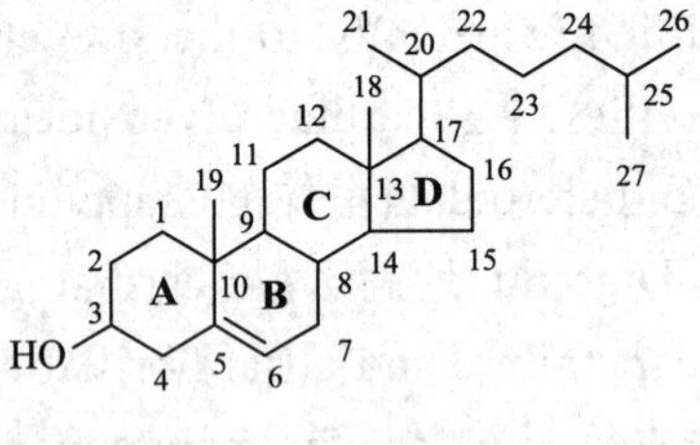

In natural steroids, the A/B ring fusion is *trans* or *cis*, or has unsaturation, either Δ^4 or Δ^5. All natural steroids have a *trans* B/C fusion. The C/D fusion is also usually *trans*, though there are notable exceptions such as the active cardiac glycosides. The stereochemistry of substituents is represented by α (on the lower face of the molecule) or β (on the upper face). Substituents on C_{10}, C_{13}, and C_{17} are usually β orientation. Ring fusions can be designated by using α or β for the appropriate bridgehead hydrogen. Steroids are classified into several groups based on the different ring fusions and side chains on C_{17} (Table 9-1).

Table 9-1   Classification of steroids

Category	Fusion of ring system			C_{17}-side chain
	A/B	**B/C**	**C/D**	
Phytosterols	*cis* or *trans*	*trans*	*trans*	hydrocarbon chain with 8–10 carbons
Bile acids	*cis*	*trans*	*trans*	pentanoic acid
C_{21}-steroids	*trans*	*trans*	*cis*	hydrocarbon chain with 2 carbons (e.g. acetyl)
Cardiac glycosides	*cis* or *trans*	*trans*	*cis*	unsaturated γ- or δ-lactone ring
Steroidal saponins	*cis* or *trans*	*trans*	*trans*	spitoketal

1.2   Color Reactions of Steroids

1.2.1   Mechanism

Steroids react with various strong acids of the Bronsted and Lewis type in anhydrous solutions to give colorful products. The mechanisms include dehydroxylation and dimerization, thereby forming a homologous series of carbonium ions.

1.2.2   Reagents

There are many color reactions for steroids, such as Lievermann-Burchard reaction, Salkowaski reaction, and Rosen-Heimer reaction. Rosen-Heimer reaction may be used to identify the nucleus of steroidal saponin and cardiac glycoside. The commonly used reagents in color reactions are listed in Table 9-2.

Table 9-2   Color reactions of steroids

Reaction	Reagent	Phenomenon
Salkowaski reaction	concentrated sulfuric acid and chloroform	The concentrated sulfuric acid layer shows red or cyan, and the chloroform layer shows green fluorescence
Liebermann-Burchard reaction (L-B for short)	concentrated sulfuric acid and acetic anhydride	The sample undergoes a series of color changes, from red, purple to blue, green, before finally fades
Rosen-Heimer reaction	trichloroacetic acid (heated to 60℃ for steroidal saponins, 100℃ for triterpenoid saponins, 90℃ for cardiac glycosides)	The sample turns purple or red

2   Cardiac Glycosides

2.1   Introduction

Steroids characterized by the highly specific and powerful action on cardiac muscles and presented as glycosides with sugars attached to the 3-position of the steroid nucleus, are named cardiac glycosides.

Many of the plants known to contain cardiac glycosides have long been used as arrow poisons [e.g. Strophanthus (羊角拗属)] or as cardiac stimulant [e.g. Digitalis (洋地黄属)], which are useful to strengthen a weakened heart and making it function more efficiently, thus are used in the treatment of congestive heart failure and cardiac arrhythmia. Because the therapeutic dose is so close to the toxic one, the dosage of them must be controlled very carefully.

In plants, cardiac glycosides are just found in angiosperms (被子植物) including monocotyledons (单子叶植物) and dicotyledons. The plant families of the Apocynaceae, Scrophulariaceae, Liliaceae, Asclepiadaceae (萝藦科), Cruciferae, Celastraceae (卫矛科), and Moraceae yield medicinal agents.

2.2 Structures and Classification

The therapeutic action of cardiac glycosides depends on the structure of the aglycone and on the type and number of sugar units attached.

2.2.1 Classification according to the Aglycone

Two types of aglycone are recognized, cardenolides (强心甾烯) [e.g. digitoxigenin (洋地黄毒苷元) from *Digitalis purpurea* (紫花洋地黄)] and bufadienolides (蟾蜍甾二烯) or scillanolide (海葱甾)[e.g. hellebrigenin (嚏根草苷元) from *Helleborus niger* (嚏根草)].

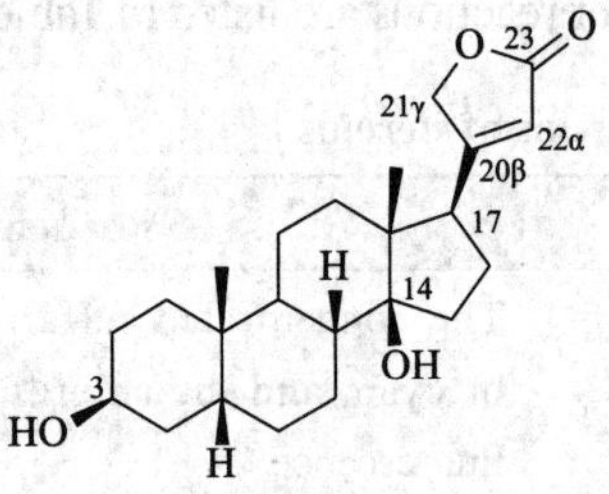

digitoxigenin
(cardenolide)

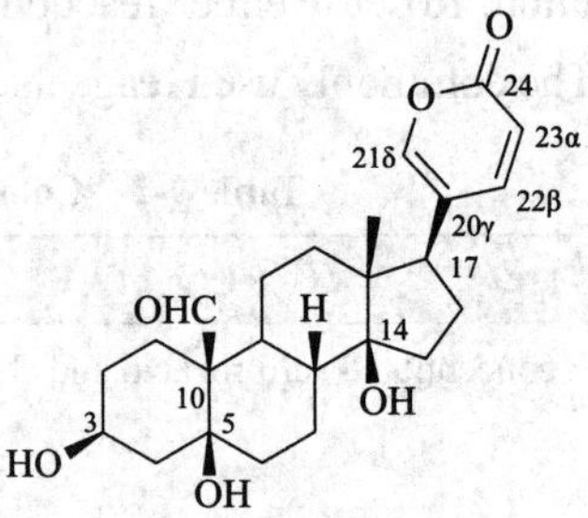

hellebrigenin
(bufadienolide/scillanolide)

(1) Cardenolides

The aglycone of cardiac glycosides bearing $\Delta^{\alpha\beta}$-γ lactone (five numbered ring) at C_{17} is classified as cardenolides. For example, purpureaglycoside (紫花洋地黄苷) A and B are from the dried leaf of the red foxglove *Digitalis purpurea* (Scrophulariaceae). Digoxin (as shown in the *introduction* part of this chapter) is the most widely used one of the cardiac glycosides prepared from *Digitalis lanata*.

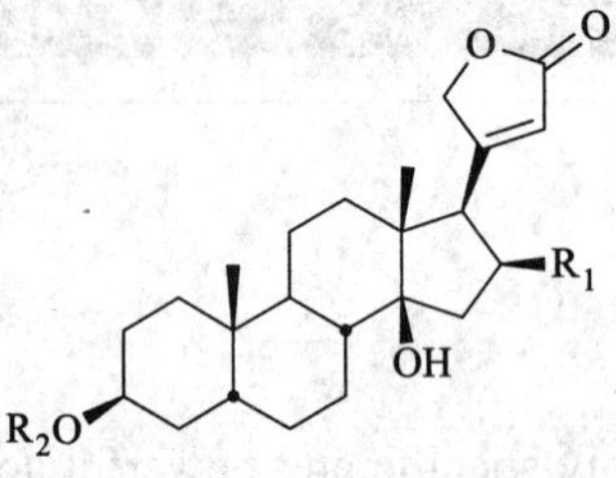

	R$_1$	R$_2$
digitoxigenin	H	H
gitoxigenin (羟基洋地黄毒苷元)	—OH	H
gitaloxigenin (吉他洛苷元)	—OCOH	H
digitoxin	H	
gitoxin (羟基洋地黄毒苷)	—OH	
gitaloxin	—OCOH	
purpureaglycoside A	H	
purpureaglycoside B	—OH	
purpureaglycoside C	—OCOH	

Ouabain (G-strophanthin) (乌本苷/G-毒毛花苷), the rhamnoside of ouabagenin (乌本苷元) from *Strophanthus gratus* (旋花羊角拗), is often employed as the biological standard in assays for cardiac activity, and is still official in many pharmacopoeias.

ouabain (G-strophanthin)

(2) Scillanolide or Bufanolide

The aglycone of cardiac glycosides bearing $\Delta^{\alpha\beta,\gamma\delta}$-δ lactone (six numbered ring) at C$_{17}$ is classified as scillanolide or bufanolide, which rarely exists in nature.

Squill (海葱) (white squill) contains scillanolides (up to 4%), principally scillaren A (海葱苷A) and pro-scillaridin A (原海葱苷A). Squill is not usually used for cardiac properties. Instead, the plant is employed for its expectorant action, while large doses cause vomiting and a digitalis-like action on the heart.

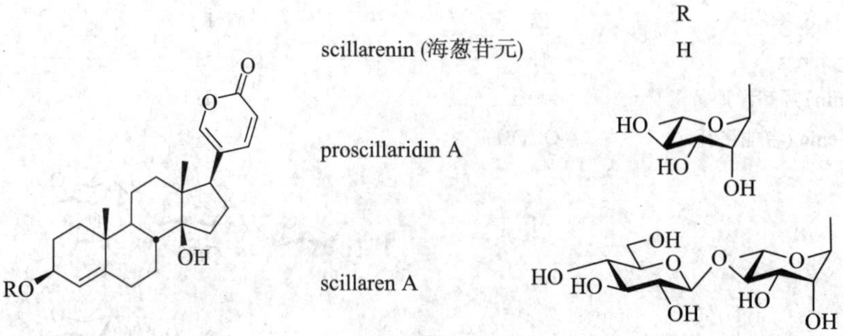

scillarenin (海葱苷元)

proscillaridin A

scillaren A

2.2.2 Classification according to the Sugar Moiety

About 20 different monosacchrides have been characterized from cardiac glycosides, and besides *D*-glucose, they are 6-deoxy- (e.g. L-fucose) or 2, 6-dideoxy- [e.g. D-digitoxose (洋地黄毒糖)] hexoses, some of which are 3-methyl ethers [e.g. D-digitalose (洋地黄糖) and D-cymarose (加拿大麻糖)].

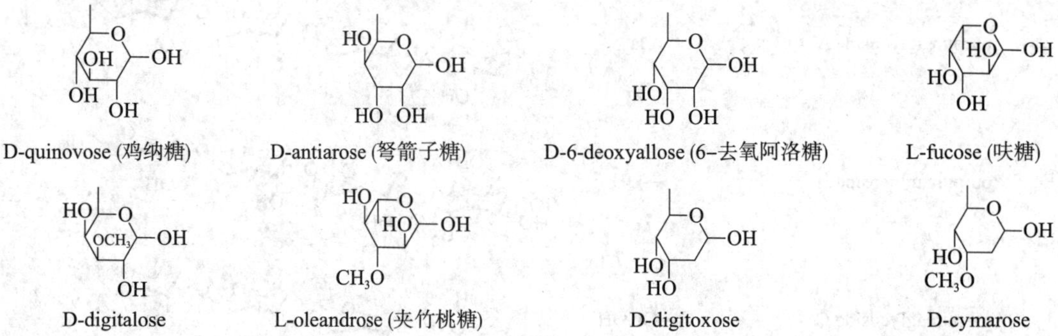

D-quinovose (鸡纳糖)   D-antiarose (弩箭子糖)   D-6-deoxyallose (6–去氧阿洛糖)   L-fucose (呋糖)

D-digitalose   L-oleandrose (夹竹桃糖)   D-digitoxose   D-cymarose

The sugar moiety of cardiac glycosides is usually oligosaccharide, while monosaccharide and disaccharide are uncommon. Thus cardiac glycosides can also be classified into three types according to the linkages of aglycone and the sugar moiety. Among these three types, type I and II are most abundant in plant.

Type I: Aglycone-(2, 6-dideoxy sugar)$_x$-(D-glucose)$_y$, e.g. purpureaglycoside A.

Type II: Aglycone-(6-deoxy sugar)$_x$-(D-glucose)$_y$, e.g. scillaren A.

Type III: Aglycone-(D-glucose)$_y$, e.g. scilliroside (红海葱苷).

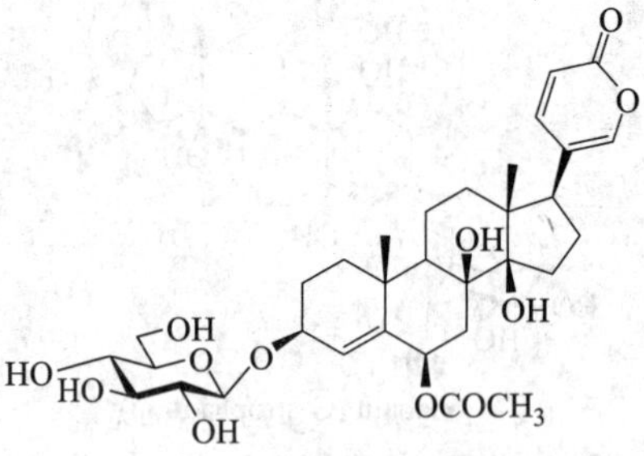

scilliroside

2.3 Relationship between Structures of Cardiac Glycosides and Their Cardiac Activities

The activity of cardiac glycosides is mainly related to the stereochemistry and substituents of the aglycones, but their toxicity is affected by the number and kind of sugars.

The fusion of A and B rings of the steroidal nucleus is either *cis* or *trans*, but the fusion of C and D rings must be *cis* to show the cardiotonic action (强心作用). The steroidal nucleus with C/D *trans*-configuration, or dehydrate aglycone do not show the cardiotonic action.

The *β*-oriented unsaturated lactone ring at C_{17} is the necessary active group. If the orientation of the lactone ring isomerizes to *α*-orientation or the lactone ring opens, the cardiotonic action is weak or lost. If the lactone ring is saturate, the cardiotonic action and the toxicity of the cardiac glycosides will decrease, which is safer and of practical value.

The *β*-oriented hydroxyl group at C_{14} (14*β*-OH) is the necessary active group. In cardenolides, when the fusion of A/B is *cis*, the 3*β*-OH is the necessary active group. But when the fusion of A/B is *trans*, the orientation of 3-OH will not affect the action. The cardiotonic action and the toxicity of the cardiac glycosides increase after the oxidization of methyl group to hydroxymethyl (羟甲基) or aldehyde group. The substituents on other positions affect the cardiotonic action of cardiac glycosides case by case.

The sugar moiety in cardiac glycosides does not have cardiotonic action, but affect their action and toxicity. For example, the glycosidation of digitoxigenin with glucose decreases the action as well as the toxicity, the longer the sugar moiety, the weaker the action. But the glycosidation of digitoxigenin with digitoxose increase the toxicity, the longer the sugar moiety, the more toxic the glycoside shows, while the glycosidation of digitoxigenin with digitoxose almost does not affect their action. The type and number of sugar affect the action and toxicity of cardiac glycoside might due to their different O/ W partition coefficient (油水分配系数). Generally, the cardiac glycosides formed by 2, 6-dideoxy sugars show stronger affinity to cardiac muscle and central nervous system than those formed by glucose. There are correlations between the cardiotonic action, toxicity, and hydrophobicity of the cardiac glycosides formed by 2, 6-dideoxy sugars. Though the cardiotonic action of the cardiac glycosides formed glucose is weaker than those contain 2, 6-dideoxy sugars, the lower toxicity guarantees the safer medicine to be developed.

2.4 Physical and Chemical Properties

2.4.1 Physical Properties

Cardiac glycosides are mostly colorless crystal or amorphous powder with optical activity. The glycosides with C_{17} *β*-orientation are bitter, while those with C_{17} *α*-orientation are not.

Cardiac glycosides are soluble in polar solvents such as water, alcohol and acetone, slightly soluble in ethyl acetate, and alcoholized chloroform, while insoluble in non-polar solvents such as ethyl ether, benzene, and petroleum ether. Meanwhile the solubility is affected by the number and type of the monosaccharides as well as the number and position of polar substituents, e. g. hydroxyl group.

2.4.2 Chemical Properties

(1) Properties of the Lactonic Ring

The lactonic ring of a cardiac glycoside encounters ring opening under the aqueous solution of KOH or NaOH and cyclizing after acidification, while in the alcoholic solvent of caustic (苛性碱), the lactonic ring isomerizes and yields a ring-opening product. The double bond in the $\Delta^{\alpha\beta}$-*γ* lactone of cardenolide delocalizes to form an active methylene at C_{22} in alcoholic alkali solvent. And the hydroxyl group at C_{14} encounters electrophilic addition on C_{20} to form the isomer (Figure 9-1).

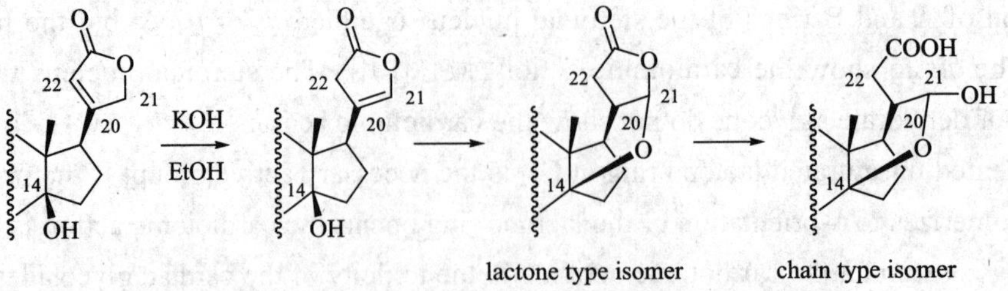

Figure 9-1　Isomerization of $\Delta^{\alpha\beta}$-γ lactone of cardenolide

The $\Delta^{\alpha\beta,\gamma\delta}$-$\delta$ lactone ring of scillanolide or bufanolide opens and encounters esterification in the alcoholic solvent of caustic, then dehydrolyzes when there is a hydroxyl group at C_{14} to form isomer (Figure 9-2).

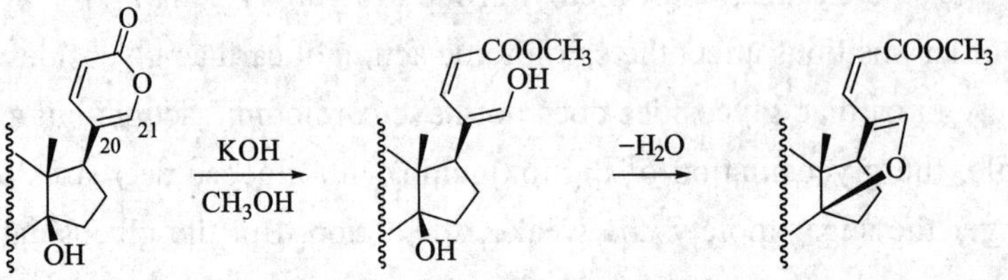

Figure 9-2　Isomerization of $\Delta^{\alpha\beta,\gamma\delta}$-$\delta$ lactone of scillanolide

(2) Hydrolysis of Cardiac Glycosides

The glycosidic linkage of a cardiac glycoside can be hydrolyzed under acidic and enzymatic conditions the same as other glycosides. Besides, its lactone ring can be hydrolyzed under alkali condition.

① Moderate Acid Hydrolysis

The glycosidic linkage formed by 2-deoxy sugar can be hydrolyzed under moderate condition. That is refluxing in 0.02–0.05mol/L HCl or H_2SO_4 for a few hours. Glycosidic linkage formed by 2-hydroxy sugar cannot be hydrolyzed under this condition. Therefore, this method can only be used for the hydrolysis of type I cardiac glycosides. For example, purpureaglycoside A yields digitoxigenin, D-digitoxose and digilanidobiose (洋地黄双糖). Digilanidobiose is a disaccharide formed by D-glucose linked at C_4 of D-digitoxose (Figure 9-3).

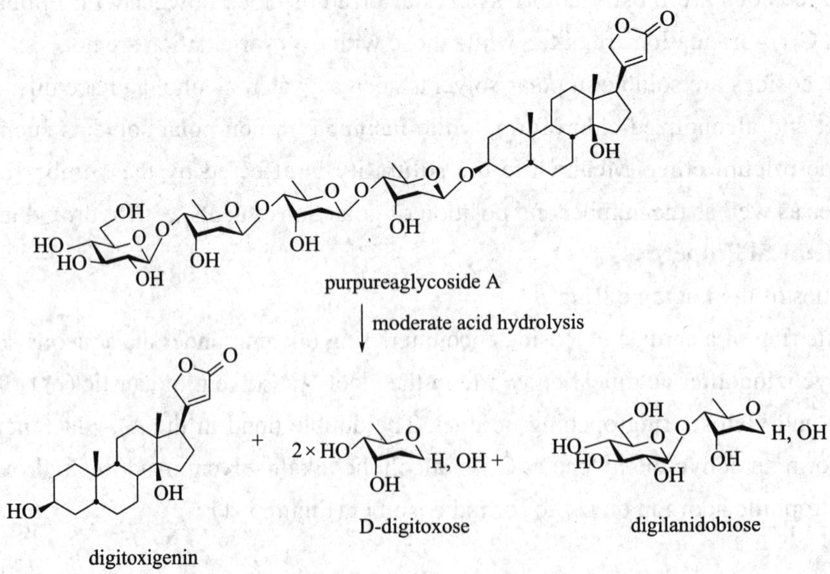

purpureaglycoside A

moderate acid hydrolysis

digitoxigenin + 2×D-digitoxose + digilanidobiose

Figure 9-3　Moderate acid hydrolysis of purpureaglycoside A

② Strong Acid Hydrolysis

The glycosidic linkage formed by 2-hydroxy sugar in cardiac glycosides can be hydrolized under strong acidic condition, i.e. 1–1.3mol/L HCl or H_2SO_4 together with heating or under pressure. However, aglycones with hydroxyl groups may dehydrate under strong acid condition and yield dehydrated aglycones. For example, gitoxin yields dehydrated aglycone under strong acid condition (Figure 9-4).

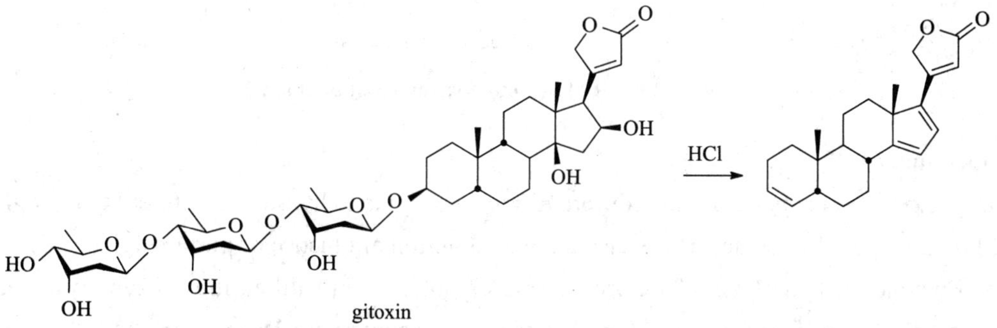

gitoxin

Figure 9-4 Strong acid hydrolysis of gitoxin

③ HCl-Acetone Hydrolysis (Mannich hydrolysis)

The cardiac glycoside reacts with acetone in the existence of hydrogen chloride under room temperature for two weeks. The 2- and 3-OH of the sugar moiety form acetonide under this condition, then the glycoside can be hydrolyzed into aglycone and sugar derivatives (Figure 9-5).

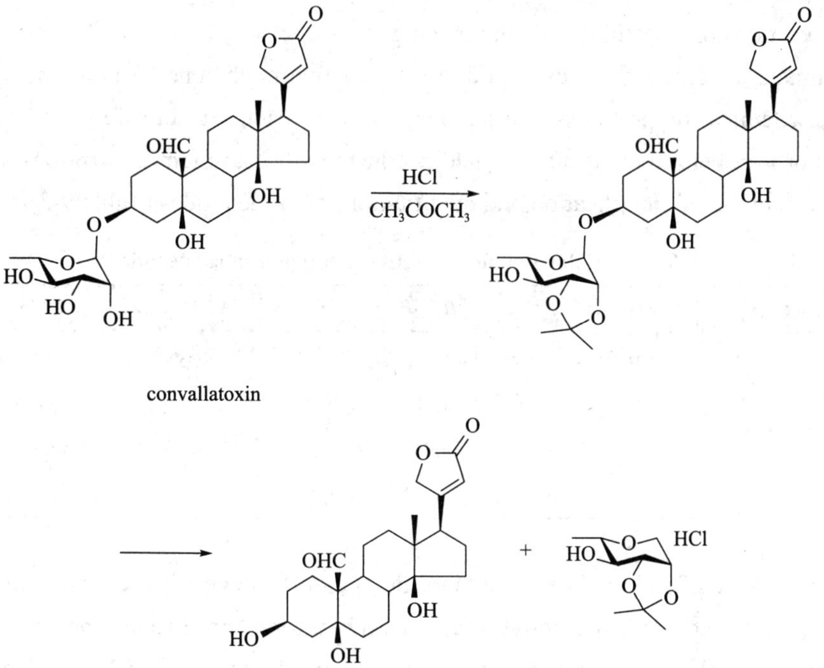

convallatoxin

strophanthidin

chloro-L-rhamnose acetonide

Figure 9-5 HCl-acetone hydrolysis of convallatoxin

This method is suitable for most cardiac glycosides with 2-hydroxyl sugar as the inner sugar moiety, but it is unsuitable for polyglycosides because they are insoluble in acetone. And aglycone containing vicinal (相邻的) hydroxyl groups will also form acetonide derivative under this condition (Figure 9-6).

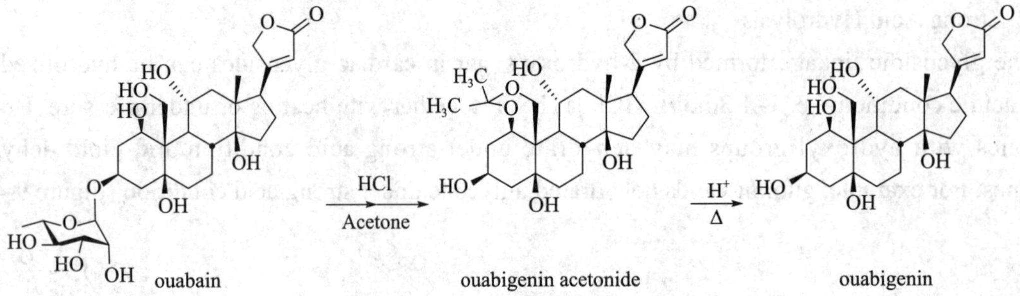

Figure 9-6   HCl-acetone hydrolysis of ouabain

④ Enzymolysis

The specificity of enzymes destines different type of enzyme to hydrolyze different type of glycosidic linkage. For example, the β-glucosidase can remove the terminal glucose of purpureaglycoside A to form digitoxin. Enzyme for hydrolyzing 2-deoxy sugar does not exist in natural, thus enzymolysis just yields secondary cardiac glycosides for those of cardiac glycosides containing 2-deoxy sugar.

(3) Color Reactions

Since the structures of cardiac glycosides contain the steroid skeleton, unsaturated lactone and 2-deoxy sugars, it can react with three types of reagents.

① Color Reactions of Steroid Skeleton

The color reactions of the steroid skeleton of cardiac glycosides are listed in Table 9-2. And the principle had explained before the Table.

② Color Reactions of Unsaturated Lactonic Ring

The unsaturated lactonic ring of cardenolide forms active methylene in alcoholic alkali solution as described in the chemical properties of the lactone, and can react with nitroferrocyanatum natrium (亚硝酰铁氰化钠) or nitrobenzene reagents to yield products with maximum absorptions at visible region. This provides the method of identification and quantitation for cardenolides (Table 9-3).

Table 9-3   Color reaction of active methylene in cardenolides

Name of the reaction	Reagent	Color	λ_{max} (nm)
Legal	Nitroferrocyanatum natrium [$Na_2Fe(NO)(CN)_5 \cdot 2H_2O$]	deep red	470
Kedde	3, 5-dinitrobenzoic acid	deep red	590
Raymond	1, 3-dinitrobenzene	mauve	620
Baljet	picric acid (2, 4, 6-trinitrophenol)	orange	490

The $\Delta^{\alpha\beta, \gamma\delta}$-δ-lactone of scillanolide or bufanolide cannot form active methylene in alcoholic alkali solvent. They cannot react with the above reagents. Therefore, these reactions are applied to differ cardenolide from scillanolide or bufanolide, exactly the $\Delta^{\alpha\beta}$-γ-lactone from the $\Delta^{\alpha\beta, \gamma\delta}$-δ-lactone.

③ Color Reactions of 2- Deoxy sugar

Cardiac glycosides containing 2-deoxy sugar may have color reactions with different reagents.

a. Keller-Kiliani Reaction (K-K reaction for short)   Dissolve the cardiac glycosides in glacial acetic acid (冰乙酸) containing Fe^{3+} [$FeCl_3$ or $Fe_2(SO_4)_3$], then add concentrated sulfuric acid along the test tube wall to let the sulfuric acid down to the bottom of the tube. Observe the color change of the acetic acid layer and the interface. The color change of the acetic acid layer is produced by 2-deoxy sugar. And the color change of the interface originates from the dehydration of aglycone by concentrated sulfuric acid. The color of the interface can be green, red, or yellow-brown based on the structure of the aglycone.

This reaction is used to identify cardiac glycosides which can be hydrolyzed under moderate acid condition to produce free 2-deoxy sugar. Purpureaglycoside A and digitoxin both contain three digitoxose moieties, but the color of the former is lighter than the latter, namely about two thirds of the latter. Purpureaglycoside A is hydrolyzed and produces two molecular of digitoxose and one molecular of digilanidobiose, and digilanidobiose is difficult to be hydrolyzed to yield digitoxose. Acetylated 2-deoxy sugar does not show color change in this reaction. So the negative results of this reaction do not indicate the absence of 2-deoxy sugar in the cardiac glycoside.

b. Ehrlich Reaction   The Ehrlich reagent is composed of *p*-dimethylaminobenzaldehyde and concentrated hydrochloric acid with the ratio of 4 : 1. Spray this reagent to the spot of cardiac glycoside on filter paper, then heat at 90 ℃ for 30 seconds. If the spot turns to red, then the existence of 2-deoxy sugar in the cardiac glycoside can be concluded.

c. Xanthydrol (呫吨氢醇) Reaction   The xanthydrol reagent is composed of glacial acetic acid solution of xanthydrol (0.1mg/ml) and concentrated sulfuric acid with the ratio of 100 : 1. This reagent reacts with 2-deoxy sugar in cardiac glycoside to turn red after heating in a water bath for 3 minutes.

d. Sodium periodate and *p*-nitroaniline reaction   This reagent is used as the TLC and PC chromogenic agent. The developed spots are firstly sprayed the aqueous solution of sodium periodate (composed of saturated water solution of sodium periodate and water with the ratio of 1 : 2). After standing for 10 minutes, *p*-nitroaniline reagent (composed of 1% *p*-nitroaniline dissolved in ethanol and concentrated hydrochloric acid with the ratio of 4 : 1) is sprayed on the spots. The deep yellow spots on the background of grayish yellow and a yellow fluorescent spot on the background of brown under UV light will indicate the existence of 2-deoxy sugar in the cardiac glycoside. The spots further turn to green after spraying 5% NaOH in methanol.

2.5   Extraction and Isolation

The cardiac glycosides from one plant always have similar structures and low abundance, and coexist with saponins, saccharides, pigments and tannins, which change the solubility of cardiac glycosides. Meanwhile, the secondary glycosides can be easily produced by enzymolysis during the storage and extraction process. Therefore, the extraction and isolation of cardiac glycosides are very difficult.

2.5.1   Extraction

Generally, cardiac glycosides are soluble in water or hydrophilic organic solvent. Methanol and 70%-80% ethanol are usually used to extract cardiac glycosides due to their high efficiency of extraction and inhibition of enzyme.

2.5.2   Isolation

Liquid-liquid partition is applied to defat. When the material is seed or contains fats or chlorophyll, petroleum ether is generally used to remove lipophilic components from the ethanol extract. Then it is extracted by mixed solvent of chloroform and methanol to produce cardiac glycoside, while the hydrophilic components are left in the water layer.

Liposoluble impurities such as chlorophyll can also be adsorbed by activated charcoal, while water-soluble impurities such as saccharides, pigments and saponins can be adsorbed by Al_2O_3. It is worth noticing that cardiac glycosides could also be adsorbed.

Adsorption chromatography is applied to isolate liposoluble monoglycoside, secondary glycoside and aglycone. The adsorbent usually used is silica gel, with eluents composed of *n*-hexane-ethyl acetate, chloroform-methanol, ethyl acetate-methanol eluting in gradient.

Partition chromatography is applied to isolate water-soluble cardiac glycosides. Silica gel, diatomite and cellulose are usually used as supported reagents, with eluents composed of ethyl acetate-methanol-water or chloroform-methanol-water eluting in gradient.

CCD and DCCC can also be used to isolate cardiac glycosides based on their different partition coefficients in immiscible solvents. For example, CCD is applied to isolate thevetin (黄花夹竹桃苷) A and B with chloroform-ethanol-water (10 : 5 : 3), the water layer is the stationary phase, while the chloroform layer is the mobile phase. Thevetin A is detected in the water layer, and thevetin B is detected in the chloroform layer after several times of partition.

thevetin A	—CHO
thevetin B	—CH₃

2.6　Identification of Cardiac Glycosides

2.6.1　Physicochemical Identification

The physicochemical identification of cardiac glycosides is based on the color reactions of steroid skeleton, unsaturated lactonic ring and 2-deoxy sugar, including L-B, Kedde, Legal, K-K, and Xanthydrol reactions etc.

The positive results of L-B and K-K reactions indicate the existence of cardiac glycosides. If positive result of Legal or Kedde reaction is also observed, the aglycone of the cardiac glycoside should be cardenolides, and the negetive result leads to scillanolide or bufanolide.

2.6.2　Chromatographic Identification

TLC is an important method for identification of cardiac glycosides. Silica gel TLC is usually used with solvents composed of chloroform-methanol-glacial acetic acid, ethyl acetate-methanol-water, dichloromethane-methanol-formamide, etc. RP-TLC is also used to identify cardiac glycosides, with methanol-water and chloroform-methanol-water as developing solvents.

The commonlly used spray reagents include: 2% 3, 5-dinitrobenzoic acid mixed with 2 M KOH (1 : 1); 1% picric acid mixed with 10% NaOH (95 : 5); 2% antimony trichloride in chloroform.

2.7　Spectroscopic Characters of Cardiac Glycosides

2.7.1　UV

The maximum absorption of cardenolides with $\Delta^{\alpha\beta}$-γ-lactone is at about 217nm (logε 4.34), and that of scillanolides or bufanolides with $\Delta^{\alpha\beta,\,\gamma\delta}$-$\delta$-lactone is at about 311nm (logε 3.13). The maximum absorption in UV spectrum is used to differentiate two types of aglycones of cardiac glycosides. Double bond conjugated with $\Delta^{\alpha\beta}$-γ lactone such as $\Delta^{16(17)}$ will shift the absorption to 270nm. Double bonds $\Delta^{8(9),\,14(15)}$ unconjugated with the lactone ring will shift the absorption to 244nm (logε 1.8). Ketone group at C_{11} or C_{12} shows weak $n \rightarrow \pi^*$ absorption at 290nm (logε 1.9).

2.7.2　IR

Unsaturated lactone ring in the aglycone of cardiac glycoside shows two absorptions in the region of 1800~1700cm^{-1}, one of which at the low wave number is ascribed to the absorption of the α, β-unsaturated carbonyl group, while the other of which at the high wave number is the frequency-doubled peak of $\delta_{\text{C-H}}$, and is enhanced by the Fermi Resonance (费米共振). The former is called normal absorption, and the latter is called abnormal absorption.

For cardenolides, the abnormal absorption changes with the solvent. Increase of the polarity of the solvent, the intensity of the abnormal absorption decreases, even disappears. But the intensity of the normal absorption does not change or even increases when the polarity of the solvent increases. For example, 3-acetyl digitoxigenin shows three absorptions in the region of 1800–1700cm^{-1} in CS_2 (1783, 1756, 1738cm^{-1}). Among them, absorption at 1738cm^{-1} is attributed to the acetyl group at C-3, and those at 1756 and 1783cm^{-1} are ascribed to the normal and abnormal absorptions of the lactone ring. The absorption at 1783cm^{-1} will change with different polarity of the solvent.

3-acetyl digitoxigenin　　　　　　**hellebrigenin**

For scillanolide or bufanolide, the two absorptions in the region of 1800–1700cm^{-1} are all smaller than that of cardenolides due to longer conjugated system. For example, hellebrigenin shows two absorptions in CHCl$_3$ at 1718 and 1740cm^{-1}. The absorption at 1718cm^{-1} is the normal absorption, and the absorption at 1740cm^{-1} is the abnormal absorption, which also decreases in polar solvent. The absorption of carbonyl group at C_{10} of hellebrigenin is also at 1718cm^{-1}, as overlapped with the normal absorption.

Therefore, IR spectrum may be used to differentiate cardenolide and bufanolide based on the absorptions and the decrease of intensity or disappearance of the abnormal absorption.

2.7.3　NMR

(1) ^{1}H-NMR

The ^{1}H-NMR is an important method in the structure identification of cardiac glycosides. The resonances of protons on the unsaturated lactonic ring are very useful for the identification of cardenolide and scillanolide or bufanolide. The protons at C_{21} of cardenolide are at δ 4.5–5.0 with peak shape of broad singlet (单峰). Sometimes, the protons couples to form an AB coupled system with peak shape of triplet (三重峰) or quartet (四重峰) (J=18Hz). The proton at C_{22} of cardenolide is a broad singlet at δ 5.6–6.0. The protons on the unsaturated lactonic ring of scillanolide or bufanolide are all alkene protons at δ 6.3–7.7. Protons at C_{22} and C_{23} split to doublet (J=10Hz) due to vicinal coupling. And the proton at C_{22} is further split to double doublet due to long-range coupling with proton at C_{21} with the coupling constant of 2Hz.

The methyl groups of C_{18} and C_{19} are singlets at about δ 1.0, the chemical shifts of which are related to the configuration of C_5 and C_{14} or the fusion of A/B and C/D ring to be exactly. If the C/D ring of cardiac glycosides is *cis* fused, the chemical shift of methyl group at C_{18} is at lower field than that of C_{19} and vice versa.

A/B *trans*, C/D *trans*
5α-H, 14α-H

A/B *trans*, C/D *cis*
5α-H, 14β-H

A/B *cis*, C/D *trans*
5β-H, 14α-H

A/B *cis*, C/D *cis*
5β-H, 14β-H

δ: chemical shift of methyl group

(2) ^{13}C-NMR

The chemical shifts of sp^3 carbons on the steriods nucleus are at δ 16–86 depending on the substituents on the carbon. When the carbon is substituted by hydroxyl group, the resonance of the carbon will shift to downfield. And the shift of the C_{18} methyl is always at higher field. The chemical shifts of sp^2 carbons on D ring of the steriods nucleus are at δ 108–161. The chemical shifts of the α, β-unsaturated lactonic carbonyl and β-carbon are at δ 171–177, which are always difficult to assign correctly. And the chemical shift of the α, β, γ, δ-unsaturated lactonic carbonyl is at δ161–162. The chemical shift of the ketonic (酮的) carbonyl is at δ 214.

The chemical shift of ^{13}C-NMR for some digitoxingen derivatives are listed as follows (Table 9-4).

Table 9-4　Chemical Shift of ^{13}C-NMR for Digitoxingen Derivatives [CDCl$_3$ -CD$_3$OD (3 : 2)]

Compound / Position	I	II	III	IV	V	VI	VII	VIII	IX	X
1	30.0	30.0	30.0	30.7	30.8	30.8	30.8	30.7	30.0	24.8
2	28.0	28.0	27.9	25.2	25.4	25.3	25.4	27.9	27.9	27.4[a]
3	66.8	66.8	66.8	71.1	71.4	71.3	71.3	66.7	66.6	67.2
4	33.5	33.5	33.4	30.7	30.8	30.8	30.8	33.5	33.3	38.1
5	35.9[a]	36.4	36.4	37.2	37.4	37.4	37.3	36.8[a]	36.4	75.3
6	27.1	27.0	26.9	26.6	26.8	26.8	26.6	26.6	26.9	27.0
7	21.6[b]	21.4[a]	21.2[a]	20.9[a]	21.6	20.6[a]	20.2[a]	24.0	21.9	18.1[b]
8	41.9	41.8	41.8	41.6	41.8	41.5	41.2	36.7[a]	41.3	42.2[c]

(continued)

Position\Compound	I	II	III	IV	V	VI	VII	VIII	IX	X
9	35.8 [a]	35.8	35.9	35.8	36.1	36.2	36.8	45.1	32.6	40.2 [c]
10	35.8	35.8	35.6	35.4	35.8	35.5	35.4	36.2	35.5	55.8
11	21.7 [b]	21.9 [a]	21.3 [a]	21.4 [a]	21.6	21.2 [a]	21.3 [a]	21.4	30.0	22.8 [b]
12	40.4	41.2	41.0	40.9	40.3	31.3	40.6	37.7	74.8	40.2
13	50.3	50.4	50.7	50.5	50.3	49.5	52.6	54.2	56.4	50.1
14	85.6	85.2	84.1	83.8	85.6	86.1	85.7	146.3 [c]	85.8	85.3
15	33.0	42.6	39.5	39.9	33.0	31.3	38.8	108.3 [d]	33.0	32.2
16	27.3	72.8	75.0	74.7	27.3	24.8	133.8	135.8 [d]	27.9	27.5 [a]
17	51.5	58.8	56.8	56.6	51.5	48.9	161.2	158.0 [c]	46.1	51.4
18	16.1	16.9	16.1	16.1	16.0	18.5	16.6	20.1	9.4	16.2
19	23.9	23.9	23.9	23.8	23.9	24.0	24.1	24.0	23.8	195.7
20	177.1 [c]	171.8 [b]	171.5 [b]	171.5 [b]	177.1 [b]	173.6 [b]	172.8 [b]	173.5 [b]	177.1 [a]	177.2 [d]
21	74.5	76.7	76.8	76.8	74.7	74.8	72.6	72.1	74.6	74.8
22	117.4	119.6	121.3	121.3	117.4	116.6	111.7	119.5	117.0	117.8
23	176.3 [c]	175.3 [b]	175.8 [b]	175.8 [b]	176.3 [b]	175.8 [b]	176.3 [b]	176.8 [b]	176.3 [a]	176.6 [d]

OCOCH₃, 21.3 ± 0.3; OCOCH₃, 171.4 ± 0.4

a~d values within column may be interchanged

I: digitoxigenin

II: gitoxigenin

III: 16-acetyl gitoxigenin

IV: 3, 16-diacetyl gitoxigenin

V: 3-acetyl digitoxigenin

VI: 3-acetyl 17β-H digitoxigenin

Ⅶ: 3-acetyl Δ^{16}-digitoxigenin

Ⅷ: Δ$^{14, 16}$-digitoxigenin

Ⅸ: digoxigenin (异羟基洋地黄毒苷元)

Ⅹ: strophanthidin (毒毛旋花子苷元)

The chemical shift of ^{13}C-NMR for some bufanolide derivatives are listed as follows (Table 9-5).

Table 9-5　Chemical shift of ^{13}C-NMR for bufanolide derivatives (CDCl$_3$)

Compound Position	I	II	III	IV	V	VI	VII	VIII	IX	X
1	24.9	29.7	29.7	31.9	31.6	29.6	29.5	29.5	23.0	20.0
2	27.3	27.8	27.9	28.5	28.3	27.7	27.5	27.9	25.4	25.8
3	66.5	66.8	66.5	64.8	64.6	66.7	64.5	64.3	64.4	63.5
4	36.6	33.2	33.2	33.7	33.5	33.4	33.0	33.6	38.0	31.8
5	73.5	35.5	35.4	37.3	37.4	35.6	35.4	36.0	28.3	28.4
6	34.9	25.7	25.7	26.9	26.5	26.5	26.0	26.8	31.0	27.0
7	23.3	20.7	20.6	21.2	21.3	21.2	20.5	20.7	19.9	19.9
8	40.2	32.4	38.8	41.0	38.9	42.0	41.3	39.2	33.6	32.9
9	38.1	39.3	37.4	40.3	39.4	35.0	34.6	45.3	38.3	36.5
10	40.3	35.9	35.5	36.2	36.7	35.2	34.8	37.0	44.7	50.6
11	21.5	21.1	20.9	66.9	73.3	21.3	20.8	213.9	20.7	20.6
12	40.0	39.4	40.4	50.3	213.4	40.7	40.2	82.0	27.3	38.7
13	47.9	45.2	45.2	48.3	62.1	47.8	48.7	53.9	44.4	44.5
14	83.4	74.4	76.9	82.8	84.1	85.2	82.6	82.1	74.2	71.6
15	31.9	59.8	59.8	32.1	31.8	32.4	39.1	33.3	59.3	59.4
16	28.4	29.5	74.6	28.2	27.6	28.5	73.5	27.2	26.8	74.4
17	49.9	47.7	49.8	49.8	40.0	50.9	55.8	45.0	46.2	48.9
18	16.8	16.8	17.2	17.7	17.3	16.7	16.8	18.2	16.5	16.7
19	16.6	23.7	23.6	23.9	23.4	23.7	23.7	24.1	64.2	207.1
20	122.7	122.2	116.1	122.3	120.8	122.7	117.3	119.8	122.0	116.0
21	149.2	149.5	151.2	149.3	150.2	148.4	151.4	150.8	150.5	152.2
22	147.3	146.9	148.3	147.2	147.1	146.9	150.1	148.1	147.4	148.5
23	114.2	115.3	113.2	114.1	114.6	115.1	111.6	113.2	114.0	112.9
24	161.3	162.0	161.4	161.3	161.1	162.4	161.2	161.2	160.9	160.8

OCOCH$_3$, 20.5 ± 0.3; OCOCH$_3$, 169.7 ± 0.4

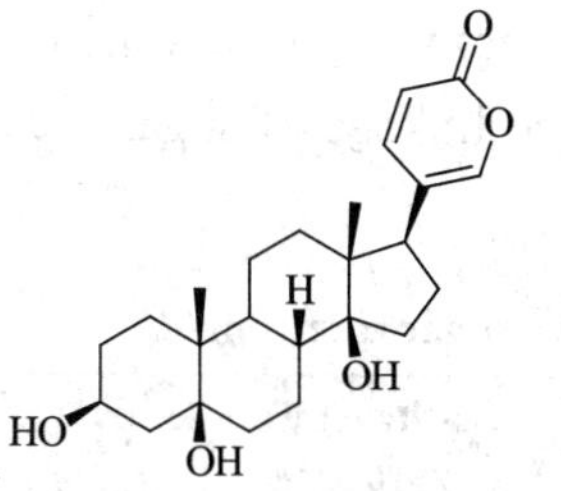

Ⅰ: telocinobufagin (远华蟾毒基)

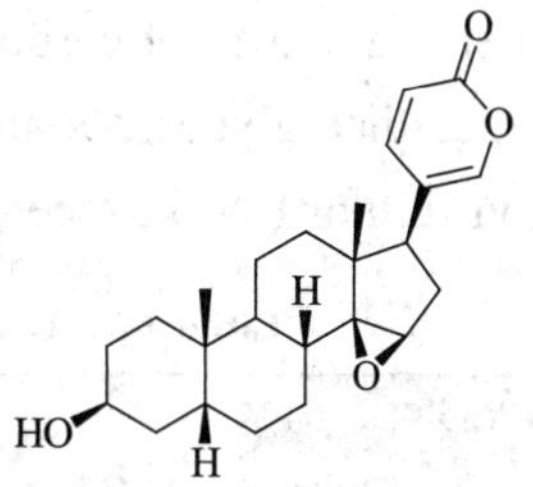

Ⅱ: resibufogenin (脂蟾毒配基)

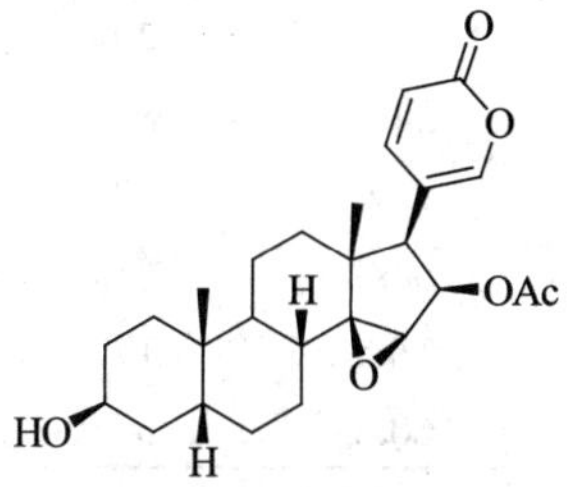

Ⅲ: cinobufagin (华蟾素)

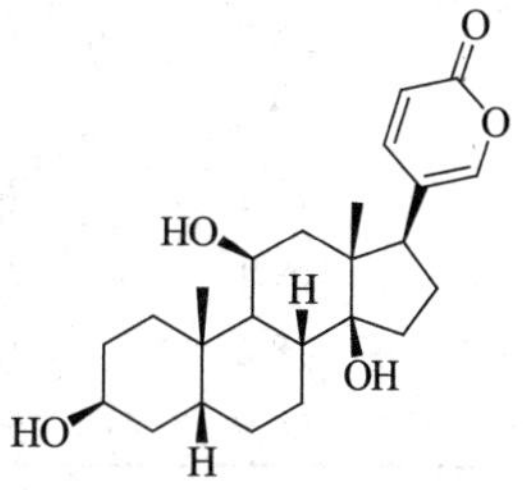

Ⅳ: gamabufotalin (蟾毒它灵)

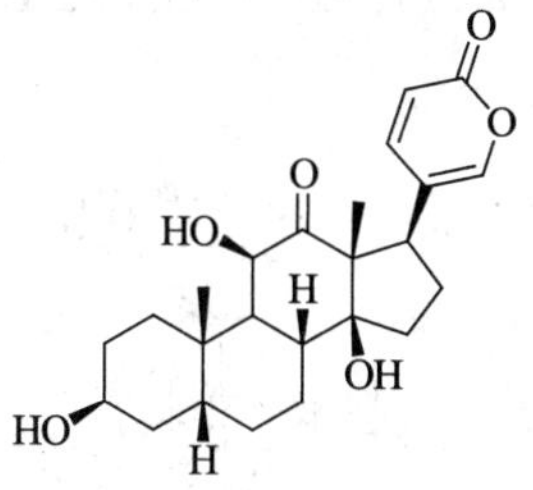

Ⅴ: arenobufagin (沙蟾毒精)

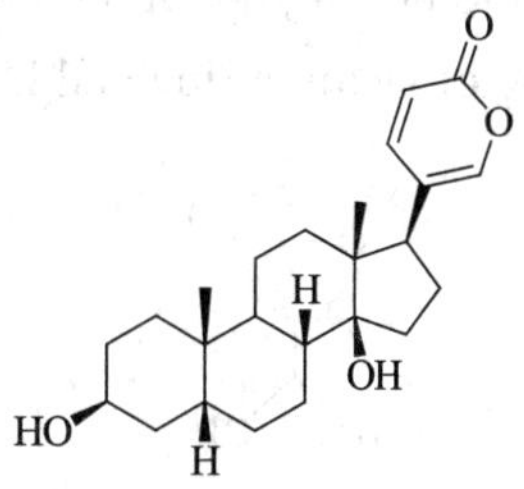

Ⅵ: bufalin (蟾蜍灵)

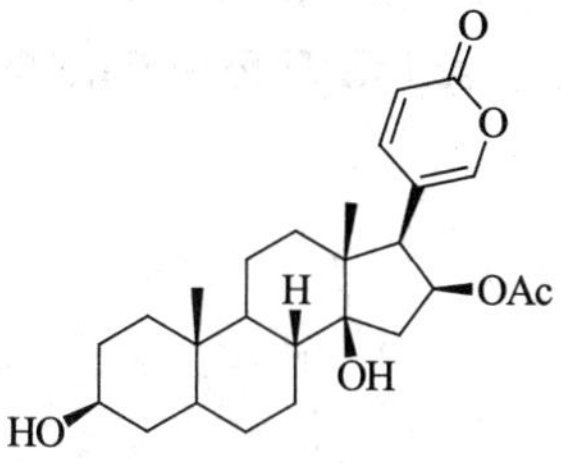

Ⅶ: bufotalin (蟾毒它灵)

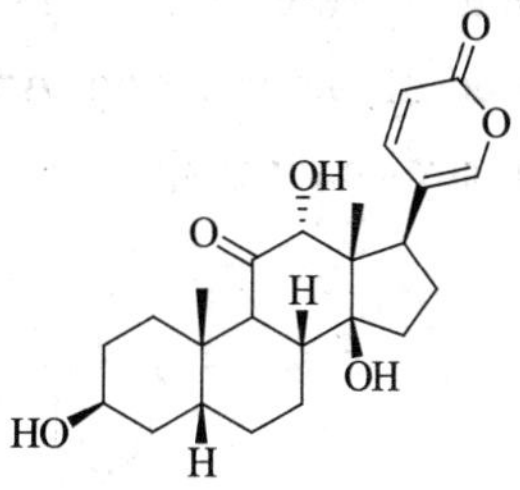

Ⅷ: pseudobufarenogin

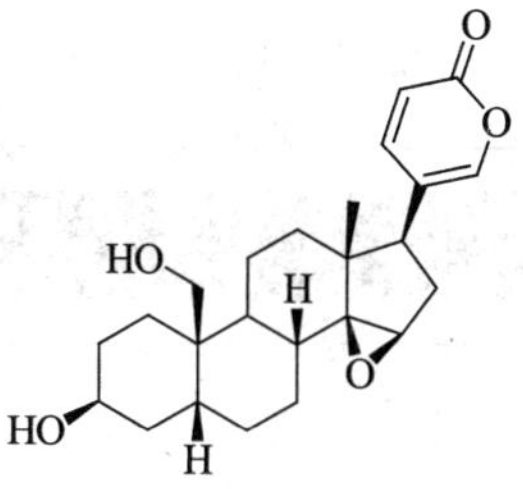

Ⅸ: resibufogenol

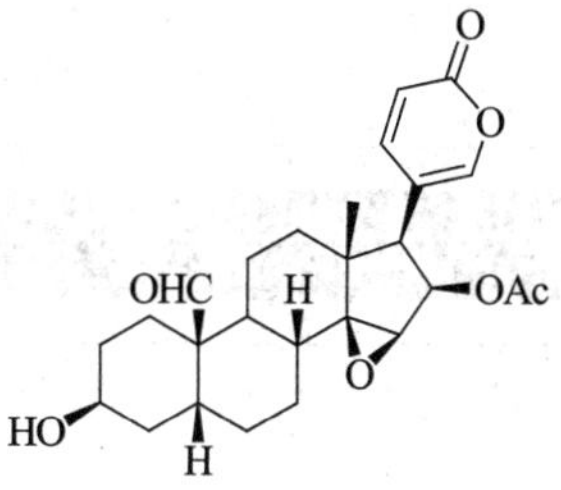

Ⅹ: 19-oxo-cinobufagin

The chemical shifts of carbons on 2, 6-dideoxy sugar, 6-deoxy sugar and methyl ethers usually occurring in cardiac glycosides are listed below (Table 9-6). The linkage of sugar moiety is settled by glycosidation shift or HMBC (see chapter 3).

Table 9-6　Chemical shift of ^{13}C-NMR for deoxy sugar (pyridine-d_5)

Compound \ Position	L-oleandrose	D-cymarose	D-diginose (地芰糖)	D-sarmentose (沙门糖)	L-thevetose (黄花夹竹桃糖)	D-digitalose	D-6-deoxy-3-methyl allose
1	95.9	97.6	98.2	97.3	98.9	103.6	104.3
2	35.8	36.4	33.1	33.6	73.8	70.9	71.6
3	79.3	78.8	79.1	80.3	84.8	85.1	85.2
4	77.1	74.0	67.0	67.9	76.6	68.7	74.6
5	69.1	71.1	71.2	69.9	68.9	71.0	68.5
6	18.6	18.9	17.6	17.5	18.5	17.4	18.4
—OCH$_3$	56.9	58.1	55.1	56.7	60.6	57.2	60.7

2.7.4　MS

The lactonic ring of cardenolides produces fragments with *m/z* 111, 124, 163, and 164 generated by lactonic ring or lactonic ring and D ring.

m/z 111　　　*m/z* 124　　　*m/z* 163　　　*m/z* 164

The lactonic ring of scillanolides or bufanolides produces fragments with *m/z* 109, 123, 135, and 136 composed of lactonic ring. And these characteristic peaks are used to differentiate the two types of aglycone of cardiac glycoside.

m/z 109　　　*m/z* 123　　　*m/z* 135　　　*m/z* 136

3　Bile Acids

3.1　Introduction

The bile acids are C_{24} steroidal acids that occur in salt form in bile, secreted into the gut to emulsify fats and encourage digestion. They act as surface active agents by virtue of their relatively hydrophobic steroid nucleus and the hydrophilic side-chain. The side chain is a valeric acid group, which is typically bound to glycine or taurine via an amide linkage.

Bile acids increase the output of bile and therefore are called choleretic. Dehydrocholic acid is especially active in this respect and increases the volume and water content of bile acid with little change in the content of bile acids. It is used to improve biliary drainage after surgery. It is administered orally. Sodium dehydrocholate is given by slow intravenous injection.

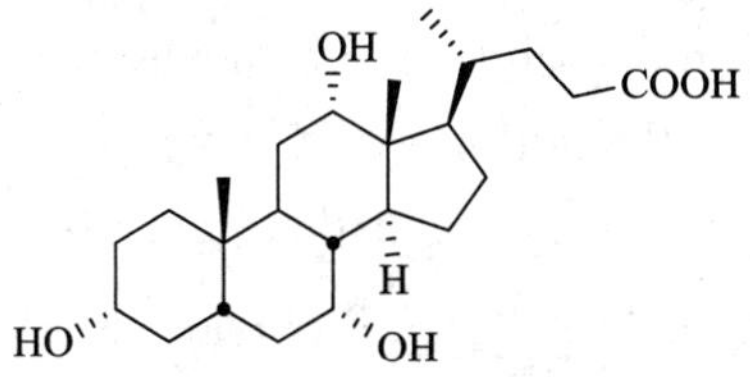

cholic acid (胆酸)

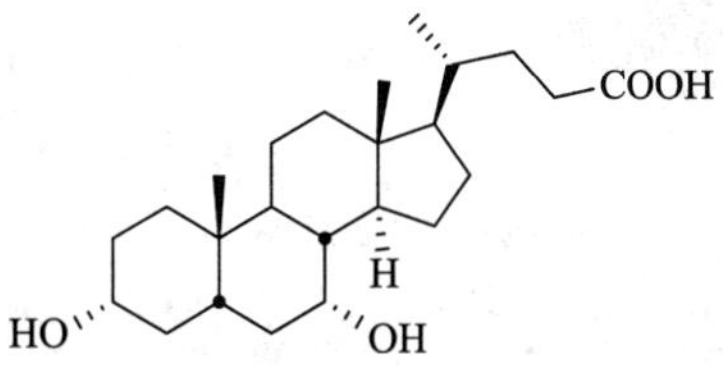

chenodeoxycholic acid

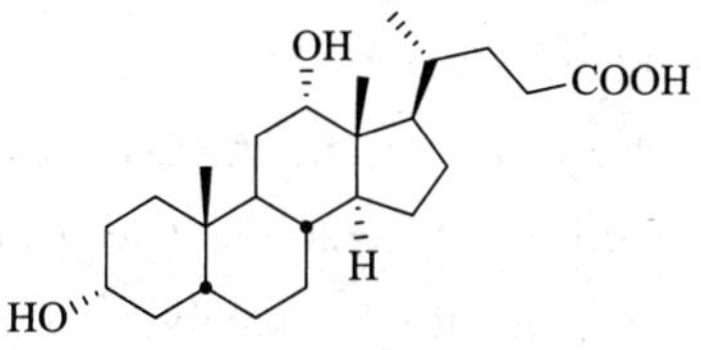

deoxycholic acid (去氧胆酸)

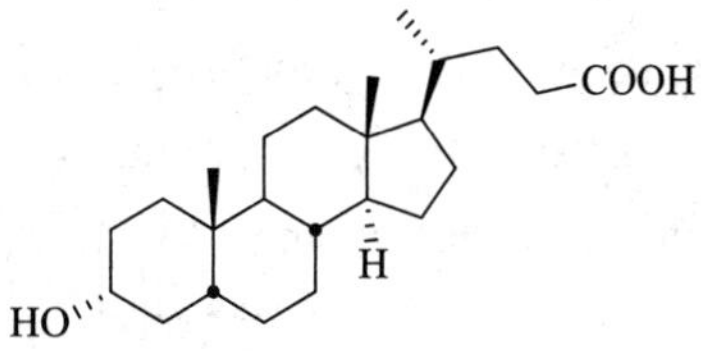

lithocholic acid (石胆酸)

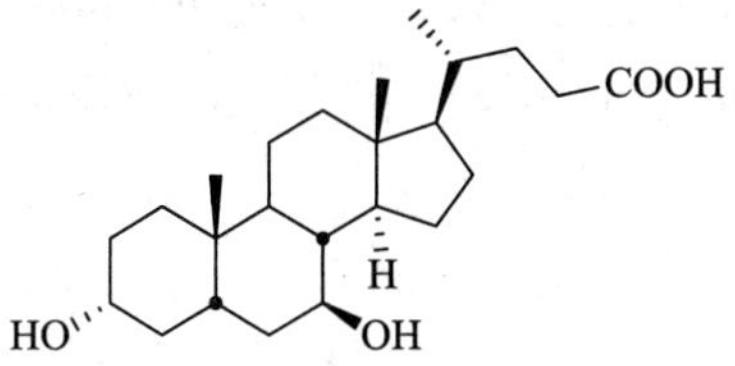

ursodeoxycholic acid

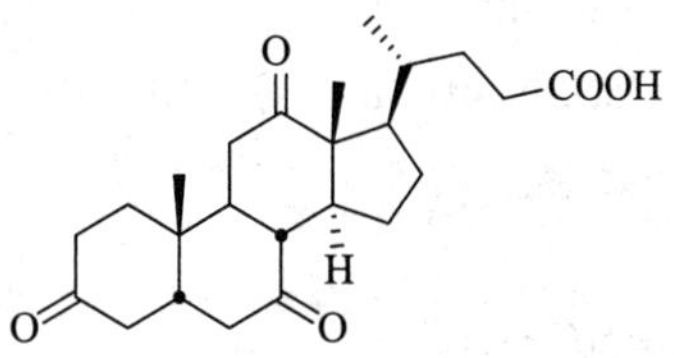

dehydrocholic acid

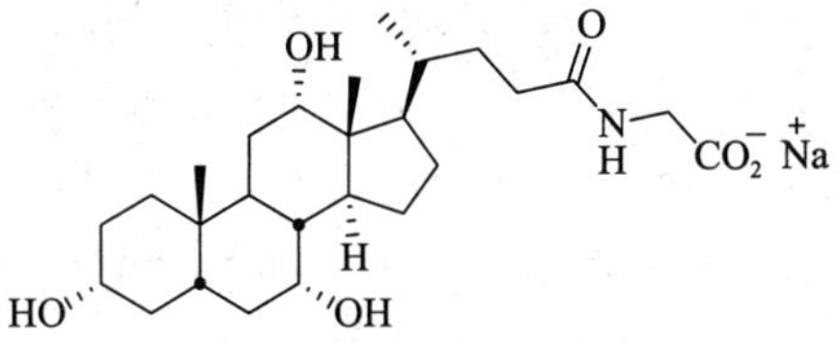

sodium glycocholate

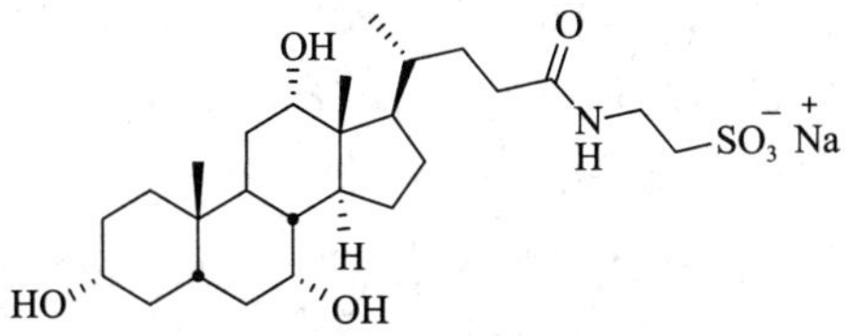

sodium taurocholate

3.2   Structure Characters

The bile acids have C_{24} cholane skeleton. The A/B, B/C, and C/D fusions are *cis*, *trans*, and *trans*, respectively. The side-chain at C-17 is valeric acid. There may be hydroxyls or ketones at C-3, C-6, C-7 and C-12, and the hydroxyl group at C-3 is α-oriented.

3.3   Main Properties

3.3.1   Acidity

Dissociated and bound bile acids are both acids, soluble in organic solvent and insoluble in water.

They are soluble in water after salifying with base. This property is used to purify bile acids.

3.3.2 Esterification

The carboxyl group of bile acids can be esterified and easily crystallize. Then these crystals are refluxed in acidic aqueous solution to get free-form bile acids. This property is also used to purify bile acids.

3.3.3 Color Reactions

(1) Pettenkofer Reaction

The reagents of this reaction are 10% sucrose solution and concentrate sulfuric acid. The sample is diluted with four times of water, then added 10% sucrose solution. Shake the mixture before add concentrate sulfuric acid along the test tube wall to let the sulfuric acid down to the bottom of the tube. Cool the tube in cold water. Then a purple layer will appear if there are bile acids in the sample. The principle of this reaction is that sucrose dehydrated by concentrate sulfuric acid to yield hydroxymethylfurfural, this product condensed with bile acids to give purple substance.

(2) Gregory Pascoe Reaction

The reagents of this reaction are 45% H_2SO_4 and 0.3% furfural (糠醛). The sample is added these reagents in the ratio of 1 : 6 : 1 (v/v/v) into a tube with cover. After shaking, the tube is put in 65℃ water bath to react for 30 minutes, then the solution turn blue if there are bile acids. The principle of this reaction is the same with Pettenkofer reaction, and it is used for the quantitative analysis of bile acids.

(3) Hammarsten Reaction

The reagent of this reaction is 20% chromic trioxide solution (dissolve 20g chromic trioxide in a little water then add acetic acid to 100ml). After heating, cholic acid turn purple, but chenodeoxycholic acid does not change color.

3.4   Identification

The identification of bile acids is achieved by color reactions above or chromatographic methods.

Silica gel TLC is widely used in the isolation and identification of bile acids. The developing solvents for free bile acids are solvent systems composed of isooctane : isoamyl ether : acetic acid : *n*-butanol-water; isooctane : acetate : acetic acid; and for combined bile acids are composed of cholorform : isopropanol: acetic acid : water; isopentanol : acetic acid : water; *n*-butanol : acetic acid : water, etc.

The spray reagents for TLC are phosphomolybdic acid, 30% sulphuric acid, or iodine.

3α-hydroxyl bile acid is selectively identified by 3α-hydroxy steroid oxidase reagent at 37℃ for 30 minutes, which is negative to 3β-hydroxyl and 3-oxo steroid, together with phenolic hydroxyl.

GC and HPLC can also be used for the identification of bile acids. Combined bile acid is hydrolyzed by alkali (e.g. 2.5mol/L NaOH) into free type, then methylated and trimethylsilylated for the carboxyl and hydroxyl groups respectively before analyzed by GC. Ursodesoxycholic acid and chenodeoxycholic acid are isolated by 3% OV-17 column with helium as carrier gas and FID detector. Due to lack of conjugated system, the detection of bile acids by UV detector on HPLC is achieved by derivation.

3.5   Extraction and Isolation

The extraction and isolation of bile acids from animal bile are shown in Figure 9-7.

Animal bile

| Saponified（皂化）by 10% NaOH

Solution

| Filtered

┌──────────────┴──────────────┐

Residue   Filtrate

| Added 30% H_2SO_4 to adjust the pH to 2–3
| Extracted with lipophilic solvent

Crude free bile acids

Figure 9-7   Extraciton and isolation of bile acids

---

4   C₂₁-Steroids

C_{21}-steroids are the steroid derivatives containing 21 carbons and are widely used in clinical trials for its anti-inflammatory, antifertility and anti-tumor activities, such as megestrol acetate and pregnenolone.

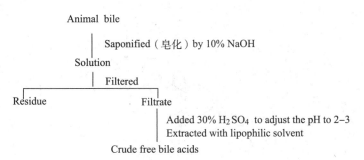

megestrol acetate   pregnenolone

C_{21}-steroids isolated from natural source have the skeleton of pregnane, may have double bonds at C-5 and C-6, carbonyl at C-20, side chain at C-17with α or β orientation.

C_{21}-steroids exist in the form of aglycone as well as glycoside in natural source. Saccharides found in C_{21}-steroid glycosides include deoxysugars, such as cymarose, oleandrose, diginose, digitoxose and thevetose, and aldohexoses, allose and glucose. The aglycone of C_{21}-steroids is classified into two groups: pregnane（Ⅰ and Ⅱ）and pseudo-pregnane derivatives（Ⅲ–Ⅶ）.

Ⅰ

Ⅱ

Ⅲ

Ⅳ

Ⅴ

Ⅵ

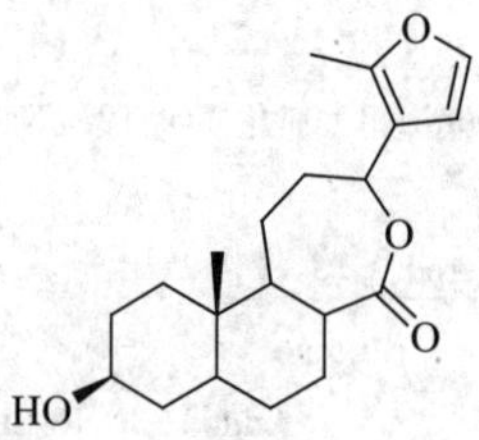

Ⅶ

C_{21}-steroids present in the plants of families of Scrophulariaceae, Apocynaceae and Ranunculaceae (毛茛科), especially Asclepiadaceae family.

5 Phytosterols

Phytosterols with 8–10 carbon-chain at C_{17}, are widely presented in plants. Phytosterols are structural components of the membranes in plants, algae, and fungi, and affect the permeability of these membranes. They also play a role in cell proliferation. Sitosterol (谷甾醇) and stigmasterol (豆甾醇) are produced commercially from soy beans and are raw materials for the semi-synthesis of medicinal steroids.

The main phytosterols in plants, fungi and algae are characterized by extra one-carbon or two-carbon substituent on the side-chain, attached to C_{24} of cholesterol. The widespread phytosterols campesterol and sitosterol are 24-methyl and 24-ethyl analogues of cholesterol, respectively. Stigmasterol contains additional unsaturation in the side-chain, a *trans*-Δ^{22} double bond, a feature seen in many phytosterols, but never in mammalian ones. The predominant sterol found in fungi is ergosterol (麦角甾醇), which has a *trans*-Δ^{22} double bond, as well as additional Δ^7 unsaturation. The most abundant sterol in brown algae is fucosterol, which demonstrates a further variant, a 24-ethylene substituent.

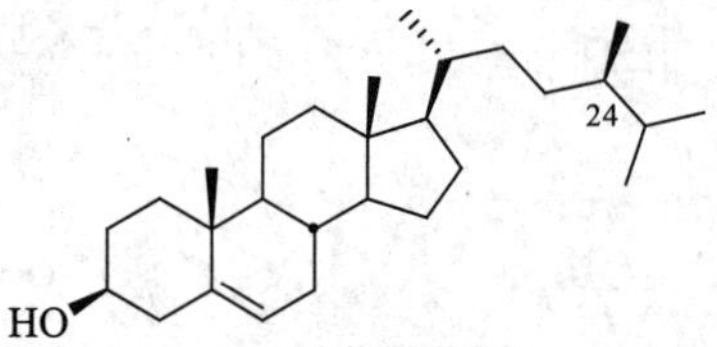

campesterol（菜油甾醇）

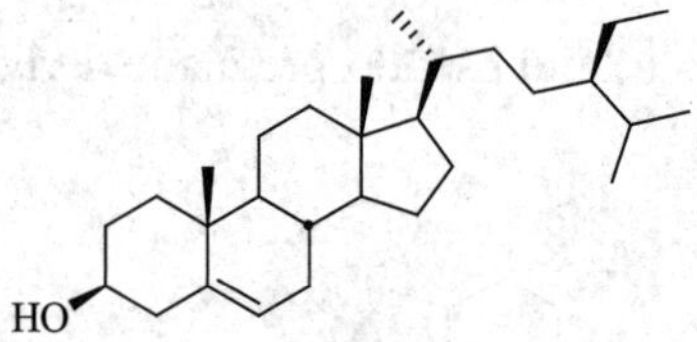

sitosterol

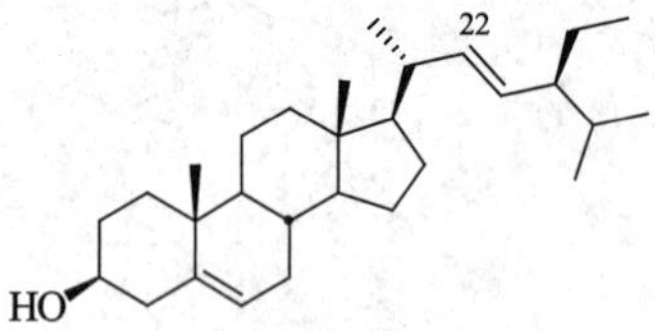

stigmasterol

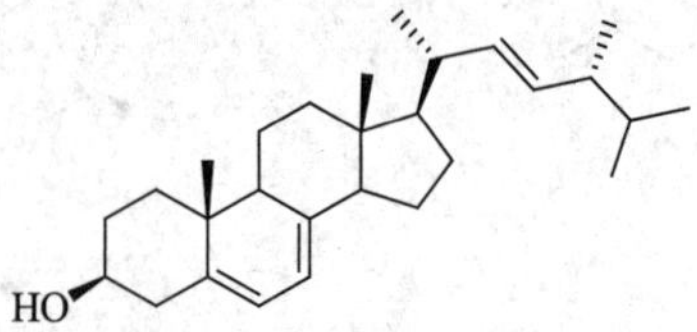

ergosterol

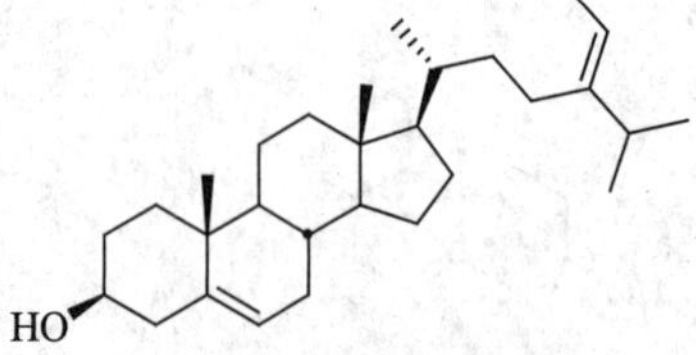

fucosterol（岩藻甾醇）

Phytosterols are found predominantly in free form, but also as esters with long-chain fatty acids [e.g. palmitic acid (棕榈酸), oleic acid (油酸), linoleic acid (亚油酸) and α-linolenic acids (亚麻酸)], as glycosides and as fatty acylated glycosides.

Phytosterols in free form are crystals with acute melting point, and soluble in organic solvents such as chloroform and ethyl ether. They can also react with acids as other steroids.

6 Examples of Chinese Herbs Containing Steroids

6.1 Periplocae Cortex (香加皮)

6.1.1 Introduction

(1) Biological Source

Periplocae Cortex is the dried root bark of *Periploca sepium* Bge. (杠柳) (Fam. Asclepiadaceae).

(2) Property, Flavor and Channels Entered

Property and Flavor: Acrid and bitter, warm, poisonous.

Channels Entered: Liver, Kidney and Heart.

(3) Actions & Indications

To relieve rheumatic conditions and tone up tendons and bones; For rheumatic arthritis with aching and weakness of the lower back and knees, palpitation, shortness of breath and edema of the lower extremities.

(4) Pharmacological Activities

The pharmacological activities associated with the Periplocae Cortex include cardiotonic action, antitumor, anti-inflammation, immunomodulation, etc. It is used to treat rheumatism and chronic congestive heart failure. The cardiac glycosides in it show toxicity similar to strophanthin.

6.1.2 Main Chemical Constituents

P. sepium Bge. distributes in province of Jilin, Inner Mongolia and Xinjiang Autonomous Regions, etc., and is recorded as *Xiangjiapi* in Chinese pharmacopia (2020 edition). It contains C_{21}-steroids, cardiac glycosides, triterpenoids, aldehydes and so on.

(1) C_{21}-steroids

The C_{21}-steroids isolated from Periplocae Cortex all belong to the pregnenolone type. The skeleton and structures of them are listed below (Table 9-7).

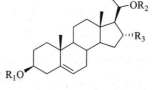

Ia   Ib

315

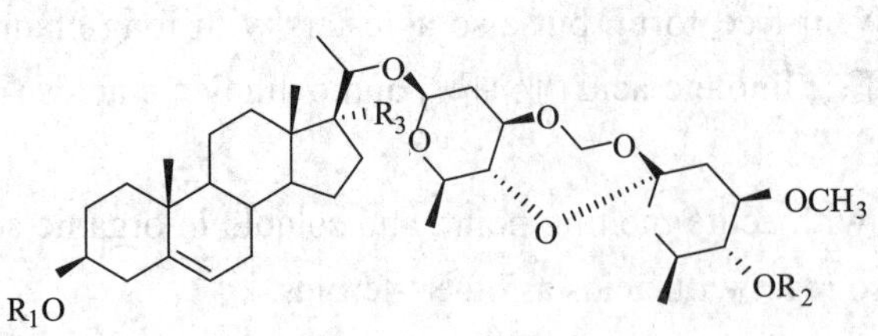

Ic

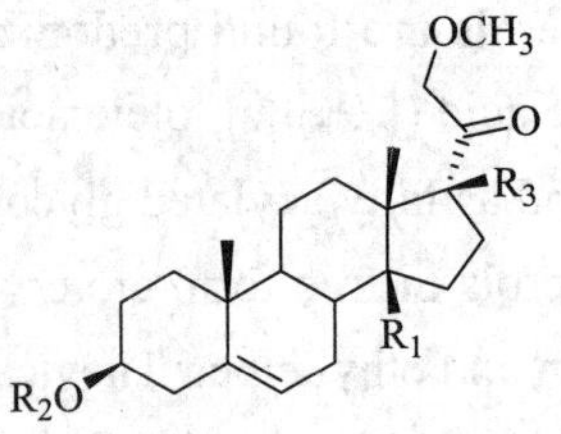

IIa

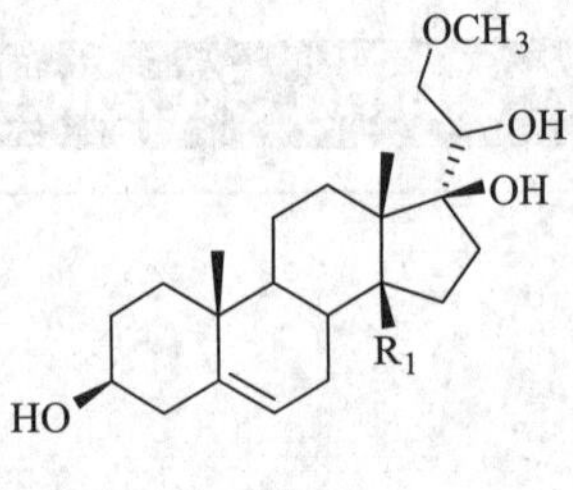

IIb

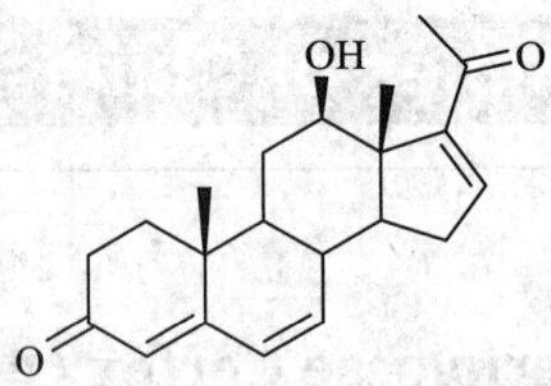

III

Table 9-7　C$_{21}$-steroids isolated from Periplocae Cortex

Type	Compound	R$_1$	R$_2$	R$_3$
Ia	glycoside E	H	β-D-can	OH
Ia	glycoside K	H	Ra	H
Ia	glycoside H$_1$	Rb	Ra	H
Ia	periplocogenin	Rc	H	OH
Ia	periplocoside F	H	Rd	OH
Ia	periplocoside L	β-D-digita	H	OH
Ia	periplocoside M	Rc	β-D-can	OH
Ia	periplocoside O	Rc	Re	OH
Ia	periploside B	Rc	β-D-can	OH
Ia	plocoside A	H	Ra	H
Ia	Δ^5-pregene-3β, 20-diol	H	H	H
Ia	Δ^5-pregene-3β, 17α, 20-triol	H	H	OH
Ia	Δ^5-pregene-3β, 20-diol 3-O-β-D-digita-(1 → 4)-β-D-cym 20-O-β-D-glc-(1 → 6)-β-D-glc-(1 → 2)-β-D-digita	Rf	Ra	H
Ia	Δ^5-pregene-3β, 20-diol 20-O-β-D-glc-(1 → 6)-β-D-glc-(1 → 6)-digita	H	Ra	H
Ia	Δ^5-pregene-3β, 20-diol 20-O-β-D-glc-(1 → 6)-β-D-glc	H	Rg	H
Ia	Δ^5-pregene-3β, 20-diol 3-O-β-D-glc -20-O-β-D-glc-(1 → 6)-β-D-glc	glc	Rg	H
Ia	Δ^5-pregene-3β, 20-diol 3-O-β-D-glc -20-O-β-D-glc	glc	glc	H
Ia	Δ^5-pregene-3β, 20-diol 3-acetyl	Ac	H	H
Ia	Δ^5-pregene-3, 17, 20-triol 20-[O-β-glucopyranosyl-(1 → 6)-O-glucopyranosyl-(1 → 4)-β-canaropyranoside]	Rh	H	OH

(continued)

Type	Compound	R_1	R_2	R_3
Ⅰa	periseoside A	Rj	H	OH
Ⅰa	periseoside B	Rg	H	OH
Ⅰa	periseoside C	glc	glc	H
Ⅰa	periseoside D	Rg	Rj	H
Ⅰb		Ac	H	H
Ⅰb	glycoside H_2	Rb	Ra	OH
Ⅰb	plocoside B	Rf	Ra	OH
Ⅰb	Δ^5-pregene-3β, 16β, 20-triol 3-(2-O-Ac-β-D-digita-(1→4)-β-D-cym) 20-β-D-glc-(1→6)-β-D-glc-(1→2)-β-D-digita	Rb	Ra	β-OH
Ⅰb	Δ^5-pregene-3β, 16α, 20-triol 20-β-D-glc-(1→6)-β-D-glc-(1→2)-digita	H	Ra	OH
Ⅰb	Δ^5-pregene-3β, 16β, 20-triol 20-β-D-glc-(1→6)-β-D-glc-(1→2)-digita	H	Ra	OH
Ⅰb	Δ^5-pregene-3β, 16α, 20α-triol	H	H	OH
Ⅰb	periseoside E	glc	glc	OH
Ⅰc	periploside A	H	Rk	OH
Ⅰc	periplocoside B	Rc	Rl	OH
Ⅰc	periplocoside C	Rc	β-D-cym	OH
Ⅰc	periplocoside D	Rc	Rr	OH
Ⅰc	Periplocoside E	H	Rk	OH
Ⅰc	Periplocoside J	H	Rs	OH
Ⅰc	periplocoside K	Rc	Rn	OH
Ⅰc	periploside C	Rc	Rk	OH
Ⅰc	periploside M	Rc	Rl	OH
Ⅰc	periploside N	Rc	β-D-cym	OH
Ⅰc	periploside D	Rc	Rm	OH
Ⅰc	periploside J	H	Rn	OH
Ⅰc	periploside E	Rc	Ro	OH
Ⅰc	periploside G	Rc	Rp	OH
Ⅰc	periploside H	H	Rp	OH
Ⅰc	periploside I	Rc	Rq	OH
Ⅰc	periploside L	H	Rq	OH
Ⅱa	21-O-methyl-Δ^5-pregnene-3β, 17β, 21-tetraol-20-one	H	H	OH
Ⅱa	21-O-methyl-Δ^5-pregnene-3β, 14β, 17β, 21-tetraol-20-one	OH	H	OH

(continued)

Type	Compound	R₁	R₂	R₃
IIa	21-*O*-methyl-Δ^5-pregnene-3β, 14β, 17β, 21-tetraol-20-one 3-[*O*-β-oleandropyranosyl-(1 → 4)-*O*-β-cym-(1 → 4)-β-cym]	OH	Ri	OH
IIa	3, 14-dihydroxy-21-methoxypregn-5-en-20-one	OH	H	H
IIb	21-*O*-methyl-Δ^5-pregnene-3β, 14β, 17β, 20, 21-pentaol	OH		
IIb	21-*O*-methyl-$\Delta^{5,14,15}$-pregnene-3β, 17β, 20, 21-tetraol	$\Delta^{14,15}$		
III	12β-hydroxy-$\Delta^{4,6,16}$-pregnene-3, 20-dione			

Ra: β-D-glc-(1 → 6)-β-D-glc-(1 → 2)-β-D-digita; **Rb:** 2-*O*-Ac-β-D-digita-(1 → 4)-β-D-cym; **Rc:** 4′, 6′-dideoxy-3′-*O*-Me-Δ^3-D-2′-hexosuloside; **Rd:** β-D-dig-(1 → 4)-β-D-cym-(1 → 4)-β-D-cym-(1 → 4)- -β-D-cym-(1 → 5)-3, 7-dideoxy-4-*O*-CH₃-α-D-glc-2-heptulo-(2 → 4)-dioxy-(1 → 3)-β-D-can; **Re:** 2-*O*-Ac-β-D-dig-(1 → 4)-β-D-cym-(1 → 4)-β-D-cym-(1 → 4)-β-D-cym-(1 → 4)-L-oleanderonic acid- δ - -lactone-(1 → 4)-3-*O*-CH₃-β-D-can; **Rf:** β-D-digita-(1 → 4)-β-D-cym; **Rg:** β-D-glc-(1 → 6)-β-D-glc; **Rh:** β-D-glc-(1 → 6)-β-D-glc-(1 → 4)-β-D-can; **Ri:** β-D-ole-(1 → 4)-β-D-cym-(1 → 4)-β-D-cym; **Rj:** β-D-glc- -(1 → 4)-β-D-digita; **Rk:** 2-*O*-Ac-β-D-digita-(1 → 4)-β-D-cym-(1 → 4)-β-D-cym-(1 → 4)-β-D-cym; **Rl:** β-D-cym-(1 → 4)-β-D-cym; **Rm:** β-D-digita-(1 → 4)-β-D-cym-(1 → 4)-β-D-cym-(1 → 4)-β-D-cym; **Rn:** β-D-digita-(1 → 4)-β-D-cym-(1 → 4)-2, 6-dideoxy-β-D-glc-(1 → 4)-β-D-digito; **Ro:** 2-*O*-Ac-β-D-digita- -(1 → 4)-β-D-cym-(1 → 4)-2, 6-dideoxy glc-β-D-digito; **Rp:** 4-*O*-Ac-β-D-cym-(1 → 4)-β-D-cym-(1 → 4)- -2, 6-dideoxy-β-D-glc-(1 → 4)-β-D-cym; **Rq:** 3-*O*-Me-2, 6-dideoxy-β-D-glc-(1 → 4)-β-D-cym-2, 6-dideoxy-β-D-glc-(1 → 4)-β-D-cym; **Rr:** β-D-digita-(1 → 4)-β-D-cym-(1 → 4)-β-D-cym-(1 → 4)-β-D-cym; **Rs:** β-D-digita-(1 → 4)-β-D-cym-(1 → 4)-β-D-can-(1 → 4)-β-D-digita

(2) Cardiac Glycosides

The cardiac glycosides isolated from Periplocae Cortex belong to cardenolide as follows.

periplogenin	R=H
peripocymarin	R=β-D-cym
periplocin	R=β-D-glc(1→4) β-D-cym
periplogenin 3-[*O*-β-glucopyranosyl-(1→4)-β-sarmentopyranoside]	R=β-D-glc(1→4) β-D-sar

xysmalogenin

(3) Triterpenoids

The triterpenoids isolated from Periplocae Cortex belong to pentacyclic trierpenoids, including β-amyrin and its acetate, oleanolic acid, α-amyrin and its acetate, lursolic acid, upeol and its acetate, hederagenin, cycloeucalenol, and 9, 19-cycloart-25-ene-3β, 24-diol.

(4) Volatile Oils

The root bark volatile oil of *Periploca sepium* is found to possess strong contact toxicity against the fruit flies, *Drosophila melanogaster* with a LD₅₀ value at 1.22μg/adult. The main component of the volatile oil is identified to be 2-hydroxy-4-methyoxy-benzaldehyde (78.8%), which contributes the aroma, followed by linalool (2.8%) and (-)-α-terpineol (2.7%).

(5) Others

Other chemicals found in Periplocae Cortex include fatty acids (palmitic acid, linoleic acid, linolenic acid, stearic acid, etc.), coumarins (scopoletin), flavonoids (baohuoside I and proanthocyandin B2) and oligosaccharides (perisaccharide A, B, C, D, E, Oligosaccharides C_1, D_2, F_1, F_2).

6.1.3　Quality Control Standards

(1) TLC Identification

Stationary Phase: Silica gel G plate.

Standard: 4-Methoxy salicylic aldehyde.

Development System: Petroleum ether (60–90℃)-acetyl acetate-glacial acetic acid (40 : 6 : 1).

Visualization: Dinitrophenylhydrazine.

(2) Tests

Water: Not more than 12.0%.

Total Ash: Not more than 10.0%.

Acid-insoluble Ash: Not more than 4.0%.

Extract (diluted ethanol): Not less than 20.0%.

(3) Assay

4-Methoxy Salicylic Aldehyde: Not less than 0.20% (HPLC).

6.2　Bufonis Venenum (蟾酥)

6.2.1　Introduction

(1) Biological Source

Bufonis venenum is the dried white secretion of the auricular and glands of *Bufo bufo gargarizans* Cantor (中华大蟾蜍) or *Bufo melanostictus* Schneider (黑眶蟾蜍).

(2) Property, Flavor and Channels Entered

Property and Flavor: Acrid, warm, toxic.

Channels Entered: Heart.

(3) Actions & Indications

To counteract toxicity, relieve pain, and restore consciousness; For carbuncles, boils, sore throat; vomiting, diarrhea, abdominal pain and delirium in heat-stroke.

(4) Pharmacological Activities

The pharmacological activities of Bufonis venenum include cardiotonic effect, anti-myocardial ischemia, anti-endotoxin shock and anti-tumor. The preparation of Bufonis venenum is applied to the anesthesia in surgery of tonsillectomy and thyroidectomy, the treatment of lung, liver and esophageal cancer, etc. Its mechanisms of anti-tumor are inducing cell apoptosis, inhibiting cell proliferation, improving differentiation, reversing drug resistance, inhibiting tumor angiogenesis and enhancing immune system, etc.

6.2.2　Main Chemical Constituents

Chemicals contained in Bufonis venenum are mainly bufanolides, bufotenines and sterols.

(1) Bufanolides

The bufanolides from Bufonis venenum are classified into bufadienolides and 20, 21-epoxy bufanolides. The structures are listed in Table 9-8. Among them, resibufogenin and cinobufagin are the chemical reference substances for Bufonis venenum in TLC identification and HPLC quantification, the total content of which is no less than 6.0%.

Table 9-8 Bufadienolides isolated from Bufonis venenum

Type	Compound	R_1	R_2	R_3	R_4	R_5	R_6	R_7	R_8	R_9
I	resibufogenin	OH	CH_3	H	H	H	H	H		
I	cinobufagin	OH	CH_3	H	H	H	OAc	H		
I	19-oxocinobufagin	OH	CHO	H	H	H	OAc	H		
I	cinobufotalin	OH	CH_3	OH	H	H	OAc	H		
I	3-oxocinobufatalin	oxo	H	OH	H	H	OAc	H		
I	19-oxocinobufotalin	OH	CHO	OH	H	H	OAc	H		
I	marinobufagin	OH	CH_3	OH	H	H	H	H		
I	desacetylcinobufotalin	OH	CH_3	OH	H	H	H	OH	H		
I	bufotalinin	OH	CHO	OH	H	H	H	H		
I	resibufagin	OH	CHO	H	H	H	H	H		
I	desacetylcinobufagin	OH	CH_3	H	H	H	H	OH	H		
I	cinobufaginol	OH	CH_2OH	H	H	H	OAc	H		
I	desacetylcinobufaginol	OH	CH_2OH	H	H	H	H	OH	H		
I	resibufaginol	OH	CH_2OH	H	H	H	H	H		
I	3β-formyl oxyresibufogenin	HCOO	CH_3	H	H	H	H	H		
I	19-oxodesacetylcinobufagin	OH	CHO	OH	H	H	H	OH	H		

(continued)

Type	Compound	R_1	R_2	R_3	R_4	R_5	R_6	R_7	R_8	R_9
I	6α-hydroxycinobufagin	OH	CH$_3$	H	OH	H	OAc	H		
I	12β-hydroxyresibufaginol	OH	CH$_2$OH	H	H	H	OH	H		
I	12β-hydroxycinobufagin	OH	CH$_3$	H	H	OH	OAc	H		
I	1β-hydroxycinobufagin	OH	CH$_3$	H	H	H	OAc	β-OH		
I	5β, 12β-hydroxycinobufagin	OH	CH$_3$	OH	H	β-OH	OAc	H		
I	cinobufagin-3-hemisuberate	a	CH$_3$	H	H	H	OAc	H		
I	cinobufagin-3-sulfate	SO$_3$H	CH$_3$	H	H	H	OAc	H		
I	cinobufagin-3-succinolylarginin ester	b	CH$_3$	H	H	H	OAc	H		
I	cinobufagin-3-glutaroyl-L-arginin	c	CH$_3$	H	H	H	OAc	H		
I	cinobufagin-3-adipoylarginin ester	d	CH$_3$	H	H	H	OAc	H		
I	cinobufagin-3-suberoylarginin ester	e	CH$_3$	H	H	H	OAc	H		
I	resibufogenin-3-sulfate	SO$_3$H	CH$_3$	H	H	H	H	H		
I	resibufogenin-3-hemisuberate	a	CH$_3$	H	H	H	H	H		
I	resibufogenin-3-hemiadipicate	g	CH$_3$	H	H	H	H	H		
I	resibufogenin-3-succinolylarginin ester	b	CH$_3$	H	H	H	H	H		
I	resibufogenin-3-suberoylarginin ester	e	CH$_3$	H	H	H	H	H		
I	resibufogenin-3-pimeloylarginine ester	f	CH$_3$	H	H	H	H	H		
I	desacetylcinobufagin-3-succinylarginin ester	b	CH$_3$	H	H	H	OH	H		
I	desacetylcinobufagin-3-hemisuberate	a	CH$_3$	H	H	H	OH	H		
I	(3β, 5β, 15β, 16β)-14, 15-epoxy-3, 5, 10, 16-tetrahydroxyl-19-norbufa-20, 22-dienolide	OH	OH	OH	H	H	OH	H		
II	14β-artebufogenin	OH	H	CH$_3$	H	H	H	H	oxo	H
II	bufalin	OH	H	CH$_3$	H	H	H	OH	H	H
II	19-oxobufalin	OH	H	CHO	H	H	H	OH	H	H
II	19-hydroxybufalin	OH	H	CH$_2$OH	H	H	H	OH	H	H
II	19-hydroxybufalin-3-sulfate	SO$_3$H	H	CH$_2$OH	H	H	H	OH	H	H
II	15-hydroxybufalin	OH	H	CH$_3$	H	H	H	OH	β-OH	H
II	12-hydroxybufalin	OH	H	CH$_3$	H	H	H	OH	H	OH
II	bufotalin	OH	H	CH$_3$	H	H	OAc	OH	H	H
II	hellebrigenol	OH	H	CH$_2$OH	OH	H	H	OH	H	H
II	hellebrigenin or bufotalidin	OH	H	CHO	OH	H	H	OH	H	H

(continued)

Type	Compound	R_1	R_2	R_3	R_4	R_5	R_6	R_7	R_8	R_9
II	desacetylbufotalin	OH	H	CH₃	H	H	OH	OH	H	H
II	desacetylbufotalin-3-sulfate	SO₃H	H	CH₃	H	H	OH	OH	H	H
II	telocinobufagin	OH	H	CH₃	OH	H	H	OH	H	H
II	telocinobufagin-3-sulfate	SO₃H	H	CH₃	OH	H	H	OH	H	H
II	gamabufotalin	OH	H	CH₃	H	OH	H	OH	H	H
II	1β-hydroxybufalin	OH	OH	CH₃	H	H	H	OH	H	H
II	5β-hydroxybufotalin	OH	H	CH₃	OH	H	OAc	OH	H	H
II	bufalin-3-hemisuberate	a	H	CH₃	H	H	H	OH	H	H
II	bufalin-3-succinolylarginine ester	b	H	CH₃	H	H	H	OH	H	H
II	gamabufotalin-3-hemisuberate	a	H	CH₃	H	OH	H	OH	H	H
II	gamabufotalin-3-adipoylarginine ester	d	H	CH₃	H	OH	H	OH	H	H
II	gamabufotalin-3-pimeloylarginine ester	f	H	CH₃	H	OH	H	OH	H	H
II	gamabufotalin-3-succinoylarginine ester	b	H	CH₃	H	OH	H	OH	H	H
II	5β-hydroxyl-14α-artebufogenin	OH	H	CH₃	OH	OH	OH	H	oxo	H
II	(16β)-16-(acetyloxy)-14-hydroxyl-bufa-5, 20, 22-trienolide	OH	H	CH₃	Δ⁵,⁶	H	OAc	H	H	H
II	(3β, 16β)-3, 16-dihydroxyl-bufa-8(14), 20, 22-trienolide	OH	H	CH₃	H	H	OH	Δ⁸,¹⁴	H	H
II	14α-artebufogenin	OH	H	CH₃	H	OH	OH	H	oxo	H
II	telocinobufagin-3-hemisuberate	a	H	CH₃	OH	H	H	OH	H	H
II	hellebrigenol-3-sulfate	SO₃H	H	CH₂OH	OH	H	H	OH	H	H
II	hellebrigenin-3-sulfate	SO₃H	H	CHO	OH	H	H	OH	H	H
III	arenobufagin	OH	H	β-OH						
III	arenobufagin-3-sulfate	SO₃H	H	β-OH						
III	arenobufagin-3-hemisuberate	a	H	β-OH						
III	1β-hydroxyl-arenobufagin	OH	OH	α-OH						
III	16-acetyl-arenobufagin	OH	H	β-OH	OAc					
IV	pseudobufarenogin	α-OH	H							
IV	bufarenogin	β-OH	H							
IV	16β-hydroxyl-pseudobufarenogin	OH	β-OH							
V	20S, 21-epoxyresibufogenin	OH								
V	20R, 21-epoxyresibufogenin	OH								
V	3-O-formyl-20R, 21-epoxyresibufogenin	HCOO								
V	3-O-formyl-20S, 21-epoxyresibufogenin	HCOO								

(continued)

Type	Compound	R₁	R₂	R₃	R₄	R₅	R₆	R₇	R₈	R₉
V	3-*O*-20S, 21-epoxyresibufogeni	=O	—							
VI	5β, 12β-12, 14-dihydroxy-11-oxobufa-3, 20, 22-trienolide	H	Δ³,⁴	—	β-OH					
VI	5β, 12α-12, 14-dihydroxy-11-oxobufa-3, 20, 22-trienolide	H	Δ³,⁴	—	α-OH					
VI	5β, 12β-12, 14-dihydroxy-11-oxobufa-2, 20, 22-trienolide	Δ²,³	—	H	β-OH					

a: OCO(CH₂)₆COOH; **b:** OCO(CH₂)₂COArg · OH; **c:** OCO(CH₂)₃COArg · OH; **d:** OCO(CH₂)₄COArg · OH; **e:** OCO(CH₂)₆COArg · OH; **f:** OCO(CH₂)₅COArg · OH; **g:** OCO(CH₂)₄COOH

Bufogargarizins A, B, C, with unprecedented carbon skeletons are isolated from the venom of *Bufo bufo gargarizans*. Isobufalin methyl ester is the ring-opening product of bufalin, which is also isolated from *Bufo bufo gargarizans*.

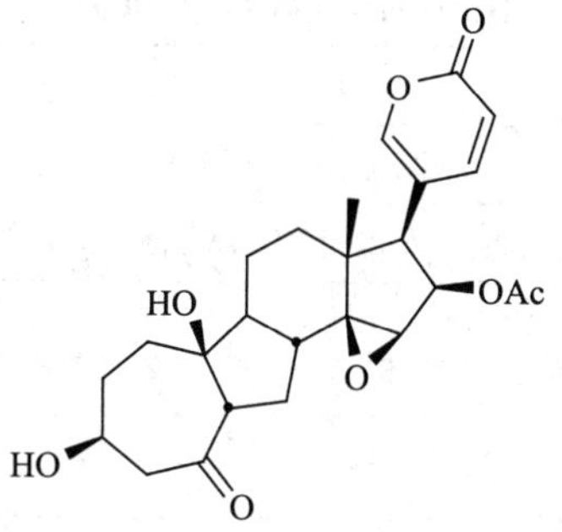

bofogargarizin A 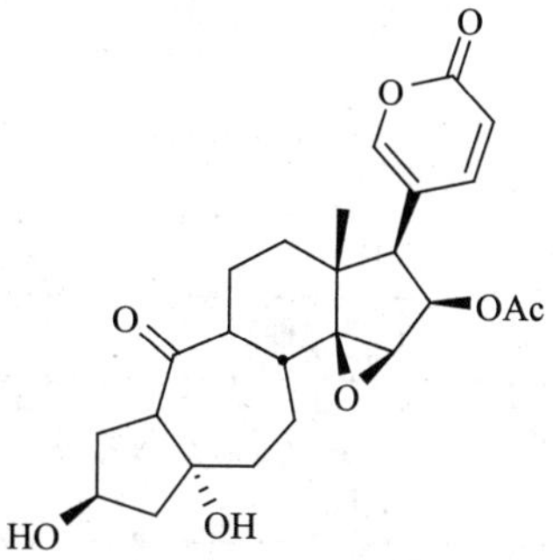   bofogargarizin B 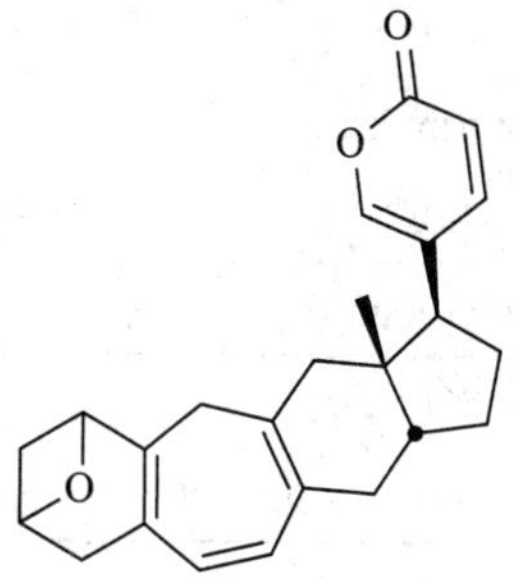   bufogargarizin C

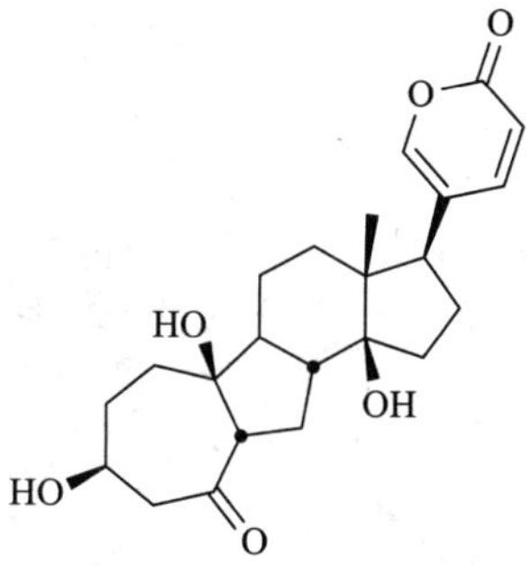

bufogargarizin 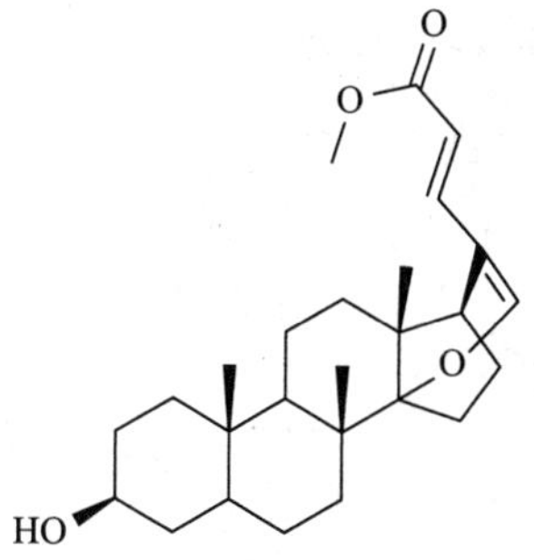   isobufalin methyl ester

(2) Bufotenines

The bufotenines from Bufonis venenum belong to indole alkaloids (Table 9-9).

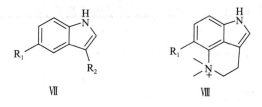

VII   VIII

Table 9-9   Indole alkaloids isolated from Bufonis venenum

Type	Compound	R_1	R_2
VII	bufotenine	OH	$CH_2CH_2N(CH_3)_2$
VII	nitrogen oxides of bufotenidine	OH	$CH_2CH_2(CH_3)_2N \rightarrow O$
VII	bufotenidine	O^-	$CH_2CH_2N^+(CH_3)_3$
VII	bufobutarginine	OH	$CH_2CH_2NH(CH_2)_2CONHCHCOOH(CH_2)_3NH(NH_2)C=NH$
VII	serotonin	OH	$CH_2CH_2NH_2$
VII	N-methyl serotonin	OH	$CH_2CH_2NHCH_3$
VII	bufobutanoic acid	OH	$CH_2CH_2NHCO(CH_2)_2COOH$
VII	bufopyramide	OH	$CH_2CH_2NH(COCH_3)CO$
VII	hufoserotonin A	OH	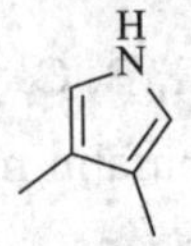 $CH_2CH_2NHCONH_2$
VII	hufoserotonin B	OH	$CH_2CH_2NHCO(CH_2)_6COOH$
VII	bufoviridine	OSO_3^-	H
VII	N'-formylserotonin	OH	CH_2CH_2NHCHO
VII	5-hydroxy-N-acetyltryptamine	OH	$CH_2CH_2NHCOCH_3$
VIII	dehydrobufotenine	O^-	
VIII	bufothionine	OSO_3^-	
VIII	dehydrobufoteinine hydrobromide	OH [VII]Br$^-$	

(3) Others

Two C_{23} steroids (bufotricosaroide A and B) and one spirostenol (螺甾烷醇) are isolated from the venom of *Bufo bufo gargarizans*.

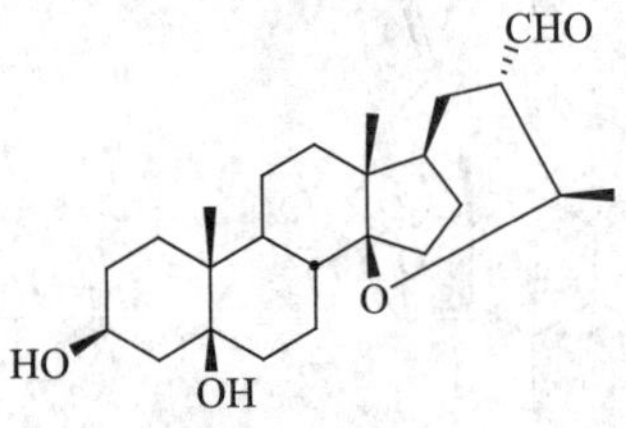

bufotricosaroide A 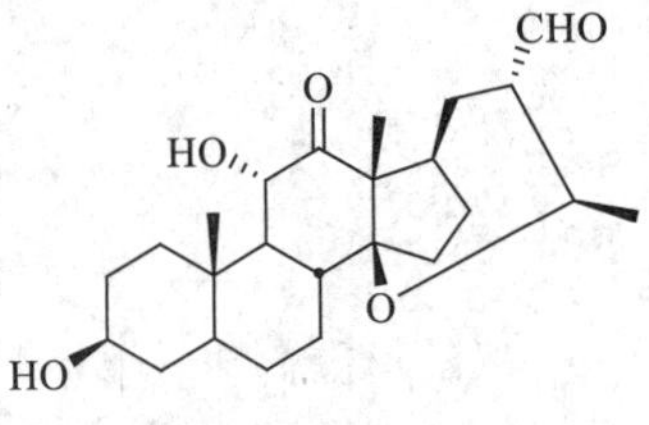   bufotricosaroide B 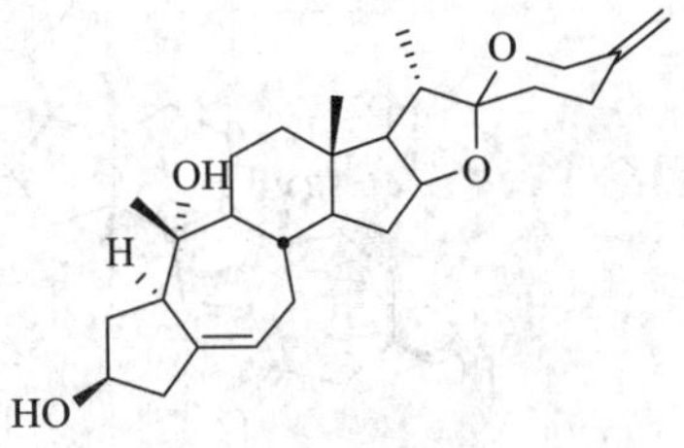   bufospirostenin A

6.2.3   Quality Control Standards

(1) TLC Identification

Stationary Phase: Silica gel G plate.

Standard: Authentic crude drug, resibufogenin, cinobufagin.

Development System: Hexane-chloroform-acetone (4 : 3 : 3).

Visualization: $10\%H_2SO_4$ in ethanol, heat until clear spots were detected.

(2) Tests

Water: Not more than 13.0%.

Total Ash: Not more than 5.0%.

Acid-insoluble Ash: Not more than 2.0%.

(3) Assay

Resibufogenin and Cinobufagin: Not less than 6.0% (HPLC).

6.3　Bovis Calculus (牛黄)

6.3.1　Introduction

(1) Biological Source

Bovis calculus is the dried gallstones of *Bos taurus domesticus* Gmelin (Fam. Bovidae).

(2) Property, Flavor and Channels Entered

Property and Flavor: Sweet, cool.

Channels Entered: Heart and Liver.

(3) Actions & Indications

To restore consciousness by reducing fire and eliminating phlegm, relieve convulsion, and counteract toxicity; For delirium in febrile diseases and stroke; infantile convulsion, epilepsy, mania; sore throat, ulcers in the mouth; carbuncles and boils.

(4) Pharmacological Activities

The pharmacological activities of Bovis Calculus are anti-pyrosis and analgesic action, anti-inflammation, anti-oxidation, free radical scavenging, anti-tumor and enhancing immune, etc.

6.3.2　Main Chemical Constituents

The chemical constituents of Bovis Calculus include bilirubin, bile acids, smooth muscle contractor (SMC), cholesterol, ergosterol, amino acids and inorganic salts. Deoxycholic acid contributes to the relaxation effect of smooth muscles, while SMC leads to the contraction of smooth muscles. Artificial Bovis Calculus is composed of bilirubin (0.7%), deoxycholic acid (15%), hyocholic acid (猪胆酸，15%), taurocholic acid (牛磺胆酸，15%), cholesterol (2%), inorganic salts (5%), and starch.

Main bile acids in Bovis Calculus are cholic acid, deoxycholic acid and lithocholic acid. The structures of them have shown before.

6.3.3　Quality Control Standards

(1) TLC Identification

① TLC Identification of bile acids

Stationary Phase: Silica gel G plate.

Standard: Cholic acid and deoxycholic acid.

Development System: Isooctane-acetyl acetate-glacial acetic acid (15∶7∶5).

Visualization: 10%H_2SO_4 in ethanol, heat until clear spots were detected, then detect under UV_{365nm} lamp.

② TLC Identification of bilirubin

Stationary Phase: Silica gel G plate.

Standard: Bilirubin.

Development System: Cyclohexane-acetyl acetate-methanol-glacial acetic acid (100∶30∶1∶1).

(2) Tests

Water: Not more than 9.0%.

Total Ash: Not more than 10.0%.

Free Bilirubin: The absorption under wavelength 453nm not higher than 0.70.

(3) Assay

Cholic Acid: Not less than 4.0% (TLC scanning method).

Bilirubin: Not less than 35% (UV-vis spectrophotometry).

词 汇 表

An Alphabetical List of Words and Phrases

A		
angiosperm	[ænˈdʒɪəlɪspəːm]	被子植物
antiarose	[ænʃɪəˈrɔz]	弩箭子糖
arenobufagin	[ərenɔbˈjuːfəgɪn]	沙蟾毒精
Asclepiadaceae		萝藦科
B		
bile acid	[baɪl][ˈæsɪd]	胆汁酸
bufadienolide	[ˌbjuːfədaɪˈenəlaɪd]	蟾蜍甾二烯，蟾二烯羟酸内酯
bufalin	[ˈbjuːflɪn]	蟾蜍灵
Bufonis Venenum		蟾酥
bufotalin	[bʌˈfəutəlɪn]	蟾毒它灵
Bufo bufo gargarizans Cantor		中华大蟾蜍
Bufo melanostictus Schneider		黑眶蟾蜍
C		
campesterol	[kæmˈpestɪrəl]	菜油甾醇
cardenolide	[kɑːˈdɪːnelaɪd]	强心甾烯，卡烯内酯
cardiac glycoside	[ˈkɑːdɪæk][ˈglaɪkəsaɪd]	强心苷
cardiotonic action	[kɑːdɪəuˈtɔnɪk][ˈækʃn]	强心作用
caustic	[ˈkɔːstɪk]	苛性碱
Celastraceae		卫矛科
chenodeoxycholic acid	[tʃenəudɪˌɔksɪˈtʃəulɪk][ˈæsɪd]	鹅去氧胆酸
cholesterol	[kəuˈləstərɔl]	胆固醇，胆甾醇
cholic acid	[ˈkəulɪk][ˈæsɪd]	胆酸
Cruciferae		十字花科
cyclopentanoperhydrophenanthrene	[saɪkləupentəˈnəupəhaɪdrəu][fəˈnænθriːn]	环戊烷骈多氢菲
cymarose	[sɪmæˈrɔz]	加拿大麻糖
D		
deoxyallose	[diːɔksɪəəˈlɔz]	去氧阿洛糖
deoxycholic acid		去氧胆酸
digilanidobiose	[dɪdʒɪlənɪdəuˈbiːəus]	洋地黄双糖
diginose	[ˈdɪdʒɪnəus]	2-去氧洋地黄糖，地芰糖

(continued)

Digitalis	[ˌdɪdʒɪˈteɪlɪs]	洋地黄属
Digitalis lanata		毛花洋地黄
Digitalis purpurea		紫花洋地黄
digitalose	[ˌdɪdʒɪˈtæləus]	洋地黄糖
digitoxigenin	[ˈdɪdʒɪˌtɔksɪˈdʒenɪn]	洋地黄毒苷元
digitoxose	[ˌdɪdʒɪˈtɔksəus]	洋地黄毒糖
digoxigenin	[dɪˈgɔksaɪdʒnɪn]	异羟基洋地黄毒苷元
digoxin	[daɪˈgɔksɪn]	地高辛
diosgenin	[daɪˈɔzdʒənɪn]	薯蓣皂苷元
E		
ergosterol	[əːˈgɔstərɔl]	麦角甾醇
F		
Fermi Resonance	[ˈfəːmi][ˈrezənəns]	费米共振
fucose	[ˈfjuːkəus]	夫糖，岩藻糖
fucosterol	[fjuːˈkɔstərɔl]	岩藻甾醇
furfural	[ˈfəːfəræl]	糠醛；呋喃甲醛
G		
gamabufotalin	[gæməbufəˈtælɪn]	蟾毒它灵
gitaloxigenin	[dʒɪtəˈlɔksɪdʒnɪn]	吉他洛苷元
gitoxigenin	[ˌdʒɪtəksɪˈdʒenɪn]	羟基洋地黄毒苷元
gitoxin	[dʒɪˈtɔksɪn]	羟基洋地黄毒苷
glacial acetic acid	[ˈgleɪʃl][əˈsiːtɪk][ˈæsɪd]	冰乙酸
H		
Helleborus niger		嚏根草
hellebrigenin	[ˌhelɪˈbraɪdʒenɪn]	嚏根草苷元
hydroxymethyl	[haɪdrɔksɪˈmeθɪl]	羟甲基
hyocholic acid		猪胆酸
K		
ketonic	[kɪˈtɔnɪk]	酮的
L		
linoleic acid	[lɪˈnəuliːk][ˈæsɪd]	亚油酸
linolenic acid	[ˌlɪnəˈlenɪk][ˈæsɪd]	亚麻酸
lithocholic acid	[ˌlɪθəˈkɔlɪk][ˈæsɪd]	石胆酸
M		
monocotyledon	[ˌmɔnəuˌkɔtɪˈliːdn]	单子叶植物
N		
nitroferrocyanatum natrium		亚硝酰铁氰化钠

(continued)

O		
O/ W partition coefficient	[pɑːˈtɪʃn][ˌkəʊɪˈfɪʃnt]	油水分配系数
oleandrose	[əʊlndˈrɔz]	夹竹桃糖
oleic acid	[əʊˈliːɪk][ˈæsɪd]	油酸
ouabagenin	[ˈuːəbɪdʒnɪn]	乌本苷元
ouabain/G-strophanthin	[wɑːˈbeɪɪn][strəʊˈfænθɪn]	乌本苷 /G– 毒毛花苷
P		
palmitic acid	[pælˈmɪtɪk][ˈæsɪd]	棕榈酸，软脂酸
Periploca sepium Bge.	[pəˈrɪpləkə][ˈsiːpɪəm]	杠柳
Periplocae Cortex		香加皮
phytosterol	[faɪˈtɔstərɔl]	植物甾醇
proscillaridin	[prəsɪlæˈraɪdɪn]	原海葱苷
proscillaridin A	[prəsɪlæˈraɪdɪn][eɪ]	原海葱苷 A
purpureaglycoside	[pəːpjuəriːglɪˈkəusaɪd]	紫花洋地黄苷
Q		
quartet	[kwɔːˈtet]	四重峰
quinovose	[ˈkwɪnəvəus]	鸡纳糖，异鼠李糖
R		
Ranunculaceae		毛茛科
resibufogenin	[rɪzɪbʌˈfəudʒnɪn]	脂蟾毒配基
S		
saponify	[səˈpɔnɪfaɪ]	使皂化
sarmentose	[sɑːˈmentəus]	沙门糖
scillanolide	[sɪˈlənɔlɪd]	海葱甾
scillaren	[sɪˈlərən]	海葱苷
scillaren A	[sɪˈlərən][eɪ]	海葱苷 A
scillarenin	[sɪˈləriːnɪn]	海葱苷元
scilliroside	[sɪlaɪˈəəusaɪd]	红海葱苷
singlet	[ˈsɪŋglət]	单峰
sitosterol	[saɪˈtɔstərəul]	谷甾醇
spirostenol		螺甾烷醇
squill	[skwɪl]	海葱
steroid	[ˈstɪərɔɪd]	甾体，甾族化合物，类固醇
steroidal	[stəˈrɔɪdəl]	甾体的，甾族化合物的，甾醇的
sterol	[ˈsterəul]	固醇，甾酮
stigmasterol	[stɪgˈmæstərɔl]	豆甾醇
strophanthidin	[strəuˈfænθɪdɪn]	毒毛旋花子苷元

(continued)

Strophanthus	[strəʊˈfænθəs]	羊角拗属
Strophanthus gratus		旋花羊角拗
T		
taurocholic acid	[tɔːrəˈkəʊlɪk][ˈæsɪd]	牛磺胆酸, 牛胆酸
telocinobufagin	[tiːləsɪnəˈbjuːfədʒɪn]	远华蟾毒基
thevetin	[ðeˈviːtɪn]	黄花夹竹桃苷
thevetose	[ðeviˈtəʊs]	黄花夹竹桃糖
triplet	[ˈtrɪplət]	三重峰
U		
ursodeoxycholic acid	[əːsɒdɪˌəʊksɪˈkəʊlɪk][ˈæsɪd]	熊去氧胆酸
V		
vicinal	[ˈvɪsɪnl]	邻近的
X		
xanthydrol	[ˈzænθɪdrɒl]	呫吨氢醇

重 点 小 结

　　甾类化合物为具有环戊烷骈多氢菲结构母核的化合物，可在无水条件、强酸作用下产生颜色变化，常用的试剂为醋酐 – 浓硫酸，即 Liebermann–Burchard 反应（L–B 反应）。甾类化合物根据其甾核 C_{17} 位取代基不同可将其分为甾体皂苷、强心苷、C_{21} 甾类、胆汁酸和植物甾醇等。其中甾体皂苷因理化性质及提取分离方法与三萜皂苷有相通之处，故在本书中将甾体皂苷和三萜皂苷合并为一章"皂苷"进行阐述。本章主要介绍强心苷、C_{21} 甾类、胆汁酸和植物甾醇。

　　强心苷为在甾核 C_{17} 位取代有不饱和内酯环的具有强心作用的甾体苷类，根据其不饱和内酯环的类型，分为强心甾烯（C_{17} 位为 $\Delta^{\alpha\beta}-\gamma$ 内酯环，甲型）和海葱甾或蟾蜍甾二烯（C_{17} 位为 $\Delta^{\alpha\beta,\ \gamma\delta}-\delta$ 内酯环，乙型）。强心苷结构中的糖除有六碳醛糖（如葡萄糖）和6- 去氧糖（如鼠李糖）外，还有 2, 6- 二去氧糖及其甲醚，因此强心苷也可根据苷元与糖的连接方式分为三种类型：Ⅰ型：苷元 –（2, 6- 二去氧糖）$_x$ –（α- 羟基糖）$_y$；Ⅱ型：苷元 –（6- 去氧糖）$_x$ –（α- 羟基糖）$_y$；Ⅲ型：苷元 –（α- 羟基糖）$_y$。强心苷的活性和毒性与其结构（如环的稠合方式、内酯环的有无及空间取向、角甲基的氧化程度等）密切相关。

　　强心苷的不饱和内酯环可在碱水中开环、酸化后环合；但在碱的醇溶液条件下，不饱和内酯环可发生异构化反应，强心甾烯类在此条件下发生双键异构化生成活性亚甲基，再与亚硝酰铁氰化钠（Legal 反应）或硝基苯类试剂生成有色产物，而海葱甾类在此条件下不产生活性亚甲基，故不发生上述颜色反应，因此 Legal 反应等可用以区分两种类型的强心苷。

　　2- 去氧糖的存在一方面影响强心苷酸水解的速率，连有 2- 去氧糖的强心苷可在温和条件下发生酸水解，而连有 2- 羟基糖的强心苷则需采用剧烈条件方可发生酸水解，此时苷元的叔醇羟基常脱水，故也可采用 HCl–acetone 法来进行苷键裂解反应；另一方面，2- 去氧糖可发生如 Keller–Kiliani（K–K）等一系列反应，因此这些反应可作为含有 2- 去氧糖的强心苷的检识反应。

　　强心苷的分离主要依靠吸附和分配色谱法。强心甾烯连有五元不饱和内酯环，故在 UV 中

λ_{max} 为 217nm；海葱甾连有六元不饱和内酯环，故 UV 中 λ_{max} 为 311nm。在 IR 谱中，不饱和内酯环在 1800~1700cm^{-1} 范围内有两个吸收峰，其中低波数的是内酯环羰基引起的吸收峰，称为正常峰；高波数的是非正常峰，其可随溶剂极性增强而减弱甚至消失。由于海葱甾连有六元不饱和内酯环，共轭体系更长，所以该类强心苷的两个吸收峰比强心甾类处于较低波数。此外，五元和六元不饱和内酯环的 NMR 特征明显，也可用于区分两种类型的强心苷。

胆汁酸是具有 24 个碳的甾醇酸类，在胆汁中以盐的形式存在。Pettenkofer 和 Gregory Pascoe 等反应可用于检识胆汁酸，其中后者用于检识生物样品中的胆汁酸更准确。

C_{21} 甾类是具有 21 个碳的甾类化合物，其在自然界既可以苷元的形式存在也可以苷的形式存在。C_{21} 甾苷类中 2- 去氧糖的存在使得部分 C_{21} 甾类 K-K 反应阳性。

植物甾醇在 C_{17} 的取代基为 8~10 个碳组成的烷烃链。植物甾醇主要以游离的形式存在，也可与长链脂肪酸成酯、与糖成苷、或与含长链脂肪酰基的糖成苷。

中药香加皮中含有 C_{21} 甾类和强心苷类化合物；蟾酥中含有具有强心活性的蟾蜍甾二烯类，但其在蟾酥中不是以苷的形式存在，而是通过 3-OH 与辛二酰精氨酸等结合成酯的形式存在；牛黄中含有胆汁酸类成分。

目 标 检 测

一、单选题

1. 属于甾体类化合物的是（   ）
   A. 蟾酥甾二烯　　　　　　　　　B. 达玛烷　　　　　　　　　　C. 羊毛脂醇
   D. 熊果酸　　　　　　　　　　　E. 薄荷醇

2. 属于强心甾型强心苷的是（   ）
   A. 蟾酥甾二烯　　　　　　　　　B. 海葱甾二烯　　　　　　　　C. 洋地黄毒苷
   D. 熊果酸　　　　　　　　　　　E. 龙胆苦苷

3. 属于 2- 去氧糖的是（   ）
   A. 葡萄糖　　　　　　　　　　　B. 鼠李糖　　　　　　　　　　C. 加拿大麻糖
   D. 呋糖　　　　　　　　　　　　E. 芸香糖

4. 属于 2,6- 二去氧糖的是（   ）
   A. 葡萄糖　　　　　　　　　　　B. 洋地黄糖　　　　　　　　　C. 洋地黄毒糖
   D. 呋糖　　　　　　　　　　　　E. 鼠李糖

5. 熊胆的特征性成分是（   ）
   A. 鹅去氧胆酸　　　　　　　　　B. 熊去氧胆酸　　　　　　　　C. 猪去氧胆酸
   D. 石胆酸　　　　　　　　　　　E. 胆酸

6. Ⅱ型强心苷的苷元和糖的连接方式是（   ）
   A. 苷元 –(D- 葡萄糖)$_x$
   B. 苷元 –(6- 去氧糖甲醚)$_x$–(D- 葡萄糖)$_y$
   C. 苷元 –(2,6- 二去氧糖)$_x$–(葡萄糖)$_y$
   D. 苷元 –(6- 去氧糖)$_x$–(葡萄糖)$_y$
   E. 苷元 –(D- 葡萄糖)$_x$–(6- 去氧糖)$_y$

7. 在温和酸水解的条件下，可水解的糖苷键是（　　　）

    A. 强心苷元 –2– 去氧糖   B. 2– 羟基糖 (1 → 4)-6– 去氧糖

    C. 强心苷元 –2– 羟基糖   D. 2– 羟基糖 (1 → 4)-2– 羟基糖

    E. 2– 羟基糖 (1 → 4)-2– 去氧糖

8. 蟾蜍甾型强心苷中 C_{17} 位上的取代基是（　　　）

    A. 醛基   B. 六元不饱和内酯环

    C. 糖链   D. 羧基

    E. 螺缩酮

9. 强心甾型强心苷的紫外最大吸收是在（　　　）

    A. 217~220nm   B. 270~280nm   C. 300~330nm

    D. 254~270nm   E. 360~415nm

10. 属于Ⅰ型强心苷的是（　　　）

    A. 苷元 –(D–葡萄糖)$_x$

    B. 苷元 –(6–去氧糖甲醚)$_x$–(D–葡萄糖)$_y$

    C. 苷元 –(2, 6–二去氧糖)$_x$–(葡萄糖)$_y$

    D. 苷元 –(6–去氧糖)$_x$–(葡萄糖)$_y$

    E. 苷元 –(D–葡萄糖)$_x$–(6–去氧糖)$_y$

二、多选题

1. 蟾酥中含有的强心苷类成分包括（　　　）

    A. 蟾酥甾二烯   B. 强心甾烯类   C. 蟾毒甾类

    D. 蟾毒萜类   E. 蟾毒色胺

2. 按苷元分类，强心苷包括（　　　）

    A. 强心甾类   B. 海葱甾类   C. Ⅰ型强心苷

    D. Ⅱ型强心苷   E. Ⅲ型强心苷

3. 强心苷常连接的糖包括（　　　）

    A. 2– 氨基糖   B. 2– 去氧糖   C. 6– 去氧糖

    D. 6– 羟基糖   E. 六碳醛糖

4. 在醇性氢氧化钠溶液中发生结构异构化的是（　　　）

    A. 强心甾型强心苷   B. 甾体皂苷

    C. 蟾蜍甾型强心苷   D. 植物甾醇

    E. 羊毛甾醇

5. 下列化合物属于甾体类的是（　　　）

    A. 甾体皂苷   B. 强心苷   C. 胆酸

    D. C_{21}– 甾   E. 羊毛脂甾醇

6. 能鉴别强心甾型强心苷的试剂是（　　　）

    A. 苦味酸   B. 3, 5– 二硝基苯甲酸

    C. 间二硝基苯   D. 氯化钠

    E. 亚硝酰铁氰化钠

7. 能鉴别强心甾型强心苷的反应是（　　　）

    A. Legal 反应   B. Feigl 反应   C. Kedde 反应

D. Bajiet 反应　　　　　　　　　　E. Raymond 反应

8. 能与呫吨氢醇反应的是（　　　）

　　A. 2- 去氧糖　　　　　　　　　　B. 2- 去氧糖苷

　　C. 所有强心甾型强心苷　　　　　　D. Ⅰ型强心苷

　　E. 2- 羟基糖

9. 能发生碱水解的是（　　　）

　　A. 强心甾型强心苷　　　　B. 海葱甾型强心苷　　　　C. 螺甾烷

　　D. 呋甾皂苷　　　　　　　E. 黄酮氧苷

10. 紫花洋地黄的温和酸水解产物为（　　　）

　　A. 苷元　　　　　　　　　B. 葡萄糖　　　　　　　　C. 洋地黄毒糖

　　D. 洋地黄双糖　　　　　　E. 加拿大麻糖

三、思考题

1. 请采用化学方法区分下列化合物

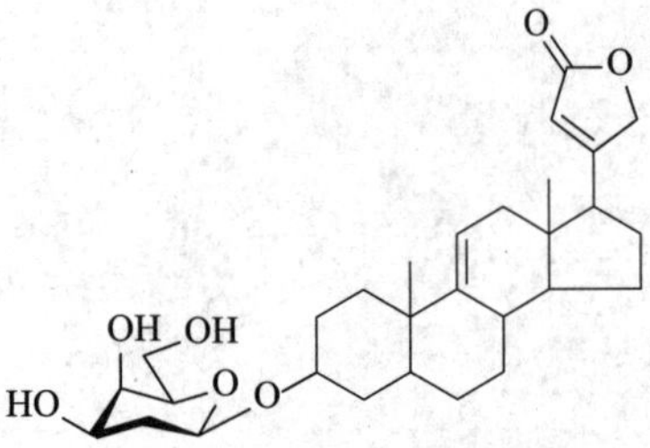

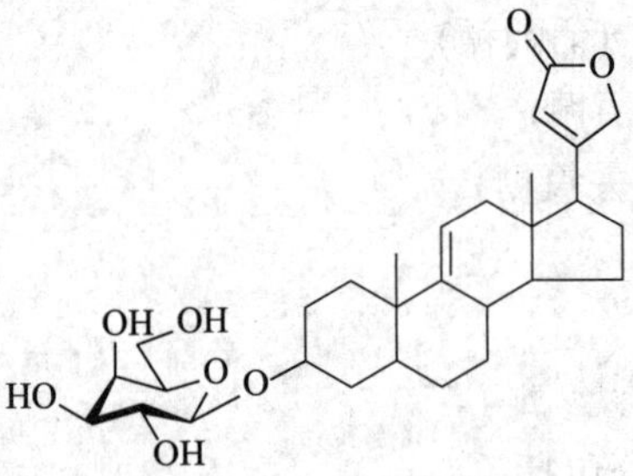

2. A、B、C、D 四个化合物均可以发生 L-B 反应，A 和 B 还可以发生 Raymond 反应，A 的 K-K 反应为阴性，B 的 K-K 反应为阳性，C 可以与 E 试剂反应，D 的 Gregory Pascoe 反应为阳性，试判断 A、B、C、D 四个化合物的类别，并说明理由。

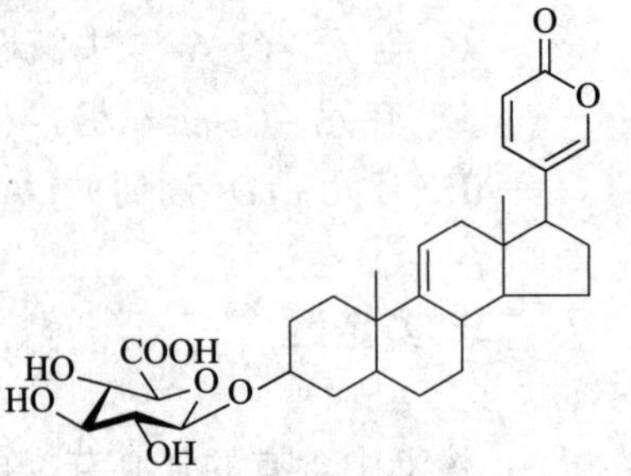

（曲　扬）

Chapter 10　Terpenoids and Volatile Oils

 学习目标

知识要求：

1. **掌握**　萜类化合物的定义及分类；萜类化合物的理化性质和检识；挥发油的定义、分类、理化性质及提取分离方法。

2. **熟悉**　萜类化合物的主要代表成分；挥发油类成分的鉴定。

3. **了解**　萜类化合物的结构测定方法和结构鉴定实例；青蒿和薄荷中主要活性成分的结构特征。

能力要求：

学会应用双键加成、羰基加成反应检识不饱和萜类化合物和含羰基的萜类化合物；学会根据具体萜类化合物和挥发油的结构特征及理化性质选择适合的提取分离方法，解决其在提取分离过程中存在的技术问题。

The term "terpenoid" (萜类) covers a large number of natural compounds and is used to mean that all these compounds have a common source of biosynthesis. Terpenoids are abundantly available in volatile oils (挥发油). Terpenoids and volatile oils are important raw materials in the daily chemical and pharmaceutical industries due to their special aroma. They also have a wide range of pharmacological effects such as antibacterial, irritating, deworming, diuretic, analgesic, anti-rheumatic, and anti-irritant. Therefore, in addition to the fragrances in the food and pharmaceutical industries, they are also used as insect repellents, pesticides, insecticides and deodorants.

1　Terpenoids

1.1　Introduction

Terpenoids may be defined as a large group of natural compounds: the derivatives of mevalonic acid (甲戊二羟酸，MVA). MVA is a key precursor in the biosynthetic pathway of terpenoids. Most of terpenoids have a general molecular formula $(C_5H_8)_n$, and their structure can be divided into isoprene units (异戊二烯单元). Therefore, terpenoids are also known as isoprenoids. In fact, these compounds are collectively called terpenes (萜烯). However, the -oid suffix is more logical than the -ene suffix, since the -ene suffix should be used for the unsaturated hydrocarbons.

A few hypotheses had been made paying attention to the biogenetic pathway of terpenoids, wherein two isoprene rules (异戊二烯法则) became dominant. One of them is "empirical isoprene rule" (经验异戊二烯法则) put forward by German Otto Wallach in 1887, which explained that terpenoids were derived from the ordered, non-head-to-tail or head-to-tail joining of isoprene units. However, with the discovery of new terpenoids, compounds *via* substantial structural rearrangements or loss of carbons during biosynthesis have been noticed. Realizing the limitation of empirical isoprene rule, Ruzicka put forward another hypothesis "biogenetic isoprene rule" (生源异戊二烯法则) in 1953, which was affirmed and accomplished as the main biogenetic pathway of terpenoids. As the latter rule described, although terpenoids are chemically built up from the union of isoprene units, isoprene is not the *in vivo* precursor. Instead, the compound actually involved is isopentenyl pyrophosphate (焦磷酸异戊烯酯，IPP), $CH_2=C(CH_3)CH_2CH_2OPP$, which is biosynthesized from acetate *via* MVA. IPP exists in living cells in equilibrium with the γ, γ-isomeric dimethylallyl pyrophosphate (焦磷酸 γ, γ-二甲基烯丙酯，DMAPP), $(CH_3)_2C=CHCH_2OPP$. Therefore, MVA is the biosynthesis precursor of terpenoids, and IPP and DMAPP are called active isoprene for their function of extending carbon chain during the biosynthesis of terpenoids. A brief demonstration of the biosynthesis of terpenoids is shown in Figure 10-1.

Terpenoids are widely found in nature, including higher plants, fungi (真菌), microorganisms, insects and marine organisms. And terpenoids are abundant in volatile oils and resins.

The structural diversity of terpenoids determines the various functions of terpenoids. Terpenoids play an important role in almost all basic processes of plant growth, development, reproduction, and defense. In addition, the role of terpenoids is not limited to nature. Many terpenoids also play an important role in human society. For example, many monoterpenes (单萜) and sesquiterpenes (倍半萜) are added as flavors to food, beverages, perfumes, soaps and other products. Some terpenes are used in industry as raw materials to make adhesives(黏合剂), coatings, emulsifiers (乳化剂) and specialty chemicals. Terpenoids are also widely used in the pharmaceutical industry. For example, camphor (樟脑) and borneol (龙脑), which belong to monoterpenoids, are used as cardiac stimulants in the clinic, and their effects are very significant. Artemisinin (青蒿素) separated from Artemisiae Annuae Herb (青蒿) is a highly effective and fast-acting antimalarial compound. It has been praised by WHO as "the only effective malaria treatment in the world at present". Paclitaxel（taxol, 紫杉醇）, a diterpene derivative (二萜类衍生物), is clinically used in the treatment of ovarian cancer, colorectal cancer, breast cancer and lung cancer with good curative effect.

1.2 Classification and Representatives of Terpenoids

Terpenoids are the largest secondary metabolites (次级代谢产物) in plants. More than 36, 000 terpenoids have been discovered, and new structures are increasing at a rate of about 1, 000 per year. Therefore, many terpenoids have different structures, showing hundreds of different carbon skeletons and different functional groups. In spite of such diversity, terpenoids are generally classified on the basis of isoprene units i.e. (C_5H_8) they contain (See Table 10-1).

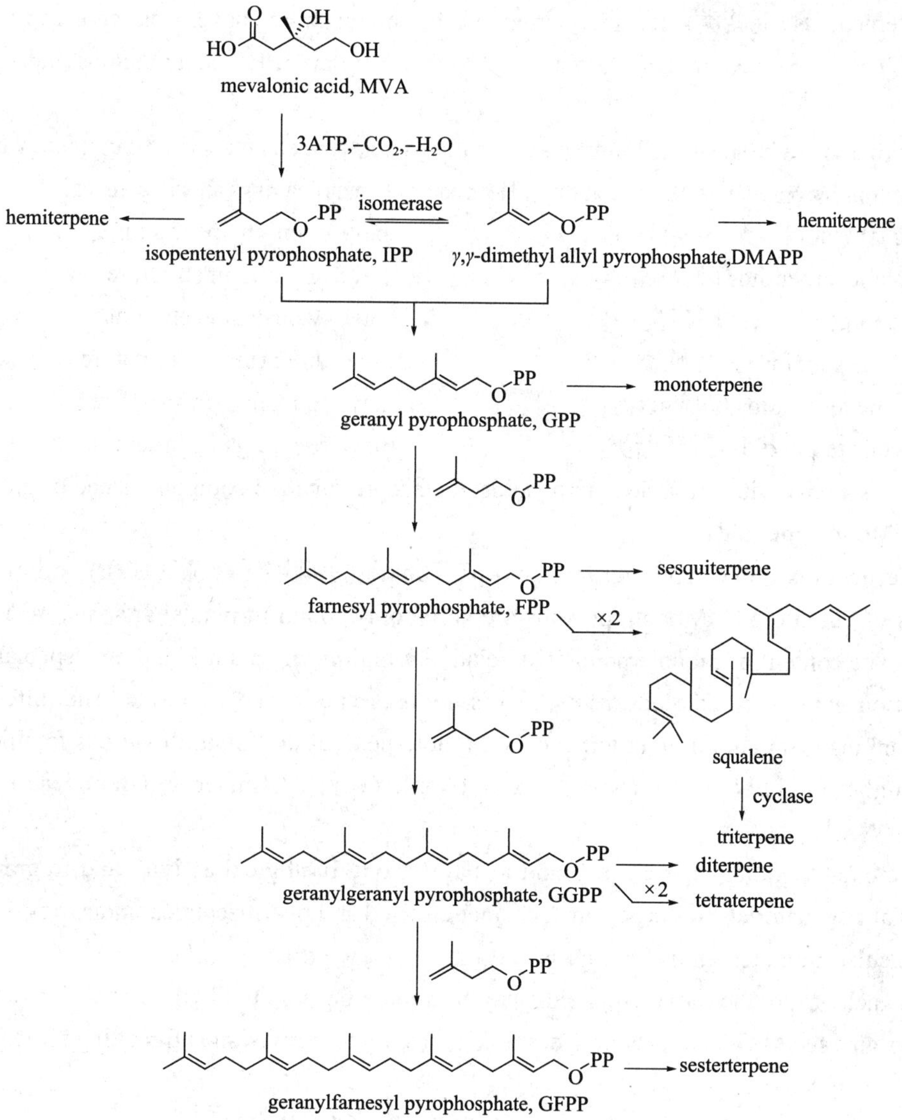

mevalonic acid, MVA

3ATP,–CO$_2$,–H$_2$O

hemiterpene ← isopentenyl pyrophosphate, IPP ⇌(isomerase) γ,γ-dimethyl allyl pyrophosphate,DMAPP → hemiterpene

geranyl pyrophosphate, GPP → monoterpene

farnesyl pyrophosphate, FPP ×2 → sesquiterpene

squalene

cyclase

triterpene
diterpene
tetraterpene

geranylgeranyl pyrophosphate, GGPP ×2

geranylfarnesyl pyrophosphate, GFPP → sesterterpene

Figure 10-1   Biosynthesis of terpenoids

Table 10-1   Classification of terpenoids

Categories	No. of isoprene units	Carbon atoms	Distribution
hemiterpene (半萜)	1	5	Woody plants
monoterpenes	2	10	Volatile oils
sesquiterpenes	3	15	Volatile oils
diterpenes (二萜)	4	20	Resins, plant latex, woody plants
sesterterpenes (二倍半萜)	5	25	Marine organism, microorganism, insects
triterpenes (三萜)	6	30	All parts of plants, resins, plant latex
tetraterpenes (四萜)	8	40	Pigments
polyterpenes (多萜)	>8	>40	Rubber

All of the above terpenoids are derived from isoprene units. In nature, few chemicals are composed of both isoprenoid and non-isoprene (非异戊二烯). And these compounds have professional names called meroterpenoids (混萜类). The meroterpenoids of natural source have been reported relatively rare, such as quinine, tea benzoquinone(vitamin K), tocopherol (vitamin E), cannabinoids and various ergot alkaloids.

Terpenoids also can be subdivided and named according to the type and number of rings (except hemiterpene). The number of rings is only limited to carbon rings. Heteroatom-containing rings are not counted.

Acyclic terpenoids (无环萜类)	have open-chain structure
Monocyclic terpenoids (单环萜类)	have one ring in structure
Bicyclic terpenoids (二环萜类)	have two rings in structure
Tricyclic terpenoids (三环萜类)	have three rings in structure
Tetracyclic terpenoids (四环萜类)	have four rings in structure
Pentacyclic terpenoids (五环萜类)	have five rings in structure

Next gives an overview of various terpenoids, their representative compounds and original herbs.

1.2.1 Monoterpenoids

Monoterpenoids come from geranyl pyrophosphate (焦磷酸香叶酯，GPP) and are important components of volatile oils. Monoterpenoids are commonly found in plants, animals, microorganisms, and insects. The content of monoterpenoids is relatively high in the plant kingdom, especially in higher plants and their parts, such as seeds, roots, leaves, inflorescence, heartwood, etc. And different parts of the same plant may contain different terpenoids. Monoterpenoids are found in various families, and their content is higher in Umbelliferae (伞形科), Camphorae (樟科), Lamiaceae, Gramineae (禾本科) and Myrtle (桃金娘科).

Many monoterpenoids have been found to have strong biological activity and fragrance, making them essential raw materials in the perfume, cosmetics, food and pharmaceutical industries.

In particular, monoterpenoids are classified into four categories: acyclic, monocyclic, bicyclic, and tricyclic. In each group, the monoterpenoids may be simple unsaturated hydrocarbons or they may have functional groups such as alcohols, aldehydes or ketones. Further division and relating representatives are summarized in Table 10-2.

Table 10-2　Types and examples of monoterpenoids

Type	Examples	Remarks
Acyclic monoterpenoids		
myrceane（月桂烷）	geraniol（香叶醇）　nerol（橙花醇）　citronellol（香茅醇）	Rose materials in perfumery industry
	geranial（香叶醛）　neral（橙花醛）	Lemon materials in perfumery industry

(continued)

Type	Examples	Remarks
Monocyclic monoterpenoids		
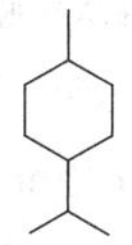 *p*-menthane （对–薄荷烷型）	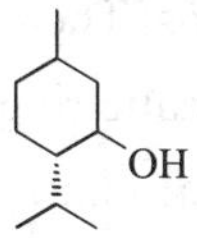 menthol（薄荷醇） 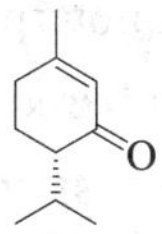　piperitone（胡椒酮） 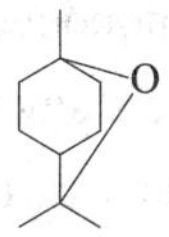　eucalyptol（桉油精）	Menthol is the main constituent of mint oil possessing weak analgesia, itching relieving and cooling effects Eucalyptol is the domain component of eucalyptus oil and used as antiseptics
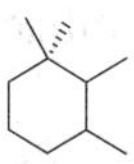 cyclogeraniane （环香叶烷型）	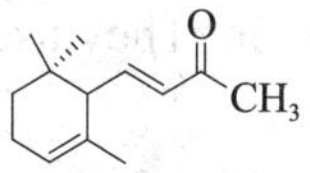 α-ionone（α–紫罗兰酮） 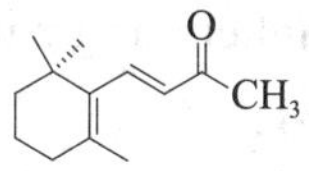　β-ionone（β–紫罗兰酮）	The former is used as perfume, while the latter is the material for synthesis of vitamin A. Dihydro-α-ionone exists in ambergris as precious perfume
irregular cases	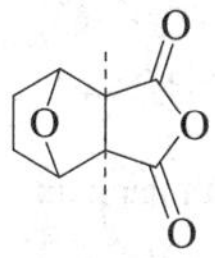 cantharidin（斑蝥素） 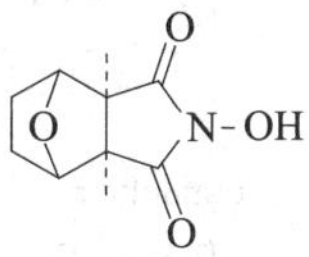　N–hydroxy-cantharidimide（N–羟斑蝥胺）	Cantharidin is the toxic agent causing dermatitis in mylabris. Its derivative *N*-hydroxy-cantharidimide shows effect on hepatocarcinoma
Bicyclic monoterpenoids		
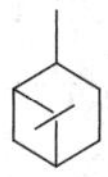 pinane （蒎烷型）	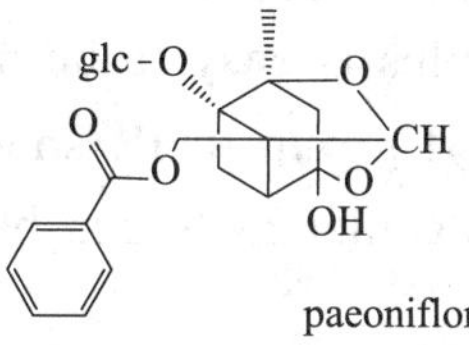 paeoniflorin（芍药苷）	It coexists in the root of *Paeonia albiflora* (白芍) with other analogs possessing sedation, analgesia and anti-inflammation activities
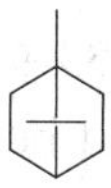 camphane （莰烷型）	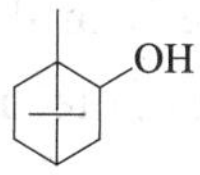 borneol 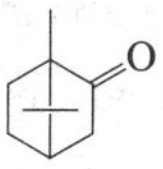　camphor	The synthetic borneol is racemic mixture and widely used in perfume, refrigerant and Chinese patent medicine
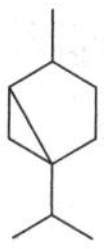 thujane （守烷）	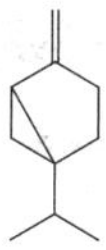 sabinene（桧烯）	It exists in the volatile oil of *Juniperus sabina* (刺柏)
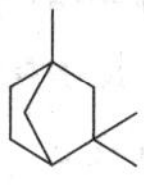 fenchane （葑烷型）	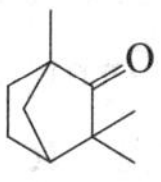 fenchone（葑酮）	It is abundant in the volatile oil of fruits of *Foeniculum vulgare* (茴香)
Tricyclic monoterpenoids		
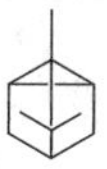 tricyclane （三环烷型）	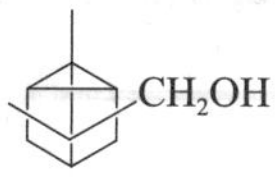 teresantalol（三环白檀醇）	It exists in the volatile oil of wood part of *Santalum album* (白檀)

337

Tropolonoids (草酚酮) and iridoids (环烯醚萜) are irregular monoterpenoids with certain special characteristics.

(1) Tropolonoids

Tropolonoids are a class of deformed monocyclic monoterpenoids. Their carbon framework does not comply with the isoprene law, and they have a seven-membered aromatic ring in the structure. Therefore, the hydroxyl and the carbonyl at the aromatic ring possess general characteristics as other phenolic hydroxyl and carbonyl respectively.

Tropolonoids restrictively distribute in some fungi, and are also found in the heartwood of Cupressaceae, such as α-thujaplicin，β-thujaplicin and γ-thujaplicin. They usually have antibacterial and anti-tumor activities. Meanwhile, they are toxic.

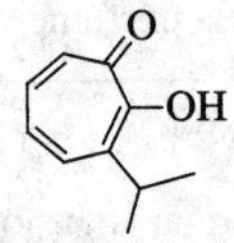

α-thujaplicin
（α-崖柏素）

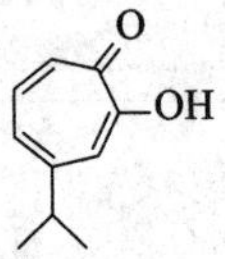

β-thujaplicin
（β-崖柏素）

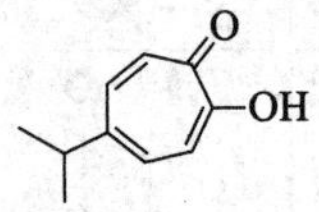

γ-thujaplicin
（γ-崖柏素）

Tropolonoids also have some special characteristics:

① The hydroxyl group on the ring shows acidity, and the acidity is between phenols and carboxylic acids. The hydroxyl group in molecules is easy to be methylated, but not easy to be acetylated. The absorption peak of the hydroxyl group in IR spectrum locates in the range of $3100\sim3200cm^{-1}$ due to the formation of intra-molecular hydrogen-bond (分子内氢键) between the hydroxyl and the carbonyl.

② The carbonyl group in the molecule is similar to the carbonyl group in a carboxylic acid, but cannot react with general carbonyl reagents. The absorption peak of the carbonyl in IR spectrum is in the range of $1600-1650cm^{-1}$ because of the formation of intra-molecular hydrogen-bond between the hydroxyl and the carbonyl.

③ Due to aromaticity, tropolonoids can form complex crystals with a variety of metal ions and show different colors, which can be used for identification. For example, copper complexes (铜络合物) are green crystals, and iron complexes (铁络合物) are red crystals.

(2) Iridoids

Iridoids are a class of derivatives of iridodial (臭蚁二醛) formed by the condensation of hydroxyl aldehydes within the molecule. Iridodial is derived from GPP, so it belongs to monoterpenoids. GPP is gradually converted into iridodial in the plant, and then forms iridoids. After the formation of iridoids, its C_4-methyl group is oxidized and decarboxylated (脱羧) to form 4-demethyliridoids（4-去甲基环烯醚萜）. The C_7-C_8 bond is broken to open the ring to form secoiridoids (裂环环烯醚萜). Iridoids, secoiridoids and 4-demethyliridoids are often combined with saccharides to form glycosides. Its biosynthetic pathway is shown in Figure 10-2. Therefore, iridoids comprise three main subtypes: iridoids, secoiridoids and 4-demethyliridoids.

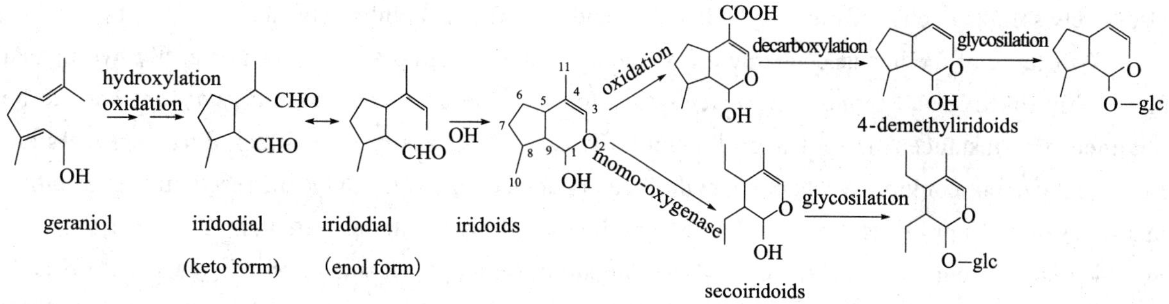

Figure 10-2　Biosynthesis of iridoid system

Iridoids are widely distributed in nature. Plant families such as Labiatae, especially Phlomis Linn (糙苏属), Stachys Linn (鼠尾草属) and Eremostachys Bunge Linn (沙穗属), Gentianaceae, Valerianaceae (败酱科) and Oleaceae, are rich sources of iridoid glycosides.

In the vast majority of natural iridoids, the hydroxyl on C-1 is usually involved in the formation of the glycoside. The double bond between C-3 and C-4 and the carboxylation of C-11 are very common. The various carbons in iridoid skeletons changing in substituents are found in nature, as displayed below.

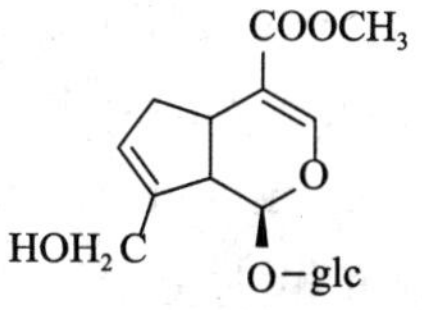

genipin-1-*O*-gentiobioside
（京尼平苷）

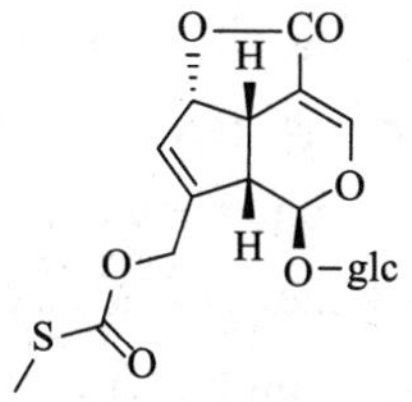

paederoside
（鸡屎藤苷）

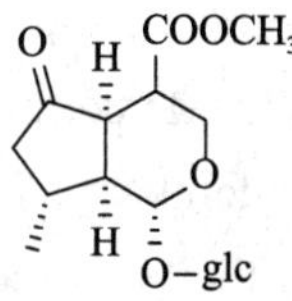

verbenalin
（马鞭草苷）

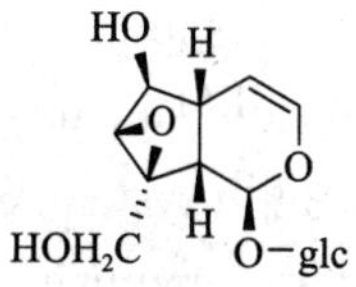

catalpol
（梓醇苷）

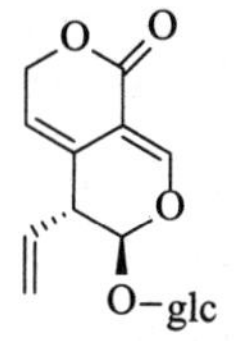

gentiopicroside
（龙胆苦苷）

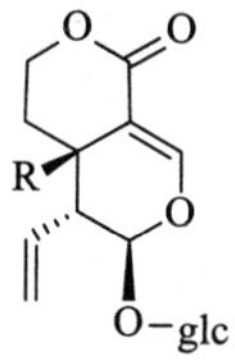

sweroside　R=H
（獐牙菜苷）

swertiamarin　R=OH
（獐牙菜苦苷）

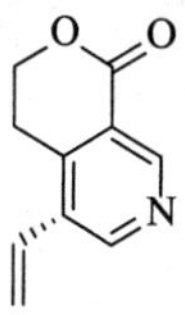

gentianine
（龙胆碱）

Other iridoids are intermediates in the biosynthesis of the indole alkaloids after the oxygen atom at 2-position was replaced by a nitrogen atom. For example, the gentianine, the product converted from gentiopicroside by reacting with ammonia (Figure 10-3).

On account of the special structure, iridoids show corresponding special characteristics as:

① Iridoids are mostly white crystals or powder, optical active and bitter.

② Not only are iridoid-glycosides easily soluble in water and methanol, soluble in ethanol, acetone and n-butanol, but

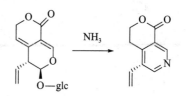

Figure 10-3　Convertion of gentiopicroside

339

also barely soluble in chloroform, ethyl ether, benzene and other lipophilic solvents.

③ Because of the hemiacetal structure of the aglycone, iridoid-glycosides can be easily hydrolyzed and highly reactive and prone to polymerization further. Therefore, aglycone crystals are hard to be obtained. For instance, the root of Rehmanniae Radix (地黄) easily turns black during precession. Because the major compound catalpol is hydrolyzed to aglycone, and the aglycone reacts further resulting in a series of black products. And it is the same as the root of Scrophulariae Radix (玄参).

④ Many regents like bases, carboxylic compounds, amino acids and so on can react with iridoids to produce different colors because of the reactivity of iridoid aglycones. It can be used to identify the existence of iridoids.

1.2.2　Sesquiterpenoids

Sesquiterpenoids are composed of three isoprene units. Therefore, they are C_{15} compounds and biosynthesized from farnesyl pyrophosphate(焦磷酸金合欢酯). They often coexist with monoterpenoids in volatile oils that the major components have a higher boiling range (250–280℃). Most of the oxygen-containing derivatives of sesquiterpenoids have strong fragrance and bioactivities. It leads them to be important materials in pharmaceutical, food and cosmetic industries. Sesquiterpenoids have a wide occurrence in nature which mainly exists in plants and microorganisms. The carbon skeleton of sesquiterpenoids has highly diverse forms compared to other terpenoids. As a consequence, the numbers of sesquiterpenoids are the top in terpenoids. Because of the remarkable biological activity, sesquiterpenoid lactones are considered more significant. They contain the α-methylene-γ-lactone (α- 亚甲基 -γ- 内酯) system. Some members of sesquiterpenoid lactones contain α,β-unsaturated carbonyls and epoxides (e.g. artemisinin). Further classification of sesquiterpenes is shown in Table 10-3.

Table 10-3　Types and examples of sesquiterpenoids

Type	Examples	Remarks
Acyclic sesquiterpenoids		
	farnesane （金合欢烯） farnesol （金合欢醇）	It is important materials in top-class perfume
Monocyclic sesquiterpenoids		
	bisabolane （没药烷） artemisinin	The major effective constituent of Artemisiae Annuae Herb has extremely remarkable anti-malaria activity, wherein the peroxide group is the pharmacophore
	germacrane （吉马烷） germacrone （吉马酮）	The active component of *Geranium macrorrhizum* (大根老鹳草) and (兴安杜鹃) act to calm panting and suppress cough

(continued)

Type	Examples	Remarks
Bicyclic sesquiterpenoids		
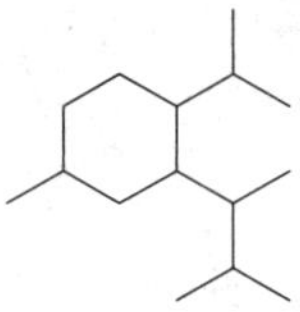 cadinane（杜松烷） gossypol（棉酚）	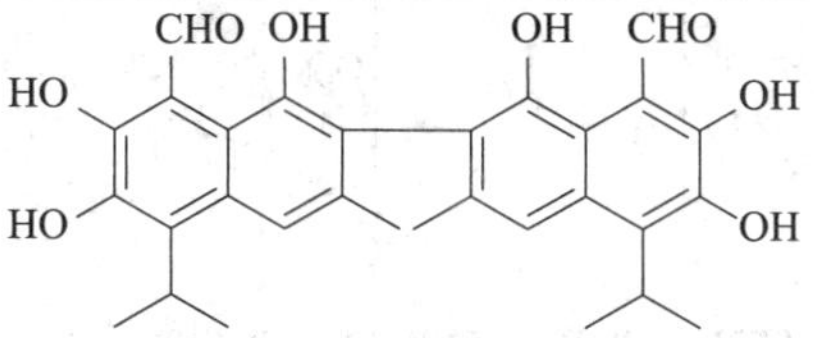	The male contraceptive principle in the seeds of cotton can alter sperm maturation, spermatozoid motility, and inactivation of sperm enzymes which is necessary for fertilization
Tricyclic sesquiterpenoids		
	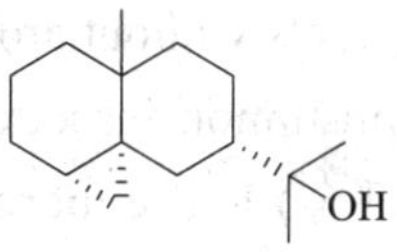 cycloeudesmol（环桉醇） 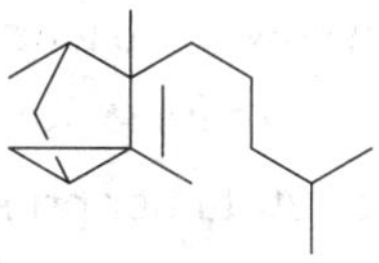　α-santalane（α−白檀醇） 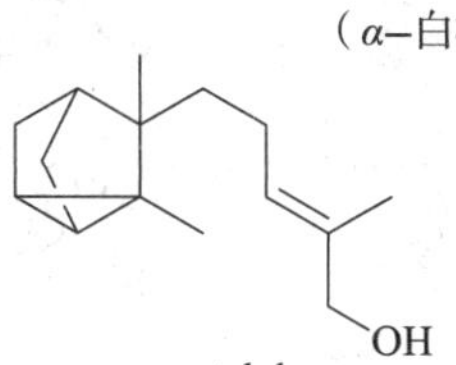　α-santalol	All the three compounds have strong antibacterial activity

Among bicyclic sesquiterpenoids fused by a five-membered ring and a seven-membered ring, aromatic derivatives can be deemed to the fusion of cyclopentadiene anion and cycloheptatriene cation which belongs to non-benzene aromatics called azulenoids (薁类化合物).

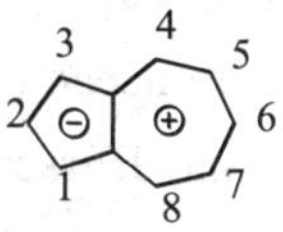

azulenoids 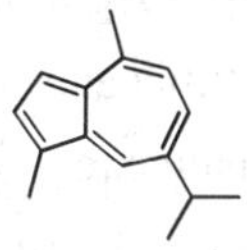　　　guaiazule

Azulenoids such as guaiazule (愈创木薁), have the following characteristics:

① Azulenoids has a high boiling point, usually at 250–300℃. During the volatile oils fractional distillation, blue, purple, or green fractions are sometimes seen at high boiling points, suggesting the possible presence of Azulenoids.

② Azulenoids are insoluble in water. But they are soluble in organic solvents and strong acids (formation of acid adducts, see Figure 10-4), and precipitate after diluted with water. Therefore, 60%–65% sulphuric acid or phosphoric acid (磷酸) may be employed as extract solvents.

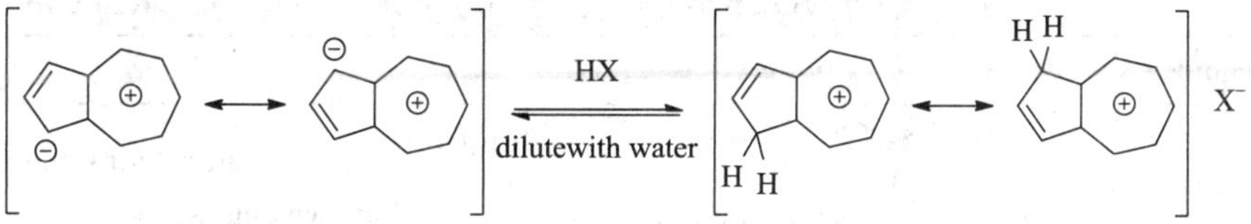

HX / dilute with water

Figure 10-4　Formation of acid adducts of azulenoids

341

③ Azulenoids can form **π**-complex (π-络合物) crystals with picric acid or trinitrobenzene reagent. The π-complex has sharp melting point. It may be used for the identification of azulenoids (Figure 10-5).

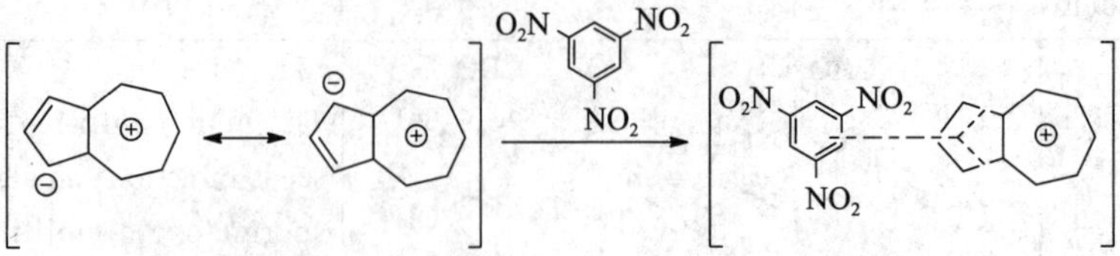

Figure 10-5　Formation of π-complex of azulenoids

④ Azulenoids have strong absorption peak within visible area 400~700nm because of the high conjugation system.

In Chinese herbs, azulenoids are mostly hydrogenated products without aromaticity and possess the structure of guaiane. Azulenoids mostly show antibacterial, anti-tumor, insecticide and other activities. For instance, curcumol (姜黄醇) from Curcumae Radix (郁金) and euparotin (泽兰苦内酯) from *Eupatorium rotundifolium* (圆叶泽兰) are anti-tumor principles.

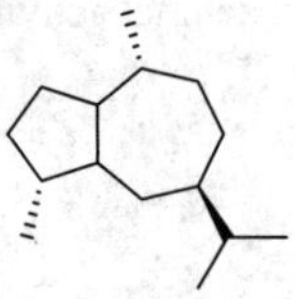

guaiane
（愈创木烷）

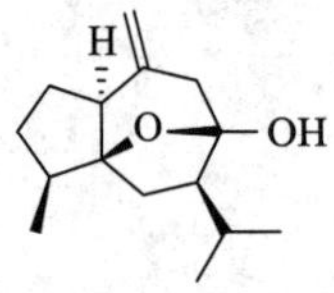

curcumol

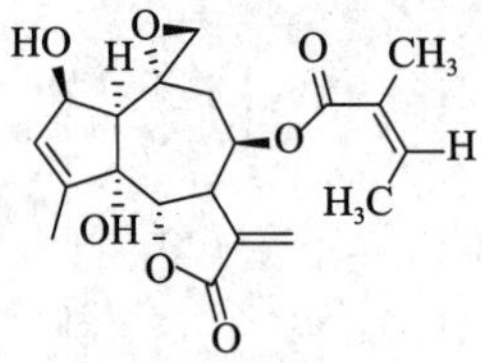

euparotin

1.2.3　Diterpenoids

Diterpenoids are C_{20} compounds including four isoprene units. Contrasting to mono or sesquiterpenoids，they are non-volatile in nature. These C_{20} natural compounds are biosynthetically originated from geranylgeranyl pyrophosphate (焦磷酸香叶基香叶酯). They exist in higher plants, fungi, insects and marine organisms. Pinaceae, Podosocarpaceae (鬼芋科) and Taxodiaceae (红豆杉科) (all conifer resins); Leguminosae, Cistaceae (茜草科) and Burseraceae (藜科) (all angiosperm resins) are the plant families rich in diterpenoids. Labiatae, Ranunculaceae and Euphorbiaceae (大戟科) are the other families containing substantial quantities of diterpenoids. They have also been found in marine animals (Coelenterates) like soft corals and sea fans. The same plant may contain different diterpenoids in different parts. The content of diterpenoids varies along with seasons.

Most of diterpenoids are considered as the defense chemicals against parasites and mechanical injury. Besides these activities, some diterpenoids have important pharmacological activities, such as taxol, gingkgolides (银杏内酯), andrographolide (穿心莲内酯), triptolide (雷公藤内酯) and so on. The examples of different types of diterpenoids are listed in Table 10-4.

Table 10-4　Types and examples of diterpenoids

Types	Examples	Remarks
Acyclic diterpenoids		
	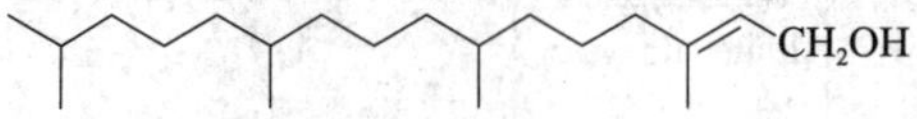 phytol (植物醇)	It is the material for synthesis of vitamin E and vitamin K_1

(continued)

Types	Examples	Remarks
Monocyclic diterpenoids		
	vitamin A (维生素A)	Animal-origin foods such as liver, meat, egg, etc. are rich in sources of vitamin A, wherein fish liver oil is the material for manufacture of natural vitamin A
Bicyclic diterpenoids		
labdane (半日花烷)	andrographolide	It is the major anti-inflammatory component of Andrographis Herbato treating diarrhea, gastroenteritis, pharyngolaryngitis, fever and so on
	ginkgolide A R_1 OH R_2 H R_3 H ginkgolide B OH OH H ginkgolide C OH OH OH ginkgolide J OH H OH ginkgolide M H OH OH (银杏内酯 A、B、C、M、J)	Ginkgolides are strong bitter principles of the root bark and leaves of *Ginkgo biloba* (银杏). They usually coexist with total flavonoids in the formulation of leaves of *Ginkgo biloba* to treat heart and cerebral vascular diseases
Tricyclic diterpenoids		
abietane (松香烷)	R_1 R_2 R_3 triptolide H H CH_3 (雷公藤甲素) tripdiolide OH H CH_3 (雷公藤乙素) triptolidenol H OH CH_3 (雷公藤内酯) 16-hydroxytriptolide H H CH_2OH (16-羟基雷公藤内酯醇)	Among the four antitumor constituents isolated from *Tripterygium wilfordii* (雷公藤), triptolide is active against breast cancer and gastric cancer; 16-hydroxytriptolide shows potent anti-inflammation, immune inhibition and male contraception activities

(continued)

Types	Examples	Remarks
taxane (紫杉烷)	taxol baccatin Ⅲ R = Ac （巴卡亭Ⅲ） 10-deacetylbaccatin Ⅲ R = H （10– 脱乙酰基巴卡亭 Ⅲ）	Taxol is one of the most successful anticancer drugs in modern times. It is isolated from the bark of *Taxus brevifolia* (红豆杉）(Taxaceae). Both the four-membered oxetane ring and the complex ester side-chain in the structure are pharmacophores. Due to the low content (ca. 0.01%–0.02%) and the slow growth of the bark, semi-synthesis from more accessible structurally related materials, such as baccatin Ⅲ and 10-deacetylbaccatin Ⅲ is currently exploited for the supply of taxol and derivatives for drug use

Tetracyclic diterpenoids

Types	Examples	Remarks
kaurane （贝壳杉烷）	stevioside (甜菊苷）	Stevioside isolated from the leaves of *Stevia rebaudianum* (甜菊) is of high saccharinity, 300 fold of sucrose and widely employed as a sweetening agent. However, owing to the carcinogenic effect, it has been forbidden to use in Western countries
phorbane （大戟烷）	phorbol （大戟醇）	The cocarcinogenic activity of phorbol consists in its diester derivatives of the two corresponding hydroxyls at C_{12} and C_{13}, wherein one ester is formed by a long-chain fatty acid, while the other is comprised of a short-chain fatty acid
grayanotoxane （木藜芦毒烷）	rhomotoxin （八厘麻毒素）	It exists in the seeds of *Rhododendron japonicum* (日本杜鹃) and possesses hypotension effect on severe hypertension and bradycardic effect on supraventricular tachycardia

1.2.4   Sesterterpenoids

The skeleton of sesterterpenoids has 25 carbons including five isoprene units. The biosynthetic precursor is geranylfarnesyl pyrophosphate (焦磷酸香叶基金合欢酯). They are discovered mainly in fungi, bracken fern(蕨类), lichens (地衣), insects and marine organisms(海洋生物). The first sesterterpenoid was discovered in 1965. The number of sesterterpenoids is the minimum among terpenoids so far.

Furanspongin-3 (呋喃海绵素–3) is a chain sesterterpenoid isolatted from the sponge. Ophiobolin A (蛇孢假壳素 A), the tricyclic sesterterpenoid separated from fungi *Ophiobulus miyabeanus* (芝麻枯) shows a wide spectrum of biological activities against bacteria, fungi and nematodes.

furanspongin-3

ophiobolin A

1.3   Physical and Chemical Properties

1.3.1   Physical Properties

Monoterpenoids and sesquiterpenoids are mainly oily liquids at room temperature, rarely crystals. They are mostly volatile and have a specific aroma. Since monoterpenoids and sesquiterpenoids are volatile, they can be extracted by steam distillation. However, diterpenoids and sesterterpeniods usually exist in the form of crystals at room temperature and are not volatile. Terpenoid glycosides are generally crystals or powder without volatility.

Because most terpenoids have strong bitterness, they are an important part of the early so-called "bitterness principle" (苦味原则). But a few terpenoids have sweet taste, such as stevioside.

Terpenoids contain chiral carbons in their structure, so they usually have optical activity.

Terpenoids are generally lipophilic, insoluble in water, soluble in methanol and ethanol, and easily soluble in lipophilic organic solvents such as ethyl acetate, ethyl ether, chloroform and benzene. Terpenoids containing carboxyl, phenolic hydroxyl and lactone are soluble in alkaline solution, such as $NaHCO_3$ and NaOH, and can be precipitated in acidic solution or soluble in lipophilic organic solvents. Therefore, this property can be used for extraction and separation.

The terpenoids glycosides are generally more polar and less soluble in lipophilic organic solvents, soluble in hot water, and easily soluble in methanol and ethanol.

From the practical point of view, it must be remembered that both isomerization (异构化) and structural re-arrangement (结构重排) of the molecule may occur quite readily under relatively mild conditions and artifact formation is always possible during extraction and isolation procedures.

1.3.2   Chemical Properties

Terpeniods with different functional groups may react accordingly. For example, terpenoids containing carbonyl (aldehydes or ketones) or double bonds (双键) may react with related reagents. And terpenoids containing hydroxyl may undergo oxidation or dehydration (脱水) reactions. In addition, during the course of the above reactions, the re-arrangement reaction (重排反应) may also occur simultaneously. The addition reaction (加成反应) is briefly introduced here. Because these products are easy to crystallize, they can be used for separation or purification, providing unsaturation for preliminary identification and preparation. These products can also be used to prepare the required derivatives.

(1) Addition to Double Bond

① Hydrogen halide (卤化氢)

The addition reaction of β-cadinene (β– 杜松烯) is shown in Figure 10-6.

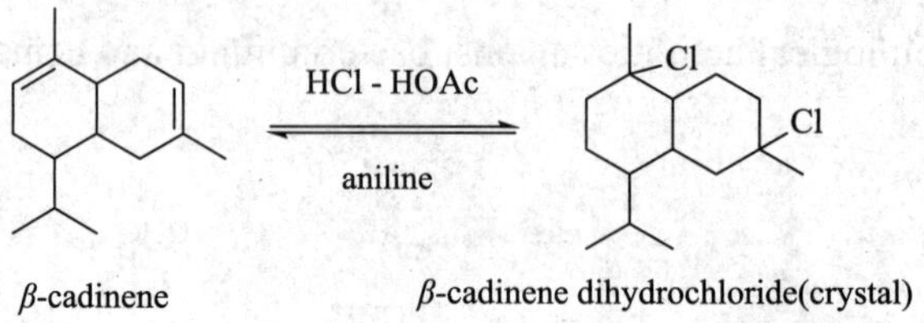

β-cadinene   β-cadinene dihydrochloride(crystal)

Figure 10-6　Addition of hydrogen halide to double bond

② Bromine

The addition reaction of bromine to double bond is shown in Figure 10-7.

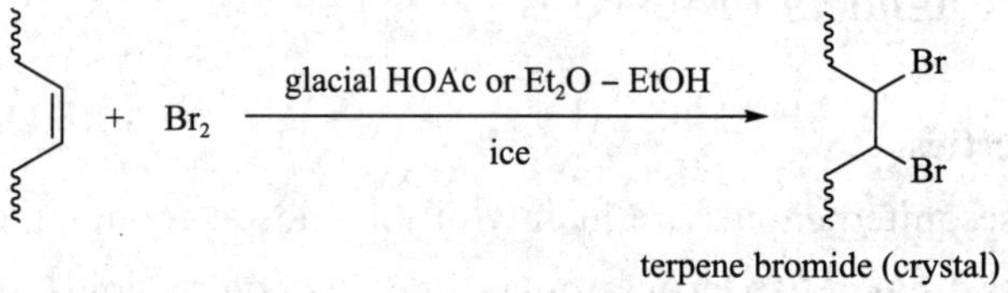

terpene bromide (crystal)

Figure 10-7　Addition of bromine to double bond

③ Nitrosyl chloride (亚硝酰氯) (Tilden reagent)

The addition reaction of nitrosyl chloride to double bond is shown in Figure 10-8.

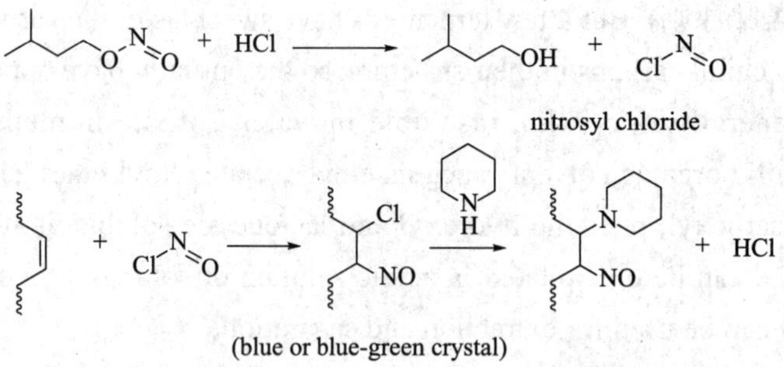

nitrosyl chloride

(blue or blue-green crystal)

Figure 10-8　Addition of nitrosyl chloride to double bond

④ Diels-Alder Reaction（Diels-Alder 反应）

The Diel-Alder reaction of conjugated double bonds is shown in Figure 10-9.

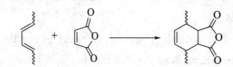

Figure 10-9　Diels-Alder reaction of conjugated double bonds

(2) Carbonyl Reactions

① Sodium Hydrosulphite (亚硫酸氢钠)

The addition reaction of carbonyl with sodium hydrosulphite is shown in Figure 10-10.

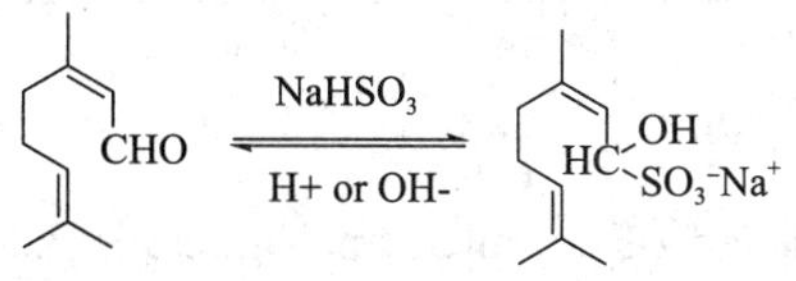

citral

Figure 10-10　Addition of carbonyl with sodium hydrosulphite

When the addition reaction is carried out for a long time or at high temperature, the reaction is irreversible, and other double bonds may also participate in the addition reaction. Therefore, we should pay attention to the control of reaction conditions.

② Girard reagent (吉拉德试剂)

Girard reagent is a type of hydrazide (酰肼) with a quaternary ammonium group (季铵基团)，and commonly used in two forms, Girard T and Girard P. The addition reactions of carbonyl with Girard reagents are shown in Figure 10-11.

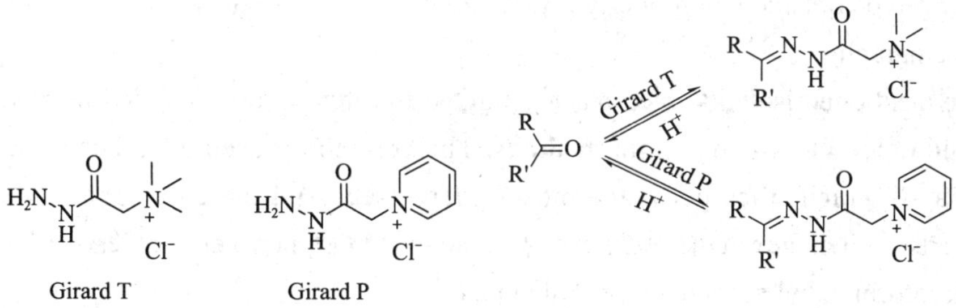

Girard T　　　　　Girard P

Figure 10-11　Addition of carbonyl with Girard reagents

1.4　Extraction and Isolation Methods

1.4.1　Extraction Methods

The extraction of terpenoids from Chinese herbs is usually based on their solubility, volatility and functional group activity. It should be noted that many external factors such as light, heat, acid, alkali and so on may cause the degradation of terpenoids.

Most of the terpenoids are extracted by methanol or ethanol, and then partitioned with various organic solvents. Except solvent extraction (溶剂萃取), steam distillation and supercritical fluid extraction are widely used for the extraction of volatile terpenoids. As regard to lipid-rich (富含油脂) or chlorophyll-rich materials, defatting with petroleum ether before extraction or after alcohol extract may be employed. Dissolve the alcohol extract in alkaline solution and precipitate with acid which may be executed in the refinement of terpenoid lactones (萜内酯), but those sensitive compounds to alkaline or acid are not appropriate to this method. The literature reports that abundant terpenoid lactones are found in petroleum ether-ethyl ether (1：1) eluent.

The extraction of terpenoid glycosides usually uses aqueous methanol or ethanol. Lipophilic impurities (脂溶性杂质) in the alcohol extract can be removed by ethyl ether, chloroform or petroleum ether. Hydrophilic impurities (水溶性杂质) can be removed with n-butanol, activated carbon or macroporous resin column after defatting. During the extraction and purification of terpene glycosides，it is necessary to prevent the cleavage of glycosidic linkages by enzymes and acids, especially the poor stability of iridoid glycosides.

1.4.2　Isolation Methods

Terpenoids are usually composed of complex analogues. In addition, isomerization often occurs in terpenoids. And it is possible to isolate pairs of isomers (such as geraniol and nerol) from plants. Therefore, the separation of terpeniods is difficult. And the separation of terpenoids can achieve better results by combining a variety of isolation methods.

(1) Isolation based on specific groups

The common specific groups in terpenoids include double bond, carbonyl, lactone, carboxyl, hydroxyl, and so on. The unsaturated hydrocarbons can be conveniently separated as their crystalline addition products with hydrochloric acid (盐酸) or hydrobromic acid (氢溴酸), or nitrosyl chloride.

(2) Crystallization

The purity of some crude extracts of terpenoids is significantly improved after appropriate treatment. For example, in the preparation of menthol, camphor and tangerine flower lactone, a single compound with high purity can be obtained by properly crystallizing the crude product.

(3) Chromatography

The above mentioned isolation methods are limited to a few terpenoids, and most separation relies on effective and quick chromatographic methods. The commonly used adsorbents are silica gel and neutral alumina, of which silica gel is the most widely used. And the corresponding eluents include lipophilic solvents such as hexane (己烷), cyclohexane (环己烷), petroleum ether, or their mixture with ethyl ether, chloroform, ethyl acetate, or even alcohols.

Another modification method is to separate terpeniods according to the number and position of double bonds. This method is using 2.5% silver nitrate solution (硝酸银溶液，$AgNO_3$) treated silica gel or aluminum. The mechanism mainly relies on the formation of a π-complex between the double bond and $AgNO_3$. Therefore, its mechanism of action depends on the number, position and conformation of the double bonds. The adsorption rules are summarized as below:

① More double bonds in π-complex, more stable, namely triene (三烯) > diene (双烯) > monoene (单烯) > saturated hydrocarbon (饱和烃).

② The conjugate degree of double bonds depends on the stability of π-complex. The π-complex with long conjugated system is more stable.

③ The π-complex with exocyclic double bond is more stable than that with intra-cyclic double bond.

④ The stability of π-complex decreases with terminal double bond, Z-double bond, and E-double bond.

⑤ The compounds without double bond have strong adsorption with high polarity.

HPLC or GC can be used for the final separation of terpenoids. For example, the separation of iridoids can be performed by HPLC or GC.

1.5　Identification

1.5.1　Physicochemical Identification

Specific reactions can be used to prove the presence or absence of certain terpenoids.

(1) Troponoids

They react positively with 1% Ferric chloride solution and dilute copper sulfate solution. However, the reaction results of other phenolic compounds are similar. Therefore, it is necessary to confirm the presence of tropolonoids together with other methods such as volatility and IR spectrum.

(2) Iridoids

They react positively with Trim-Hill reagent (10ml acetic acid, 1ml 0.2% $CuSO_4 \cdot 5H_2O$ in water and 0.5ml con. HCl) and Shear reagent (con. HCl∶aniline = 1∶15). In addition, iridoids are easily affected by acid or alkali and produce different colors.

(3) Azulenoids

They react positively with Sabety reaction (5% Br_2 in chloroform) and Ehrlich reagent (p-Dimethylaminobenzaldehyde-con. H_2SO_4) (对－二甲胺基苯甲醛－浓硫酸试剂).

1.5.2　Chromatography Identification

Because all terpenoids, except carotenoids (类胡萝卜素), are colorless and there is no sensitive universal reagent for them, It is usually difficult to detect on a micro-scale. Their testing usually relies on the relatively non-specific characteristics of TLC plates. Generally used spraying reagents include H_2SO_4-ethanol, vanillin-H_2SO_4 (香兰素－浓硫酸), anisaldehyde-H_2SO_4 (茴香醛－浓硫酸), antimony chloride (氯化锑) and phosphomolybdic acid,etc. These reagents are strong oxidants reacting with most of the compounds without selectivity to generate conjugated system, thus, corresponding colors occur. More reagents can be used to detect terpeniods with double bonds and ketone groups. For example, Br_2 vapor can detect terpeniods with double bonds, and 2, 4-dinitrophenyl hydrazine (2,4–二硝基苯肼) can detect those with ketone groups.

Terpenoids can be identified by comparing their retention times (t_R) on HPLC or GC to the corresponding standard reference. HPLC-MS and GC-MS are now used to greatly speed up the identification of terpenoids and improve the research level. Because most terpenoids give characteristic fragmentation patterns comparing the measured spectra with those in the standard library, most terpenoids can be identified.

1.6　Structure Determination

Terpenoids have so many structural types that common rules for spectral data are difficult to be concluded. Furthermore, terpenoids are mostly alicyclic compounds (脂环类化合物) and because the cyclohexane ring is usually distorted in the so-called 'chair' form, different geometric conformations are possible, relying on the substitution around the ring. The stereochemistry of the cyclic terpenoids is therefore highly complex and often difficult to determine. However, iridoids have fixed structural types with peculiar spectral characteristics as follows.

1.6.1　UV

Iridoids substituted by carboxyl (—COOH) or ester group (—COOR) at C-4 possess chromophore of α, β-unsaturated carbonyl, so they display strong absorption in the range of 230–240nm (log ε ≈ 4). If they are tested in 0.01M NaOH solution, the maximum absorption peak will move to long wavelength by 30–40nm. Such a shift can be attributed to the formation of enol anion (烯醇阴离子). An example is shown in Figure 10-12.

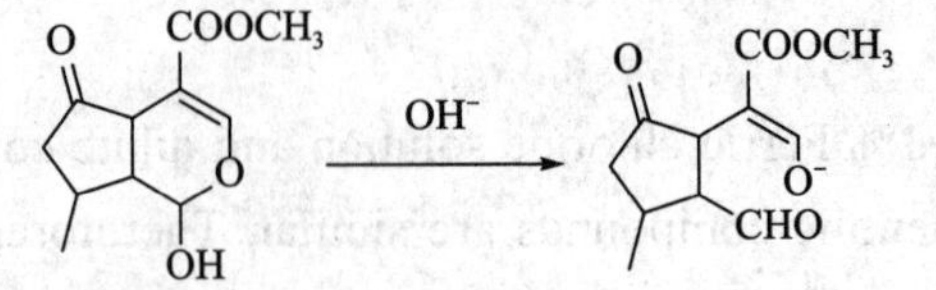

verbenalol
(240nm)

enol anion
(271nm)

Figure 10-12   Formation of enol anion form of verbenalol

1.6.2   IR

The IR spectrum of iridoids can give some useful structural information as below (Table 10-5).

Table 10-5   IR spectrum characters of iridoids

Structural character	Absorption (cm⁻¹)
Vinyl group (—CH=CH$_2$) in seco-iridoids	990 and 910
4-COOR	1680 or 1710
Double bond in enol ether	1640
Carbonyl at cyclopentane moiety	1740 (1710–1750)
Epoxy at cyclopentane moiety	1250 and 830–890

1.6.3 ^{1}H-NMR

The chemical shift of acetal H-1 is between δ4.5 – 6.2, which is similar to sugar. The coupling constant (耦合常数) between H-1 and H-9 determines the stereochemical properties of the dihydropyran ring (二氢吡喃环).

When $J_{1,9}$ is small (0–3Hz), it suggests H-1 is equatorial and –OH (or –OR) at C-1 is axial, and thus C-1 will orientate upwards. If $J_{1,9}$ is large (7–10Hz), the case is on the contrary and C-1 will orientate downwards.

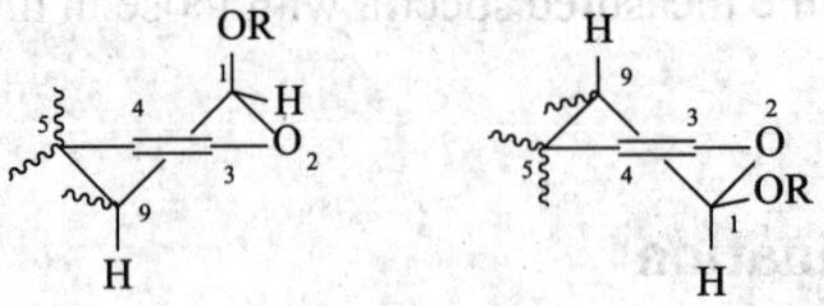

$J_{1,9}$ = 0–3Hz

$J_{1,9}$ = 7–10Hz

The chemical shift of H-3 can be used to determine the substitution of C-4. When C-4 is substituted by –COOR, the chemical shift of H-3 will shift to downfield at δ 7.3–7.7. When C-4 is replaced by -CH$_3$ or –CH$_2$OR, the chemical shift of H-3 will locate at δ 6.0 – 6.2 and δ 6.28 – 6.6, respectively. Due to the long-range coupling between H-3 and H-5, a small coupling constant ($J_{3,5}$ = 0–2Hz) may be observed in the spectrum measured on a high resolution instrument. If there is no substituents at C-4, the chemical shift of H-3 will appear at δ ca. 6.5 ($J_{3,4}$ = 6–8Hz).

If 10-CH$_3$ is linked to saturate C-8, its signal will locate at δ 1.1–1.2 (3H, d, $J_{8,10}$ = 6Hz). When C-8 is unsaturated, 10-CH$_3$ will locate at δ ca. 2.0 (3H, s or br. s). The signal of methyl in –COOCH$_3$ locates at δ 3.7–3.9 (3H, s).

1.6.4　^{13}C-NMR

The chemical shift of C-1 appears at δ 95 – 104, which is similar to the anomeric carbon of sugar. The chemical shifts of C-3 and C-4 occur at δ 139 – 155 and δ 102 – 111, respectively. The other signals depend on the substitution at individual carbons.

1.6.5　ORD

Iridoids with cyclopentanone (环戊酮) moiety generally show strong negative Cotton effect, which is used to confirm the existence of carbonyl and stereochemistry of the structure.

2　Volatile Oils

2.1　Introduction

Volatile oils, also known as essential oils, are a general term for oily liquids with volatility and water-insoluble, which usually obtained by steam distillation from plant. Most volatile oils have an aromatic odor, so they are also called aromatic oils (芳香油).

The plant sources of volatile oils are extensive, mainly in seed plants, especially aromatic plants, such as Asteraceae, Rutaceae (芸香科), Apiaceae, Lamiaceae, Zingiberaceae (姜科), Piperaceae (樟科) and so on. The distribution of volatile oils in plant body varies with species, some of which are distributed in the whole plant, some of which are concentrated in one organ like root, rhizome, leaf, flower, fruit or seed. Volatile oils are stored in various tissues and organs of the plant, such as glandular trichomes (腺毛), oil chambers (油室), secretory cells (分泌细胞), epidermal cells (上皮细胞) or resin canals (树脂道).

Volatile oils have diverse biological activities and are widely used in clinical applications, such as carminatives (anise oil) (茴香油), anthelmintic (chenopodium oil) (土荆芥油), diuretic (sandalwood oil, turpentine oil) (檀香油、松节油), antipyretic (volatile oil of bupleurum) (柴胡挥发油), sedative (ginger oil) (生姜油), local anesthetic (clove oil) (丁香油), and antibacterial agent (bergamot oil) (香柠檬油), etc. In addition, volatile oil is also an important raw material in the perfume industry, daily food industry and chemical industry.

2.2　Composition

The compositions of volatile oils are relatively complex, and one volatile oil often consists of dozens to hundreds of compounds. For example, nearly 300 compounds have been detected in Bulgarian rose oil. There are four types of components in volatile oils, including terpenoids, aromatic compounds, aliphatic compounds and other compounds, among which terpenoids are the most common.

2.2.1　Terpenoids

The terpenoids in the volatile oil are mainly monoterpenes, sesquiterpenes and their oxygen-containing derivatives. The oxygen-containing derivatives are mostly the main components with strong biological activity or aromatic odor. For example, pinene accounts for about 80% of turpentine oil, peppermint oil (薄荷油) contains 80% of menthol, and 50% of camphor exists in camphor oil (樟脑油).

pinene　　　　menthol　　　　camphor

2.2.2　Aromatic compounds

The aromatic compounds are second only to terpenoids in volatile oils. The aromatic compounds in volatile oils are mostly small molecules, most of which are phenylpropanoid derivatives with C_6-C_3 skeleton. For instance, clove oil contains 85% of eugenol (丁香酚), and anethole (茴香脑) account for 50%–80% of anise oil.

thymol　　　　eugenol　　　　anethole

2.2.3　Aliphatic compounds

Small aliphatic compounds often exist in volatile oils, and some volatile oils often contain small molecules of alcohols, aldehydes and acid compounds. For example, ***n***-nonyl alcohol (正壬醇), decanoyl acetaldehyde (癸酰乙醛) and panaxynol (人参炔醇) are found in the volatile oils of tangerine peel, *houttuynia cordata* and ginseng, respectively.

n-nonyl alcohol　　　　decanoyl acetaldehyde

panaxynol

2.2.4　Other compounds

Besides the above 3 types of compounds, some Chinese herbs can decompose volatile components through steam distillation, which is also called volatile oils, such as mustard oil (芥子油), protoanemonin, garlic oil (大蒜油), etc. They exist in the form of glycosides in plants, and the aglycones after enzymatic hydrolysis are distilled out with water vapor to form volatile oils. For example, black mustard oil is allyl isothiocyanate (异硫氰酸烯丙酯) produced by glucosinolate hydrolysis by mustard enzyme, protoanemonin is a substance produced by hydrolysis of ranunculin, and garlic oil is a substance produced by enzymatic hydrolysis of garlic amino acids, such as allicin (大蒜辣素).

protoanemonin　　　　allyl isosulfocyanate　　　　allicin

2.3　Physical and Chemical Properties

2.3.1　Characteristics

Volatile oils are normally colorless or light yellow oily liquid, while few of them show colors. For example, mugwort leaf oil is blue-green (including azulenoids) and cassia oil (桂皮油) is red-brown. Some components in high content may crystalize from volatile oil at low temperature.

They possess characteristic and spicy odors, and some of them are smelly. The odor may indicate the quality of volatile oils. Aromatic volatile oils are usually used as pharmaceutical correctant (矫味药).

2.3.2　Volatility

Volatile oils can volatilize at room temperature spontaneously without persistent oil spot, which can be easily distinguished from fatty oil.

2.3.3　Solubility

Volatile oils are insoluble in water, but easily soluble in various organic solvents, such as petroleum ether, ethyl ether, carbon disulfide, grease, etc. It can be completely dissolved in high-concentration ethanol, while only partially dissolved in low-concentration ethanol.

2.3.4　Physical Constants

The bp. of volatile oils is generally between $70 - 300\,^\circ\!C$. Most volatile oils are lighter than water, while a few of them, such as clove oil and cinnamon oil, are heavier than water. The relative density is normally in the range of $0.850 - 1.065$. Almost all volatile oils are optically active, with specific rotations in the range of $+97^\circ - 117^\circ$, and they have high refractive indexes of $1.43 - 1.61$.

2.3.5　Stability

The volatile oil will gradually oxidize and denature in contact with air and light, which will increase its relative density, darken its color, lose its original fragrance, and form a resin-like substance, so that it can no longer be distilled with water vapor. Therefore, volatile oils should be stored in brown bottles, filled, tightly sealed and kept in a cool place at low temperature.

2.4　Extraction and Isolation Methods

2.4.1　Extraction Methods

(1) Hydro-distillation

This method is a classic method for extracting volatile oils from Chinese herbs. The medicinal materials can be soaked in water and then directly heated for distillation. Alternatively, the medicinal materials are placed on a perforated partition, and when the steam generated by the heated water at the bottom and passes through the medicinal materials, the volatile oils are simultaneously distilled out with the steam. Then collect the distillates and separate the oil layer after cooling. If the oil and water in the distillate are not stratified, the method of salting out can be used to promote the precipitation of volatile oil, or the primary distillate can be redistilled, and then the volatile oil can be extracted with a low-boiling organic solvent after salting out.

This method has the advantages of simple equipment, easy operation, low cost, high extraction rate, etc. However, the extraction temperature of this method is high, so the volatile oils with thermal instability cannot be extracted by the method.

(2) Solvent Extraction

This method uses low-boiling organic solvents, such as petroleum ether (30–60℃), carbon disulfide, carbon tetrachloride, benzene and so on, to extract volatile oils by continuous reflux or cold dipping. Then the crude volatile oils can be obtained by vacuum distillation, but there are many fat-soluble impurities, such as resin, grease, wax, chlorophyll, etc. In order to obtain more pure volatile oils, the crude volatile oils can be distilled re-distilled. Another method is to dissolve the extract with hot ethanol, leave it to cool, filter out the precipitates, and evaporate ethanol, because the solubility of ethanol for fat-soluble impurities decreases with temperature.

(3) SFE

CO_2 supercritical fluid extraction (CO_2-SFE) is mostly used to extract aromatic volatile oils, which has the advantages of preventing oxidation and pyrolysis and improving quality of volatile oils. The aroma of the volatile oils obtained by this method is the same as that of the raw materials, so it is obviously superior to other methods in this respect, such as the application in the extraction of orange peel oil, lemon oil, osmanthus oil and vanillin.

(4) Greases Absorption Method (油脂吸收法)

Greases generally have the property of absorbing volatile oils, so they are often used to extract valuable volatile oil like rose oil and jasmine oil. Greases absorption method is divided into cold absorption method and warm soak absorption method. The greases after absorbing the volatile oils can be directly used in the perfume industry. Alternatively, essential oils can be obtained by adding anhydrous ethanol for stirring and then evaporating the ethanol under reduced pressure.

(5) Press Method (压榨法)

This method is suitable for the extraction of fresh and volatile oil-rich raw materials, such as the peel of fresh tangerine, mandarin and lemon. The medicinal materials are torn, mashed, cold-pressed, and then left to stand or separated by a centrifuge to obtain the oil layer as the crude volatile oils. The volatile oil obtained by this method can keep the original fresh fragrance, but it may dissolve the non-volatile substances in the raw materials. For example, lemon oils often contain chlorophyll from raw materials, causing it to be green.

2.4.2 Isolation Methods

(1) Freeze Crystallization

The volatile oils are kept below 0℃ to precipitate crystals. If no crystals are precipitated, the temperature can be reduced to −20℃ and left to crystallize. Then the crystals were taken out and recrystallized to get pure products. The method is simple in operation, but most of the volatile oil can't be crystallized after freezing.

(2) Fractionation Method

The components of volatile oil are mostly monoterpenoids and sesquiterpenoids. Although their structures and physical properties are similar, the boiling points of each component are different due to the difference in the number of carbon atoms, double bonds and oxygen-containing functional groups in the molecule. This can be used as a basis for separation. The bp. ranges of some terpenoids are listed in Table 10-6.

Table 10-6　bp. ranges of some terpenoids

Terpenoids	Range of bp. at normal pressure (℃)
Semi-terpene	ca. 130
Bicyclic monoterpene with a double bond	150 – 170
Monocyclic monoterpene with two double bonds	170 – 180
Acyclic monoterpene with three double bonds	180 – 200
Oxygenated monoterpene	200 – 230
Sesquiterpene and its oxygenated derivative	230 – 300

According to the different boiling points of each component in the volatile oil, fractionation can be used for isolation. In order to prevent volatile oil from being damaged by heat during fractionation, vacuum fractionation is usually used. Each fraction is still a mixture, and further distillation or freezing, recrystallization, chromatography and other methods are required to obtain a single compound.

(3) Chromatography Method

① Adsorption chromatography

Among the chromatography methods, silica gel and alumina adsorption column chromatography are the most widely used method. The separation of volatile oils is usually combined with fractionation and adsorption column chromatography because of their complicated compositions. Generally, the fraction is dissolved in petroleum ether or hexane, and then applied to a silica gel or alumina adsorption column. The eluent is mostly composed of petroleum ether or hexane, mixed with ethyl acetate in different proportions.

② Silver nitrate complex chromatography

There are many isomers of terpenoids in volatile oil, and many of them are only different in the number or position of double bonds. Therefore, they can be separated according to the difficulty and stability of forming complex between double bond and silver nitrate (硝酸银). Silver nitrate-silica gel or silver nitrate-alumina column chromatography and thin layer chromatography are commonly used for separation. The relationships between adsorption and structure are as follows: firstly, the more double bonds, the stronger the adsorption and the harder elution. Secondly, the adsorption of *cis*-form is stronger than that of *trans*-form. Thirdly, when the number of double bonds is the same, the adsorption of terminal double bond is stronger. Lastly, among the compounds without double bond, the higher the polarity, the stronger the adsorption. For example, Asarum volatile oil is passed through a 20% silver nitrate-silica gel column and eluted with benzene-ethyl ether (5 : 1). The compounds were eluted from the column in the following order: α-asarone, β -asarone and euasarone.

③ Other chromatography methods

Gas chromatography is a very effective method for studying the composition of volatile oils. In particular, the gas chromatography-mass spectrometry (GC-MS) can be used to separate and identify many components in volatile oils simultaneously.

Besides the above isolation methods, chemical separation has been widely used in early days, because terpenoids are treated with corresponding solutions or reagents according to the characteristics of various functional groups.

2.5 Identification

2.5.1 Physicochemical Identification

(1) Determination of Physical Constants

Important physical constants for identification of volatile oils include relative density, specific rotation, refractive index, etc.

(2) Determination of Chemical Constants

Key indicating parameters comprise of the following three values:

① Acid Value

It is the milligrams of potassium hydroxide consumed to neutralize free acidic components in 1g of the volatile oil. It indicates the content of free carboxyl acids and phenols in the volatile oil.

② Ester Value

It is the milligrams of potassium hydroxide consumed for the hydrolysis of esters in 1g of the volatile oil. It indicates the content of esters in the volatile oil.

③ Saponification Value

It is the milligrams of potassium hydroxide consumed for the neutralization and saponification of free acidic components and esters in 1 g of the volatile oil. It represents the content of free carboxyl acids and phenols along with esters in the volatile oil. In fact, the saponification value is the sum of the acid value and the ester value.

Identification of functional groups is usually performed by treating volatile oils with corresponding reagents which is based on the characteristics of various groups, such as acids or alkalines, phenols, carbonyls, unsaturated compounds, azulenoids and lactones, etc.

2.5.2 Chromatography Identification

(1) TLC

Silica gel is a commonly used absorbent. The development systems are composed of strong lipophilic solvents like petroleum ether, hexane, cyclohexane, or their mixtures with benzene, ethyl acetate. Presence of volatile oils can be detected by spraying either universal or specific reagents. The commonly used reagents for the detection of volatile oils are summarized in Table 10-7.

Table 10-7 Commonly used chromogenic reagents for the detection of volatile oils

Reagent	Color	Types of compounds
1% vanillin–con. H_2SO_4	Different colors (at 105℃)	Various compounds
$HONH_2 \cdot HCl–FeCl_3$	Red	Esters
0.05% Bromophenol blue (in ethanol)	Yellow spots in blue background	Carboxyl acids
Ammonium ceric nitrate	Brown spots in yellow background	Alcohols
KI–glacial acetic acid–starch	Blue	Peroxides
2% Aqueous $KMnO_4$	Yellow–brown	Unsaturated compounds
2, 4-Dinitrophenylhydrazine	Yellow	Carbonyls
Bromine vapor	Red	Double bonds

(2) GC

GC has been widely applied for qualitative or quantitative analysis of volatile oils. Comparison the component's retention time (t_R) in the sample with the standard references under the same chromatographic condition may determine the presence or content of the component in the sample. In addition, GC-MS is now widely used for the rapid separation and accurate detection of volatile oils. The individual compounds separated by GC are measured subsequently online by MS, and the structures of compounds may be provided by comparison their MS spectra with those in the data library automatically. Note that in most cases, internal standard usually selected from aliphatic hydrocarbons (*n*-alkanes containing $C_8 - C_{24}$, e.g. *n*-nonane) is required to be spiked into the sample solution.

3   Examples of Chinese Herbs Containing Terpenoids and Volatile Oils

3.1   Artemisiae Annuae Herba (青蒿)

3.1.1   Introduction

(1) Biological Source

Artemisiae Annuae Herba is the dried aerial part of *Artemisia annua* L. (Fam. Compositae).

(2) Property, Flavor and Channels Entered

Property and Flavor: Cold; Bitter, pungent.

Channels Entered: Liver, Gallbladder.

(3) Actions & Indications

To clear deficiency heat, relieve steaming bone, interrupt malaria, release summer heat, abate jaundice. For warm pathogen damaging yin, fever at night and cool in the morning, steaming bone and consumptive fever, yin deficiency fever, fever induced by summer pathogen, malaria, dampness-heat jaundice.

(4) Pharmacological Activities

The most famous pharmacological activity of Artemisiae Annuae Herba is anti-malaria. The active principle artemisinin is of high therapeutic values in treating malaria, especially chloroquine-resistant *Plasmodium falciparum* and the cerebral infections. Moreover, artemisinin significantly inhibits humoral immunity and facilitates cellular immunity. Artemisinin can also slow down heart rate, suppress cardiac contractility and lower coronary flow. The volatile oil of Artemisiae Annuae Herba possesses significant antibacterial activity and induces apoptosis in human hepatoma cell lines, and it is also used clinically to treat neurodermitis, fungal infection and so on.

3.1.2   Main Chemical Constituents

Artemisiae Annuae Herba is the main component of the Chinese antimalaria prescription (qing-hao-bie-jia-tang), which is a decoction of Artemisiae Annuae Herba and turtle shell. From 1965 to 1970, more than five thousand plants have been screened using animal malarial tests. It was found that the alcoholic extract of *A. annua* was one of the most active samples against mice malaria (*Plasmodium berghai*), and the active compound, artemisinin, was isolated. Artemisinin is a sesquiterpenoid. Artemisiae Annuae Herba contains sesquiterpenoids, volatile oils, flavonoids, phenylpropanoic acids and other type of compounds.

(1) Sesquiterpenoids

Artemisinin (*1*) is a sesquiterpene lactone containing a rare peroxide linkage which appears to be essential for activity. The plant of *A. annua* has been found to produce as much as 1.4% artemisinin, but the yield is normally very much less, typically 0.05% – 0.2%. Apart from one or two low-yielding species, the compound has not been found in any other species of the genus *Artemisia* (about 400 species). Small amounts (about 0.01%) of the related peroxide structure artemisitene (*2*) are also present in *A. annua*, though this has a lower antimalarial activity. The most abundant sesquiterpenoids in the plant are artemisinic acid (*3*, arteannuic acid, typically 0.2% – 0.8%), and lesser amounts (0.1%) of arteannuin B (*4*, qinghaosu-II). Fortunately, the artemisinic acid content may be converted chemically into artemisinin by a relatively straightforward and efficient process.

Owing to its poor solubility in water or oil, artemisinin is difficult to prepare as a clear solution for parenteral administration. The suspended injection of artemisinin causes localized pain at the injection area. Most brain malaria patients went into a coma, and the intravenous administration form is the best choice. Therefore, structural modification of artemisinin may be a better way to find new anti-malaria derivatives with low toxicity for clinical use.

Artemisinin contains peroxy, lactone and acetal functional groups in its structure. Most chemical reactions may attack the peroxy group first, but in converting the peroxy to the deoxyartemisinin derivative (*5*), which loses anti-malarial activity. Reduction of artemisinin with NaBH$_4$ reduces its 12-carbonyl group to a hydroxyl group and forms two isomers, α-dihydroartemisinin (*6*) and β-dihydroartemisinin (*6*). Both the α and β forms show four-fold antimalarial activity and can be further reacted to prepare their ether, ester, and other derivatives. The lipid-soluble artemether (*7*) and arteether (*8*), and the water soluble artesunic acid (*9*) and artelinic acid (*10*), were designed for in severe malaria cases. For dihydroartemisinin is a more active antimalarial than artemisinin and appears to be the main metabolite of these drugs (*5 – 8*) in the body, these artemisinin derivatives have increased activity compared with artemisinin, and the chances of infection recurring are also reduced. Currently, the World Health Organization (WHO) recommends the following artemisinin-based oral combination therapies for the treatment of malaria: artemether and lumefantrine; sodium artesunic acid and amodiaquine; sodium artesunic acid and mefloquine; and sodium artesunic acid and sulfadoxine-pyrimethamine. Artemisone (*11*), a new semi-synthetic thiomorpholine dioxide derivative of dihydroartemisinin, is currently in clinical trials. Chemically, these agents are quite unlike any other class of current antimalarial agent, are well tolerated with no major side-effects, and so far no drug resistance is evident. As new analogues are introduced, they may well provide an important group of drugs in the fight against this life-threatening disease.

Deoxyartemisinin (*5*)　　Dihydroartemisinin α-(*6*)　　Dihydroartemisinin β-(*6*)　　Artemether (*7*)

Arteether (*8*)　　Artesunic acid (*9*)　　Artelinic acid (*10*)　　Artemisone (*11*)

Currently, artemisinin-based antimalarial therapies remain too expensive to be afforded by those in the developing countries who need this most, due to low yields from the plant of origin, *Artemisia annua* L., and also due to the high cost of the specialized processing involved in the purification of this compound. In order to solve this problem, artificial compound arterolane (*12*) was designed. It is a totally synthetic 1, 2, 4-trioxolane developed from the artemisinin template that shows potent antimalarial activity and is currently in clinical trials.

arterolane (*12*)

(2) Volatile Oils

Dozens of compounds have been identified from the volatile oil of *A. annua* in various habitats. Goel and coworkers had characterized 93 compounds from the volatile oil of stem, leaves, flowers and root of India originated *A. annua*. Great differences exist in components of volatile oils of *A. annua* collected from different habitats, but there are some common compounds such as camphor, 1, 8-cineole, artemisia ketone, seltnene, camphene, caryophyllene, pinene and so on.

(3) Flavonoids

Five flavonoids apigenin, luteolin, 5, 7, 4'-trihydroxy-6, 3', 5'-trimethoxyflavone, eupatilin and casticin have been isolated from Artemisiae Annuae Herba for the first time. Sixteen flavonoids are characterized by LC-DAD-ESI-MS[n] from methanol extract of Artemisiae Annuae Herba including apigenin-6, 8-di-C-glucoside, apigenin-6-C-arabinosyl-8-C-glucoside, mearnsetin-glucoside, apigenin-6-C-rhamnosyl-8-C-glucoside, quercetin-rhamnosyl-glucoside, apigenin-8-C-glucoside, 3, 5-dihydroxy-6, 7, 4'-trimethoxyflavone, apigenin-6-C-glucosyl-8-C-pentoside, mearsetin-diglucoside, 3-hydroxy-6, 7, 4'-trimethoxyflavone, quercetin-glucoside, apienin-6-C-glucosyl-8-C-rhamnoside, 3, 5-dihydroxy-6, 7, 3', 4'-tetramethoxyflavone and isorhamnetin-glucoside.

apigenin　　　　　　luteolin　　　　　5,7,4'-trihydroxy-6,3',5'-
　　　　　　　　　　　　　　　　　　trimethoxyflavone

eupatilin   casticin

(4) Phenylpropanoic Acids

Derivatives of quinic acid are characterized by LC-DAD-ESI-MS^n from methanol extract of Artemisiae Annuae Herba including 5-caffeoylquinic acid, 3-caffeoylquinic acid, 1-feruoyl-5-caffeoylquinic acid, 3, 4, 5-tricaffeoylquinic acid, 4, 5-dicaffeoylquinic acid, 3, 4-dicaffeoylquinic acid, 1-caffeoyl-5-feruoylquinic acid, 5-feruoylquinic acid, 3, 4-diferuoylquinic acid, 3, 5-5-diferuoylquinic acid, 4, 5-diferuoylquinic acid, etc.

(5) Others

Other constituents found in Artemisiae Annuae Herba include scopoletin, fatty acids, sterols, amino acids and so on.

3.1.3   Quality Control Standards

(1) TLC Identification

Stationary Phase: Silica gel plate.

Standard: Artemisinin.

Development System: Petroleum ether-ether (4 : 5).

Visualization: After spraying the solution of 10% H_2SO_4-ethanol containing 2% vanillin, heat to 105 ℃ until spots are clear, and visualize under 365nm UV light.

(2) Tests

Water: Not more than 14.0%.

Total Ash: Not more than 8.0%.

Extract (anhydrous ethanol): Not less than 1.9%.

3.2   Menthae Haplocalycis Herba (薄荷)

3.2.1   Introduction

(1) Biological Source

Menthae Haplocalycis Herba is the dried aerial part of *Mentha haplocalyx* Briq. (Fam. Labiatae).

(2) Property, Flavor and Channels Entered

Property and Flavor: Cool; Pungent.

Channels Entered: Lung, Liver.

(3) Actions & Indications

To disperse wind-heat, clear and smooth head and eyes, smooth the throat, promote eruption, smooth the liver to move qi. For common cold caused by wind-heat, early onset of wind-warmth disease, headache, red eyes, mouth sore, throat impediment, rubella, measles, distension and oppression in the chest and the hypochondrium.

(4) Pharmacological Activities

The volatile oil of Menthae Haplocalycis Herba (mint oil) as the major active principle has been intensively investigated and reported in pharmacological activities. The pharmacological activities include antibacterial, anti-inflammation, pain relieving, as well as anti-oxidation, etc. The main compound menthol in mint oil has short local analgesic effect. It has effects of inhibition of the growth and propagation of fungi and two subtypes (HSV21 and HSV22) of HSV. The flavonoids from Menthae Haplocalycis Herba are responsible for antioxidant activity.

3.2.2   Main Chemical Constituents

Menthae Haplocalycis Herba grows in most provinces of China, but is mainly cultivated in the south area of Changjiang River, especially in Jiangsu and Zhejiang provinces. Volatile oils and flavonoids are the major components of the aerial parts of *M. Haplocalyx*. China is the major exporter of high-quality menthol and mint oil. In addition, other constituents such as organic acids, sterols and amino acids are also included.

(1) Volatile Oils

The term "mint oil" refers to the volatile oil of *M. haplocalyx* and is the main active principle. Due to the widespread and great difference in growing conditions, the types and contents of constituents in the volatile oil vary with the varieties, habitat and collection time. Generally, the content of volatile oil in the fresh leaves of cultivated *M. haplocalyx* is about 0.8% – 1.0%, and of 1.3% – 2.0% in the dried stems and leaves. The chemical components of mint oil are complicated, which are mainly monoterpenoids and the corresponding oxygen-containing derivatives, and non-terpenoid aromatic or aliphatic compounds as well, e.g. menthol, menthone, neomenthol, menthyl acetate, piperitone, linalool, linalyl acetate, 1, 8-cineole, carvone, limonene and the like. It is reported that nearly fifty compunds have been characterized from mint oil.

l-menthol	*d*-neomenthol	menthone	menthyl acetate

piperitone	carvone	limonene	1,8-cineole

The quality of mint oil is mainly determined on the content of *l*-menthol, which is generally more than 50% up to 85%. There are 3 chiral carbons in the molecules of menthol, which should have 8 stereoisomers theoretically, however, only *l*-menthol and *d*-neomenthol have been found naturally occurring in mint oil.

(2) Flavonoids

Twenty flavonoids have been reported in Menthae Haplocalycis Herba. They are menthoside, isoraifolin, luteolin-7-*O*-glucoside, naringenin-7-*O*-glucoside, eriocitrin, tilianine, 5, 6, 4′-trihydroxy-7, 8-dimethoxyflavone, 5, 6-dihydroxy-7, 8, 3′, 4′-tetramethoxyflavone, acacetin, 5, 3′-dihydroxy-6, 7, 8, 4′-tetramethoxyflavone, 5-hydroxy-6, 7, 3′, 4′-tetra-methoxyflavone, buddleoside, diosmin,

5, 4′-dihydroxy-7-methoxyflavone, luteolin, 5, 6-dihydroxy-7, 8, 4′-trimethoxyflavone, and 5, 4′-dihydroxy-6, 7, 8-trimethoxyflavone. The accumulation of flavonoids varies with different growth phases.

(3) Others

Other constituents found in Menthae Haplocalycis Herba involve organic acids such as rosmarinic acid (0.156%), salvianolic acid, caffeic acid, lithospermic acid, formic acid and so on, triterpenoids including oleanolic acid, usrolic acid, buddlejasaponin. Amino acids and sterols are also included in Menthae Haplocalycis Herba.

3.2.3　Quality Control Standards

(1) TLC Identification

Stationary Phase: Silica gel G plate.

Standard: Authentic crude drug; menthol.

Development System: Toluene-acetyl acetate (19 : 1).

Visualization: After spraying the mixed solution of vanillin and sulphuric acid-ethanol (1 : 4) and heating at 100℃ until spots are clear, visualize in visible light.

(2) Tests

Leaves: Not less than 30%.

Water: Not more than 15.0%.

Total Ash: Not more than 11.0%.

Acid-insoluble Ash: Not more than 3.0%.

(3) Assay

Volatile oils: Not less than 0.80%.

词　汇　表

An Alphabetical List of Words and Phrases

A		
abietane	[æ'baɪətən]	松香烷
acyclic terpenoids	[eɪ'saɪklɪk]['tə:pi:nɔɪdz]	无环萜类
addition reaction	[ə'dɪʃn][rɪ'ækʃn]	加成反应
adhesives	[əd'hi:sɪvz]	黏合剂
alicyclic compounds	[ælɪ'saɪklɪk]['kɔmpaundz]	脂环类化合物
allicin	['æləsɪn]	大蒜辣素
andrographolide	[ændrəug'ræphɔlɪd]	穿心莲内酯
anethole	['ænəθəul]	茴香醚、茴香脑
anisaldehyde-H_2SO_4	[ænaɪ'zældɪhaɪd]	茴香醛－浓硫酸
antimony chloride	['æntɪməni]['klɔ:raɪd]	氯化锑
Artemisiae Annuae Herb		青蒿
artemisinin	[ɑ:tɪmɪ'saɪnɪn]	青蒿素
azulenoids	['æzjulɪˌnɔɪdz]	薁类化合物

(continued)

allyl isothiocyanate	[ˈæləl] [ˌɪsəʊθɪəʊˈsɪəneɪt]	异硫氰酸烯丙酯
anise oil	[ˈænɪs][ɔɪl]	茴香油
aromatic oils	[ærəˈmætɪk][ɔɪlz]	芳香油
B		
baccatin	[ˈbækətɪn]	巴卡亭
biogenetic isoprene rule	[baɪəʊdʒeˈnetɪk][ˈaɪsəpriːn][ruːl]	生源异戊二烯法则
bisabolane	[bizæˈbəulən]	没药烷
bitterness principle	[ˈbɪtənɪs][ˈprɪnsəpl]	苦味原则
borneol	[ˈbɔːnɪɔl]	冰片，龙脑
bracken fern	[ˈbrækən][fəːn]	蕨类
Burseraceae		藜科
bergamot oil	[ˈbəːgəmɔt][ɔɪl]	香柠檬油
C		
cadinane	[ˈkeɪdɪnæn]	杜松烷
β-cadinene		β- 杜松烯
camphane	[ˈkæmfeɪn]	莰烷型
camphor	[ˈkæmfə]	樟脑
Camphorae		樟科
camphor oil	[ˈkæmfə][ɔɪl]	樟脑油
cantharidin	[kænˈθærɪdɪn]	斑蝥素
carotenoids	[ˈkærəutiːnɔɪdz]	类胡萝卜素
catalpol	[kæˈtælpɔl]	梓醇苷
Cistaceae		茜草科
citronellol	[ˌsɪtrəˈnelɔːl]	香茅醇
π-complex	[ˈkɔmpleks]	π- 络合物
copper complex	[ˈkɔpə][ˈkɔmpleks]	铜络合物
correctant	[kəˈrektənt]	矫味药
coupling constant	[ˈkʌplɪŋ][ˈkɔnstənt]	耦合常数
Curcumae Radix		姜黄温郁金
curcumol	[kəˈkjuːmɔl]	姜黄醇
cycloeudesmol	[saɪkˈluːdzml]	环桉醇
cyclogeraniane		环香叶烷
cyclohexane	[ˌsaɪkləʊˈhekseɪn]	环己烷
cyclopentanone	[saɪkləʊˈpentənəun]	环戊酮
cassia oil	[ˈkæsɪə][ɔɪl]	桂皮油
chenopodium oil		土荆芥油
clove oil	[kləuv][ɔɪl]	丁香油

(continued)

D		
10-deacetylbaccatin	[ˈdiːsɪtɪlbəkeɪtɪn]	10– 脱乙酰基巴卡亭 Ⅲ
decarboxylated	[ˌdiːkɑːˈbɔksəleɪtɪd]	脱羧
dehydration reactions	[ˌdiːhaɪˈdreɪʃn][riˈækʃənz]	脱水
4-demethyliridoids		4– 去甲基环烯醚萜
diene	[ˈdaɪiːn]	双烯
dihydropyran ring	[diːhaɪdrəˈpɪəræn][rɪŋ]	二氢吡喃环
2, 4-dinitrophenyl hydrazine	[daɪnaɪtrəuˈfenɪl][ˈhaɪdrəziːn]	2,4– 二硝基苯肼
diterpene derivative	[daɪtəˈpiːn][dɪˈrɪvətɪv]	二萜类衍生物
diterpenes	[daɪtəˈpiːnz]	二萜
double bonds	[ˈdʌbl][bɔndz]	双键
E		
empirical isoprene rule	[ɪmˈpɪrɪkl][ˈaɪsəpriːn]	经验异戊二烯法则
emulsifiers	[ɪˈmʌlsɪfaɪəz]	乳化剂
enol anion	[ˈiːnəul][ˈænaɪən]	烯醇阴离子
epidermal cells		上皮细胞
Eremostachys Bunge Linn		沙穗属
eucalyptol	[ˌjuːkeˈlɪptɔl]	桉精油
eugenol	[ˈjuːdʒɪnɔl]	甲基丁香酚
euparotin	[juːˈpærɔtɪn]	泽兰苦内酯
Eupatorium rotundifolium		圆叶泽兰
Euphorbiaceae		大戟科
F		
farnesane	[ˈfɑːrnɪzæn]	金合欢烯
farnesol	[ˈfɑːnɪsəul]	金合欢醇
farnesyl pyrophosphate	[ˈfɑːrnsɪl] [ˌpaɪrəuˈfɔsfeɪt]	焦磷酸金合欢酯
fenchane	[ˌfentʃeɪn]	葑烷型
fenchone	[ˈfenkəun]	葑酮
Foeniculum vulgare		茴香
fungi	[ˈfʌŋgəs]	真菌
furanspongin-3		呋喃海绵素 –3
G		
genipin-1-*O*-gentiobioside	[dʒeˈnaɪpɪn][ˈdʒentiːəubaɪəsaɪd]	京尼平苷
gentianine	[ˈdʒeʃənɪn]	龙胆碱
gentiopicroside, gentiopicrin	[dʒentaɪɔpaɪkˈrəusaɪd],[dʒenˈtaɪɔpaɪkrɪn]	龙胆苦苷
geranial	[dʒɪˈreɪnɪəl]	香叶醛

(continued)

geraniol	[dʒɪˈreɪɪɔl]	香叶醇
Geranium macrorrhizum		大根老鹳草
geranylfarnesyl pyrophosphate (GFPP)		焦磷酸香叶基金合欢酯
geranylgeranyl pyrophosphate (GGPP)		焦磷酸香叶基香叶酯
geranyl pyrophosphate (GPP)	[ˈdʒerənɪl][ˌpaɪrəuˈfɔsfeɪt]	焦磷酸香叶酯
germacrane	[ˈdʒəːməkreɪn]	吉马烷
germacrone	[ˈdʒəːməkrəun]	吉马酮
Ginkgo biloba		银杏
Girard reagent		吉拉德试剂
gossypol	[ˈgɔsɪˌpɔl]	棉酚
Gramineae		禾本科
grayanotoxane		木藜芦毒烷
greases absorption method	[ˈgriːsɪs][əbˈsɔːpʃn][ˈmeθəd]	油脂吸收法
guaiane	[ˈgjuəɪən]	愈创木烷
guaiazule		愈创木薁
garlic oil	[gɑːlɪk][ɔɪl]	大蒜油
glandular trichome	[ˈglændjulə][ˈtrɪkəum]	腺毛
ginger oil	[ˈdʒɪndʒə][ɔɪl]	生姜油
H		
hemiterpene	[ˌhemɪˈtəːpiːn]	半萜
hexane	[hekˈseɪn]	己烷
hydrazide	[ˈhaɪdrəzaɪd]	酰肼
hydrobromic acid	[ˌhaɪdrəuˈbrəumɪk][ˈæsɪd]	氢溴酸
hydrochloric acid	[ˌhaɪdrəuˈklɔrɪk][ˈæsɪd]	盐酸
hydrogen halide	[ˈhaɪdrəudʒən][ˈhælaɪd]	卤化氢
hydrophilic impurities	[ˌhaɪdrəˈfɪlɪk][ɪmˈpjuərɪtɪs]	水溶性杂质
16-hydroxytriptolide	[haɪˈdrɔksɪˈtrɪptəulaɪd]	16-羟基雷公藤内酯醇
I		
intra-molecular hydrogen bond	[ˈɪntrə][məˈlekjələ][ˈhaɪdrədʒən][bɔnd]	分子内氢键
α-ionone	[ˈaɪəˌnɔn]	α-紫罗兰酮
β-ionone	[ˈaɪəˌnɔn]	β-紫罗兰酮
iridodial	[ɪərɪˈdəudɪəl]	臭蚁二醛
iridoids	[ɪərɪˈdɔɪdz]	环烯醚萜类
iron complexes	[ˈaɪən][ˈkɔmpleksɪz]	铁络合物
γ, γ-isomeric dimethylallyl pyrophosphate, DMAPP	[ˌaɪsəˈmerɪk][daɪmeθɪlæˈlɪl][paɪrəuˈfɔsfeɪt]	焦磷酸γ, γ-二甲基烯丙酯
isomerization	[aɪˌsɔməraɪˈzeɪʃn]	异构化

(continued)

isopentenyl pyrophosphate, IPP	[ˌaɪsəuˈpəntənəl][ˌpaɪrəuˈfɒsfeɪt]	焦磷酸异戊烯酯
isoprene rules	[ˈaɪsəpriːn][ˈruːlz]	异戊二烯法则
isoprene units	[ˈaɪsəpriːn][ˈjuːnɪts]	异戊二烯单元
J		
Juniperus sabina		刺柏
K		
kaurane	[kauˈreɪniː]	贝壳杉烷
L		
labdane	[ˈlæbdeɪn]	半日花烷
lichens	[ˈlaɪkənz]	地衣
lipid-rich	[ˈlɪpɪd][rɪtʃ]	富含油脂的
lipophilic impurities	[ˌlɪpəˈfɪlɪk][ɪmˈpjuərɪtɪs]	脂溶性杂质
M		
Menthae Haplocalycis Herba		薄荷
menthol	[ˈmenθɒl]	薄荷醇
meroterpenoids	[ˈmerəutəpiːnɔɪdz]	混源萜类
α-methylene-γ-lactone	[ˈmeθɪliːn][ˈlæktəun]	α-亚甲基-γ-内酯
mevalonic acid (MVA)		甲戊二羟酸
monocyclic terpenoids	[mɒnəˈsaɪklɪk][ˈtəːpiːnɔɪdz]	单环萜类
monoene	[məˈnəun]	单烯
monoterpene	[ˌmɒnəˈtəːpiːn]	单萜
myrceane	[maɪrˈsiːn]	月桂烷
Myrtle	[ˈməːtl]	桃金娘科
mustard oil	[ˈmʌstəd][ɔɪl]	芥子油
N		
neral	[ˈniːræl]	橙花醛
nerol	[ˈnɪərul]	橙花醇
N-hydroxy-cantharidimide	[haɪˈdrɒksɪ][ˈkænθærɪdɪmaɪd]	N-羟基斑蝥胺
nitrosyl chloride	[ˈnaɪtrəsɪl][ˈklɔːraɪd]	亚硝酰氯
non-isoprene	[nʌnˈaɪsəpriːn]	非异戊二烯
n-nonyl alcohol	[ˈnɒnɪl][ˈælkəhɒl]	正壬醇
O		
ophiobolin A	[əfiːəuˈbəlɪn]	蛇孢假壳素 A
Ophiobulus miyabeanus		芝麻枯
oil chambers	[ɔɪl][ˈtʃeɪmbəz]	油室
P		
paclitaxel	[ˌpæklɪˈtæksəl]	紫杉醇，红豆杉醇

(continued)

paederoside	[pedə'rəusaɪd]	鸡屎藤苷
Paeonia albiflora		白芍
paeoniflorin		芍药苷
panaxynol	[pæ'næksɪnɒl]	人参炔醇
p-Dimethylaminobenzaldehyde-con. H₂SO₄	[daɪmeθɪlæmɪənəuben'zældɪhaɪd]	对 – 二甲胺基苯甲醛 – 浓硫酸试剂
Phlomis Linn		糙苏属
phorbane	['fɔ:beɪn]	大戟烷
phorbol	['fɔ:bɒl]	大戟醇
phosphoric acid	[fɒs'fɒrɪk]['æsɪd]	磷酸
phytol	['faɪtɒl]	植物醇
pinane	['paɪneɪn]	蒎烷
Piperaceae		樟科
piperitone	[pɪ'perɪtəun]	薄荷酮，胡椒酮
p-menthane	['menθeɪn]	对 – 薄荷烷型
Podosocarpaceae		鬼芋科
polyterpenes		多萜
press method	[pres]['meθəd]	压榨法
peppermint oil	['pepə'mɪnt][ɔɪl]	薄荷油
Q		
quaternary ammonium group	[kwə'tə:nərɪ][ə'məunɪəm][gru:p]	季铵基团
R		
re-arrangement reaction	[rɪə'reɪndʒmənt][rɪ'ækʃn]	重排反应
Rehmanniae Radix	[rɪ'mænɪi:]['reɪdɪks]	地黄
Rhododendron dauricum		兴安杜鹃
Rhododendron japonicum	[ˌrəudə'dendrən][dʒə'pɒnɪəkm]	日本杜鹃
rhomotoxin	[rəuməu'tɒksɪn]	八厘麻毒素
Rutaceae		芸香科
resin canals	['rezɪn][kə'næl]	树脂道
S		
sabinene	[sæbaɪ'ni:n]	桧烯，香桧烯，刺柏烯
α-santalane	['sæntəleɪn]	α– 白檀醇
α-santalol	['sæntəlɒl]	α– 白檀醇
Santalum album	['sæntələm]['ælbəm]	白檀
saturated hydrocarbon	['sætʃəreɪtɪd][ˌhaɪdrə'kɑ:bən]	饱和烃
Scrophulariae Radix	['skrɒfju'leəlɪə]['reɪdɪks]	玄参
secoiridoids		裂环环烯醚萜

(continued)

secondary metabolites	['sekəndrɪ][meˈtæbəblaɪts]	次级代谢产物
sesquiterpene	[ˌseskwɪˈtəːpiːn]	倍半萜
sesterterpene	[sestəːtəˈpiːn]	二倍半萜
silver nitrate, AgNO₃	['sɪlvə]['naɪtreɪt]	硝酸银
silver nitrate solution	['sɪlvə]['naɪtreɪt][səˈluːʃn]	硝酸银溶液
sodium hydrosulphite	['səudiːəm][ˌhaɪdrəuˈsʌlfaɪt]	亚硫酸氢钠
solvent extraction	['sɔləvnt][ɪkˈstrækʃn]	溶剂萃取
Stachys Linn	['steɪkɪs][lɪn]	鼠尾草属
Stevia rebaudianum		甜菊
stevioside	['stiːvɪəsaɪd]	甜菊苷
sweroside	[swəˈrəusaɪd]	獐芽菜苷
swertiamarin	['swətaɪəmɑːrɪn]	獐芽菜苦苷
sandalwood oil	['sændlwud][ɔɪl]	檀香油
secretory cells	[sɪˈkriːtərɪ]['selz]	分泌细胞
structural re-arrangemnet	['strʌktʃərəl][rɪəˈreɪndʒmənt]	结构重排
T		
taxane	['tæksæn]	紫杉烷
Taxodiaceae		红豆杉科
Taxus brevifolia		红豆杉
teresantalol	[təreˈzæntəlɔl]	三环白檀醇（对檀香醇/檀油醇）
terpenes	[təˈpiːnɪz]	萜烯
terpenoid	['təːpənɔɪd]	萜类
terpenoid lactones	['təːpənɔɪd]['læktəunz]	萜内脂
tetracyclic terpenoids	[ˌtetrəˈsaɪklɪk]['təːpiːnɔɪdz]	四环萜类
tetraterpenes	[tetreɪtəˈpiːnɪz]	四萜
thujane	['θjuːdʒeɪn]	守烷型
tricyclane	[traɪˈsaɪkleɪn]	三环烷型
tricyclic terpenoids	[traɪˈsaɪklɪk]['təːpiːnɔɪdz]	三环萜类
triene	['traɪɪːn]	三烯
tripdiolide	['trɪpdɪəlɪd]	雷公藤乙素
Tripterygium wilfordii		雷公藤
triptolide	['trɪptɔlɪd]	雷公藤甲素，雷公藤内酯
triptolidenol	['trɪptɔlɪdɪnəl]	雷公藤内酯
triterpenes	[traɪtəˈpiːnɪz]	三萜
tropolonoids		草酚酮
α-thujaplicin	[θjuːˈdʒæplɪsɪn]	α– 崖柏素
β-thujaplicin	[θjuːˈdʒæplɪsɪn]	β– 崖柏素

(continued)

γ-thujaplicin	[θjuː'dʒæplɪsɪn]	γ– 崖柏素
turpentine oil	['təːpentiːn]['ɔɪl]	松节油
U		
Umbelliferae	[ʌmbelɪfə'riː]	伞形科
V		
Valerianaceae		败酱科
vanillin-H_2SO_4	[və'nɪlɪn]	香兰素 – 浓硫酸
verbenalin	[vəː'benəlɪn]	马鞭草苷
vitamin A	['vɪtəmɪn]	维生素 A
volatile oil	['vɔlətaɪl]['ɔɪl]	挥发油
volatile oil of bupleurum		柴胡挥发油
Z		
Zingiberaceae		姜科

重 点 小 结

　　萜类化合物是由甲戊二羟酸衍生而成，根据分子结构中异戊二烯单元的数目将萜类分为单萜、倍半萜、二萜、二倍半萜、三萜等。其中，单萜和倍半萜是挥发油的重要组成成分。

　　单萜根据是否成环以及成环数目，分为链状单萜、单环单萜、双环单萜等。其中草酚酮和环烯醚萜是特殊的单萜衍生物。

　　倍半萜根据是否成环以及成环数目，分为链状倍半萜、单环倍半萜、双环倍半萜等。其中，奥类化合物是一类具有芳环骨架的特殊倍半萜。

　　萜类的物理性质包括性状、溶解性、旋光性。化学性质包括加成反应、氧化反应、脱氢反应等，重点掌握萜类化合物的双键和羰基的加成反应。含有双键的萜类化合物可以与卤化氢、溴水、亚硝酰氯发生加成反应，生成结晶性的加成物，可用于含有双键的萜类化合物的检识、分离和纯化；含有羰基的萜类化合物可以与亚硫酸氢钠、吉拉德试剂发生加成反应，可用于含有羰基的萜类化合物的检识、分离和纯化。

　　萜类化合物的提取方法有：溶剂提取法、碱提酸沉法、吸附法。萜类化合物的分离方法有：结晶法、利用特殊官能团进行化学分离、柱色谱法等。其中，对于含有双键的萜类化合物，可用硝酸银－硅胶、硝酸银－氧化铝柱色谱分离。硝酸银络合柱色谱法的分离原理是硝酸银与双键形成 π– 络合物进行络合吸附，分子中双键的数目、位置、立体结构的不同，其络合程度及络合稳定性不同，利用此差异可以分离。络合稳定性顺序：末端双键 ＞ 顺式双键 ＞ 反式双键。

　　挥发油也称精油，是存在于植物中的一类具有挥发性、可随水蒸气蒸馏、与水不相混溶的油状液体的总称。挥发油大多具有芳香气味，所以又称为芳香油。

　　构成挥发油的成分可分为萜类化合物、芳香族化合物、脂肪族化合物和其他类化合物（有些中药经水蒸气蒸馏分解出的挥发性成分）四类，其中以萜类化合物为多见。

　　挥发油的理化性质包括性状、挥发性、溶解性、物理常数和不稳定性。挥发油与空气及光线接触，常会逐渐氧化变性，使之相对密度增加，颜色变深，失去原有香味，并能形成树脂样物质，不能再随水蒸气而蒸馏。因此，产品应贮存于棕色瓶内，装满、密塞，并在阴凉处低温保存。

挥发油的提取方法包括水蒸气蒸馏法、溶剂提取法、CO_2超临界流体萃取法、油脂吸收法和压榨法等，其中水蒸气蒸馏法是提取挥发油最常用的方法，但对热不稳定的挥发油不能用此法。

挥发油的分离方法包括冷冻析晶法（析脑）、分馏法、色谱法和化学法等，其中色谱法又分为吸附色谱法、硝酸银络合色谱法、气相色谱法等。掌握硝酸银络合色谱法的色谱行为。

挥发油的鉴定可测定相对密度、比旋度及折光率等物理常数，酸值、酯值、皂化值等化学常数，也可用 TLC、GC、GC-MS，其中 GC 已广泛用于挥发油的定性和定量分析。

青蒿中含有倍半萜、黄酮、挥发油等类型的成分，其中倍半萜中的青蒿素是主要的抗疟有效成分，过氧基是青蒿素分子中的抗疟活性基团。薄荷中主要含挥发油类成分，薄荷油的质量优劣主要依据其中薄荷醇（薄荷脑）含量的高低而定。

目 标 检 测

题库

一、单选题

1. 单萜类化合物分子中有（   ）个碳原子
   A. 5　　　　　　　　　　　B. 10　　　　　　　　　　　C. 15
   D. 20　　　　　　　　　　　E. 以上都不是

2. 由甲戊二羟酸途径衍生出的化合物类型是（   ）
   A. 黄酮类　　　　　　　　　B. 有机酸类　　　　　　　　C. 生物碱类
   D. 萜类　　　　　　　　　　E. 醌类

3. 青蒿素属于（   ）
   A. 单萜　　　　　　　　　　B. 倍半萜　　　　　　　　　C. 二萜
   D. 二倍半萜　　　　　　　　E. 以上都不是

4. 非含氧的开链萜烯的分子通式是（   ）
   A.（C_5H_8）$_n$　　　　　　　B.（C_6H_8）$_n$　　　　　　　C.（C_5H_{10}）$_n$
   D.（C_6H_{10}）$_n$　　　　　　　E. 以上都不是

5. 组成萜类的基本结构单元是（   ）
   A. 异戊二烯　　　　　　　　B. 苯丙素　　　　　　　　　C. 2- 苯基色原酮
   D. 甲戊二羟酸　　　　　　　E. 以上都不是

6. 挥发油的（   ）往往是其品质优劣的重要标志
   A. 色泽　　　　　　　　　　B. 气味　　　　　　　　　　C. 比重
   D. 溶解度　　　　　　　　　E. 比旋度

7. 挥发油的酸值是指（   ）
   A. 中和 1g 挥发油中酸性成分所消耗氢氧化钾的毫克数
   B. 水解 1g 挥发油中所含的酯类需要的氢氧化钾的毫克数
   C. 皂化 1g 挥发油所消耗氢氧化钾的毫克数
   D. 皂化值与酯值之和
   E. 挥发油中酚类成分的含量指标

8. 区别油脂与挥发油，一般可采用（   ）

　　A. 升华试验　　　　　　　　　B. 泡沫试验　　　　　　　　C. 油斑试验

　　D. 溶血试验　　　　　　　　　F. 沉淀实验

9. 挥发油显绿色、蓝色或紫色可能含有（　　　　）

　　A. 芳香醛类　　　　　　　　　B. 脂肪族类　　　　　　　　C. 含氮化合物

　　D. 薁类　　　　　　　　　　　F. 含氧化合物

10. 在青蒿素的结构中，具有抗疟活性必备的基团是（　　　　）

　　A. 羰基　　　　　　　　　　　B. 过氧基　　　　　　　　　C. 内酯环

　　D. C_{10} 位 H 的构型　　　　　E. 以上皆不是

二、多选题

1. 组成挥发油的萜类成分有（　　　　）

　　A. 单萜　　　　　　　　　　　B. 倍半萜　　　　　　　　　C. 二萜

　　D. 二倍半萜　　　　　　　　　E. 三萜

2. 碱溶酸沉法适用于分离（　　　　）

　　A. 具有内酯结构的萜类　　　　　B. 具有酚羟基结构的萜类

　　C. 具有羧基的萜类　　　　　　　D. 具有羰基的萜类

　　E. 具有双键的萜类

3. 环烯醚萜苷的性质是（　　　　）

　　A. 具有较强酸性　　　　　　　　B. 易被酸水解

　　C. 与 Trim-Hill 试剂呈阳性反应　　D. 易溶于水

　　E. 可与氨基酸发生反应

4. 关于萜的描述正确的是（　　　　）

　　A. 异戊二烯的聚合物及衍生物　　B. 开链萜烯符合通式（C_5H_8）$_n$

　　C. 可按异戊二烯单元的数目进行分类　　D. 无其他杂原子

　　E. 易溶于水

5. 属于萜类性质的是（　　　　）

　　A. 多具手性碳　　　　　　　　　B. 易溶于水　　　　　　　　C. 溶于醇

　　D. 易溶于亲脂性有机溶剂　　　　E. 都具有挥发性

6. 挥发油主要成分包括（　　　　）

　　A. 纤维素化合物　　　　　　　　B. 脂肪族化合物　　　　　　C. 芳香化合物

　　D. 萜类化合物　　　　　　　　　E. 一些中药经水蒸气蒸馏而分解出的挥发性物质

7. 挥发油在下列哪种条件下易变质（　　　　）

　　A. 高温　　　　　　　　　　　　B. 低温　　　　　　　　　　C. 暴露空气中

　　D. 光照　　　　　　　　　　　　E. 密封

8. 挥发油具有的性质有（　　　　）

　　A. 难溶于水　　　　　　　　　　B. 易溶于水　　　　　　　　C. 升华性

　　D. 挥发性　　　　　　　　　　　E. 能水蒸气蒸馏

9. 提取挥发油可采用的方法为（　　　　）

　　A. 水蒸气蒸馏法　　　　　　　　B. 溶剂提取法　　　　　　　C. 压榨法

　　D. 超临界流体萃取法　　　　　　E. 升华法

10. 分离挥发油可采用的方法为（　　　　）

A. 分馏法　　　　　　　B. 色谱法　　　　　　　C. 透析法

D. 化学法　　　　　　　E. 冷冻法

三、思考题

1. 常见萜类化合物可以分成哪些类型? 请列举含有各类型萜的常见中药。

2. 挥发油应如何保存? 为什么?

3. 青蒿素是哪类化合物? 具有何生物活性? 如何增强其生物活性?

4. 常采用什么方法对挥发油进行定性定量分析? 该方法有何优点?

（潘晓丽　辛　萍）

Chapter 11   Saponins

 学习目标

知识要求：

1. 掌握 皂苷的定义及主要理化性质；皂苷的提取与分离方法。

2. 熟悉 皂苷的分类及皂苷元主要类型的波普特征鉴别方法；人参、柴胡、甘草和麦冬的主要化学成分、提取和检识方法。

3. 了解 皂苷的水解方法、水解产物；人参、柴胡、甘草和麦冬的功能与主治，药理活性，质量标准等。

能力要求：

熟练掌握皂苷的提取分离方法及基本操作技能，能根据不同的皂苷类型及所具有的性质设计合理的提取分离步骤和方案；学会采用化学反应方法初步检识皂苷的存在及区分皂苷的类型；学会根据重要波谱特征判断皂苷的结构类型。

1   Introduction

Saponins (皂苷) are a group of glycosides which, even at low concentration, produce a frothing in aqueous solution and upon hydrolysis they yield an aglycone known as a sapogenin (皂苷元), either steroid or triterpenoid. The name saponin was from the Latin "*sapo*" (soap) and plant materials containing saponins were originally used for cleaning clothes.

Saponins are widely distributed in nature, especially in the higher plants including the families: Rosaceae, Caryophyllaceae, Sapindaceae, Dioscoreaceae, Polygalaceae, Campanulaceae, Araceae, Liliaceae, Scrophulariaceae, Leguminosae, Araliaceae and Rhamnaceae, etc.

Most of the plants containing saponins have medicinal and commercial values. Saponins have a wide range of pharmacological activities, such as anticancer, antibacterial, antiviral, anti-inflammatory and antifertility activities. Saponins are active constituents of Chinese herbs such as Ginseng Radix et Rhizoma, Glycyrrhizae Radix et Rhizoma (甘草), Bupleuri Radix (柴胡), Platycodonis Radix (桔梗) and Ophiopogonis Radix (麦冬) etc.

2 Structural Characters and Classification

Depending on the sapogenin, saponins are firstly classified into two main groups: triterpenoid saponins and steroidal saponins. The former is widely distributed in nature, especially in many dicotyledon families, while the latter is less widely distributed in nature. They are found in many monocotyledon families such as Dioscoreaceae, Agavaceae and Liliaceae.

Saccharides generally presented in saponins are mainly D-xylose, D-ribose, D-glucose, D-mannose, L-arabinose, L-rhamnose, L-fucose, D-glucuronic acid and D-galacturonic acid, etc.

According to the number of monosaccharides in saponins, saponins are further classified into monosaccharide saponins, disaccharide saponins and trisaccharide saponins, etc.

Based on the number of position in which saccharides joined to sapogenin, saponins are further classified into monodesmosidic saponins (单糖链皂苷), bisdesmosidic saponins (双糖链皂苷) and tridesmosidic saponins (三糖链皂苷), etc.

The secondary glycosides of saponins produced by hydrolysis or enzymolysis from primary glycosides are called prosapogenins (次皂苷). Saponins with ester bond are called ester saponins (酯皂苷).

2.1 Steroidal Saponins

2.1.1 Structural Characters

Steroidal saponins are glycosides which contain steroidal aglycone group and saccharide moiety in nature. Their aglycones are C_{27} sterols in which the side-chain of cholesterol has undergone modification to produce a spiroketal (螺缩酮). The basic skeleton is spirostane (螺甾烷).

spirostane

There are six rings in the structure, among them ring E joins ring F by spiroketal style directly to form the spirostane. In general, rings A and B are fused through *trans* or *cis* configuration; but rings B/C and C/D are always fused through *trans* styles.

Pertaining to the rings E and F in spirostane, the C-20, C-22, and C-25 are chiral carbon atoms. Among them, the configuration of C-20 is *S* type, and C-22 is *R* type. However, there are two stereoisomers as of the position of C-25. When the chemical bond of the methyl group at C-25 position is upright bond (axial bond) above the plane of the ring F, the configuration of C-25 is *S* type, also known as

L type or neo type, herein it is called spirostane. Conversely, when the bond of the methyl group at C-25 position is flat bond (equatorial bond) below the F ring plane, the configuration of C-25 is *R* type, also known as *D* type or *iso* type, herein it is called isospirostane (异螺甾烷). Spirostane and isospirostane are stereoisomers, often co-occur in the plant. Type 25*R* is more stable than type 25*S*, but type 25*S* can be easily transformed into type 25*R*.

There are some hydroxyl groups in steroidal sapogenins, and the most common one is connected at C-3 and the configuration of this hydroxyl group is mostly *β*. Except C-9 and quaternary carbons, the other positions may also be substituted by hydroxyl groups. There are also carbonyl and double bonds in the structures, and carbonyl is mostly occurring at C-12. This is the required substituent for the synthesis of adrenal cortex hormones. The double bonds are mostly located at Δ^5 and $\Delta^{9(11)}$ and less at $\Delta^{25\,(27)}$.

In general, the saccharide moiety in steroidal saponins commonly includes D-glucose, D-galactose, D-xylose, L-rhamnose and L-arabinose. In addition, L-fucose and D-cymarose also occur, and there are 6-deoxy-D-glucose (D-quinovose) and 6-deoxy-D-galactose in the starfish saponins. Saccharides are mostly connected with the aglycone at C-3 to form glycosides, and are also at other positions such as C-1 and C-26, etc. The modes of connection are the line-chain, branched-chain or disaccharides chain.

Steroidal saponins do not contain any carboxyl group. They are neutral. Therefore, steroidal saponins are also called neutral saponins. Conversely, some of triterpenoid saponins contain carboxyl group and are acidic. Therefore, acidic saponins must be triterpenoid saponins.

2.1.2　Classifications

According to the configurations of C-25 in spirostane and the cyclic states of ring F, steroidal saponins are classified into four types: spirostanol (螺甾烷醇), isospirostanol (异螺甾烷醇), furostanol (呋甾烷醇) and ***pseudo***-spirostanol (变形螺甾烷醇) types, respectively. Examples are listed in Table 11-1.

Table 11-1　Four types of steroidal saponins and related examples

Type	Example
spirostanol	timosaponin (知母皂苷) A–Ⅲ
isospirostanol	dioscin (薯蓣皂苷）

(continued)

Type	Example
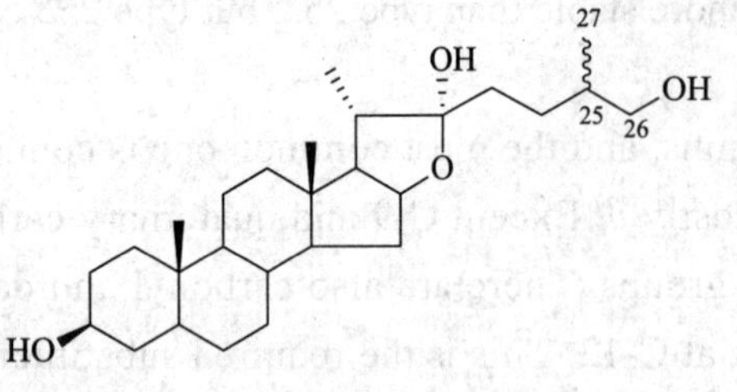 furostanol	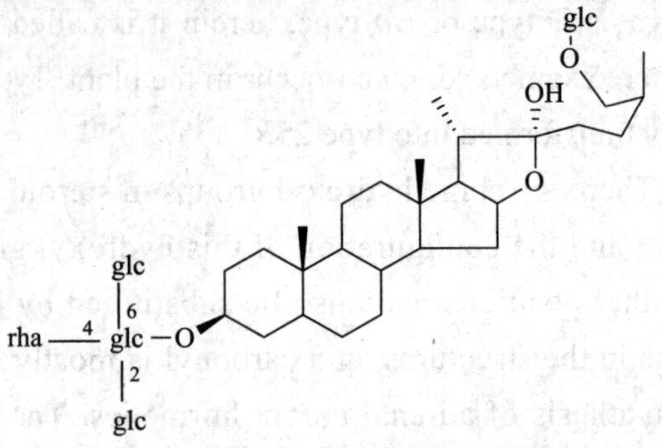 sarsaparilloside (原菝葜皂苷）
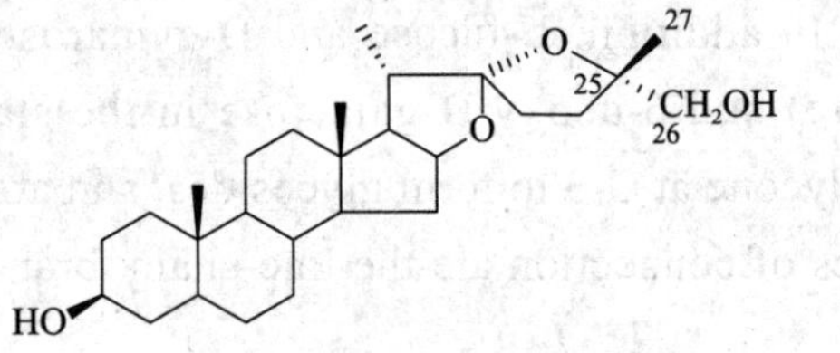 *pseudo*-spirostanol	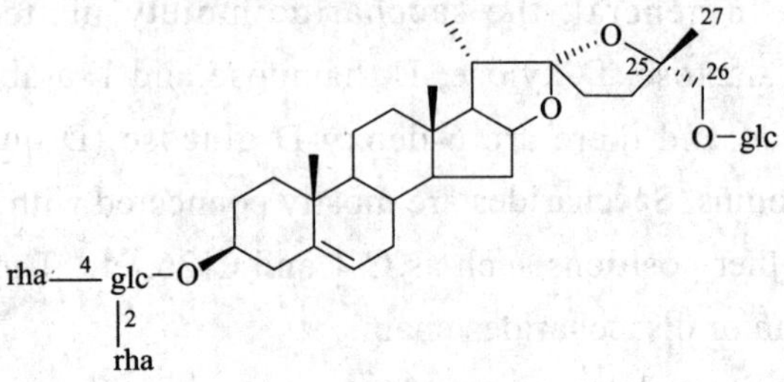 aculeatiside (颠茄皂苷) A

Saponins of the furostanol type are that they are derived from the broken F ring. In the molecule of the furostanol type saponins, besides C-3 or other positions, the hydroxyl group at C-26 also generally forms glycosides, but the glycosidic linkage at C-26 is easily hydrolyzed by enzymes. After removing the glucose connected at C-26, it becomes monodesmosidic saponins and the ring F formed. Then it will transform to either the spirostanol or isospirostanol type. For example, parillin (菝葜皂苷) from Smilax aristolochiaefolia (菝葜属) belongs to monodesmosidic saponin of the spirostanol type. It comes from sarsaparilloside coexisted in the plant. Sarsaparilloside is a bisdesmosidic saponin of the furostanol type and easily hydrolyzed by *β*-glucosidase to lose the glucose at C-26 and to form parillin. It is shown in Figure 11-1.

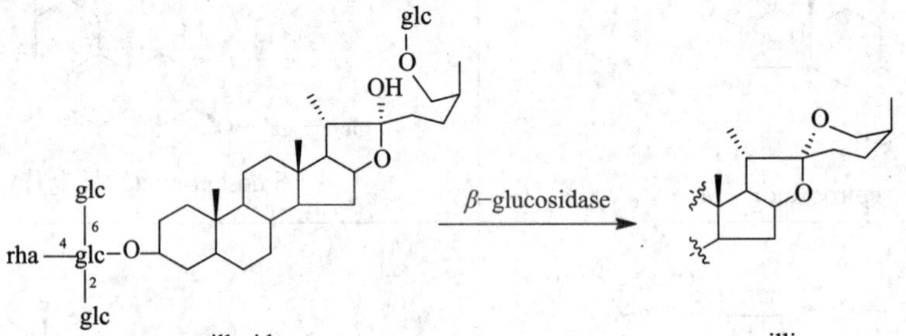

$$\xrightarrow{\beta\text{-glucosidase}}$$

sarsaparilloside

parillin

Figure 11-1   Hydrolysis of sarsaparilloside

Saponins of the *pseudo*-spirostanol type are that the F ring is the furan ring. This type of saponins is less found in nature, and the hydroxyl group at C-26 is a primary alcohol (—RCH₂OH) and always connected with glucose to form glucosides. After removing glucose by acidic hydrolysis, the F ring of a *pseudo*-spirostanol type saponin is rapidly rearranged to form a pyran ring and transform to either a spirostanol or isospirostanol type. For example, aculeatiside A from ***Solanum aculeatissimum*** (刺茄) is a bisdesmosidic saponin of nuatigenin. After acidic hydrolysis, an isospirostanol type sapogenin, isonuatigenin, is yielded (Figure 11-2).

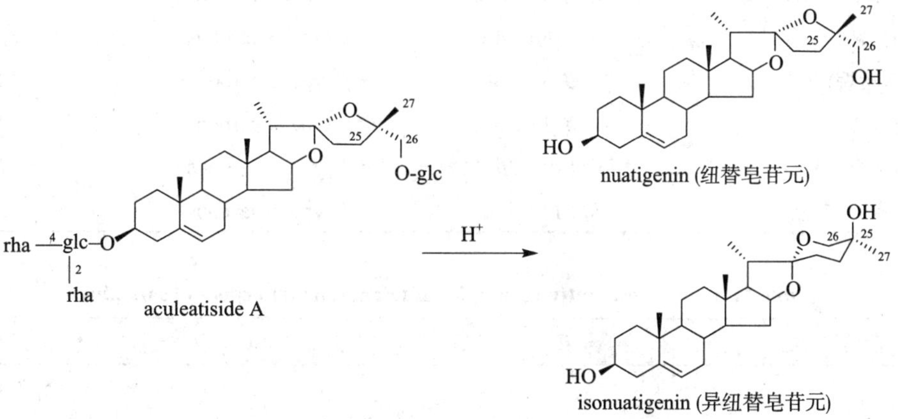

nuatigenin (纽替皂苷元)

aculeatiside A

isonuatigenin (异纽替皂苷元)

Figure 11-2　Acidic hydrolysis of aculeatiside A

In recent 10 years, many novel steroidal saponins have been found. For example, *l*-dehydrotrillenogenin, the derivatives of steroidal saponins, has no methyl at C-13.

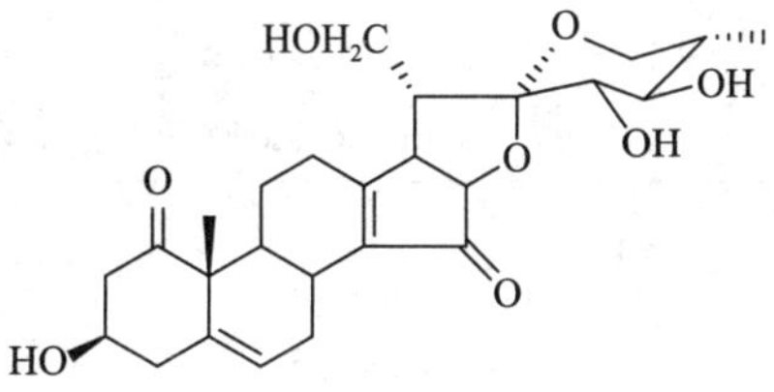

l-dehydrotrillenogenin

2.2　Triterpenoid Saponins

2.2.1　Structural Characters

Triterpenoid saponins are glycosides formed by triterpene aglycone and saccharides. Aglycones are triterpene derivatives generally containing 30 carbon atoms.

Many of triterpenoid saponins possess carboxyl groups at position 4, 17 or 20 of the aglycone, so they are often referred to as acidic saponins. Most of them are alcohol glycosides, but there are also ester glycosides. The latter is also known as ester saponins.

2.2.2　Classifications

According to the nature of aglycone, triterpenoid saponins are categorized into two groups: tetracyclic triterpenoid saponins and pentacyclic triterpenoid saponins.

(1) Tetracyclic Triterpenoid Saponins

Tetracyclic triterpenoid saponins are widely distributed in plants, bacteria, algae, as well as some animals. Structural features of the major types of tetracyclic triterpenoid saponins and representative examples are shown in Table 11-2 and Table 11-3.

Table 11-2 Structural features of the major types of tetracyclic triterpenoid saponins

Type	Methyl	C-17 side chain	C-20 configuration
Lanostane (羊毛脂烷)	$10\beta, 13\beta, 14\alpha$	β type, 8 carbons	R
Euphane (大戟烷)	$10\beta, 13\alpha, 14\beta$	α type, 8 carbons	R
Dammarane (达玛烷)	$10\beta, 8\beta, 14\alpha$	β type, 8 carbons	S, R
Protostane (原萜烷)	$10\beta, 8\alpha, 14\beta$	β type, 8 carbons	S
Meliacane (楝烷)	$10\beta, 13\alpha, 8\beta$	α type, 4 carbons	S
Cycloartane (环菠萝蜜烷)	$10\text{-CH}_2\text{-}9, 13\beta, 14\alpha$	β type, 8 carbons	R
Cucurbitane (葫芦素烷)	$9\beta, 13\beta, 14\alpha$	β type, 8 carbons	R

Table 11-3 Representative examples of tetracyclic triterpenoid saponins

Type	Example
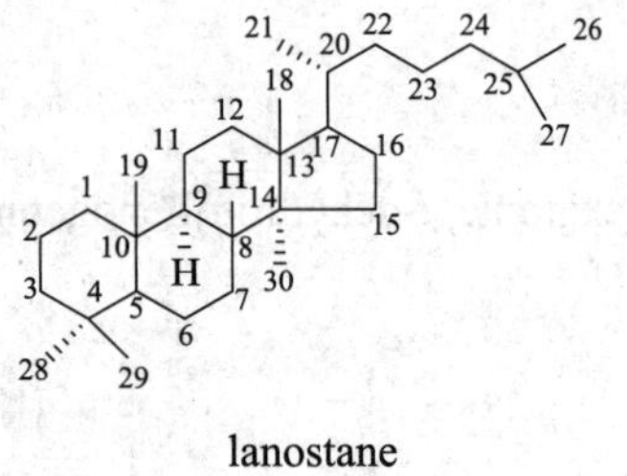 lanostane	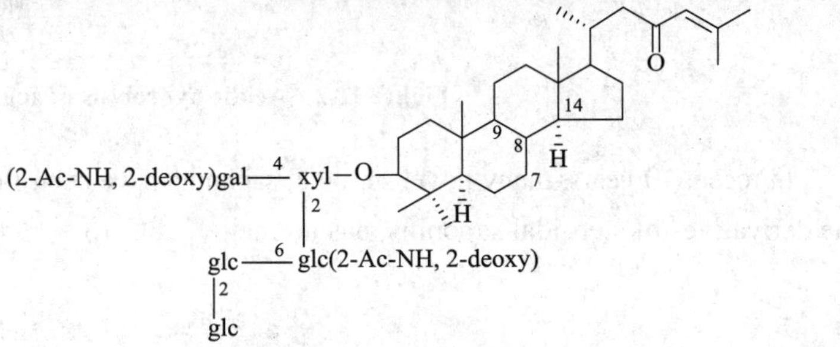 (2-Ac-NH, 2-deoxy)gal —4— xyl—O... glc —6— glc(2-Ac-NH, 2-deoxy), glc sarasinosides A$_1$ (Δ^8), A$_2$ ($\Delta^{7,9(11)}$) and A$_3$ ($\Delta^{8,14}$)
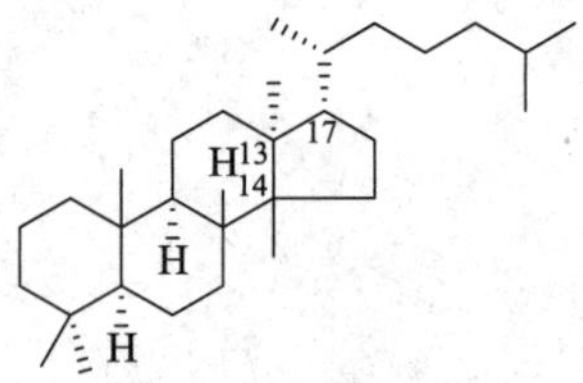 euphane	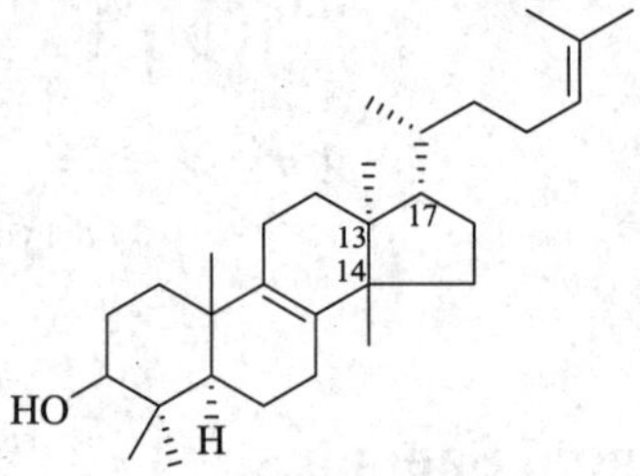 euphol (大戟醇)
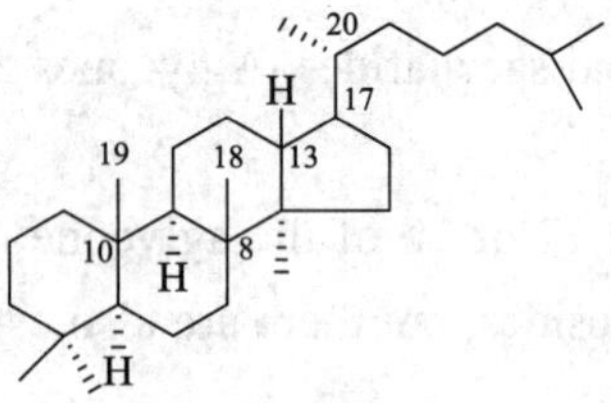 dammarane	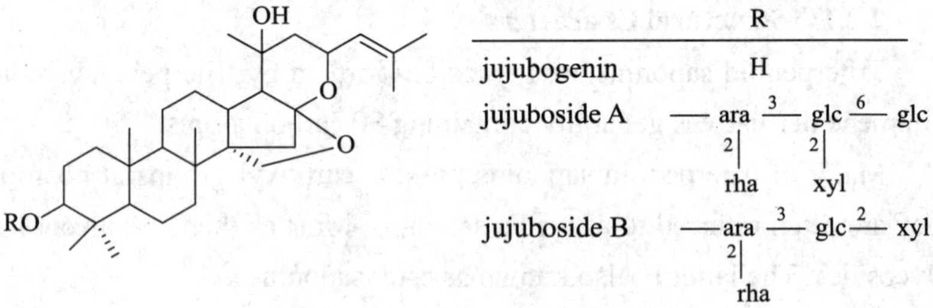 jujuboside (酸枣仁皂苷) A and B
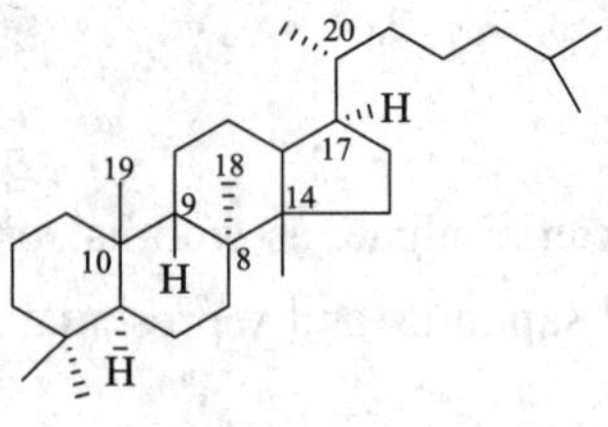 protostane	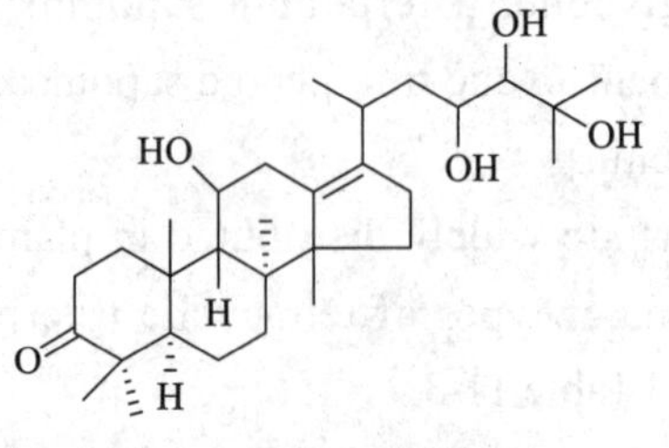 alisol (泽泻萜醇) A 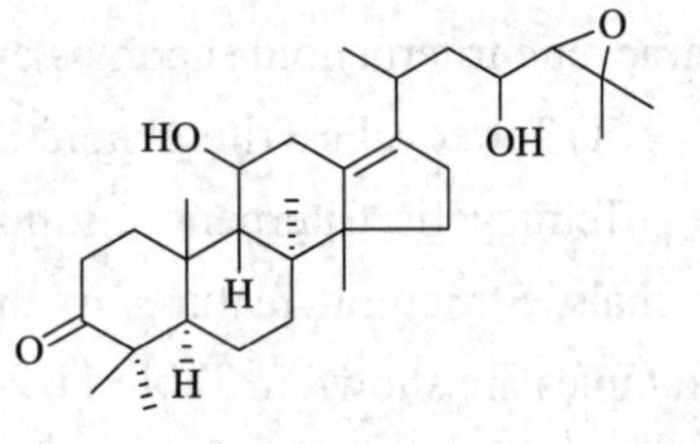 alisol B

(continued)

Type	Example
meliacane	chuanliansu (川楝素) · · · isochuanliansu (异川楝素)
cycloartane	astragenol (黄芪醇) · · · astragalosides (黄芪苷)
cucurbitane	mogroside (罗汉果甜素) V

For the cycloartane example:

	R₁	R₂	R₃
cycloastragenol	H	H	H
astragaloside I	xyl(2,3-diAc)	glc	H
astragaloside V	glc(1—2)xyl—	H	glc
astragaloside VII	xyl	glc	glc

(2) Pentacyclic Triterpenoid Saponins

Pentacyclic triterpenoid saponins are more common in nature, and the main structure types of pentacyclic triterpenoid saponins are oleanane, ursane, lupane, friedelane, fernane, isofernane, hopane, isohopane and other types. Structure features of the major types of pentacyclic triterpenoid saponins and representative examples are shown in Table 11-4 and Table 11-5.

Table 11-4　Structure features of the major types of pentacyclic triterpenoid saponins

Type	Methyl	C-4 substituent	C-20 substituent	Other substituent
Oleanane (齐墩果烷)	10β, 8β, 14α, 17β	two methyl	two methyl	—
Ursane (乌苏烷、熊果烷)	10β, 8β, 14α, 17β	two methyl	20α-methyl	19β-methyl

(continued)

Type	Methyl	C-4 substituent	C-20 substituent	Other substituent
Lupane (羽扇豆烷)	10β, 8β, 14α, 17β	two methyl	—	19α-isopropyl
Friedelane (木栓烷)	9β, 14β, 13α, 17β	4β, 5β-methyl	two methyl	—
Fernane (羊齿烷)	10β, 13α, 14β, 17α	two methyl	—	22α-isopropyl
Isofernane (异羊齿烷)	10β, 13β, 14α, 17β	two methyl	—	22β-isopropyl
Hopane (何帕烷)	10β, 8β, 14α, 18α	two methyl	—	22α-isopropenyl
Isohopane (异何帕烷)	10β, 8β, 14α, 18α	two methyl	—	22α-isopropyl
Other type	Ring C is the seven-membered ring, ring E is the six-membered ring			

Table 11-5　Representative examples of pentacyclic triterpenoid saponins

Type	Example
Oleanane	esculentosides A, B, C, D
ursane	ursolic acid (熊果酸)　sanguisoubin (地榆皂苷) B (R=H)　sanguisoubin E (R=3-Ac–glc)
lupane	23-hydroxy-betulinic acid (白桦脂酸)　pulsatiloside A　pulsatiloside B　pulsatiloside (白头翁苷) A and B

	R_1	R_2	R_3
esculentic acid	H	H	H
esculentoside A	OH	Me	—xyl(4—1)—glc
esculentoside B	OH	Me	—xyl
esculentoside C	H	Me	—xyl(4—1)—glc
esculentoside D	OH	Me	—glc

23-hydroxy-betulinic acid (白桦脂酸)　R_1=R_2=H

pulsatiloside A　R_1=—ara(2–1)–glc(4–1)–glc
R_2=H

pulsatiloside B　R_1=—ara(2–1)–glc(4–1)–glc
R_2=—glc(6–1)–glc(4–1)–rha

(continued)

Type	Example
friedelane	tripterygone (雷公藤酮)
fernane	arundoin (芦竹素)
isofernane	cylindrin (白茅素)
hopane	diploptene (里白烯)
isohopane	hydroxyhopanone (羟基何帕酮)
others	lycoclavanin (石松素)　　　　lycoclavanol (石松醇)

3 Physical and Chemical Properties

3.1 Physical Properties

3.1.1 Characteristics

Most of saponins are colorless or white amorphous powder. They are not easy to crystallize, while most of sapogenins are crystal. Saponins commonly can absorb moisture. Most of them are bitter, acrid, which may strongly irritate human mucosa.

3.1.2 Melting Point and Optical Activity

Sapogenins have fixed melting point, and those containing a carboxyl group have higher melting point. For example, the melting point of oleanolic acid is 308–310℃. The melting points of sapogenins commonly increase with the number of hydroxyl groups in the molecules. Saponins have the higher melting point too, but some of them are decomposed before melting. The decomposition point measured mostly is at 200–350℃.

Both saponins and sapogenins have optical activities.

3.1.3 Solubility

Saponins are soluble in water and easily dissolve in hot water, dilute alcohol, hot methanol and hot ethanol. They are insoluble in petroleum ether, benzene, chloroform, ethyl ether and acetone. In general, saponins can easily dissolve in *n*-butanol containing water or amyl alcohol, so they are often used for extracting saponins from aqueous solution.

Sapogenins are usually insoluble in water, but can dissolve in organic solvents, such as methanol, ethanol, petroleum ether, benzene, chloroform and ethyl ether.

Saponins have the ability of assisting dissolution and can promote the solubility of other constituents in water. When saponins are hydrolyzed into secondary glycosides, the solubility in water will be decreased and may easily dissolve in acetone and ethyl acetate.

3.1.4 Foaming Character

The aqueous solution of saponins upon shaking can produce persistent foam and the foam does not disappear by heating. This is because saponins can reduce the surface tension of aqueous solution, so saponins can also be used as a cleaning agent or emulsifier.

The surface activity of saponins is related to the proportion of lipophilicity moiety to hydrophilicity moiety in the molecules. When the proportion of the two moieties is appropriate, it has excellent effect of the surface activity. If the proportion is imbalanced, the surface activity of the saponins will be weaker or disappear. For example, glycyrrhizin (甘草皂苷) aqueous solution after shaking has little amount of foam.

3.2 Chemical Properties

3.2.1 Color Reactions

Saponins can react with various strong, moderately strong or Lewis acids to give colorful products under anhydrous condition. It is similar to steroids (Table 11-6).

Table 11-6　Color reactions of saponins

Reaction	Reagent	Steroidal saponins	Triterpenoid saponins
Salkowaski reaction	Con. H_2SO_4	Red	Red
Liebermann-Burchard reaction	Con. H_2SO_4 and Ac_2O	Green	Red
Tschugaeff reaction	$ZnCl_2$ and CH_3COCl	Purplish-red	Purplish-red
Rosen-Heimer reaction	25% CCl_3COOH	Purple or red (60℃)	Purple or red (100℃)
Kahlenberg reaction	20% $SbCl_5/CHCl_3$	Blue, gray blue, gray purple, or other colors (60–70℃)	Blue, gray blue, gray purple, or other colors (60–70℃)

3.2.2　Precipitation Reactions

The aqueous solution of saponins can generate precipitation reactions with lead salt, barium salt, and copper salt, etc. Ammonium sulfate, lead acetate or other neutral salts can precipitate acidic saponins (refers to acidic triterpenoid saponins), however neutral saponins (refers to steroidal saponins) can only be precipitated by basic lead acetate or barium hydroxide.

3.2.3　Hydrolysis of Saponins

Saponins can be hydrolyzed by many methods, such as acidic hydrolysis, enzymatic hydrolysis, acetyl hydrolysis and Smith degradation. By selecting an appropriate method of hydrolysis or controlling the specific condition of hydrolysis, the reaction can produce saccharides and aglycone (complete hydrolysis) or secondary glycoside, prosapogenin (partly hydrolysis).

(1) Acidic Hydrolysis

The easiness of acidic hydrolysis of saponins is related to the structure of aglycone and saccharides. Therefore, for saponins containing more than two saccharide chains, different secondary saponins can be obtained by changing the hydrolysis conditions.

During the acidic hydrolysis of saponins, the sapogenins of some triterpenoid saponins are easy to have dehydration, double bond transposition, cyclization and other structure variation reactions. In this case, the original sapogenin cannot be obtained. In order to get the original sapogenin, two-phase acidic hydrolysis, enzymatic hydrolysis and Smith degradation can be used.

(2) Acetylation and Hydrolysis (Acetolysis)

Under the catalysis of BF_3, the full acetylated oligosaccharides and full acetylated aglycone can be obtained from the full acetylated compounds of saponins by using acetic anhydride to make the glycosidic linkage cleavage.

(3) Smith Degradation

Due to the milder condition of Smith degradation, many unstable sapogenins under the acidic hydrolysis can be obtained by this method, for example ginsenosides (人参皂苷) hydrolysis.

(4) Enzymatic Hydrolysis

Some saponins are unstable under the conditions of acid or alkali, and can be easily damaged by $NaIO_4$ degradation. Then enzymes will be a good choice to hydrolyze them. The hydrolysis of Astragalus saponins is an example. In recent years, the enzymatic hydrolysis method has become the most popular method for saponins hydrolysis.

(5) Hydrolysis of Glycosides of Uronic Acid

In addition to conventional methods, some special methods, such as the photolysis method, four lead acetate-acetic anhydride method, acetic anhydride-pyridine method and microbial transformation method, etc., should be used for the hydrolysis of uronic acid saponins that are difficult to be hydrolyzed by acid.

(6) Hydrolysis of Ester Saponins

Saponins containing ester glycosidic linkage can be hydrolyzed by alkaline. In general, ester glycosidic linkage of saponins can be cleaved in NaOH aqueous solution or 5N ammonia.

Lithium iodide (LiI) hydrolysis method can also be used for the hydrolysis of ester saponins. Saponins are refluxed with LiI in methanol solution of 2, 6-dimethyl pyridine. The advantage of this method is that the reaction only makes ester glycosidic linkage broken, while the other glycosidic linkages and other acyl groups in the molecule are not affected. The oligosaccharide chain joined the aglycone in the form of ester glycosidic linkage can be quantitatively cleaved, and the oligosaccharide structure will be unchanged. Then the secondary saponin and the oligosaccharide can be obtained by the chromatography method, and their structures can be identified respectively. This is very helpful for the structure analysis of a complex saponin.

3.2.4 Hemolysis

The aqueous solution of saponins can mostly destroy red blood cells by hemolysis and it is toxic, so saponins are also called sapotoxins (皂毒类). By intramuscular injection, the aqueous solution of saponins can easily cause tissue necrosis, but oral administration does not lead to any hemolysis.

Hemolysis index can be used for indicating the hemolysis degree of different saponins. It refers to the lowest concentration of the saponins that can cause the red blood cell completely dissolved in certain conditions (isotonic, buffer and constant temperature). For example, the hemolysis index (M) of glycyrrhizin is 1:4000, while the hemolysis index of dioscin is 1:400000.

Hemolysis of saponins is because most saponins can combine with cholesterol on the red blood cell wall to form the insoluble complexes. When the aqueous solution of saponins encountered with red blood cells, the precipitate of insoluble complexes will be formed on the wall of red cells. The precipitate can destroy normal permeability of the red blood cells, make osmotic pressure inside the cells increase, and lead to hemolysis phenomenon. But not all saponins can destroy red blood cells and generate hemolysis phenomenon. For example, the total ginsenosides have no hemolysis, but after isolation, type B and type C of ginsenosides have significant hemolysis, while type A of ginsenosides has anti-hemolysis.

It is worth noting that some other constituents in extract solution of Chinese herbs also have hemolysis, such as resin, fat and volatile oils in some plants. In this case, to determine whether hemolysis is due to saponins, further purification is needed, and the cholesterol precipitation method can also be used. If the filtrate of the solution containing precipitate has no hemolysis phenomenon, and after dissolution of the precipitate it has hemolytic activity, this indicates hemolysis is caused by saponins.

4　Extraction and Isolation Methods

4.1　Extraction Methods

4.1.1　Extraction of saponins with Alcohols

Alcohols (ethanol or methanol) are commonly used for the extraction of saponins. The process is shown in Figure 11-3.

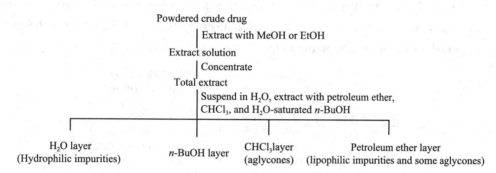

Figure 11-3　General extraction procedure of total saponins from crude drugs

4.1.2　Extraction of Sapogenins with Organic Solvents

Sapogenins can be extracted with organic solvents. In laboratory, crude saponins are commonly extracted first and then hydrolyzed by acid to yield sapogenins. At last sapogenins are subsequently extracted with organic solvent from the hydrolysis solution. In industry, the plant materials are directly hydrolyzed in acidic solution, and then the hydrolysis solution is filtered, and the residue after washing and drying is extracted with organic solvent to get the sapogenins.

4.1.3　Extraction of Acidic Saponins with Alkali Aqueous Solution

Acidic saponins can be extracted by alkali aqueous solution, and then precipitated with acid to obtain acidic saponins.

4.2　Isolation Methods

4.2.1　Solvent Precipitation

Saponins are insoluble in ethyl ether or acetone, but soluble in methanol or ethanol. The procedure is: Dissolve the mixture containing saponins in a small amount of methanol or ethanol; Dropwise ethyl ether or acetone or ethyl ether-acetone (1:1) to the solution until the precipitate of saponins has been produced. The first precipitate obtained from the solution often contains impurities. Therefore, after being filtered to remove the impurity precipitate, to continue adding ethyl ether to the solution, the following precipitate will be total saponins.

The gradient solvent precipitation method can also be used by gradually reducing the solvent polarity. Then different polarity saponins can be precipitated in batches for the separation. This method is simple. But it is difficult to separate them completely to obtain pure compounds.

4.2.2 Cholesterol Precipitation

Saponins can combine with cholesterol to form insoluble complexes. The complexes of triterpenoid saponins are unstable compared with the complexes of steroidal saponins. This property can be used for the separation of saponins: The crude saponins are dissolved in a small amount of ethanol. Then, add cholesterol saturated ethanol solution until the precipitate of the complexes has no longer been produced. Afterwards, slightly heating is needed. After filtration, the precipitate is washed with water, alcohol and ethyl ether, respectively, to remove sugars, pigments, fat and free cholesterol. After the precipitate (insoluble complex) is dried, reflux the precipitate with ethyl ether. Cholesterol will dissolve in ethyl ether, but saponins cannot dissolve in ethyl ether. At last, the residues are the released saponins after filtration to remove the solution.

4.2.3 Chromatography Method

Saponins are hydrophilic and often co-occurring with other polar impurities. There is little difference between them in structure, so it is difficult to obtain a pure saponin with the above methods. The chromatography method is commonly used for isolation of saponins. In general, multiple chromatography methods are applied for isolation of saponins (Figure 11-4).

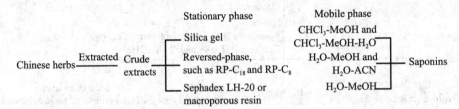

Figure 11-4　General chromatography isolation methods for saponins

5　Identification

5.1　Physicochemical Identification

Color reactions, foaming test and hemolysis test are used to identify saponins (Table 11-7).

Table 11-7　Physicochemical identification of saponins

Test	Reagent or condition	Positive results
Foaming	Strongly shaking the aqueous solution of samples	Producing persistence foam (over 15min)
Liebermann-Burchard reaction	Con. H_2SO_4 + Ac_2O	Showing red color (for triterpenoid saponins) Showing green color (for steroidal saponins)
Rosen-Heimer reaction	25% CCl_3COOH	Showing purple or red color (for triterpenoid saponins heated to 100℃, for steroidal saponins heated to 60℃)
Molish reaction	5% α-Naphthol Con. H_2SO_4	Forming a purple ring between two layers
Hemolysis	0.9% Physiological saline 2% Red cell suspension	Turning clear to turbid

5.2　Chromatography Identification

TLC is an important method for the identification of saponins. Silica gel TLC is usually used with developing solvent systems of chloroform-methanol-water (65:35:10, lower layer), *n*-butanol-acetic acid-water (4:1:5, upper layer), ethyl acetate-*n*-butanol-water (4:5:1, upper layer), ethyl acetate-acetic acid-water (8:2:1), ethyl acetate-pyridine-water (3:1:3), etc. RP-TLC is also used with methanol-water or acetonitrile-water as eluents.

For sapogenins and low polar saponins, cyclohexane-ethyl acetate (1:1), benzene-chloroform, benzene-methanol or benzene-acetone (1:1), chloroform-ethyl acetate (1:1), chloroform-methanol or chloroform-acetone (95:5) is used as the developing solvent system.

For acidic saponins, a small amount of formic acid or acetic acid can be added into the developing solvent system to improve the separation.

The commonly used spray reagents for TLC are trichloroacetic acid, 10% sulfuric acid ethanol solution, phosphomolybdic acid, antimony pentachloride and vanillin-sulfuric acid, etc. After spraying and heating, different saponins or sapogenins will present different colors.

6　Structure Determination

The spectroscopic method is mainly used for the structure determination of saponins. The 2D-NMR and X-ray crystal diffraction analysis methods can be used for the structure determination of novel skeleton and complex structures.

6.1　UV

6.1.1　Steroidal Saponins

Most steroidal saponins do not have the conjugated system, so there is no long wave-length absorption in their UV spectrum. But if the isolated double bonds, carbonyl group, and α, β-unsaturated ketones or conjugated double bonds presented in the structure, they can generate absorption in UV spectrum. In addition, when steroidal sapogenins react with concentrate sulfuric acid, an absorption at 270–275nm will appear. It may be caused by the E and F rings of the steroidal sapogenins.

6.1.2　Triterpenoid Saponins

Most of triterpenoid saponins do not produce UV absorption, but for the compounds of oleanane type having the structure with double bonds, the UV spectrum can be used to determine the type of double bond. The Maximum absorption and related structure feature are listed in Table 11-8.

Table 11-8　UV absorptions of the oleanane type triterpenoid saponins

Structure feature	Maximum absorption (nm)
Isolate C=C	205–250 (weak)

(continued)

Structure feature	Maximum absorption (nm)
C=C—C=O	242–250
C=C—C=C in one ring	285
C=C—C=C in two rings	240, 250, 260
11-oxo, Δ^{12}	248–249 (18β-H, *i.e.*, D/E *cis*)
	242–243 (18α-H, *i.e.*, D/E *trans*)

6.2 IR

The IR characters of different types of saponins are shown in Table 11-9.

Table 11-9   IR characters of different types of saponins

Types of saponins		Characters of IR (cm^{-1})	
Steroidal	Spirostanol (25*S*)	980(A), 920(B), 900(C), 860(D)	B>C
	Isospirostanol (25*R*)		B<C
Triterpenoid	Oleanane type	A area: 1392–1355	A area has 2 peaks but B has 3 peaks
	Ursane type	B area: 1330–1245	A and B areas both have 3 peaks

6.3 MS

6.3.1 Steroidal Sapogenins

The EI-MS fragmentation of steroidal sapogenins is very typical, with a strong basic peak at *m/z* 139, a moderate intensity fragment at *m/z* 115, and a weak ion at *m/z* 126. The fragmentation pathway is shown in Figure 11-5.

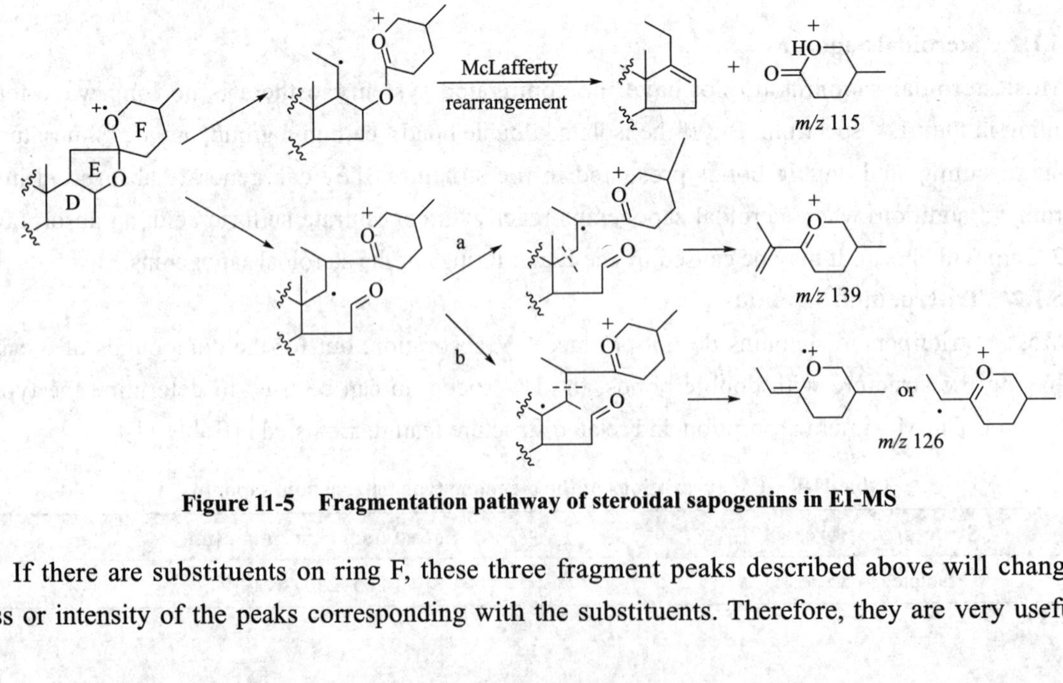

Figure 11-5   Fragmentation pathway of steroidal sapogenins in EI-MS

If there are substituents on ring F, these three fragment peaks described above will change the mass or intensity of the peaks corresponding with the substituents. Therefore, they are very useful for identification of the substitution on ring F.

In addition, in EI-MS spectra there are also a series of fragments (c–h) of steroidal skeleton or the skeleton plus ring E (Figure 11-6). The mass to charge ratio (*m/z*) of these characteristic fragments can be used to identify the aglycones of saponins, the property, number and position of the substituents.

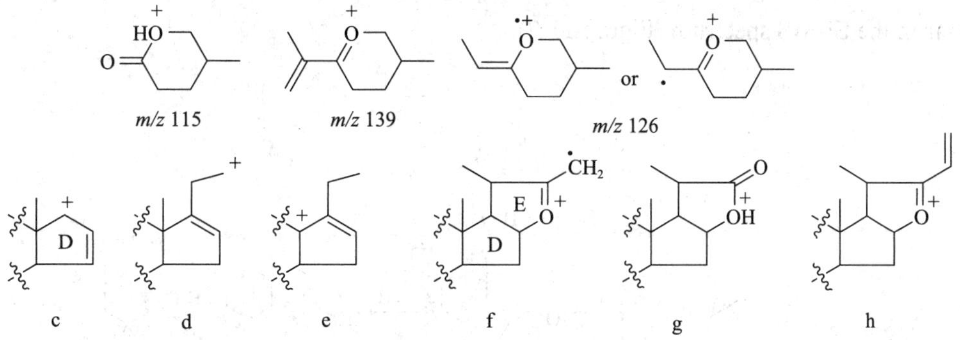

m/z 115   *m/z* 139   *m/z* 126

c   d   e   f   g   h

Figure 11-6   Main fragments of steroidal sapogenins in EI-MS

6.3.2   Steroidal Saponins

FD-MS is applicable in determination of the molecular weight and saccharides connected sequence of steroidal saponins. For example, FD-MS spectrum of compound Balanitin-1 provide the following data: *m/z* 1053 (base peak), 1031, 907, 885, 745, 723, 601, 538 and 415. From the data of *m/z* 1053 [M+Na]$^+$ and 1031 [M+H]$^+$, it can be inferred that the molecular weight is 1030. The fragment peaks at *m/z* 907 [M+Na–146]$^+$ and 885 [M+H–146]$^+$ indicate the loss of a deoxy hexose (rha). The fragment peaks at *m/z* 745 [M+Na–146–162]$^+$ and 723 [M+H–146–162]$^+$ indicate that the above fragments further lose a hexose (glc), and the fragment peaks at *m/z* 601 [M+Na–452]$^+$ is that the *quasi*-molecular ion peak lose two molecules of deoxy hexose and one molecule of hexose. Then the fragment peak at *m/z* 415 [aglycone+H]$^+$ belongs to the fragment of aglycone. Therefore, the number, types and order of the connections of the saccharides and aglycone in the molecule have been inferred.

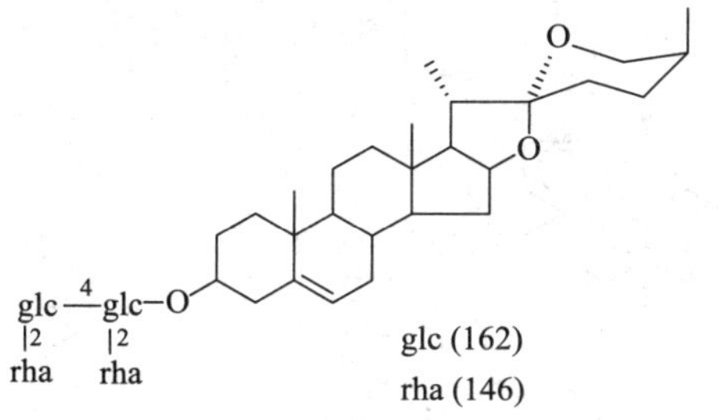

glc $\overset{4}{-}$ glc $-$ O   glc (162)
|2 |2
rha   rha   rha (146)

balanitin-1 (MW=1030)

Although FD-MS has provided more detailed information of the ion fragments in the high mass range, it can't give the information about the structural fragments of the aglycone part. While FAB-MS in addition to giving out the information of the molecular weight and saccharide fragments, particularly it can provide the information of fragments of aglycone in the low mass area, and can also give the information of corresponding anion mass spectrometry. Therefore, FAB-MS can not only determine the molecular weight, the number and order of the saccharides, but infer the aglycone types from the aglycone fragments. It is an effective method for the structural determination of steroidal saponins.

6.3.3 Triterpenoid Sapogenins

(1) Oleanane-12-ene (Ursane-12-ene) Type

There are the molecular ion peak (M^+) and fragments of losing CH_3, OH, or COOH in the EI-MS spectra. Due to the double bond at the C-12 in the molecules, with cyclohexene structure, the reverse Diels-Alder (RDA) cleavage of ring C occurs and the fragments containing A and B rings or D and E rings appear in the EI-MS spectrum (Figure 11-7).

Figure 11-7　RDA cleavage of oleanane-12-ene (ursane-12-ene) type sapogenins in EI-MS

(2) Lupane Type

There are M-43 and the characteristic fragment of losing isopropyl group in the EI-MS spectrum of lupane type sapogenins (Figure 11-8).

Figure 11-8　Characteristic fragment of lupane type sapogenins in EI-MS

6.3.4 Triterpenoid Saponins

FD-MS and FAB-MS both can give the information of *quasi*-molecular ion of saponins, *i.e.*, $[M+H]^+$, $[M+Na]^+$, $[M+K]^+$ or $[M-H]^-$,*etc.*, and also can give the information of the fragments about losing oligosaccharide moieties or monosaccharide of saponins as well as the corresponding fragments of the saccharide moiety.

For example, the structure of saponin X is oleanane-3-*O*-β-D-glucosyl-(1 → 4)-*O*-β-D-glucosyl-

$(1 \rightarrow 3)$-O-α-L-rhamnosyl-$(1 \rightarrow 2)$-O-α-L-arabinoside, its FAB-MS spectrum shows the *quasi*-molecular ion at m/z 1081 [M+Na]$^+$, and the fragments at m/z 919 [(M+Na)-162]$^+$, 757 [(M+Na)-162-162]$^+$, 611 [(M+Na)-162-162-146]$^+$ and 479 [(M+Na)-162-162-146-132]$^+$ (Figure 11-9). The above data not only show its molecular weight, but also can infer the order of connection between monosaccharides.

In addition, the secondary ion mass spectrometry (SI-MS), time of flight mass spectrometry (TOF-MS),

Figure 11-9   Fragmentation of saponin X in FAB-MS

electrospray ionization mass spectrometry (ESI-MS), and laser desorption mass spectrometry (LD-MS) have also been successfully applied to identify the structure of saponins.

6.4   NMR

NMR is a well-established and the most commonly used method for structure determination of saponins. The chemical shifts and multiplicity of signals corresponding to particular atoms and their coupling with other atoms within the molecules allow for easy identification of the aglycone structure, the pattern of glycosylation, and the identity of the saccharide moiety.

6.4.1 ^{1}H-NMR

(1) The ^{1}H-NMR Characteristics of Steroidal Saponins

Steroidal sapogenins have the characteristic peaks of four methyl groups at 18, 19, 21 and 27 positions in the high field. The proton signals of 18-CH$_3$ and 19-CH$_3$ are singlet, the former occurring at higher field, and the signals of 21-CH$_3$ and 27-CH$_3$ are doublet, the latter occurring at higher field. If there is a substitute of hydroxyl group at C-25, the 27-CH$_3$ shows as a singlet peak and shifts to downfield. The H-16 and H-26 are the protons with oxygen on the same carbon, occurring at downfield, which is easy to be identified. The chemical shifts of the protons on other carbon atoms are similar, overlapping each other and not easy to be identified.

The chemical shift of α-orientation (25R) 27-CH$_3$ (δ_H 0.7) is smaller than that of β-orientation (25S) 27-CH$_3$ (δ_H 1.1). In addition, the chemical shift signals of the two protons on C-26 are similar in the 25R isomer, but different in the 25S isomer. Therefore, the proton signals of 27-CH$_3$ and C-26 can be used to distinguish the 25R and 25S isomers.

(2) The ^{1}H-NMR Characteristics of Triterpenoid Saponins

In the high field region of the ^{1}H-NMR spectrum, a number of singlet peaks of the methyl groups are the major features of triterpenoid sapogenin. The characteristic signals of triterpenoid sapogenin are shown in Table 11-10.

Table 11-10   Characteristic signals of triterpenoid sapogenins in ^{1}H-NMR

Types of methyl group	Chemical shift (δ_H)
Quaternary carbon-CH$_3$	0.60–1.50 (s)
C=C—CH$_3$	1.63–1.80 (s)
O=C—CH$_3$	1.82–2.07 (s)

(continued)

Types of methyl group	Chemical shift (δ_H)
$O=C-O-CH_3$	3.6 (s)
6-Deoxy sugar (6-CH$_3$)	1.4–1.7 (d, $J = 5.5$–7.0Hz)
Ursane type 29-CH$_3$ and 30-CH$_3$	0.8–1.0 (d, $J \approx 6$Hz)
C=CH	4.3–6.0
HO—CH	3.2–4.0
AcO—CH	4.0–5.5

In the saccharide moiety of saponins, the anomeric proton signal is generally easy to be recognized. Its coupling constants can be used to determine the configuration of glycosidic linkage (Referring to Chapter 3).

6.4.2 ^{13}C-NMR

(1) ^{13}C-NMR Characteristics of Steroidal Saponins

Generally, if there is a hydroxyl group on carbon atom of steroidal sapogenin, the chemical shift value of the carbon will shift 40–45 downfield. If the hydroxyl group forms a glycoside linkage with a saccharide, the carbon will show a glycosidic shift of 6–10 downfield. The chemical shift values of C=C are in the range of 115–150. If C-16 and C-20 are linked to oxygen, their chemical shifts will be at δ_C 80 and 109, respectively. The chemical shift values of the four methyl groups at C-18, 19, 21 and 27 are less than C-20.

For different types of steroidal sapogenins, the chemical shifts of C-22 are significantly different. In general, the signals of C-22 of spirostanol, furostanol and *pseudo*-spirostanol occur at δ_C 109.5, 90.3 and 120.9, respectively.

(2) ^{13}C-NMR Characteristics of Triterpenoid Saponins

The ^{13}C-NMR spectrum is valuable to determine the structures of triterpenoid saponins. In ^{13}C- NMR spectra, the signals of angular methyl groups on the triterpenoid skeleton generally occur in the δ_C 8.9–33.7 range. Among them the signals of the 23-CH$_3$ and 29-CH$_3$ with equatorial-bond appear at *ca.* δ_C 28.0 and 33.0, respectively. The signals of the carbons linked to oxygen in the sapogenins and saccharides are at *ca.* δ_C 60.0–90.0, the anomeric carbon of a saccharide is at *ca.* δ_C 90.0–112.0. The olefinic carbon is at *ca.* δ_C 109.0–160.0, and the carbonyl carbon is at *ca.* δ_C 170.0–220.0.

The application of ^{13}C-NMR in determination of the types of triterpenoid sapogenins and the C-20 configuration of the sapogenin in ginsenosides are shown in Table 11-11 and Table 11-12.

Table 11-11   Determination of oleanane, ursane, lupane types

Types of triterpenoid sapogenin	Characteristics of ^{13}C NMR	Chemical shift (δ_C)
Oleanane	6 quaternary carbons (C-4, 8, 10, 14, 17, 20)	37.0–42.0
Ursane	5 quaternary carbons (C-4, 8, 10, 14, 17)	37.0–42.0
Lupane	5 quaternary carbons (C-4, 8, 10, 14, 17)	37.0–42.0
	terminal double bond $\Delta^{20(29)}$	110, 150

Table 11-12   Determination of the C-20 configuration of the sapogenin of ginsenosides

Configuration of C-20	Chemical shifts (δ_c)					
	C-13	C-16	C-17	C-20	C-21	C-22
20*S*	47.7	26.6	53.6	74.0	26.8	34.8
20*R*	48.5	26.4	49.9	74.6	21.8	42.3

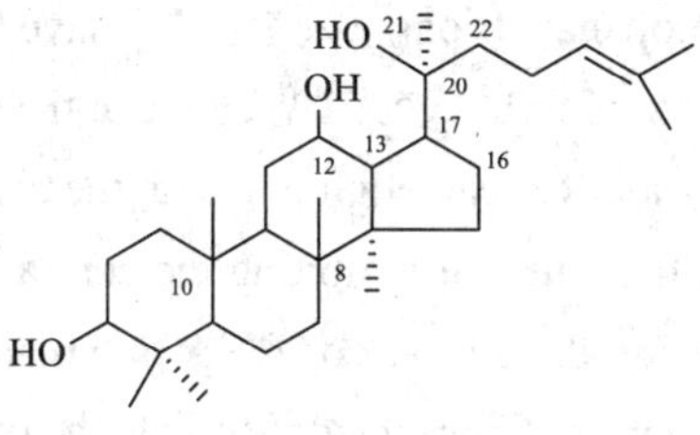

20(*S*)-protopanaxadiol

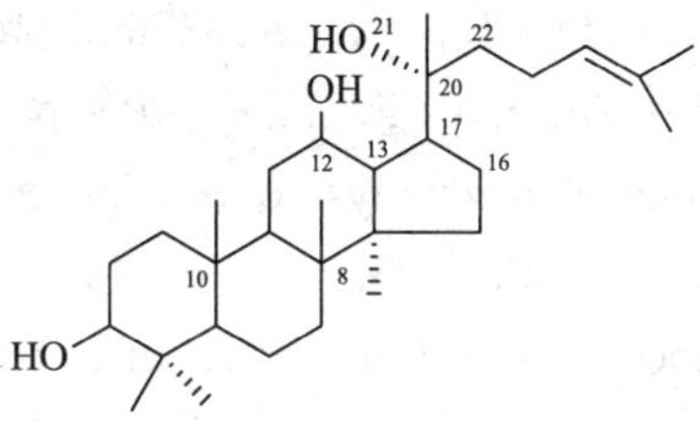

20(*R*)-protopanaxadiol

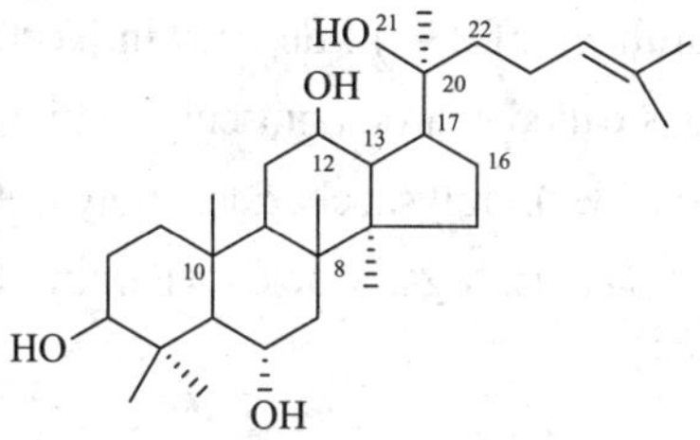

20(*S*)-protopanaxatriol

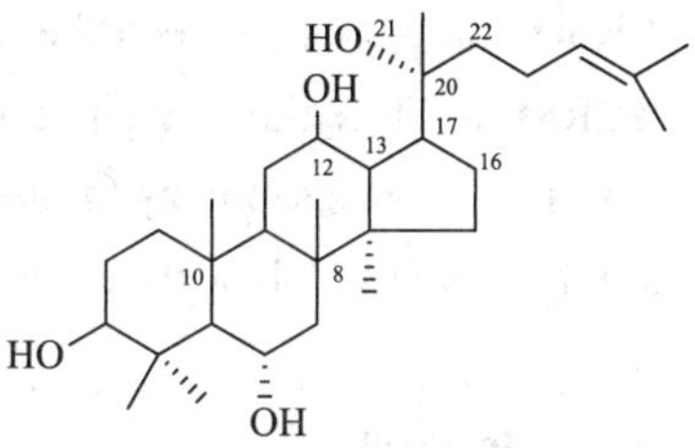

20(*R*)-protopanaxatriol

7   Examples of Chinese Herbs Containing Saponins

7.1   Ginseng Radix et Rhizoma (人参)

7.1.1   Introduction

(1) Biological Source

Ginseng Radix et Rhizoma is the dried root and rhizome of Panax ginseng C. A.Mey. (人参) (Fam. Araliaceae).

(2) Property, Flavor, and Channels Entered

Property and Flavor: Mild warm; Sweet, Mild bitter.

Channels Entered: Spleen, Lung, Heart, and Kidney.

(3) Actions & Indications

Tonify the original qi greatly, resume pulse and secure collapse, tonify the spleen and replenish kidney, engender fluid and nourish blood, tranquilize the mind and replenish wisdom. For collapse caused by body deficiency, cold limbs and faint pulse, low appetite caused by spleen deficiency, dyspnea and cough caused by lung deficiency, thirsty caused by body fluid damage, internal heat and wasting-thirst, deficiency of qi and blood, fright palpitations and insomnia, frail caused by long-term illness, impotence and uterine coldness.

(4) Pharmacological Activities

The pharmacological activities associated with Ginseng Radix et Rhizoma include anti-fatigue, anti-stress, anti-tumor, anti-inflammation, anti-radiation, reducing blood sugar, promoting the synthesis of proteins and nucleic acids, promoting the secretion of pituitary gonadotropin, promoting the growth and development, protecting the liver, myocardium, and the function of adrenal cortex, improving the biological membrane permeability, the immunity, memory, and delaying aging, etc.

The ginsenosides of type B derived from 20(*S*)-protopanaxatriol (原人参三醇) have hemolysis effect, but the ginsenosides of type A derived from 20(*S*)-protopanaxadiol (原人参二醇) have anti- hemolysis effect, and the total ginsenosides have no hemolysis effect. Ginsenoside Rg_1 can slightly excite the central nervous system and have the effect of anti-fatigue. Ginsenoside Rb_1 has the effect of inhibiting the central nervous system and sedation. Also, ginsenoside Rb_1 has the effect of increasing the activity of RNA polymerase, but ginsenoside Rc has the effect of inhibiting the activity of RNA polymerase. Ginsenoside Rh_2 has the effect of reversing the cancer cells and can be used as an anticancer drug, but its content in ginseng is very low.

7.1.2　Main Chemical Constituents

Ginseng Radix et Rhizoma grows between the latitudes of 33–48 degrees in Northeast Asia including China, Korea, Japan, and Russia. The cultivated ginseng is called "garden ginseng", while the wild is known as "mountain ginseng". Ginseng contains saponins (ginsenosides), polysaccharides, polyacetylenes, volatile oils, sterols, flavonoids, alkaloids, proteins, polypeptides, amino acids, organic acids, vitamins, trace elements, etc.

(1) Ginsenosides

① Structure and Classification

Ginsenosides are the major effective constituents in ginseng. The content of total ginsenosides in the root of ginseng is about 3%, and the content in fibrous root is more than that in the taproot. The root, rhizome, stem, leaf, flower and fruit of ginseng all contain a variety of ginsenosides. Up to now more than fifty ginsenosides have been isolated from different parts of the plant material.

Ginsenosides can be classified into 3 types according to the structure of aglycone: A (protopanaxadiol type, PPD), B (protopanaxatriol type, PPT) and C (oleanolic acid type). In addition, some ginsenosides belong to types A or B, but their side chains on the aglycone have some changes, so they are grouped as other types of ginsenosides and will be introduced below.

Moreover, it is found that acyl group substituted ginsenosides also present in ginseng. If the acetyl group substituted on C-6 of the terminal saccharide of the saccharide chain on C-3 of the aglycone, they are called acetyl ginsenosides. If there is a malonyl (forming a half ester) at the same position, they are called malonyl ginsenosides.

a. Type A - Protopanaxadiol Type (PPD)　According to the configuration of C-20 of the aglycone, they are classified into two types: 20(*S*)-protopanaxadiol and 20(*R*)-protopanaxadiol. Their structures are shown below.

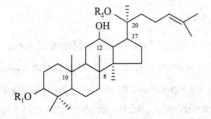

20(*S*)-protopanaxadiol (R_1=R_2=H)

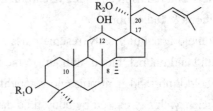

20(*R*)-protopanaxadiol (R_1=R_2=H)

The detailed ginsenosides of protopanaxadiol type are listed in Table 11-13.

Table 11-13　Protopanaxadiol type ginsenosides

Compound	R₁	R₂	C-20 configuration
Ginsenoside Ra₁	—glc(2 → 1)—glc	—glc(6 → 1)—ara(p)(4 → 1)—xyl	*S*
Ginsenoside Ra₂	—glc(2 → 1)—glc	—glc(6 → 1)—ara(f)(2 → 1)—xyl	*S*
Ginsenoside Ra₃	—glc(2 → 1)—glc	—glc(6 → 1)—glc(3 → 1)—xyl	*S*
Ginsenoside Rb₁	—glc(2 → 1)—glc	—glc(6 → 1)—glc	*S*
Ginsenoside Rb₂	—glc(2 → 1)—glc	—glc(6 → 1)—ara(p)	*S*
Ginsenoside Rb₃	—glc(2 → 1)—glc	—glc(6 → 1)—xyl	*S*
Ginsenoside Rc	—glc(2 → 1)—glc	—glc(6 → 1)—ara(f)	*S*
Ginsenoside Rd	—glc(2 → 1)—glc	—glc	*S*
20(*S*)-ginsenoside Rg₃	—glc(2 → 1)—glc	—H	*S*
20(*R*)-ginsenoside Rg₃	—glc(2 → 1)—glc	—H	*R*
Ginsenoside F₂	—glc	—glc	*S*
Ginsenoside Rh₂	—glc	—H	*S*
20(*R*)-ginsenoside Rh₂	—glc	—H	*R*
Quinquenoside R₁	—glc(2 → 1)—glc(6)—Ac	—glc(6 → 1)—glc	*S*
Ginsenoside Rs₁	—glc(2 → 1)—glc(6)—Ac	—glc(6 → 1)—ara(p)	*S*
Ginsenoside Rs₂	—glc(2 → 1)—glc(6)—Ac	—glc(6 → 1)—ara(f)	*S*
Malonyl-ginsenoside Rb₁	—glc(2 → 1)—glc(6)—Ma	—glc(6 → 1)—glc	*S*
Malonyl-ginsenoside Rb₂	—glc(2 → 1)—glc(6)—Ma	—glc(6 → 1)—ara(p)	*S*
Malonyl-ginsenoside Rc	—glc(2 → 1)—glc(6)—Ma	—glc(6 → 1)—ara(f)	*S*
Malonyl-ginsenoside Rd	—glc(2 → 1)—glc(6)—Ma	—glc	*S*
Notoginsenoside R₄	—glc(2 → 1)—glc	—glc(6 → 1)—glc(6 → 1)—xyl	*S*

　　b. Type B - Protopanaxatriol Type (PPT)　According to the configuration of C-20 of the aglycone, they are classified into two types: 20(*S*)-protopanaxatriol and 20(*R*)-protopanaxatriol. Their structures are shown below.

20(*S*)-protopanaxatriol (R₁=R₂=H)　　　　　20(*R*)-protopanaxatriol (R₁=R₂=H)

The detailed ginsenosides of protopanaxatriol type are listed in Table 13-14.

Table 11-14　Protopanaxatriol type ginsenosides

Compound	R₁	R₂	C-20 configuration
Ginsenoside Re	—glc(2 → 1)—rha	—glc	*S*
Ginsenoside Rf	—glc(2 → 1)—glc	—H	*S*
20-gluco-ginsenoside Rf	—glc(2 → 1)—glc	—glc	*S*
Ginsenoside Rg₁	—glc	—glc	*S*

(continued)

Compound	R_1	R_2	C-20 configuration
Ginsenoside Rg_2	—glc(2→1)—rha	—H	*S*
20(*R*)-ginsenoside Rg_2	—glc(2→1)—rha	—H	*R*
Ginsenoside Rh_1	—glc	—H	*S*
20(*R*)-ginsenoside Rh_1	—glc	—H	*R*
Ginsenoside F_1	—H	—glc	*S*
Ginsenoside F_3	—H	—glc(6→1)—ara(p)	*S*
Ginsenoside F_5	—H	—glc(6→1)—ara(f)	*S*
Notoginsenoside R_1	—glc(2→1)—xyl	—glc	*S*
Koryoginsenoside R_1	—glc(2→1)—Bu	—glc	*S*

c. Type C - Oleanolic Acid Type   Ginsenoside-Ro belongs to this type. The aglycone is oleanolic acid.

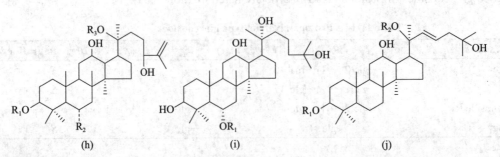

ginsenoside-Ro

Other types ginsenosides are listed in Table 11-15.

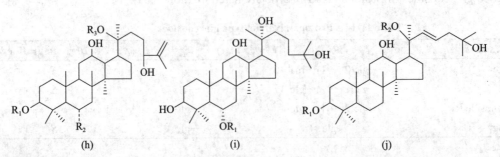

(a)   (b)   (c)   (d)

(e)   (f)   (g)

(h)   (i)   (j)

Table 11-15   Other types Ginsenosides

Compound	Skeleton	R₁	R₂	R₃
Ginsenoside Rh₃	(a)	—glc		
Isoginsenoside Rh₃	(c)	—glc		
Ginsenoside Ia	(b)	—glc	—glc	
Ginsenoside Rg₅	(c)	—glc—glc		
Ginsenoside F₄	(d)	—glc—rha		
Ginsenoside Rh₄	(d)	—glc		
Ginsenoside La	(e)	—glc	—glc	
20(21)-dehydroxylation-ginsenoside Rg₂	(f)	—glc—rha		
Ginsenoside F6a	(g)	—glc—glc	—H	—glc
Majoroside F₄	(g)	—glc	—H	—glc
Ginsenoside L9bc	(h)	—H	—OH	—glc—ara(f)
Majoroside F₂	(h)	—glc	—OH	—glc
Ginsenoside M7cd	(h)	—H	—OH	—glc
25-hydroxyl-ginsenoside Rg₂	(i)	—glc—rha		
Koryoginsenoside R₂	(j)	—glc—glc	—glc—glc	

② Hydrolysis of Ginsenosides

When ginsenosides of types A or B are hydrolyzed by an acid, the real original sapogenins cannot be obtained in the products. This is because the aglycones of ginsenosides are not very stable. During the acidic hydrolysis, isomerization and cyclization of the side chain will occur, and the panaxadiol or panaxatriol will be produced. The reaction process is shown in Figure 11-10.

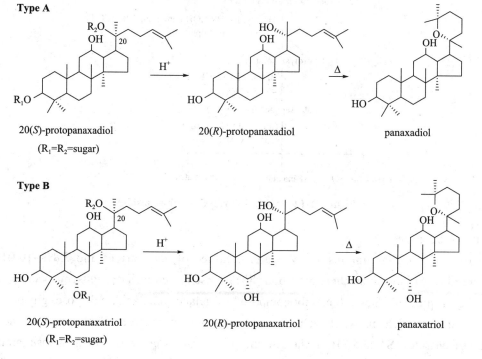

Figure 11-10   Acidic hydrolysis of ginsenosides types A and B

In order to get original sapogenins, an appropriate method of hydrolysis, such as enzymatic hydrolysis or Smith degradation, should be used for hydrolysis of ginsenosides.

③ Extraction and Isolation of Ginsenosides

The extraction and isolation procedure of ginsenosides is shown in Figure 11-11.

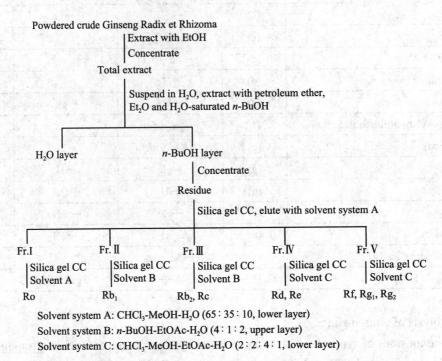

Solvent system A: $CHCl_3$-MeOH-H_2O (65 : 35 : 10, lower layer)
Solvent system B: n-BuOH-EtOAc-H_2O (4 : 1 : 2, upper layer)
Solvent system C: $CHCl_3$-MeOH-EtOAc-H_2O (2 : 2 : 4 : 1, lower layer)

Figure 11-11　Extraction and isolation procedure of ginsenosides

The acid hydrolysis of ginsenosides is shown in Figure 11-12.

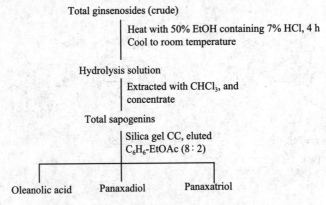

Figure 11-12　Acidic hydrolysis of ginsenosides

(2) Polysaccharides

The root of ginseng contains 38.3% water-soluble polysaccharides and 7.8%–10.0% alkaline polysaccharides. Among them there are about 80% ginseng starch, 20% ginseng pectin and a small amount of glycoprotein. They are mainly composed of galacturonic acid, galactose, glucose, arabinose and a small amount of rhamnose as well as unknown pentose derivatives. There are two kinds of acidic heteropolysaccharides, SA and SB, in the ginseng pectin. SA is composed of galactose, arabinose and rhamnose in molar ratio of 4.7:2.6:1, and contains 26% galacturonic acid. SB is composed of galactose, arabinose and rhamnose in molar ratio of 3.3:1.8:1, and contains 76% galacturonic acid.

7.1.3　Quality Control Standards

(1) TLC Identification

Stationary Phase: Silica gel plate.

Standard: Authentic crude drug; Ginsenoside-Rb_1, Re, and Rg_1 (Chemical Reference Substance, CRS).

Development System: Chloroform-acetyl acetate-methanol-water (15:40:22:10) (Stand below 10℃, lower layer).

Visualization: Spray the solution of 10.0% sulfuric acid in ethanol, heat to 105℃ until spots are clear. Sun light and 365nm UV light.

(2) Tests

Water: Not more than 12.0%.

Total Ash: Not more than 5.0%.

(3) Assay

Total of ginsenoside-Rg_1 and Re: Not less than 0.30% (HPLC).

Ginsenoside-Rb_1: Not less than 0.20% (HPLC).

7.2　Glycyrrhizae Radix et Rhizoma (甘草)

7.2.1　Introduction

(1) Biological Source

Glycyrrhizae Radix et Rhizoma is the dried root and rhizome of Glycyrrhiza uralensis Fisch. (甘草), Glycyrrhiza inflata Bat. (胀果甘草), or Glycyrrhiza glabra L. (光果甘草) (Fam. Leguminosae).

(2) Property, Flavor and Channels Entered

Property and Flavor: Neutral; Sweet.

Channels Entered: Heart, Lung, Spleen, and Stomach.

(3) Actions & Indications

Tonify spleen and qi, clear heat and remove toxin, dispel phlegm and suppress cough, relax spasm and relieve pain, and moderate drug actions. For spleen-stomach weakness, fatigue and lack of strength, palpitation and shortness of breath, cough and profuse sputum, painful spasm in the stomach duct, abdomen and limbs, swelling abscess, sore and toxin, reduce the other drugs' toxic and drastic action.

(4) Pharmacological Activities

The pharmacological activities associated with Glycyrrhizae Radix et Rhizoma include anti-ulcer, anti-allergy, anti-inflammation, prevention of hepatitis, tumor, and HIV, etc.

Glycyrrhizin and glycyrrhetinic acid (甘草次酸), the major effective constituents of Glycyrrhizae Radix et Rhizoma, have the biological activity like adrenocorticotropic hormone (ACTH), clinical as anti-inflammatory drugs, and used in the treatment of gastric ulcer, but only 18β-H-glycyrrhetinic acid has ACTH-like effect. The 18α-H-glycyrrhetinic acid has no such biological activity. In addition, glycyrrhizic acid ammonium salt (diammonium glycyrrhizinate), glycyrrhizin cysteine ester and glycyrrhizin hemisuccinate are also clinically-used as drugs. The pharmacological study also finds that except for resisting allergic reaction, glycyrrhizin can enhance nonspecific immune effect and resist acute injury due to CCl_4 on the liver.

7.2.2 Main Chemical Constituents

Glycyrrhizae Radix et Rhizoma is mainly produced in Gansu, Shanxi, Qinghai, Xinjiang, Hebei, Jilin, Liaoning, Heilongjiang, Neimenggu and Ningxia, etc. It contains saponins, flavonoids, polysaccharides, coumarins, alkaloids, etc. Saponins are the major effective constituents and the content is about 5%–11%.

(1) Triterpenoid Saponins

More than 60 triterpenoid saponins have been isolated from the plants of Glycyrrhiza genus. Most of them are the derivatives of pentacyclic triterpenoids. The skeleton of aglycone belongs to oleanane. The aglycone is mostly 3β-hydroxy-oleanane. The saponins are generally 3β-hydroxyl-oxygen-glucoside. The saccharide moieties are mostly D-glucuronic acid or D-glucose.

The major effective constituents in Glycyrrhizae Radix et Rhizoma are glycyrrhizin (also known as glycyrrhizic acid) and its aglycone is glycyrrhetinic acid. Glycyrrhizin is composed of aglycone (18β-glycyrrhetinic acid) and 2 molecules of glucuronic acid. Glycyrrhizin can be hydrolyzed into 2 molecules of glucuronic acid and 1 molecule of glycyrrhetinic acid by 5% dilute H_2SO_4 solution at 110–120℃ under pressure (Figure 11-13). The crystallized glycyrrhizin from the glacial acetic acid is a colorless and columnar crystals, with melting point about 220℃ (decomposition) $[\alpha]_D^{27} +46.2°$, and soluble in hot dilute ethanol, almost insoluble in ethanol or ethyl ether. Its aqueous solution has a faint foaming and hemolysis properties.

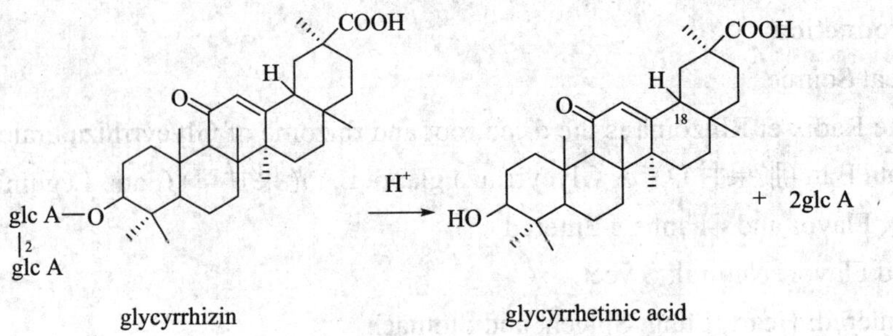

Figure 11-13 Hydrolysis of glycyrrhizin

There are two types of glycyrrhetinic acid. One is that the configuration of D/E ring is *cis* fused (18β-H), needle crystals, melting point 256℃, $[\alpha]_D^{20} +86°$ (ethanol); the other is its isomer, the D/E ring is *trans* fused (18α-H), i.e., 18-α-glycyrrhetinic acid, also known as uralenic acid, small flaky crystals, melting point 283℃, $[\alpha]_D^{20} +140°$ (ethanol). The two crystals are both soluble in ethanol or chloroform.

Besides glycyrrhizin and glycyrrhetinic acid in Glycyrrhizae Radix et Rhizoma, there are also ural-saponin (乌拉尔甘草皂苷) A and B, glycyrrhizin A_3, B_2, C_2, D_3, E_2, F_3, G_2, H_2, J_2, K_2, and a variety of triterpenoids.

① Preparation of Ammonium Salt of Glycyrrhizic Acid

The preparation of ammonium salt of glycyrrhizic acid is shown in Figure 11-14.

② Preparation of Monopotassium Glycyrrhizinate

Glycyrrhizic acid is not easy to be refined. It needs to be made to the potassium salt and then can be further refined. The methods are shown in Figure 11-15.

③ Preparation of Glycyrrhetinic Acid

The Preparation procedure of glycyrrhetinic acid is shown in Figure 11-16.

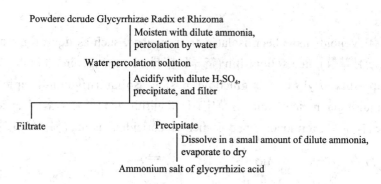

Figure 11-14   Preparation of ammonium salt of glycyrrhizic acid

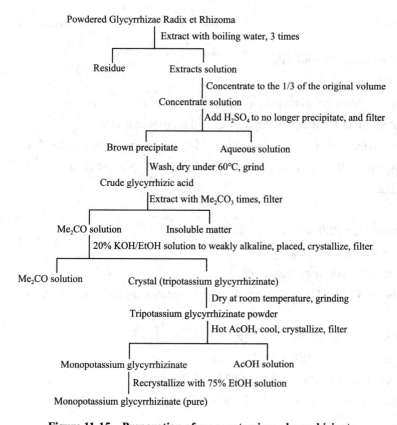

Figure 11-15   Preparation of monopotassium glycyrrhizinate

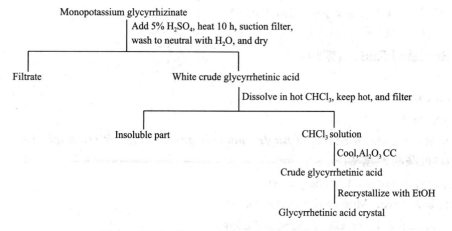

Figure 11-16   Preparation of glycyrrhetinic acid

(2) Flavonoids

More than 70 flavonoids have been isolated from *gancao*, such as liquiritin, isoliquiritin (异甘草苷), neoliquiritin (新甘草苷), neoisoliquiritin (新异甘草苷), liquiritigenin (甘草素)-7, 4′-diglucoside, liquiritigenin-4′-apiofuranosyl (1 → 2) glucopyranoside, isoliquiritigenin-4′-apiofuranosyl(1 → 2) glucopyranoside, liquiritigenin, licoricidin (甘草定), isoliquiritigenin (异甘草素), isolicoflanonol (异甘草黄酮醇), licoricone (甘草酮), formononetin, 5-*O*-methyllicoricidin, ononin (刺芒柄花苷), etc.

liquiritigenin   liquiritin   isoliquiritin

7.2.3   Quality Control Standards

(1) TLC Identification

Stationary Phase: Silica gel plate (made with 1.0% NaOH).

Standard: Authentic crude drug; Glycyrrhizic acid ammonium salt.

Development System: Acetyl acetate-formic acid-glacial acetic acid-water (15:1:1:2).

Visualization: Spray the solution of 10.0% sulfuric acid in ethanol, heat to 105℃ until spots are clear, 365nm UV light.

(2) Tests

Water: Not more than 12.0%.

Total Ash: Not more than 7.0%.

Acid-insoluble Ash: Not more than 2.0%.

Heavy Metals and Other Harmful Elements: Pb ≤ 5 ppm, Cd ≤ 0.3 ppm, As ≤ 2 ppm, Hg ≤ 0.2 ppm, Cu ≤ 20 ppm.

Pesticide Residue of the Organic Chloride:

Benzene hexachloride (Total BHC) ≤ 0.2 ppm

Dichlorodiphenyltrichloroethane (Total DDT) ≤ 0.2 ppm

Pentachloronitrobenzene (Quintozene, PCNB) ≤ 0.1 ppm

(3) Assay

Liquiritin: Not less than 0.50% (HPLC).

Glycyrrhizic Acid: Not less than 2.0% (HPLC).

7.3   Bupleuri Radix (柴胡)

7.3.1   Introduction

(1) Biological Source

Bupleuri Radix is the dried root of ***Bupleurum chinense*** DC. (北柴胡) or ***Bupleurum scorzonerifolium*** Willd (狭叶柴胡, 南柴胡).

(2) Property, Flavor and Channels Entered

Property and Flavor: Mild cold; Pungent, bitter.

Channels Entered: Liver, Gallbladder, and Lung.

(3) Actions & Indications

Disperse and reduce fever, soothe the liver to resolve depression, upraise yang qi. For common cold with fever, alternating chills and fever, distending pain in the chest and the hypochondrium, menstrual irregularities, prolapse of uterine and rectum.

(4) Pharmacological Activities

Saikosaponins (柴胡皂苷) have the effects of anti-inflammation, anti-tumor, antivirus, and regulating endocrine and immune system, protecting the liver and kidney. Saikosaponin a and d have the effects of anti-inflammation and reducing serum cholesterol and triglyceride. Saikosaponin a and saikogenin A have the effects of sedation and removal of heat on experimental animals.

7.3.2　Main Chemical Constituents

Bupleurum chinense DC. chiefly grows in the provinces of Liaoning, Gansu and Hebei. Bupleurum scorzonerifolium Willd mainly yields in the provinces of Hubei, Jiangsu and Sichuan. Bupleuri Radix contains triterpenoid saponins, flavonoids, lignans, coumarins, volatile oils, polysaccharides, *etc.* The total saponins are the major effective components of Bupleuri Radix.

(1) Saikosaponins

① Structure and Classification

Nearly 100 triterpenoid saponins have been isolated from the Bupleurum genus plants. The structures are mostly the derivatives of pentacyclic triterpenes. The skeleton of aglycone belongs to oleanane, and the aglycone is divided into seven types. They are listed in Table 11-16. The examples of saikosaponins are listed in Table 11-17.

Table 11-16　Aglycone types of saikosaponins

Type	Structure of the aglycone
I	olean-13, 28-epoxy-11-ene
II	olean-11, 13(18)-diene
III	olean-12-ene
IV	olean-9(11), 12-diene
V	olean-12-en-28-carboxylic acid
VI	olean-11, 13(18)-dien-30-carboxylic acid
VII	olean-18-ene

Table 11-17　Examples of saikosaponins and their structures

Type	Saikosaponin	Structure	R₁	R₂	R₃
I	saikosaponin a, c, d, e	saikogenin E	H	β-OH	H
		saikosaponin c	H	β-OH	glc (6→1) glc (4→1) rha
		saikosaponin e	H	β-OH	fuc (3→1) glc
		saikogenin F	OH	β-OH	H
		saikosaponin a	OH	β-OH	fuc (3→1) glc
		saikogenin G	OH	α-OH	H
		saikosaponin d	OH	α-OH	fuc (3→1) glc

(continued)

Type	Saikosaponin	Structure
II	saikosaponin b_1, b_2	
III	saikosaponin b_3, b_4, f	
IV	saikosaponin g	
V	rotundioside A, B, C	
VI	saikosaponin v	
VII	bupleuroside XIII	

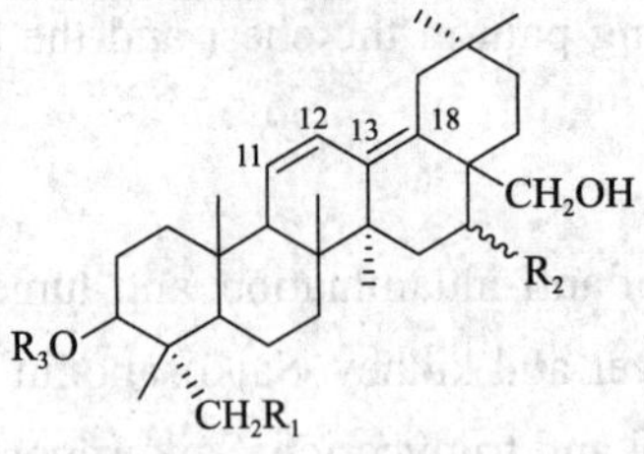

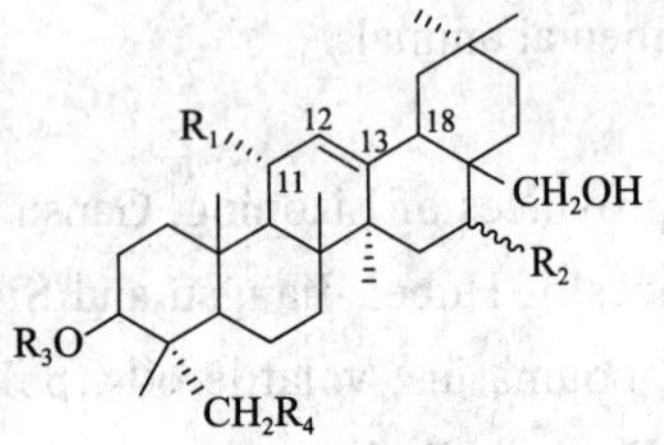

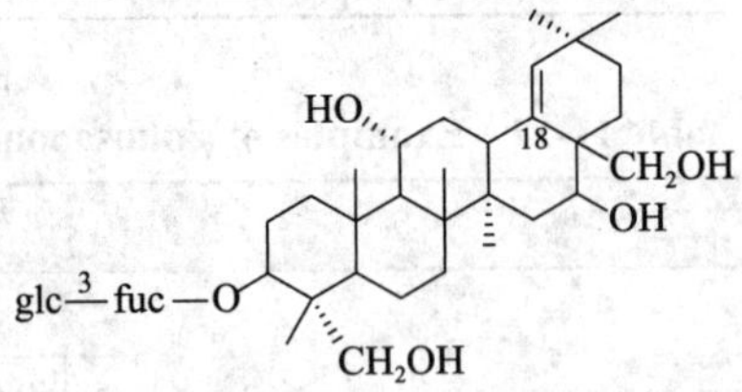

Type II

	R_1	R_2	R_3
saikogenin A	OH	β-OH	H
saikosaponin b_1	OH	β-OH	fuc(3→1)glc
saikogenin D	OH	α-OH	H
saikosaponin b_2	OH	α-OH	guc(3→1)glc
saikogenin C	H	β-OH	H

Type III

	R_1	R_2	R_3	R_4
saikosaponin b_3	OCH_3	β-OH	fuc(3→1)glc	OH
saikosaponin b_4	OCH_3	α-OH	fuc(3→1)glc	OH
longispinogenin	H	β-OH	H	H
saikosaponin f	H	β-OH	glc(6→1)glc ↓4 rha	H

Type IV

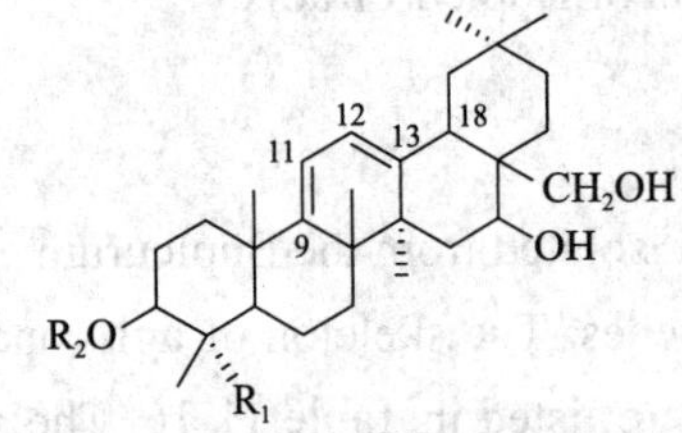

	R_1	R_2
saikogenin B	CH_3	H
saikosaponin g	CH_2OH	—fuc(3→1)glc

Type V

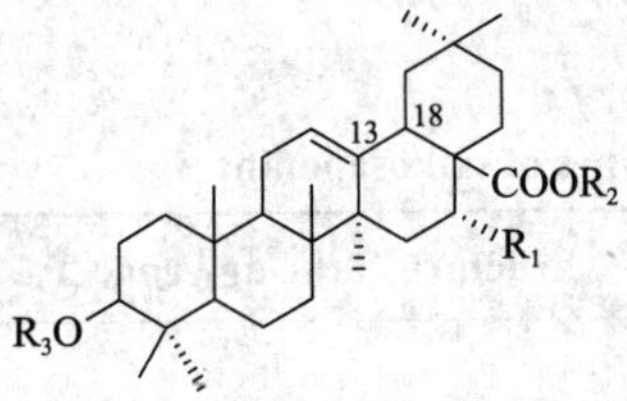

	R_1	R_2	R_3
rotundioside A	α-OH	—glc(6→1)glc(2→1)glc(6→1)glc	SO_3H
rotundioside B	H	—glc(6→1)glc(2→1)glc(6→1)glc	SO_3H
rotundioside C	H	—glc(2→1)glc(2→1)glc(6→1)glc	SO_3H

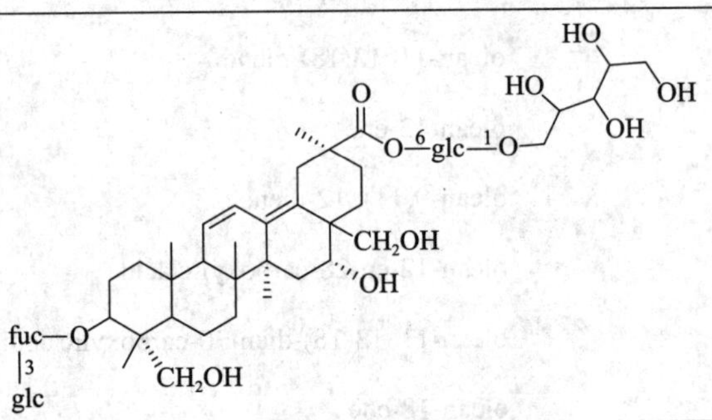

In type I, saikogenins E, F, and G have 13, 28-ether bond, and they are the real aglycones of saikosaponins. The corresponding saponins are saikosaponin a, c, d, e, and their acetyl derivatives. Among them, saikosaponins a and d are the chemical reference substances for Bupleuri Radix to be identified.

The 13, 28-epoxy compounds are unstable. Under the acidic condition, the 13, 28-epoxy bond can be broken to generate artifacts, such as saikogenin A, B, C and D (Figure 11-17). Saikosaponin b₁, b₂, b₃ and b₄ are formed from saikosaponin a, d in the extracting process. Therefore, to control the condition of extraction and purification, neutral is very important for keeping the original structures of saikosaponins. In general, pyridine is added to the solvent to avoid acids presented in the plant to damage the 13, 28-epoxy bond during the extraction process.

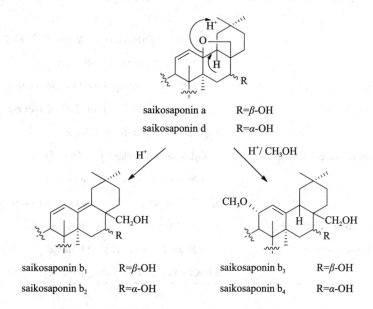

saikosaponin a   R=β-OH
saikosaponin d   R=α-OH

saikosaponin b₁   R=β-OH
saikosaponin b₂   R=α-OH

saikosaponin b₃   R=β-OH
saikosaponin b₄   R=α-OH

Figure 11-17   Damage of saikosaponins a and d

② Extraction and Isolation of Saikosaponins

The extraction and isolation procedure of saikosaponins is shown in Figure 11-18.

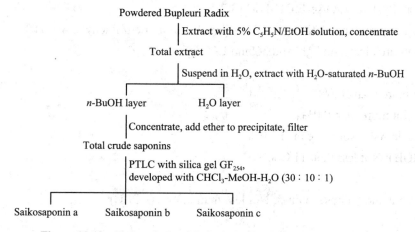

Powdered Bupleuri Radix
| Extract with 5% C₅H₅N/EtOH solution, concentrate
Total extract
| Suspend in H₂O, extract with H₂O-saturated n-BuOH
n-BuOH layer   H₂O layer
| Concentrate, add ether to precipitate, filter
Total crude saponins
| PTLC with silica gel GF₂₅₄, developed with CHCl₃-MeOH-H₂O (30 : 10 : 1)
Saikosaponin a   Saikosaponin b   Saikosaponin c

Figure 11-18   Extraction and isolation procedure of saikosaponins

(2) Flavonoids

Many kinds of flavonoids have been isolated from Bupleuri Radix. Some of them are listed in Table 11-18.

Table 11-18   Flavonoids from Bupleuri Radix

Flavonoids	Structure
Kaempferol	3, 5, 7, 4'-tetrahydroxy-flavone
Kaempferol-7-rhamnoside	3, 5, 7, 4'-tetrahydroxy-flavone-7-O-rha
Kaempferol-3, 7-double-rhamnoside	3, 5, 7, 4'-tetrahydroxy-flavone-3-O-rha-7-O-rha
Kaempferol-3-O-α-L-arabino-furanosyl-7-O-α-L-rhamnopyranoside	3, 5, 7, 4'-tetrahydroxy-flavone-3-O-ara-7-O-rha
Rutin	3, 5, 7, 3', 4'-pentahydroxy-flavone-3-O-rha(1 → 6)-O-glc
Quercetin	3, 5, 7, 3', 4'-pentahydroxy-flavone
Isorhamnetin (异鼠李素)	3, 5, 7, 4'-tetrahydroxy-3'-methoxy-flavone
Isorhamnetin-3-O-glucoside	3, 5, 7, 4'-tetrahydroxy-3'-methoxy-flavone-3-O-glc
Puerarin (葛根素)	7, 4'- dihydroxy-isoflavone-8-glc
7, 4'-dihydroxy-isoflavone-7-O-β-D-glucoside	7, 4'-dihydroxy-isoflavone-7-O- β -D-glc
Saikochromonic acid	5, 6-dihydroxy-2-carboxyl-chromone
Narcissin	3, 5, 7, 4'-tetrahydroxy-3'-methoxy-flavone-3-O-rha(1 → 6)-O-glc
Kaempferol-3-O- α -L-arabinofuranoside	3, 5, 7, 4'-tetrahydroxy-flavone-3-O-ara
7-hydroxy-2, 5-di-methyl-chromone	7-hydroxy-2, 5-di-methyl-chromone
Saikochrome A	2-hydroxymethyl-5-hydroxyl-7-methoxy-tetrahydrogen-chromone

7.3.3   Quality Control Standards

(1) TLC Identification

Stationary Phase: Silica gel plate.

Standard: Authentic crude drug; Saikosaponin-a and saikosaponin-d.

Development System: EtOAc-EtOH-H$_2$O (8:2:1).

Visualization: Spray the solution of 2.0% p-dimethylaminobenzaldehyde in 40.0% sulfuric acid, heat to 60℃ until spots are clear, sun light and 365nm UV light.

(2) Tests

Water: Not more than 10.0%.

Total Ash: Not more than 8.0%.

Acid-insoluble Ash: Not more than 3.0%.

Extract (EtOH): Not less than 11.0%.

(3) Assay

Saikosaponin-a and Saikosaponin-d: Not less than 0.30% (HPLC).

7.4   Ophiopogonis Radix (麦冬)

7.4.1   Introduction

(1) Biological Source

Ophiopogonis Radix is the dried root tuber of Ophiopogon japonicus (L.f) Ker-Gawl. (麦冬) (Fam. Liliaceae).

(2) Property, Flavor and Channels Entered

Property and Flavor: Mild cold; Sweet, Mild bitter.

Channels Entered: Heart, Lung, and Stomach.

(3) Actions & Indications

Nourish yin and engender body fluid, moisten the lung and clear the heart. For dry cough caused by lung dryness, cough caused by yin consumptive disease, thirst caused by fluid consumption, throat impediment and sore throat, internal heat wasting-thirst, insomnia caused by vexation, constipation caused by intestinal dryness.

(4) Pharmacological Activities

The pharmacological activities associated with Ophiopogonis radix include improving the animal's tolerance to anoxia, improving microcirculation of the coronary artery, reducing blood sugar, anti-arrhythmia, enhancing immune function, etc.

7.4.2　Main Chemical Constituents

Ophiopogonis Radix grows mainly in Zhejiang, Sichuan and Jiangsu, Guizhou, Yunnan, Guangxi, Anhui, Hunan, Hubei and Henan of China. It contains saponins, flavonoids, polysaccharides, sterols, volatile oils, etc.

(1) Ophiopogonins (麦冬总皂苷)

① Structure and Classification

Saponins are one of the major effective constituents of Ophiopogonis Radix. More than 40 steroidal saponins have been isolated from different plants of the Ophiopogon genus, for example, ophiopogonin (麦冬皂苷) B, B′, C, C′, D, D′, E, F, and G (Table 11-19, 11-20). Their aglycones are ruscogenin (鲁斯可皂苷元) and diosgenin. Saponins F and G are of the furostanol type. Saccharides in these saponins are mostly fucose, rhamnose, xylose, arabinose and glucose, etc. Some of these saccharides have the sulfonic acid group substitution. Glycosidations are at the C-1, C-3 and C-26 positions in the molecules.

Table 11-19　Main aglycone types of saponins from the Ophiopogon genus

Type	Structure	Type	Structure
I	 25(*S*)-ruscogenin	III	 diosgenin
II	 ruscogenin	IV	 ophiopogonin

(continued)

Type	Structure	Type	Structure
V		X	
VI	pennogenin (偏诺皂苷元)	XI	
VII	neoruscogenin (新鲁斯可皂苷元)	XII	
VIII		XIII	yamogenin
IX		XIV	

Table 11-20　Main steroidal saponins from Ophiopogon japonicus

Saponins	Type	R₁	R₂
Ophiopogonin A	II	$R_1 = Ac(1 \rightarrow 3_{rha})rha(1 \rightarrow 2)fuc$—	$R_2 = H$
Ophiopogonin B	II	$R_1 = rha(1 \rightarrow 2)fuc$—	$R_2 = H$

(continued)

Saponins	Type	R₁	R₂
Ophiopogonin C	II	$R_1 = Ac$—$rha(1 \rightarrow 2_{fuc})xyl(1 \rightarrow 3_{fuc})fuc$—	$R_2 = H$
Ophiopogonin D	II	$R_1 = rha(1 \rightarrow 2_{fuc})xly(1 \rightarrow 3_{fuc})fuc$—	$R_2 = H$
Ophiopogonin B′	III		$R_2 = Ac(1 \rightarrow 4_{rha})rha(1 \rightarrow 2_{glc})xly(1 \rightarrow 3_{glc})glc$—
Ophiopogonin C′ (Glycoside B)	III		$R_2 = rha(1 \rightarrow 2)glc$—
Ophiopogonin D′	III		$R_2 = rha(1 \rightarrow 2_{glc})xly(1 \rightarrow 3_{glc})glc$—
Ophiopogonin E	VI	$R_1 = H$	$R_2 = xyl(1 \rightarrow 4)glc$—
Glycoside C	III		$R_2 = rha(1 \rightarrow 2_{glc})glc(1 \rightarrow 4_{glc})glc$—
Glycoside D	XI	$R_1 = glc$—	$R_2 = rha(1 \rightarrow 2)glc$—
Glycoside E	II	$R_1 = SO_3M(1 \rightarrow 4_{ara})rha(1 \rightarrow 2_{ara})ara$—	$R_2 = H$
Glycoside F	XI	$R_1 = glc$—	$R_2 = glc(1 \rightarrow 4_{glc})rha(1 \rightarrow 2_{glc})glc$—
Glycoside G	X	$R_1 = SO_3M(1 \rightarrow 4_{ara})rha(1 \rightarrow 2_{ara})ara$—	$R_2 = H$
Ophiopogonin F	XI	$R_1 = glc(1 \rightarrow 2)glc$—	$R_2 = xyl(1 \rightarrow 4_{glc})rha(1 \rightarrow 2_{glc})glc$—
Ophiopogonin G	XI	$R_1 = glc(1 \rightarrow 6)glc$—	$R_2 = xyl(1 \rightarrow 4_{glc})rha(1 \rightarrow 2_{glc})glc$—
Ophiopojaponin A	VI	$R_1 = H$	$R_2 = Ac(1 \rightarrow 2_{rha})rha(1 \rightarrow 2_{glc})xyl(1 \rightarrow 3_{glc})glc$—
Ophiopojaponin B	IX		$R_2 = rha(1 \rightarrow 2)glc$—
Ophiopojaponin C	IV	$R_1 = H$	$R_2 = rha(1 \rightarrow 2_{glc})xly(1 \rightarrow 4_{glc})glc$—

② Extraction and Isolation of Ophiopogonins

Ophiopogonins in Ophiopogon japonicus are similar and are strong water-soluble, so the extraction and isolation are very difficult. The procedure is shown in Figure 11-19.

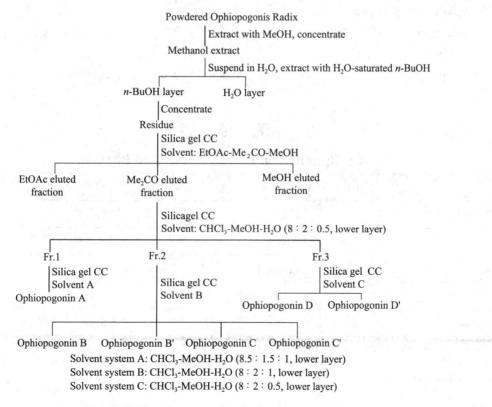

Figure 11-19　Extraction and isolation procedure of ophiopogonins

(2) Flavonoids

Many flavonoids have been isolated from Ophiopogonis Radix. They are ophiopogonone (麦冬黄酮) A, B, ophiopogonanone (麦冬黄烷酮) A, B, methylophiopogonone (甲基麦冬黄酮) A, B, methylophio-pogonanone (甲基麦冬黄烷酮) A, B, etc.

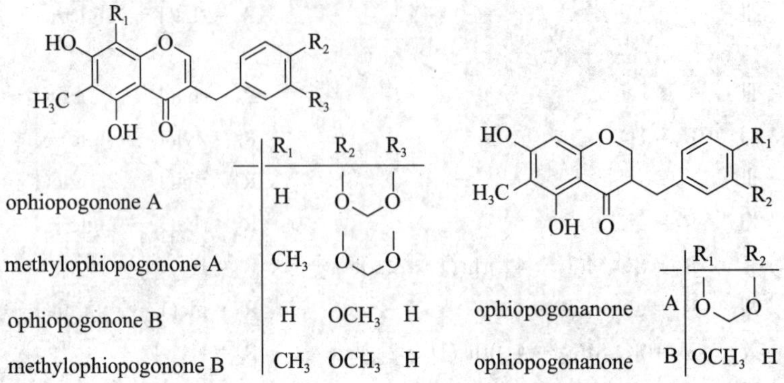

	R_1	R_2	R_3
ophiopogonone A	H	O	O
methylophiopogonone A	CH_3	O	O
ophiopogonone B	H	OCH_3	H
methylophiopogonone B	CH_3	OCH_3	H

		R_1	R_2
ophiopogonanone	A	O	O
ophiopogonanone	B	OCH_3	H

7.4.3 Quality Control Standards

(1) TLC Identification

Stationary Phase: Silica gel GF$_{254}$ plate.

Standard: Authentic crude drug.

Development System: Methylbenzene-methanol-glacial acetic acid (80∶5∶0.1).

Visualization: 365nm UV light.

(2) Tests

Water: Not more than 18.0%.

Total Ash: Not more than 5.0%.

Extract (water): Not less than 60.0%.

(3) Assay

Total Ophiopogonins Counted by Ruscogenin: Not less than 0.12% (spectrophotometry method).

词 汇 表

An Alphabetical List of Words and Phrases

A		
aculeatiside		颠茄皂苷
alisol	[əlɪˈsɔl]	泽泻萜醇
arundoin	[ɑːˈrʌndɔɪn]	芦竹素
astragalosides	[æstrəɡəˈləusaɪdz]	黄芪苷
astragenol		黄芪醇
B		
bisdesmosidic saponins		双糖链皂苷
Bupleuri radix		柴胡

(continued)

Bupleurum chinense DC.		北柴胡
Bupleurum scorzonerifolium Willd.		狭叶柴胡，南柴胡
C		
chuanliansu		川楝素
cucurbitane	[kju:'kə:bɪtən]	葫芦素烷
cycloartane	[saɪk'lɔ:tæn]	环木菠萝烷
cylindrin	[sə'lɪndrɪn]	白茅素
D		
dammarane	['dæməreɪn]	达玛烷
dioscin	['daɪəusɪn]	薯蓣皂苷
diploptene	[dɪp'lɔpti:n]	里白烯
E		
ester saponin	['estə] ['sæpənɪn]	酯皂苷
euphane	[ju:'feɪn]	大戟烷
euphol	['ju:fɔl]	大戟醇
F		
fernane	[fə:'neɪn]	羊齿烷
friedelane	['fraɪdi:lən]	木栓烷
furostanol	[fuə'rɔstænɔl]	呋甾烷醇
G		
ginsenoside	[gɪnse'nəusaɪd]	人参皂苷
glycyrrhetinic acid	[ˌglaɪsɪrɪ'tɪnɪk]['æsɪd]	甘草次酸
Glycyrrhiza glabra L		光果甘草
Glycyrrhiza inflate Bat.		胀果甘草
Glycyrrhiza uralensis Fisch.		甘草
Glycyrrhizae radix et rhizoma		甘草
glycyrrhizin	[glɪ'kə:raɪzɪn]	甘草皂苷
H		
hopane	['həupən]	何帕烷
hydroxyhopanone	[haiˌdrɔksi'həupənəun]	羟基何帕酮
I		
isochuanliansu	[aɪsətʃwɑ:nlɪəns'ju:]	异川楝素
isofernane	[aɪsəfə'neɪn]	异羊齿烷
isohopane	[aɪsəu'hɔpən]	异何帕烷
isolicoflanonol		异甘草黄酮醇
isoliquiritigenin	[aɪsəlɪkwɪə'rɪtaɪdʒnɪn]	异甘草素
isoliquiritin	['aɪsəlɪkwɪərɪtɪn]	异甘草苷

(continued)

isonuatigenin	[aɪsnjueɪˈtɪdʒnɪn]	异纽替皂苷元
isorhamnetin	[aɪsəˈhæmnɪtɪn]	异鼠李素
isospirostane		异螺甾烷
isospirostanol	[aɪsɔspaɪəˈrɔstænol]	异螺甾烷醇
J		
jujuboside	[dʒuːdʒʌˈbəusaɪd]	酸枣仁皂苷
L		
lanostane	[ˈlænəsteɪn]	羊毛脂烷
licoricidin	[lɪkərɪˈsaɪdɪn]	甘草定
licoricone	[lɪkəriˈkəun]	甘草酮
liquiritigenin	[lɪkwɪəˈrɪtaɪdʒnɪn]	甘草素
lupane	[ljuːˈpeɪn]	羽扇豆烷
lycoclavanin	[lɪkəukleɪˈvænɪn]	石松素
lycoclavanol	[lɪkəukleɪˈvænɔl]	石松醇
M		
meliacane		楝烷
methylophiopogonanone	[miːθɪləˈfaɪɔpɔgənənən]	甲基麦冬黄烷酮
methylophiopogonone		甲基麦冬黄酮
mogrosides	[mɔgˈrəusaɪdz]	罗汉果甜素
monodesmosidic saponins	[ˌmɔnəuˈdɪsməusaɪdɪk][sæˈpɔnɪnz]	单糖链皂苷
N		
neoisoliquiritin	[niːˈəuaɪsəlɪkwɪərɪtɪn]	新异甘草苷
neoliquiritin	[niːˈɔlɪkwɪərɪtɪn]	新甘草苷
neoruscogenin	[nɪəˈrəskəudʒnɪn]	新鲁斯可皂苷元
nuatigenin	[njueɪˈtɪdʒnɪn]	纽替皂苷元
O		
oleanane	[əulˈnɑːn]	齐墩果烷
ononin	[ˈɔnəunɪn]	刺芒柄花苷
Ophiopogon japonicus (L.f.) Ker Gawl.		麦冬
ophiopogonanone	[əˈfaɪɔpɔgənənən]	麦冬黄烷酮
ophiopogonin	[əˈfaɪɔpɔgənɪn]	麦冬皂苷
ophiopogonins	[əˈfaɪɔpɔgənɪnz]	麦冬总皂苷
Ophiopogonis radix		麦冬
ophiopogonone	[əfaɪɔpɔˈgɔnəun]	麦冬黄酮
P		
Panax ginseng C.A.Mey		人参
parillin	[pəˈrɪlɪn]	菝葜皂苷

(continued)

pennogenin	[peˈnɔdʒənɪn]	偏诺皂苷元
Platycodonis radix		桔梗
prosapogenins	[ˈprəuzæpədʒnɪnz]	次皂苷
protopanaxadiol	[prəutɔpənækseɪˈdaɪəl]	原人参二醇
protopanaxatriol	[prəutɔpənækseɪtˈraɪəl]	原人参三醇
protostane	[prəuˈtəstæn]	原萜烷
pseudo-spirostanol	[ˈsju:dəu][spaɪəˈrɔstænɔl]	变形螺甾烷醇
puerarin	[ˈpju:rərɪn]	葛根素
pulsatiloside	[pʌlsəˈtɪləusaɪd]	白头翁苷
R		
ruscogenin	[rʌsˈkəudʒnɪn]	鲁斯可皂苷元
S		
saikosaponin	[saɪkəuzæˈpəunɪn]	柴胡皂苷
sapogenin	[ˈsæpədʒenɪn]	皂苷元
saponin	[ˈsæpənɪn]	皂苷
sapotoxin	[ˌsæpəˈtɔksɪn]	皂毒类
sanguisoubin		地榆皂苷
sarsaparilloside	[sɑ:spərɪˈləusaɪd]	原菝葜皂苷
Smilax aristolochiaefolia		菝葜属
Solanum aculeatissimum		刺茄
spiroketal	[spaɪəˈrəukɪtl]	螺缩酮
spirostane	[spaɪəˈrɔstæn]	螺甾烷
spirostanol	[spaɪəˈrɔstænɔl]	螺甾烷醇
T		
timosaponin	[tɪməuzæˈpəunɪn]	知母皂苷
tridesmosidic saponins		三糖链皂苷
tripterygone	[trɪptərɪˈgɔn]	雷公藤酮
U		
uralsaponin	[juərəlsæˈpɔnɪn]	乌拉尔甘草皂苷
ursane	[əːˈseɪn]	乌苏烷
ursolic acid	[əːˈsɔlɪk][ˈæsɪd]	熊果酸，乌索酸

重点小结

皂苷是苷元为三萜或甾类化合物的一类糖苷。皂苷的分类如下：

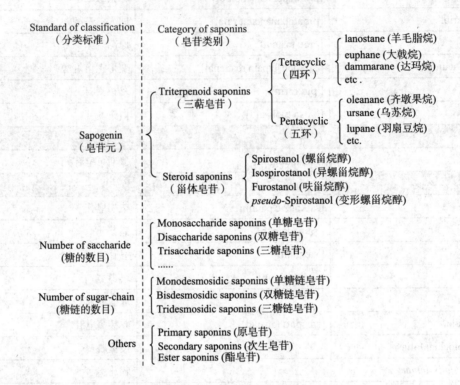

Standard of classification （分类标准）	Category of saponins （皂苷类别）	
Sapogenin （皂苷元）	Triterpenoid saponins （三萜皂苷）	Tetracyclic （四环）: lanostane (羊毛脂烷), euphane (大戟烷), dammarane (达玛烷), etc.
		Pentacyclic （五环）: oleanane (齐墩果烷), ursane (乌苏烷), lupane (羽扇豆烷), etc.
	Steroid saponins （甾体皂苷）	Spirostanol (螺甾烷醇), Isospirostanol (异螺甾烷醇), Furostanol (呋甾烷醇), pseudo-Spirostanol (变形螺甾烷醇)
Number of saccharide (糖的数目)	Monosaccharide saponins (单糖皂苷), Disaccharide saponins (双糖皂苷), Trisaccharide saponins (三糖皂苷)......	
Number of sugar-chain (糖链的数目)	Monodesmosidic saponins (单糖链皂苷), Bisdesmosidic saponins (双糖链皂苷), Tridesmosidic saponins (三糖链皂苷)	
Others	Primary saponins (原皂苷), Secondary saponins (次生皂苷), Ester saponins (酯皂苷)	

皂苷的物理性质：①多为白色或乳白色无定形粉末；没有固定熔点，加热至200~350℃下常分解；②一般可溶于水，易溶于热水、甲醇、乙醇和正丁醇，不溶于丙酮、乙醚、三氯甲烷及苯；③皂苷是很强的表面活性剂，其水溶液振摇后能产生持久性（15分钟）的肥皂样泡沫，加热也不消退；④皂苷结构中均含有手性碳，因此均具有光学活性。

皂苷的化学性质：①沉淀反应，包括与胆甾醇和与金属盐（醋酸铅、氢氧化钡）的沉淀；②颜色反应（Liebermann-Burchard反应、Rosen-Heimer反应等）；③不破坏皂苷元的水解方法有两相酸水解、Smith降解和酶解；④溶血性，大多数皂苷能与红细胞膜上胆甾醇结合生成不溶于水的复合物，破坏了红细胞的通透性，使得红细胞内渗透压升高，而引发溶血现象。

皂苷的提取：一般用醇提取，总提物分散在水中，用亲脂性溶剂（如三氯甲烷）萃取除去亲脂性杂质，然后用水饱和正丁醇萃取，减压蒸干，即可得总皂苷。也可用醇提取－丙酮或乙醚沉淀法得到总皂苷。皂苷元的提取：一般直接将药材进行两相酸水解，得到总皂苷元。

皂苷的分离：①沉淀法，包括梯度沉淀和胆甾醇沉淀；②色谱法，包括吸附色谱（如硅胶、氧化铝、反相硅胶），HPLC，大孔树脂（纯水洗脱糖，10%~30%乙醇水洗脱极性皂苷，50%乙醇水洗脱极性较弱的皂苷），葡聚糖凝胶LH-20（分子量大的皂苷被先洗脱下来）等。

皂苷的检识反应：①泡沫反应；②Liebermann-Burchard反应，甾体皂苷呈现绿色，三萜皂苷则呈现红色；③Rosen-Heimer反应，甾体皂苷加热到60℃呈现紫色或红色，三萜皂苷加热到100℃呈现紫色或红色；④Molish反应阳性；⑤溶血作用。还可用硅胶TLC检识，常用的显色剂有25%三氯乙酸、10%硫酸－乙醇、5%磷钼酸、5%香草醛－硫酸。

皂苷的结构测定：①紫外光谱，甾体皂苷元加浓硫酸，其 UV 最大吸收波长在 270~275 nm；②红外光谱，螺甾烷醇型甾体皂苷中 B 带强度大于 C 带，异螺甾烷醇型甾体皂苷中 B 带强度小于 C 带。三萜皂苷的 A 带在 1392~1355 cm^{-1}，齐墩果烷型三萜皂苷中 A 带有两个峰，乌苏烷型三萜皂苷中 A 带有三个峰；③质谱，甾体皂苷元的质谱中均出现一个很强的 m/z 139 的基峰和中等强度的 m/z 115 碎片峰及一个很弱的 m/z 126 的辅助离子峰；④ ^{1}H-NMR，螺甾烷醇型甾体皂苷 C_{27}-CH_3 的化学位移为 1.1 ppm，异螺甾烷醇型甾体皂苷 C_{27}-CH_3 的化学位移为 0.7 ppm；⑤ ^{13}C-NMR，螺甾烷醇型甾体皂苷 C_{22} 的化学位移为 109.5 ppm，呋甾烷醇型甾体皂苷 C_{22} 的化学位移为 90.3 ppm，变形螺甾烷醇型甾体皂苷 C_{22} 的化学位移为 120.9 ppm；三萜皂苷元中齐墩果烷型含有六个季碳原子信号，乌苏烷型含有五个季碳原子信号，羽扇烷型含有五个季碳原子信号，其末端碳碳双键的化学位移为 110 ppm 和 150 ppm。

人参皂苷的结构分类和性质：A 型，皂苷元为 20(S)-原人参二醇（达玛烷型），种类最多，具有抗溶血性质；B 型，皂苷元为 20(S)-原人参三醇（达玛烷型），具有溶血性质；C 型，皂苷元为齐墩果酸，种类最少，具有溶血性质。人参总皂苷不溶血。C 型结构中 C_{28} 为羧基，因此水溶性最大，A 型水溶性次之，B 型因含有糖的数目较少且是去氧糖，水溶性最小。

甘草皂苷元结构为齐墩果烷型，C_{30} 为羧基，甘草皂苷的 3 位连接两个葡萄糖醛酸，因此也称甘草酸，又因具有甜味，也称甘草甜素。甘草皂苷较难进行酸水解，一般 10% 的硫酸需要加热 24 小时，或 5% 的硫酸加热加压，可以水解得到甘草次酸和乌拉尔甘草次酸，还有两分子的葡萄糖醛酸。甘草中也含有黄酮苷类成分，如甘草苷、异甘草苷。

柴胡皂苷元也属于齐墩果烷型；柴胡皂苷 a, c, d, e 为原生皂苷，在 13 和 28 位含有环氧醚键，不稳定，酸性条件下，环氧醚键断裂得到次生皂苷元。为了得到原生皂苷，在提取时通常加入 5% 吡啶以中和药材中的酸性。

目 标 检 测

题库

一、单选题

1. 下列不符合甾体皂苷元结构特点的是（　　　）
    A. 含 A、B、C、D、E、F 六个环　　　B. E 环和 F 环以螺缩酮形式连接
    C. 分子中常含羧基，又称酸性皂苷　　　D. 甾体皂苷元共有 27 个碳原子组成
    E. C-3 位常有羟基取代

2. 可用于分离呋甾烷醇皂苷和三萜皂苷的方法是（　　　）
    A. 正丁醇提取法　　　　　　B. 明胶沉淀法　　　　　　C. 胆甾醇沉淀法
    D. 乙醇沉淀法　　　　　　E. 分段沉淀法

3. 溶剂沉淀法分离皂苷是利用总皂苷中各皂苷的（　　　）
    A. 在乙醇中溶解度不同　　　B. 极性不同　　　　　　C. 分子量大小不同
    D. 酸性强弱不同　　　　　　E. 糖的数目不同

4. 极性较大的三萜皂苷分离多采用（　　　）
    A. 氧化铝吸附柱色谱　　　　B. 硅胶吸附柱色谱　　　　C. 硅胶分配柱色谱
    D. 聚酰胺柱色谱　　　　　　E. Sephadex LH-20

5. 皂苷具溶血作用的原因为（　　　）

医药大学堂
WWW.YIYAODXT.COM

A. 与细胞壁上胆甾醇生成沉淀 B. 具有表面活性

C. 具有甾体母核 D. 多为寡糖苷，亲水性强

E. 极性较大

6. 甾体皂苷不具有的性质是（   ）

A. 可溶于水、正丁醇 B. 醋酸铅产生沉淀

C. 表面活性与溶血 D. 苷键可被酶、酸、碱水解

E. 与胆甾醇形成沉淀

7. 不符合皂苷通性的是（   ）

A. 分子较大，多为无定形粉末 B. 大多有溶血作用

C. 水溶液振摇后能产生泡沫 D. 有显著而强烈的甜味

E. 没有固定的熔点

8. 属于齐墩果烷衍生物的是（   ）

A. 原人参二醇 B. 雪胆甲素 C. 甘草次酸

D. 乌苏酸 E. 原人参三醇

9. 可以作为皂苷纸色谱显色剂的是（   ）

A. 醋酐－浓硫酸试剂 B. 三氯化铁－冰醋酸试剂

C. 三氯醋酸试剂 D. 香草醛－浓硫酸试剂

E. 氯化锌－乙酰氯试剂

10. 有关柴胡皂苷叙述错误的是（   ）

A. 属于三萜皂苷 B. 酸性条件下稳定

C. 结构类型为齐墩果烷型 D. 柴胡皂苷 a, c, d, e 是原皂苷

E. 原皂苷结构中有环氧醚键

11. 从水溶液中萃取皂苷类最好用（   ）

A. 三氯甲烷 B. 正丁醇 C. 乙醚

D. 乙醇 E. 苯

12. 有关人参皂苷叙述错误的是（   ）

A. C 型是齐墩果酸的双糖链苷

B. 人参皂苷的原始苷元应是 20（S）－原人参二醇和 20（S）－原人参三醇

C. A 型、B 型苷元是达玛烷型衍生物

D. A 型、B 型有溶血作用，C 型有抗溶血作用

E. 总皂苷没有溶血作用

二、多选题

1. 皂苷在下列哪些溶剂中溶解度较大（   ）

A. 热水 B. 含水稀醇 C. 热乙醇

D. 乙醚 E. 苯

2. 可用于皂苷元显色反应的试剂是（   ）

A. 醋酐－浓硫酸 B. 冰醋酸－乙酰氯 C. 苦味酸钠

D. 三氯醋酸 E. 五氯化锑

3. 属于四环三萜皂苷元结构的是（   ）

A. 羽扇豆烷 B. 羊毛脂甾烷 C. 达玛烷

医药大学堂
WWW.YIYAODXT.COM

D. β- 香树脂烷   E. 齐墩果烷

4. 有关甘草皂苷叙述正确的是（　　　）

 A. 酸性皂苷   B. 可用作食品工业甜味剂

 C. 又称甘草次酸   D. 属于五环三萜皂苷结构

 E. 在植物中多以盐的形式存在

5. 皂苷多具有下列哪些性质（　　　）

 A. 吸湿性   B. 发泡性   C. 味苦而辛辣

 D. 刺激性   E. 溶血性

6. 精制皂苷时，先将粗皂苷溶于甲醇或乙醇，然后加何溶剂可使皂苷析出（　　　）

 A. 乙醚   B. 水   C. 正丁醇

 D. 丙酮   E. 乙醚：丙酮（1：1）

7. 可以区分皂苷和皂苷元的反应是（　　　）

 A. Molish 反应   B. α- 萘酚 – 浓硫酸反应   C. 醋酐 – 浓硫酸反应

 D. 碱性苦味酸反应   E. 三氯甲烷 – 浓硫酸反应

8. 《中国药典》规定的人参质量控制成分为（　　　）

 A. 人参皂苷 Rb$_1$ B. 人参皂苷 Rg$_1$ C. 人参皂苷二醇

 D. 人参皂苷 Re   E. 人参总皂苷

9. 具有溶血性质的苷类化合物是（　　　）

 A. 黄酮苷   B. 强心苷   C. 三萜皂苷

 D. 甾体皂苷   E. 甘草苷

10. 提取皂苷最常用的方法是（　　　）

 A. 稀醇提取，正丁醇萃取法   B. 碱提取 – 酸沉淀法

 C. 铅盐沉淀法   D. 稀醇提取 – 大孔树脂吸附法

 E. 胆甾醇沉淀法

11. 分离皂苷时，常用的色谱法有（　　　）

 A. 硅胶吸附色谱法   B. HPLC 法   C. 硅胶分配色谱法

 D. 大孔树脂色谱法   E. Sephadex LH-20 色谱法

12. 检识皂苷类成分的化学反应有（　　　）

 A. Liebermann-Burchard 反应   B. Rosen-Heimer 反应

 C. Gibbs 反应   D. Kedde 反应

 E. Molish 反应

三、思考题

1. 简述皂苷常用的提取分离方法有哪些？

2. 如何用显色反应来区分三萜皂苷和甾体皂苷？

3. 如何通过理化方法确定某中药是否含有皂苷？请给予说明。

（马　涛　王继彦）

Chapter 12   Other Constituents

 学习目标

知识要求：

1. 掌握 脂肪酸的定义、分类、结构特点和主要理化性质。

2. 熟悉 脂肪酸、氨基酸的识别和提取分离方法。

3. 了解 有机含硫化合物、蛋白质、酶和矿物药的定义和主要理化性质；大蒜的主要有效成分结构特征。

能力要求：

学会应用常用显色反应检识氨基酸；学会应用结合氨基酸的具体结构特征选择适合的提取分离方法。

1 Fatty Acids

1.1   Introduction

Fatty acids (脂肪酸) are defined as the aliphatic monocarboxylic acids (一元脂肪羧酸) that can be liberated by hydrolysis from naturally occurring fats and oils. They generally present in plants and animals as esters. They are active components of Chinese herbs and they may be used to synthesize other active compounds.

Fatty acids are widely presented in Chinese herbs, mostly existing in leaves and fruits of such plants as Erio-botryae Folium (枇杷叶), Artemisiae Scopariae Herba, Mume Fructus (乌梅), Lonicerae Japonicae Flos, etc.

1.2   The Structure Characters and Classification

Fatty acids in nature are commonly straight chain and possess an even number of carbon atoms. The number of carbon atoms may be from 4 to 30, or even more. But those with 16 or 18 carbons are the most common.

Fatty acids can be classified into saturated fatty acids (饱和脂肪酸) and unsaturated fatty acids (不饱和脂肪酸) (including monounsaturated and polyunsaturated fatty acids) according to the number of double-bond in the molecules. In virtually all cases, the stereochemistry of the double bond is *Z* (*cis*).

Saturated fatty acids contain no double-bond. They can accelerate the absorption of cholesterol in human

医药大学堂
WWW.YIYAODXT.COM

418

bodies, so that cholesterols in blood rise up and deposit on vessel wall, finally developing to vascular sclerosis.

Monounsaturated fatty acids (单不饱和脂肪酸) only possess one double-bond in molecules and are the main components of fat in terrestrial animals.

Polyunsaturated fatty acids (多不饱和脂肪酸) in plant oils usually possess two or three double-bonds, while those in fat of marine animals are commonly comprised of four or more double-bonds.

The main polyunsaturated fatty acids include linoleic acid (亚油酸), α-linolenic acid（α– 亚麻酸）, γ-linolenic acid（γ–亚麻酸）, arachidonic acid (花生四烯酸), eicosapentaenoic acid (二十碳五烯酸) (EPA), doesahexaenoic acid (二十二碳六烯酸) (DHA), etc. Among them, linoleic acid and α-linolenic acid cannot be synthesized in human body and required to be provided from diet. Linoleic acid can convert into arachidonic acid and γ-linolenic acid in human body, and then other polyunsaturated fatty acids can be synthesized from them. Arachidonic acid is the key material for synthesize prostaglandins which is important for regulating the contraction and relaxation of smooth muscles. Therefore, linoleic acid and α-linolenic acid are called essential fatty acids (必需脂肪酸). Moreover, polyunsaturated fatty acids can be easily emulsified, transported and metabolized. They act as the role of reducing blood fat and cholesterol, decreasing atherosclerosis, restraining the growth of cancer cells and promoting the growth of brains. Common fatty acids in natural are listed in Table 12-1.

linoleic acid

α-linolenic acid

γ-linolenic acid

Table 12-1   Common fatty acids in nature

Category	Fatty acid	Structure abbreviation	Source
Saturated	butyric (丁酸)	4 : 0	plants and animals
	caproic (hexanoic) (己酸)	6 : 0	
	caprylic (octanoic) (辛酸)	8 : 0	
	capric (decanoic) (癸酸)	10 : 0	
	lauric (月桂酸)	12 : 0	
	myristic (豆蔻酸)	14 : 0	
	palmitic (棕榈酸)	16 : 0	
	stearic (硬脂酸)	18 : 0	
	arachidic acid (花生酸)	20 : 0	
	behenic (二十二烷酸)	22 : 0	
	lignoceric (木蜡酸)	24 : 0	

(continued)

Category	Fatty acid	Structure abbreviation	Source
Saturated	cerotic (蜡酸)	26 : 0	plants and animals
	montanic (二十八烷酸)	28 : 0	
	melissic (蜂花酸)	30 : 0	
Monounsaturated	palmitoleic (棕榈油酸)	16 : 1 (9c)	terraneous animals
	oleic (油酸)	18 : 1 (9c)	
	cis-vaccenic (顺 – 十八碳烯酸)	18 : 1 (11c)	
	gadoleic (顺 – 二十碳 –9– 烯酸)	20 : 1 (9c)	
	erucic (芥酸)	22 : 1 (13c)	
	nervonic (顺 –15– 二十四碳烯酸)	24 : 1 (15c)	
Polyunsaturated	linoleic	18 : 2 (9c, 12c)	plants
	α -linolenic	18 : 3 (9c, 12c, 15c)	
	γ -linolenic	18 : 3 (6c, 9c, 12c)	
	arachidonic	20 : 4 (5c, 8c, 11c, 14c)	marine animals
	eicosapentaenoic (EPA)	20 : 5 (5c, 8c, 11c, 14c, 17c)	
	docosapentaenoic (DPA) (二十二碳五烯酸)	22 : 5 (7c, 10c, 13c, 16c, 19c)	
	docosahexaenoic (DHA)	22 : 6 (4c, 7c, 10c, 13c, 16c, 19c)	

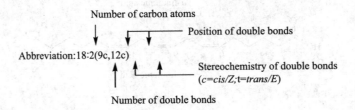

1.3 Physicochemical Properties

Fatty acids with eight or less carbon atoms are liquid at room temperature. However, the fatty acids with more carbon atoms are solid. Fatty acids are insoluble in water, soluble in hot ethanol, acetone, ethyl acetate, chloroform, ethyl ether, cyclohexane, etc. They contain carboxyl group, so they can form salts with bases.

Fatty acids may become rancid when stored in air for a long time and the change is called rancidity (酸败). Fatty acids have positive color reactions with some reagents. The reactions are listed in Table 12-2.

Table 12-2　Color reactions of fatty acids

Reaction	Reagent	Color
Bromphenol blue (溴酚蓝)	0.1% bromphenol blue solution of ethanol/water (70 : 30)	yellow spot in blue background
Br_2-CCl_4	2% Br_2/CCl_4	color of solution disappearing

(continued)

Reaction	Reagent	Color
Potassium permanganate (高锰酸钾)	1% $KMnO_4$	color of solution disappearing
KIO_3-KI	2% KI and 4% KIO_3, 0.1% starch solution	blue

1.4   Extraction and Isolation Methods

1.4.1   Extraction

CO_2-SFE can be used to extract fatty acids at the pressure of 0.1–5 kPa and the temperature of 35–45℃. Ethyl ether, petroleum ether and cyclohexane can also be used to extract fatty acids.

1.4.2   Isolation

Distillation method can be used to isolate or purify fatty acids. It is often adopted with urea crystallization method together.

The total fatty acids are added into acetone, cooled below −25℃, stirred, filtered and concentrated to give EPA and DHA with higher concentration. This is acetone freezing method (丙酮冷凝法).

The esters of total fatty acids can be transferred into fatty acid salts by adding sodium hydroxide solution in ethanol, cooled and then give the crystal of salts of saturated and monounsaturated fatty acids. Addition of acid into the filtrate gives free polyunsaturated fatty acids. This method is suitable for industrial production.

Chromatography method is necessary for the isolation of fatty acids with similar structures.

2   Organic Sulphur Compounds

2.1   Introduction

Sulfur (硫) is the essential element of all organisms. Organic sulfur compounds (有机硫化物) such as amino acids, vitamins, coenzyme A, polypeptides and proteins act as many crucial roles in organisms.

In Chinese herbs, secondary metabolites containing sulfur occur few, though they possess important biological activities. For example, potassium myronate (芥子苷) possesses potent antibiosis and killing-insect effect. Both allitridin (大蒜新素) and rorifone (旱菜素) possess remarkable anti-bacterial action.

2.2   Organic Sulphur Compounds from Chinese Herbs

On behalf of the natural *S*-glycoside, potassium myronate is a series of glucosides which sulfur atom is presented as glycosidic atom. They usually present in plant as a salt, and the structure can be expressed by the general formulae below. Sinigrin from *Brassica nigra* is potassium salt. Beside potassium salt (钾盐), sinalbin from *Sinapis alba* is a quaternary ammonium salt with sinapine (芥子碱).

General formulae of myronate potassium

sinigrin

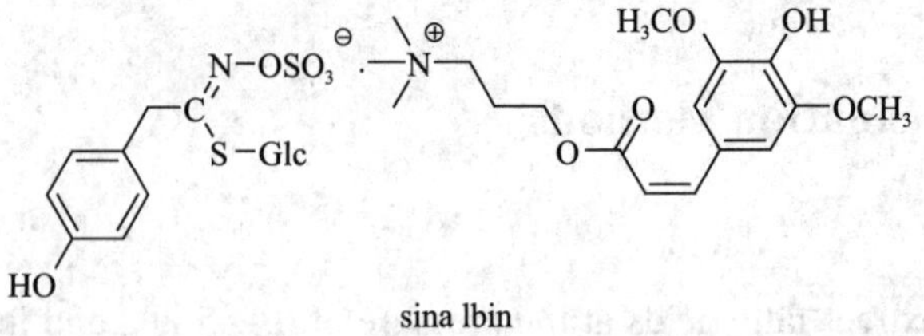

sina lbin

Under neutral condition, potassium myronate is hydrolyzed by myrosinase into glucose and thiohydroximic acid (硫代羟肟酸), the latter finally transferring into isothiocyanate with strong odour (Figure 12-1).

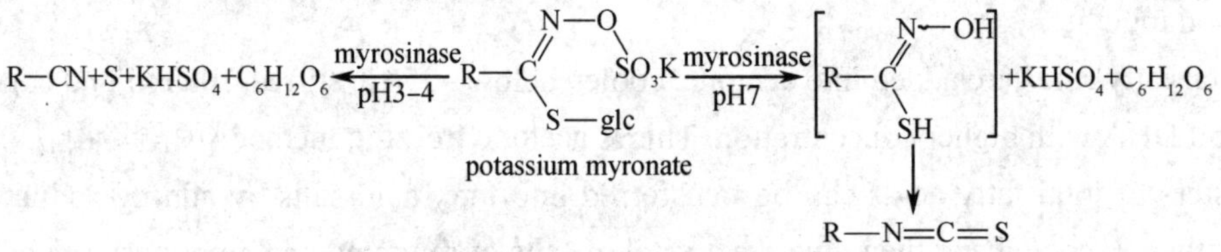

Figure 12-1   Hydrolysis of potassium myronate

3   Amino Acids, Proteins and Enzymes

3.1   Amino Acids

3.1.1   Introduction

Amino acids contain both a basic amino group and an acidic carboxyl group. According to the relative positions of amino group and carboxyl group, amino acids can be classified into three types: α-, β- and γ-amino acids. Among them, the α-amino acid is the major one and the elementary units to construct proteins. Amino acids can also be classified into three series according to the number of amino group and carboxyl group in molecules. They are neutral amino acids (中性氨基酸), acidic amino acids (酸性氨基酸) and basic amino acids (碱性氨基酸). The number of carboxyl groups is equal to that of amino groups in neutral amino acids. Accordingly, carboxyl groups are more than amino groups in acidic amino acids, and it is opposite in basic amino acids.

Most of amino acids are the primary units consisting of proteins and essential to human bodies, so they are also defined as essential amino acids (必需氨基酸). An essential amino acid is one that cannot be synthesized from other available sources, and therefore must be supplied as part of the diet. Eight amino acids (i.e. lysine, tryptophan, phenylalanine, methionine, threonine, leucine, isoleucine and valine) are generally regarded as essential, with two others, histidine and arginine (精氨酸), being essential only for children.

Amino acids are common in Chinese herbs and have particular bioactivities. For example, quisqualic acid (使君子氨酸) from Quisqualis Frutus (使君子) and kainic acid (海人草氨酸) from Caloglossa Leprieuii (鹧鸪菜) have anthelminthic (驱虫) activity; cucurbitine (南瓜子氨酸) from Cucurbitae Semen (毛边南瓜子) may be used as the treatment of filariasis (丝虫病) and schistosomiasis (血吸虫病); asparagine (天门冬素) from Asparagi Radix (天冬) and Scrophulariae Radix can relieve cough and asthma; dencichine (三七素) from Notoginseng Radix et Rhizoma (三七) shows hemostasis (止血) effect.

3.1.2　Physicochemical Properties

Amino acids are colorless crystals with high melting point. They are soluble in water but insoluble in ethyl acetate, ethyl ether and chloroform etc.

Amino acids contain both an acidic and a basic group. They can dissolve in base as well as in acid, and transfer into salts, depending on the circumstances. So they are called amphoteric compounds (两性化合物). Undergoing an intra-molecular acid-base reaction (分子内酸碱反应), amino acids may exist primarily in internal salts (内盐), the form of a dipolar ion, or zwitterions (两性离子).

In aqueous solution, the amino group or carboxyl group in amino acids can be ionized as a base or acid. In strong acid solution (low pH), an amino acid is protonated and exists primarily as a cation. But in base solution (high pH), an amino acid is deprotonated and exists primarily as an anion. Thus, at certain intermediate pH value, the amino acid can be exactly balanced between anionic and cationic forms and exist primarily as the neutral, dipolar zwitterions. This pH is called isoelectric point (pI, 等电点).

At the isoelectric point, amino acids exist as internal salts so that its solubility is minimum and can be precipitated from water. Different amino acids have different pI. Therefore, amino acids can be separated by adjusting the pH of buffer solution.

$$
\begin{array}{ccccc}
\underset{\underset{NH_3^+}{|}}{\overset{\overset{COOH}{|}}{R-CH}} & \underset{+H^+}{\overset{-H^+}{\rightleftharpoons}} & \underset{\underset{NH_3^+}{|}}{\overset{\overset{COO^-}{|}}{R-CH}} & \underset{-OH^-}{\overset{+OH^-}{\rightleftharpoons}} & \underset{\underset{NH_2}{|}}{\overset{\overset{COO^-}{|}}{R-CH}}
\end{array}
$$

3.1.3　Identification

(1) Physicochemical Identification

Ninhydrin reaction (茚三酮反应): Take 1ml test solution, add 2-3 drops of 0.2% ninhydrin solution, mix, boil in water bath for 5 minutes, cool. If it shows blue or violet, it indicates that amino acids, peptides or proteins are presented in the test solution.

Isatin reaction (吲哚醌反应): Drop test solution onto filter paper, dry and spray indole-dione reagent (吲哚醌试液) (1g 1H-indole-2, 3-dione dissolve in 100ml acetone, add 10ml glacial acetic acid), bake it for 5 minutes. Different amino acids show various colors.

Folin reaction (福林试剂反应): Take 0.5ml test solution, add Folin reagent [0.02g 1, 2-naphtho-quinone-4-sulfonic acid sodium (1, 2- 萘醌 –4– 磺酸钠), dissolve in 100ml of 5% sodium carbonate solution (碳酸钠溶液), match just before used] 0.5ml, standing for 3 minutes. Then different amino acids show various colors.

(2) Chromatographic Identification

TLC: Development solvent systems: *n*-butanol-acetic acid-water (4∶1∶5, upper layer), *n*-butanol-formic acid-water (15∶3∶2), chloroform-methanol-17% ammonium water (2∶2∶1), phenol-water (3∶1).

PC: Development solvent systems: *n*-butanol-acetic acid-ethanol-water (4∶1∶1∶2), methanol-water- pyridine (20∶20∶4), water saturated phenol. Two-dimensional development system is *n*-butanol-acetic acid-water (3∶1∶1) and phenol-water (3∶1).

Spray reagents: Ninhydrin reagent (at 110℃ to give purple, several amino acids such as proline, kainic acid to give yellow); Isatin reagent (different colors); Folin reagent (different colors).

3.1.4　Extraction and Isolation Methods

Generally, amino acids can be extracted with water or dilute alcohol, then precipitation at isoelectric points. Ion exchange chromatography and electrophoresis are usually used in the isolation of amino acids.

Ion exchange chromatography is widely used in isolation of amino acids. On cation exchange resin, adsorption abilities of acidic amino acids and hydroxyl amino acids are weakest. Neutral amino acids are stronger. And amino acids containing aromatic ring are further stronger. Basic amino acids show the most strong adsorption abilities. Moreover, amino acids of big molecules are greater than the small ones. Citrate buffer solution and sodium acetate buffer solution are frequently used eluents. Adjusting the buffer to pH 3.28, 4.30 and 6.71 respectively, acidic amino acids, neutral amino acids and basic acids can be eluted from the resin in turn.

3.2　Proteins and Enzymes

3.2.1　Introduction

Proteins are amino acid polymers in which the amino acid units are joined together by peptide bonds. Enzymes (酶) are proteins possessing catalytic capability. Enzymes show maximum activity between 35℃ to 40℃.

Many plant original proteins are found to have pharmacological activities. For example, trichosanthin (天花粉蛋白) from the root of *Trichosanthes kirilouii* Maxim. or *Trichosanthes rosthornii* Harms being remedies of malignancy hydatidiform (恶性葡萄胎) and chorioepithelioma (绒膜上皮癌). Papain (木瓜蛋白酶) from Carica Papaya (番木瓜) can drive out intestinal parasite (肠内寄生虫). Amylase (淀粉酶) from Hordei Fructus Germinatus (麦芽) is often used in treatment of dyspepsia (消化不良).

3.2.2　Physicochemical Properties

Proteins are macromolecules (大分子) with molecular weights often above 10, 000. The higher may be about 10, 000, 000. Proteins are water-soluble, but insoluble in organic solvents. Concentrated alcohol can precipitate them. The water solution of proteins is colloid (胶体). Proteins are unable to penetrate semipermeable membrane (半透膜). Proteins are easily denatured due to heat, changes of pH value, treatment of organic solvents or by ultraviolet radiation (紫外线照射).

Proteins are amphoteric in nature and exhibit characteristics of zwitterions and isoelectric point like amino acids. Proteins can be separated by electrophoresis depending on their isoelectric points and the pH value of the buffer.

In water solution, proteins can be precipitated by high-concentration solution of ammonium sulfate or sodium chloride and this process is reversible. But heating or reacting with acids or bases or metal salts will precipitate proteins or enzymes permanently, which is irreversible.

Proteins can be hydrolyzed by an acid, base or enzyme.

3.2.3　Identification

Generally used reactions for identification of proteins are listed in Table 12-3.

Table 12-3   Generally used reactions for identification of proteins

Reaction	Reagent or condition	Result
Precipitation	Boiling or 1ml 5% ammonium sulfate	Precipitate
Biuret reaction (双缩脲反应)	40% NaOH, 1% $CuSO_4$	Purple

4   Minerals

4.1   Introduction

Minerals have a long history in clinical applying like medicinal plants in China. Twenty two minerals are recorded in Chinese Pharmacopeia 2020 edition. Their compositions generally are inorganic compounds.

4.2   Examples of Minerals

Some examples of minerals are listed in Table 12-4.

Table 12-4   Some examples of minerals

Example	Main composition	Action
Gypsum fibrosum (石膏)	$CaSO_4 \cdot 2H_2O$	To remove heat, quench fire, ease the mind, and relieve thirst
Alumen (白矾)	$KAl(SO_4)_2 \cdot 12H_2O$	To counteract toxicity, kill parasites, arrest discharges, and relieve itching by external use; to arrest bleeding, relieve diarrhea, and dispel wind-phlegm by internal administration
Natrii Sulfas (芒硝)	$Na_2SO_4 \cdot 10H_2O$	To relax bowels and purge heat, remove fire and cause subsidence of swelling
Stalactitum (钟乳石)	$CaCO_3$	To warm the lung, relieve asthma, and inhibit acid secretion
Talcum (滑石)	$Mg_3(Si_4O_{10})(OH)_2$	To relieve dysuria, eliminate summer-heat and damp, and arrest discharges and promote healing of sores
Pyritum (自然铜)	FeS_2	To eliminate blood stasis, promote healing of fracture and relieve pain
Realgar (雄黄)	As_2S_2	To counteract toxicity, to kill parasites, and cure malarial
Cinnabaris (朱砂)	HgS	To cause sedation and counteract toxicity

5　Examples of Chinese Herbs Containing Organic Sulphur Compounds

Allii Sativi Bulbus (大蒜)

5.1.1　Introduction

(1) Biological Source

Allii Sativi Bulbus is the bulb of *Allium sativum* L. (Fam. Liliaceae) .

(2) Property, Flavor and Channels Entered

Property and Flavor: Pungent (辛); warm.

Channels Entered: The Spleen, Stomach and Lung.

(3) Actions & Indications

To counteract toxicity, relive swelling, kill parasites, and stop dysentery (痢疾); For carbuncle (痈) and sores ulceration, mange (疥癣), lung tuberculosis (肺痨), pertussis (顿咳), enterorrhea (泄泻), dysentery.

(4) Pharmacological Activities

Allii Sativi Bulbus exhibits pharmacological activities such as prevention and cure of cardiovascular (心血管) diseases, anti-pathogenic microorganism, anti-tumor, antihypertensive (降压), relaxing smooth muscle, lowering cholesterol and plasma lipids, etc. The extract of Allii Sativi Bulbus shows antibacterial and antifungal activity in a broad range. Allicin is the main contributor to antimicrobial activities. Allicin is also the active anthelminthic constituent.

5.1.2　Main Chemical Constituents

The chemical constituents of Allii Sativi Bulbus include sulfur-volatiles (含硫挥发物), thiosulfinates, amino acids, peptides, *S*-glycosides and allinases (蒜氨酸酶). Sulfur compounds are the most important constituents reported from it. It has been estimated that cysteine sulfoxides, e.g. alliin (蒜氨酸) and the non-volatile γ-glutamylcysteine peptides (谷氨酰半胱氨肽类) make up more than 82% of the total sulfur content of Allii Sativi Bulbus. The thiosulfinates (e.g. allicin), ajoenes (阿焦烯) (e.g. *trans*-ajoene, *cis*-ajoene) and sulfides, e.g. diallyldisulfide (二烯丙基二硫), diallyltrisulfide (二烯丙基三硫), however, are not naturally occurring compounds. They are degradation (降解) products from the naturally occurring cysteine sulfoxide, alliin. The main chemical constituents from Allii Sativi Bulbus are listed in Table 12-5.

Table 12-5　Main chemical constituents from Allii Sativi Bulbus

Type	Name	Structure
Sulfur volatiles	diallyltrisulfide, allitridin (大蒜新素，大蒜素)	H_2C —S—S—S— CH_2
	diallylsulfide (二烯丙基硫醚)	H_2C —S— CH_2
	methylallyldisulfide (甲基烯丙基二硫)	H_2C —S—S— CH_3
	methylallyltrisulfide (甲基烯丙基三硫)	H_2C —S—S—S— CH_3

(continued)

Type	Name	Structure
Sulfur volatiles	diallyldisulfide	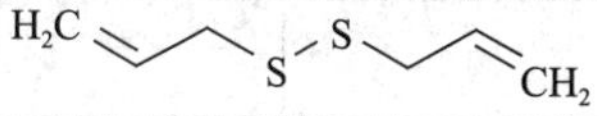
	diallyltetrasulfide (二烯丙基四硫)	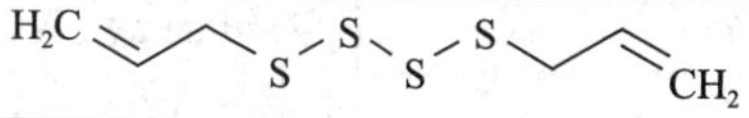
	trans-ajoene (反– 阿焦烯)	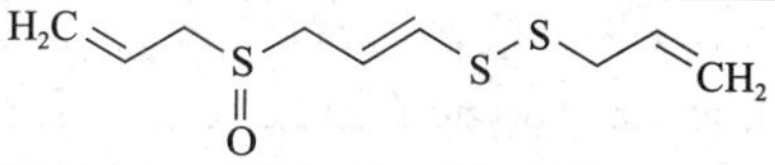
	cis-ajoene (顺– 阿焦烯)	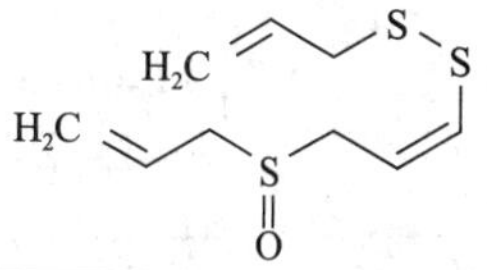
Thiosulfinates	diallylthiosulfinate (二烯丙基硫亚磺酸盐), allicin	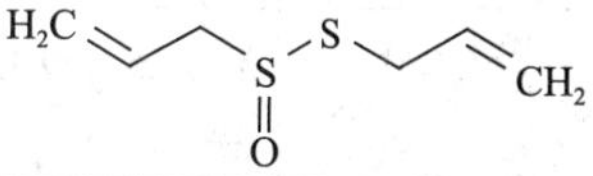
	1-propenylallylthiosulfinate (丙烯烯丙基硫代亚砜)	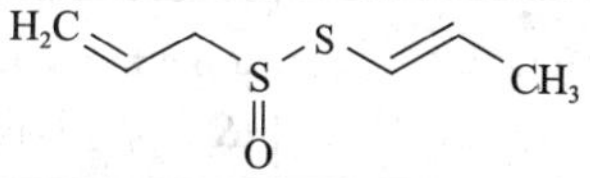
	ally-1-propenylthiosulfinate (烯丙丙烯基硫代亚砜)	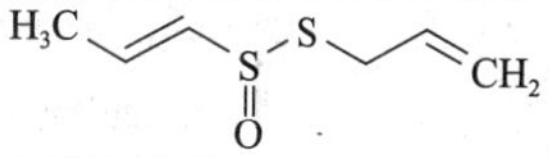
	methylallylthiosulfinate (甲基烯丙基硫代亚砜)	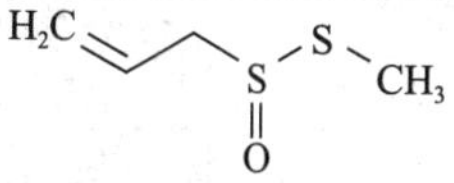
	allylmethylthiosulfinae (烯丙基甲基硫代亚砜)	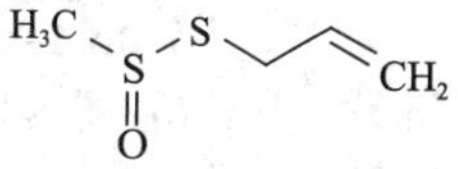
	methyl-1-propenylthiosulfinate (甲基丙烯基硫代亚砜)	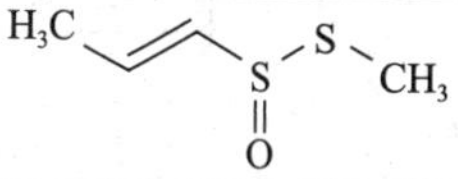
	Dimethylthiosulfinate (二甲基硫代亚砜)	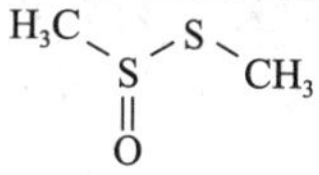
γ-L-glutamyl peptides	γ-L-glutamyl-L-cysteine (γ–L– 谷氨酰 –L– 半胱氨酸)	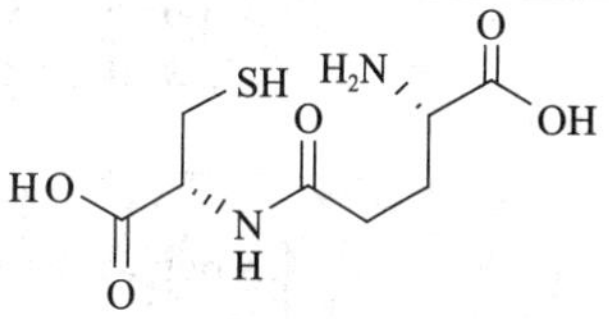
	γ-L-glutamyl-*S*-methly-L-cysteine (γ–L– 谷氨酰 –*S*– 甲基 –L– 半胱氨酸)	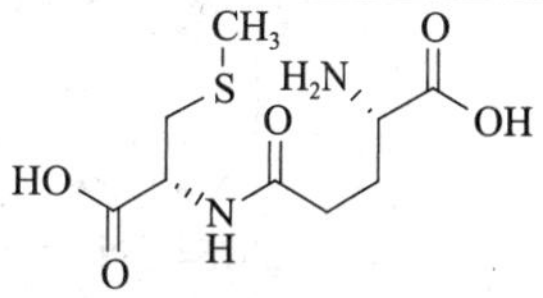
	γ-L-glutamyl-*S*-methyl-L-cysteisulfoxide (γ–L– 谷氨酰 –*S*– 甲基 –L– 半胱亚砜)	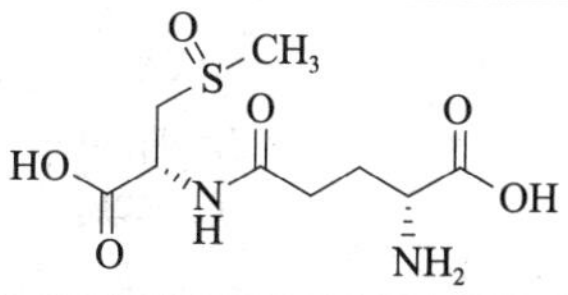
	γ-L-glutamyl-*S*-allylmercapto-L-cysteine (γ–L– 谷氨酰 –*S*– 烯丙基硫基 –L– 半胱氨酸)	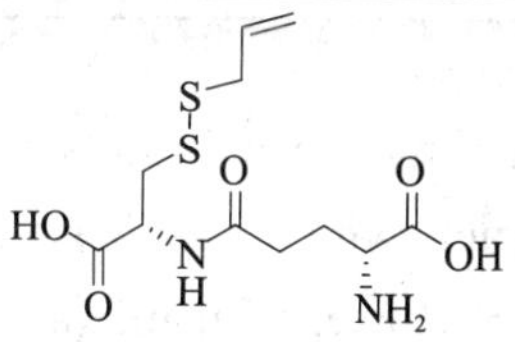

427

(continued)

Type	Name	Structure
γ-L-glutamyl peptides	γ-L-glutamyl-S-allyl-L-cysteine (γ–L– 谷氨酰 –S– 烯丙基 –L– 半胱氨酸)	
	γ-L-glutamyl-S-(*trans*-l-propenyl)-L-cysteine ［γ–L– 谷氨酰 –S–(反–l–丙烯基)–L– 半胱氨酸］	
S-alkyl-L-cysteine derivatives	alliin,S-ally-L-cysteinsulfoxide (蒜氨酸)	
	S-methylcysteinsulfoxide (S– 甲基半胱氨酸亚砜)	
	cycloalliin (环蒜氨酸)	
	S-ally-L-cysteine (S– 烯丙基 –L– 半胱氨酸)	
	S-propenyl-L-cysteine (S– 丙烯基 –L– 半胱氨酸)	
	S-propyl-L-cysteine (S– 丙基 –L– 半胱氨酸)	
	S-butyl-L-cysteine (S– 丁基 –L– 半胱氨酸)	
	S-allymercapto-L-cysteine (S– 烯丙基硫基 –L– 半胱氨酸)	
	S-methylmercapto-L-cysteine (S– 甲基硫基 –L– 半胱氨酸)	

When the garlic bulb is crushed, minced, or other processed, alliin is released from compartments and interacts with the alliinase in adjacent vacuoles. Hydrolysis and immediate condensation of the reactive intermediate, allylsulfenic acid (烯丙基次磺酸), forms allicin. Allicin is unstable and will undergo additional reactions to form other derivatives depending on environmental and processing conditions.

Extraction of garlic cloves with ethanol at 0℃ gives alliin. Extraction with ethanol and water at 25℃ leads to allicin and no alliin. And steam distillation converts the alliin totally to diallyl sulfides. Therefore, different products of Allii Sativi Bulbus have different components (Table 12-6).

Table 12-6　Main components of different products of Allii Sativi Bulbus

Products	Main Components
Bulbs	alliin, allitridin
Dry powder	alliin, allitridin
Volatile oils	diallyl sulfide, diallyl disulfide, diallyl trisulfide and diallyl tetrasulfide
Oil macerate	2-vinyl-[4*H*]-1, 3-dithiin, 3-vinyl-[4*H*]-1, 3-dithiin, *trans*-ajoene and *cis*-ajoene

5.1.3　Quality Control Standards

(1) TLC Identification

Stationary Phase: Silica gel plate.

Standard: Allitridin.

Development System: *n*-Hexane.

Visualization: Iodine vapor.

(2) Tests

Total Ash: Not more than 2.0%.

Extract (water): Not less than 63.0%.

(3) Assay

Allitridin: Not less than 0.15% (HPLC).

词　汇　表

An Alphabetical List of Words and Phrases

A		
acetone freezing method	['æsɪtəun]['fri:zɪŋ]['meθəd]	丙酮冷凝法
acidic amino acids	[ə'sɪdɪk]['æmɪnəu]['æsɪdz]	酸性氨基酸
ajoene	[əd'ʒi:n]	阿焦烯
aliphatic monocarboxylic acid	[ˌælə'fætɪk]['mɔnəukɑ:bɔk'sɪlɪk]['æsɪd]	一元脂肪羧酸
alliin	['ælɪɪn]	蒜氨酸
allinase	['ælɪɪneɪs]	蒜氨酸酶
Allii Sativi Bulbus		大蒜
allitridin		大蒜新素
allyl	['æləl]	烯丙基
allylmercapto		烯丙基巯基
allylmethylthiosulfinae		烯丙基甲基硫代亚砜
allylsulfenic acid		烯丙基次磺酸

(continued)

ally-1-propenylthiosulfinate		烯丙丙烯基硫代亚砜
alumen	[əˈluːmen]	白矾
amphoteric compounds	[ˌæmfəˈterɪk][ˈkɔmpaundz]	两性化合物
amylase	[ˈæmɪleɪz]	淀粉酶
anthelminthic	[ˌænθelˈmɪntɪk]	驱虫剂；驱肠虫的
antihypertensive	[ˈæntiːhaɪpəˈtensɪv]	降压药；抗高血压的
arachidic acid	[ɑːræˈkɪdɪk][ˈæsɪd]	花生酸，二十烷酸
arachidonic acid	[ærəkɪˈdɔnɪk][ˈæsɪd]	花生四烯酸
arginine	[ˈɑːdʒɪnɪn]	精氨酸
asparagine	[əsˈpærədʒiːn]	天冬酰胺
Asparagi Radix	[əsˈpærɪdʒiː][ˈreɪdɪks]	天冬
B		
basic amino acid	[ˈbeɪsɪk][ˈæmɪnəu][ˈæsɪd]	碱性氨基酸
behenic acid		二十二烷酸
biuret reaction	[bjəˈreɪt][riˈækʃn]	双缩脲反应
bromphenol blue	[brɔmˈfiːnɔl][bluː]	溴酚蓝
butyric acid	[bjuːˈtɪrɪk][ˈæsɪd]	丁酸
C		
Caloglossa Leprieuii		鹧鸪菜
capric acid	[ˈkæprɪk][ˈæsɪd]	癸酸
caproic acid	[kəˈprəuɪk][ˈæsɪd]	己酸
caprylic acid	[kəˈprɪlɪk][ˈæsɪd]	辛酸
carbuncle	[ˈkɑːbʌŋkl]	痈
cardiovascular	[ˌkɑːdɪəuˈvæskjulə]	心血管的
Carica Papaya	[ˈkærɪkə][pəˈpaɪə]	番木瓜
cerotic acid	[sɪˈrɔtɪk][ˈæsɪd]	蜡酸
chorioepithelioma	[ˌkəurɪəuˌepɪθiːlɪˈəumə]	绒癌
cinnabaris		朱砂
colloid	[ˈkɔlɔɪd]	胶体
Cucurbitae Semen		毛边南瓜子
cucurbitine	[kjuːˈkəːbɪtiːn]	南瓜子氨酸
cycloalliin	[saɪkləuˈlɪɪn]	环蒜氨酸
cysteine	[ˈsɪstɪn]	半胱氨酸
cysteisulfoxide		半胱亚砜
D		
decanoic acid		癸酸
degradation	[ˌdegrəˈdeɪʃn]	降解
dencichine	[dənsɪˈtʃaɪn]	三七素

(continued)

diallyldisulfide	[daɪrəlɪldaɪˈsʌlfaɪd]	二烯丙基二硫
diallylsulfide		二烯丙基硫醚
diallyltetrasulfide		二烯丙基四硫
diallylthiosulfinate	[dɪəlɪlθɪːəuˈsʌlfɪneɪt]	二烯丙基硫亚磺酸盐
diallyltrisulfide		二烯丙基三硫
dimethylthiosulfinate		二甲基硫代亚砜
docosapentaenoic acid		二十二碳五烯酸
doesahexaenoic acid		二十二碳六烯酸
dyspepsia	[dɪsˈpepʃə]	消化不良
dysentery	[ˈdɪsəntri]	痢疾
E		
eicosapentaenoic acid		二十碳五烯酸
enterorrhea	[entərɔˈrɪə]	泄泻
enzyme	[ˈenzaɪm]	酶
Eriobotryae Folium		枇杷叶
erucic acid		芥酸
essential amino acids	[ɪˈsenʃl][ˈæmɪnəu][ˈæsɪdz]	必需氨基酸
essential fatty acids	[ɪˈsenʃl][ˈfæti][ˈæsɪdz]	必需脂肪酸
F		
fatty acid	[ˈfæti][ˈæsɪd]	脂肪酸
filariasis	[ˌfɪləˈraɪəsɪs]	丝虫病
Folin reaction		福林试剂反应
G		
gadoleic acid		顺－二十碳 –9– 烯酸
glutamyl	[ˈgluːtəmɪl]	谷氨酰
γ-glutamylcysteine peptides		谷氨酰半胱氨肽类
gypsum fibrosum	[ˈdʒɪpsəm][ˈfaibrəsəm]	石膏
H		
hemostasis	[ˌhiːməˈsteɪsɪs]	止血，止血法
hexanoic acid	[heksəˈnɔɪk][ˈæsɪd]	己酸
Hordei Fructus Germinatus		麦芽
I		
indole-dione reagent		吲哚醌试液
internal salts	[ɪnˈtəːnl][sɔːlts]	内盐
intestinal parasite	[ˌɪntesˈtaɪnl][ˈpærəsaɪt]	肠内寄生虫
intra-molecular acid-base reaction	[ˈɪntrə][məˈlekjələ][ˈæsɪd][beɪs][riˈækʃn]	分子内酸碱反应
isatin reaction	[ˈaɪsətɪn][riˈækʃn]	吲哚醌反应

431

(continued)

isoelectric point	[ˌaɪsəuɪˈlektrɪk][pɔɪnt]	等电点
K		
kainic acid	[ˈkaɪnɪk][ˈæsɪd]	红藻氨酸
L		
lauric acid	[ˈlɔːrɪk][ˈæsɪd]	月桂酸
lignoceric acid	[ˌlɪgnəuˈserɪk][ˈæsɪd]	二十四烷酸，木蜡酸
linoleic acid	[lɪˈnəuliːk][ˈæsɪd]	亚油酸
linolenic acid	[ˌlɪnəˈlenɪk][ˈæsɪd]	亚麻酸
lung tuberculosis	[lʌŋ][tjuːˌbəːkjuˈləusɪs]	肺痨
M		
macromolecules	[mækrɔməˈlekjuːlz]	大分子
malignancy hydatidiform	[məˈlɪgnənsɪ][haɪˈdeɪtɪdɪːfɔːm]	恶性葡萄胎
mange	[meɪndʒ]	疥癣
melissic acid		蜂花酸
methylallyldisulfide		甲基烯丙基二硫
methylallylthiosulfinate		甲基烯丙基硫代亚砜
methylallyltrisulfide		甲基烯丙基三硫
methyl-1-propenylthiosulfinate		甲基丙烯基硫代亚砜
monounsaturated fatty acids	[ˌmɔnəʌnˈsætʃəˌreɪtɪd][ˈfæti][ˈæsɪd]	单不饱和脂肪酸
montanic acid	[mɔnˈtænɪk][ˈæsɪd]	二十八烷酸
Mume Fructus		乌梅
myristic acid	[mɪˈrɪstɪk][ˈæsɪd]	豆蔻酸
N		
1,2-naphthoquinone-4-sulfonic acid sodium	[ˈnæfθəkwɪˈnəun][sʌlˈfɔnɪk][ˈæsɪd][ˈsəudiːəm]	1,2- 萘醌 -4- 磺酸钠
Natrii Sulfas		芒硝
nervonic acid		15- 二十四碳烯酸
neutral amino acids	[ˈnjuːtrəl][ˈæmɪnəu][ˈæsɪdz]	中性氨基酸
ninhydrin reaction	[nɪnˈhaɪdrɪn][riˈækʃn]	茚三酮反应
Notoginseng Radix et Rhizome	[nəuˈtɔdʒɪnseŋ][ˈreɪdɪks][et][[ˈraɪzəum]	三七
O		
octanoic		辛酸
oleic acid	[əuˈliːɪk][ˈæsɪd]	油酸
organic sulfur compounds	[ɔːgænɪk][ˈsʌlfə][ˈkɔmpaundz]	有机硫化物
P		
palmitic acid	[pælˈmɪtɪk][ˈæsɪd]	棕榈酸，软脂酸
palmitoleic acid	[pælˈmaɪtəuleɪk][ˈæsɪd]	棕榈油酸

(continued)

papain	[pə'peɪɪn]	木瓜蛋白酶
pertussis	[pə'tʌsɪs]	顿咳
polyunsaturated fatty acid	[ˌpɒlɪʌn'sætʃəreɪtɪd]['fætɪ]['æsɪd]	多不饱和脂肪酸
potassium myronate	[pə'tæsɪəm]['maɪrəneɪt]	芥子苷 / 黑芥子苷钾盐
potassium permanganate	[pə'tæsɪəm][pə:'mæŋgəneɪt]	高锰酸钾
potassium salt	[pə'tæsɪəm][sɔ:lt]	钾盐
propenyl		丙烯基
1-propenylallylthiosulfinate		丙烯烯丙基硫代亚砜
pungent	['pʌndʒənt]	辛辣的，刺激性的
pyritum		自然铜
Q		
quisqualic acid	[kwɪs'kwɔ:lɪk]['æsɪd]	使君子氨酸
Quisqualis Frutus		使君子
R		
rancidity	[ræn'sɪdɪtɪ]	酸败
realgar	[rɪ'ælgə]	雄黄
rorifone	[rɔ:rɪf'wʌn]	旱菜素
S		
saturated fatty acids	['sætʃəreɪtɪd]['fætɪ]['æsɪd]	饱和脂肪酸
schistosomiasis	[ˌʃistəsə'maiəsis]	血吸虫病
semipermeable membrane	['semɪ'pə:mɪəbl]['membreɪn]	半透膜
sinapine	['sɪnəpɪn]	芥子碱
sodium carbonate solution	['səudi:əm]['kɑ:bəneɪt][sə'lu:ʃn]	碳酸钠溶液
stalactitum		钟乳石
stearic acid	[stɪ'ærɪk]['æsɪd]	硬脂酸
sulfur	['sʌlfə]	硫
sulfur-volatiles	['sʌlfə]['vəlætəli:z]	含硫挥发物
S-ally-L-cysteinsulfoxide		蒜氨酸
S-methylcysteinsulfoxide		S– 甲基半胱氨酸亚砜
T		
talcum	['tælkəm]	滑石
thiohydroximic acid	[ˌθaɪəuˌhaɪdrəu'sɪmɪk]['æsɪd]	硫代羟肟酸
thiosulfinates	[ˌθaɪəu'sʌlfɪneɪt]	硫代亚磺酸酯
trichosanthin	[ˌtraɪkəu'sænθɪn]	天花粉蛋白
U		
ultraviolet radiation	[ˌʌltrə'vaɪələt][ˌreɪdɪ'eɪʃn]	紫外线照射
unsaturated fatty acids	[ʌn'sætʃəreɪtɪd]['fætɪ]['æsɪd]	不饱和脂肪酸

(continued)

V		
vaccenic acid		十八碳烯酸
Z		
zwitterions	[ˈtsvɪtəraɪənz]	两性离子

重点小结

脂肪酸为脂肪族一元羧酸，通常以酯类形式存在于动植物中。自然界中以直链脂肪酸为常见，碳原子数为偶数，碳数以 16 或 18 最为常见。根据分子中双键的数目不同，分为饱和脂肪酸和不饱和脂肪酸。饱和脂肪酸不含双键，能加速人体对胆固醇的吸收、并沉积在血管壁上，最终发展为血管硬化。不饱和脂肪酸又分为单不饱和脂肪酸和多不饱和脂肪酸。天然不饱和脂肪酸中的双键均为 Z 型（顺式）。植物油来源的多不饱和脂肪酸通常有 2~3 个双键，而海洋动物来源的多不饱和脂肪酸中则有 4 个或更多的双键。多不饱和脂肪酸主要包括亚油酸、α- 亚麻酸、γ- 亚麻酸、花生四烯酸、二十碳五烯酸等，其中亚油酸和 α- 亚麻酸被称为必需脂肪酸。多不饱和脂肪酸易于乳化、运输和代谢，具有降低血脂和胆固醇、减少动脉粥样硬化、抑制癌细胞生长和促进大脑生长的作用。

中药中的有机含硫化合物具有重要的生物活性。如芥子苷具有显著的抗菌和杀虫效果；大蒜新素和旱菜素具有显著的抗菌作用。中药中的有机含硫化合物多以硫苷形式存在。如黑芥子苷、白芥子苷等。在中性条件下，芥子苷可由芥子苷酶水解为葡萄糖和硫代羟肟酸并最终转化为异硫氰酸酯。

氨基酸是分子中同时含有氨基和羧基的物质。根据氨基和羧基的相对位置不同，可分为 α-、β- 和 γ- 氨基酸。按照氨基酸的氨基和羧基数量不同，氨基酸也可分为中性氨基酸、酸性氨基酸和碱性氨基酸。氨基酸在中药中很常见，具有特殊的生物活性。如中药使君子中的使君子氨酸和鹧鸪菜中的海人草氨酸有驱虫作用，毛边南瓜子中的南瓜子氨酸有治丝虫病和血吸虫病的作用，天冬、玄参和棉根中的天门冬素有镇咳和平喘作用，三七中的三七素具有止血作用。氨基酸常用茚三酮反应、吲哚醌反应和 Folin 试剂检识。通常氨基酸可以使用等电点法、离子交换色谱法和电泳法进行分离。

蛋白质分子中的氨基酸残基由肽键连接，形成含有多达几百个氨基酸残基的多肽链。酶是具有催化活性的蛋白质。近年来，发现许多植物来源的蛋白质具有很强的生物活性，如天花粉蛋白具有中期妊娠引产的功效，并可用于治疗恶性葡萄胎和绒癌；番木瓜中的木瓜蛋白酶可驱除肠内寄生虫；麦芽中的淀粉酶常用于食积不消。蛋白质为大分子物质，分子量多在 1 万以上，高的可达 1000 万左右，可溶于水，难溶于有机溶剂。其水溶液具有胶体特性，不能透过半透膜，此性质可用于蛋白质分离纯化。蛋白质分子两端有氨基和羧基，具有两性和等电点。在水溶液中，蛋白质可被高浓度的硫酸铵或氯化钠溶液盐析而沉淀，此性质可逆。当蛋白质被加热或与酸、碱等作用时，则变性而失去活性。蛋白质在酸、碱、酶等作用下可逐步水解，最终产物为各种氨基酸。

矿物药在中医临床应用历史悠久，从《神农本草经》起，历代本草均有记载。矿物药主要成分为无机化合物，所含有机质甚微，但是具有各种各样的作用，例如石膏清热泻火，朱砂安神，赤石脂收敛等。

目 标 检 测

一、单选题

1. 水溶液加热产生沉淀的化合物是（　　）
 A. 低聚糖   B. 氨基酸   C. 甾醇
 D. 蛋白质   E. 苯丙酸

2. 蛋白质分子两端有氨基和羧基，具有两性和（　　）
 A. 电离点   B. 等电点   C. 等势点
 D. 水溶性   E. 等电性

3. 下列不属于脂肪酸的是（　　）
 A. 长链饱和脂肪酸   B. 长链不饱和脂肪酸   C. 芥酸
 D. 苯甲酸   E. 棕榈油酸

4. 下列化合物中属于必需氨基酸的是（　　）
 A. 海人草氨酸   B. 南瓜子氨酸   C. 使君子氨酸
 D. 三七素   E. 组氨酸

5. 氨基酸分子内的氨基和羧基可相互作用而生成（　　）
 A. 苷   B. 络合物   C. 内盐
 D. 氢键   E. 内酯

6. 天然游离氨基酸的提取多是采用（　　）等溶剂进行提取
 A. 三氯甲烷或乙醚   B. 水或稀醇   C. 丙酮或丁醇
 D. 乙酸乙酯或三氯甲烷   E. 乙醚或乙酸乙酯

7. 芥子苷类化合物在中性条件下被芥子苷酶水解，生成葡萄糖和硫代羟肟酸，后者经转位最后产生（　　），具有强烈的辛辣味
 A. 异硫氰酸酯   B. 异硫酸氰酯   C. 氢氰酸
 D. 大蒜素   E. 大蒜新素

8. 在阳离子交换树脂上，下列氨基酸中吸附力最弱的是（　　）
 A. 含芳香环的氨基酸   B. 含长链烃基的氨基酸   C. 中性氨基酸
 D. 碱性氨基酸   E. 酸性氨基酸

9. 矿物药在中医临床应用历史悠久，从（　　）起，历代本草均有记载
 A.《神农本草经》   B.《日华子诸家本草》   C.《重广英公本草》
 D.《唐本草》   E.《本草纲目》

10. 麦芽中的淀粉酶具有的作用是（　　）
 A. 抑菌   B. 止咳平喘   C. 治疗消化不良
 D. 杀虫   E. 抑制病毒

二、多选题

1. 分离氨基酸时，可以使用的方法有（　　）

A. 等电点法　　　　　　　　B. 离子交换树脂法　　　　C. 成盐法
D. 电泳法　　　　　　　　　E. 加热法

2. 下列化合物中，属于氨基酸的有（　　　）
A. 使君子氨酸　　　　　　　B. 海人草氨酸　　　　　　　C. 三七素
D. 天门冬素　　　　　　　　E. 东莨菪碱

3. 根据不同的分类原则，氨基酸可以分为（　　　）
A. 酸性氨基酸　　　　　　　B. 碱性氨基酸　　　　　　　C. 中性氨基酸
D. α- 氨基酸　　　　　　　　E. 以上均可以

4. 以下关于氨基酸的叙述，正确的是（　　　）
A. 为两性化合物
B. 在水溶液中可被离子化
C. 可用加热沸腾法鉴别
D. 调节溶液 pH 可实现分离
E. 在等电点时，分子以内盐形式存在，溶解度最大

5. 下列方法中，蛋白质可用哪些方法进行检识（　　　）
A. 加热法　　　　　　　　　B. 成盐法　　　　　　　　　C. 显色法
D. 冷凝法　　　　　　　　　E. 沉淀法

6. 下列物质中，可以使用离子交换法进行分离的有（　　　）
A. 生物碱　　　　　　　　　B. 氨基酸　　　　　　　　　C. 甾醇
D. 木脂素　　　　　　　　　E. 脂肪酸

7. 下列化合物中，含有硫原子的有（　　　）
A. 芥子碱　　　　　　　　　B. 大蒜新素　　　　　　　　C. 黑芥子苷
D. 白芥子苷　　　　　　　　E. 秦皮苷

8. 关于氨基酸的性质，下列叙述不正确的有（　　　）
A. 茚三酮反应可使氨基酸呈色
B. 可以使用乙酸乙酯或三氯甲烷提取
C. 在强碱溶液中，氨基酸主要以阳离子形式存在
D. 可用水提法提取总氨基酸
E. 在水溶液中，其分子中的羧基和氨基可以离子化，为不可逆反应

9. 离子交换树脂法分离氨基酸时，常用的洗脱液有（　　　）
A. 磷酸氢钠缓冲液　　　　　B. 柠檬酸钠缓冲液　　　　　C. 枸橼酸钠缓冲液
D. 碳酸氢钠缓冲液　　　　　E. 醋酸钠缓冲液

10. 下列物质中，属于中药矿物药的有（　　　）
A. 滑石　　　　　　　　　　B. 芒硝　　　　　　　　　　C. 钟乳石
D. 五灵脂　　　　　　　　　E. 雄黄

三、思考题

1. 简述脂肪酸的结构特点和分类。
2. 什么是氨基酸的等电点？如何利用等电点性质对不同的氨基酸进行分离？

（柴慧芳）

岗位对接

中药化学是在中医药理论和临床用药经验指导下，运用现代科学理论和技术等研究中药化学成分的一门学科。中药化学的核心知识是中药用于防治疾病的物质基础——化学成分，是中药中具有防病治病作用的化学成分，因此中药中的化学成分是反映中药临床疗效和评价中药质量的重要组成部分。

中医临床治疗疾病的物质基础是中药的化学成分，具体地说，应该是指中药所含的各化学成分类型及其之间含量的比例。中药化学成分变化贯穿中药质量形成的全过程，包括中药（中药材、饮片和中成药）生产、经营和使用（包装、储存、运输、调剂和指导合理用药等），因此中药化学成分的变化直接影响中药质量。

执业中药师是以对中药药品质量负责、保征人民用药安全有效为基本准则，是提供中药药品服务的直接参与者和指导者。执业中药师应当对保证中药药品服务质量负责，在执业范围内负责对中药质量的监督和管理，严格执行《药品管理法》及国家有关中药的研究、生产、经营、使用的各项法律、法规和政策。中药质量贯穿中药生产、经营和使用等领域，因此执业中药师只有掌握了中药化学知识，才能在执业活动过程中管控中药质量，确保中药质量"安全、有效、稳定、可控"，满足患者需要。

中药化学知识是执业中药师必备的中药学专业知识的重要组成部分，根据国家对中药执业药师考试大纲要求，对接执业中药师的岗位职责与执业活动的需要，要求较为全面地掌握中药化学基础理论知识和常用中药的有效成分结构特征及其质量控制的标志物等。学习过程应该以"化学结构"为核心，以"绪论"为基础，以"化学结构－理化性质"为主线，全面复习与重点掌握。

中药执业药师岗位要求对**中药化学研究对象**，尤其是中药化学有效成分需要掌握，特别是有效成分与无效成分之间的划分是相对的。中药化学研究对象是中药化学成分，其有效成分是指具有生物活性、能防病治病的化学成分，如麻黄碱、甘草皂苷、芦丁、大黄素等；无效成分是指没有生物活性和防病治病作用的化学成分，如淀粉、树脂、叶绿素等。两者的划分也是相对的。一方面，随着科学的发展和人们对客观世界认识的提高，一些过去被认为是无效成分的化合物，如某些多糖、多肽、蛋白质和油脂类成分等，现已发现它们具有新的生物活性或药效，如鹧鸪氨酸（驱虫）；天花粉蛋白（引产）；茯苓多糖、猪苓多糖（抗肿瘤）等。

对**中药化学成分的一般研究方法**需要掌握中药化学成分的常见提取和分离方法及其优缺点。**常用提取方法**包括浸渍法、渗漉法、煎煮法、回流提取法和连续回流提取法。浸渍法特点是适用于遇热易破坏或挥发性成分及含淀粉、黏液质、果胶较多的中药，但提取时间长、效率低、易发霉、体积大等。渗漉法特点是提取效率高、不加热、不破坏成分，但提取时间长、体积大。煎煮法是必须使用水为溶剂的提取方法，对挥发性和加热易破坏成分不适用。回流提取法提取效率高，但不适用遇热易破坏的成分，且溶剂消耗大。连续回流提取法的提取效率高、节省溶剂，且操作简单，但不适用遇热破坏的成分。另外还有水蒸气蒸馏法提取，适用于具有挥发性的有效成分提取；升华法提取具有升华性的成分，如樟树中的樟脑，茶叶中的咖啡因；超声提取法是利用超声波产生强烈的空化效应和搅拌作用提取中药化学成分；超临界流体萃取法（SFE）最常用的超临界流体是二氧化碳，该法优点是低温下提取，对亲脂性小分子化合物提取效果好，对"热敏性"成分尤其适用，但对极性大化合物提取效果较差，设备造价高。

中药化学成分的分离与精制，可根据不同原理分离：物质溶解度的差别、物质在两相溶剂中分配比的不同、物质的吸附性差别、物质分子大小的差别、物质解离程度的不同、物质的沸点高低不同等。

根据物质溶解度差别进行分离：一是结晶及重结晶，其原理是利用混合物中各成分在溶剂中溶解度的差异，其中选择合适的溶剂是关键，溶剂要求一般高温对结晶物质溶解度大，低温溶解度小，同时对杂质的溶解度或者很大（待重结晶物质析出时，杂质仍留在母液中）或者很小（待重结晶物质溶解度在溶剂里，过滤除去杂质）。结晶化合物的纯度判断方法包括：晶形均匀、色泽一致、熔点明确且熔距敏锐（1~2℃）；色谱采用三种以上展开剂展开，呈单一斑点；还有高效液相色谱、质谱、核磁共振等方法。二是利用两种以上不同溶剂极性的差异分离，有水提醇沉法，沉淀多糖、蛋白质等；醇提水沉法，除去树脂、叶绿素等亲脂性杂质。三是利用酸碱性进行分离，有酸提碱沉法，用于生物碱提取分离；碱提酸沉法，用于酚、酸类成分的提取分离。

根据物质在两相溶剂中的分配比不同进行分离：一是液–液萃取法，利用混合物中各成分在互不相溶的两相溶剂中的分配系数 K 不同而达到分离；二是，液–液分配柱色谱法，包括正相分配色谱和反相分配色谱，前者固定相极性大于流动相极性，固定相常为氰基（—CN）与氨基（—NH），后者固定相极性小于流动相极性，固定相常为石蜡油、$RP-C_2$、$RP-C_8$ 和 $RP-C_{18}$。

根据物质的吸附性差别进行分离：一是物理吸附，吸附特点是无选择性，过程可逆，应用最广；常用固定相有极性吸附剂（硅胶和氧化铝）和非极性吸附剂（活性炭）；极性表示分子中电荷对称程度，极性强弱与偶极矩、极化度、介电常数有关。若是吸附柱色谱用于物质分离应注意：尽可能选用极性小的溶剂装柱和溶解样品；酸性物质分离用硅胶为固定相，碱性物质分离用氧化铝为固定相；柱色谱流动相选择参考 TLC 组分 R_f 达到 0.2~0.3 时的溶剂。二是聚酰胺柱色谱，吸附原理是氢键吸附；要注意的是聚酰胺不溶于水及常用有机溶剂，对碱性稳定，对酸（尤其是无机酸）稳定性较差；其吸附规律为：酚羟基数目越多吸附力越强；酚羟基所处的位置易于形成分子内氢键，则吸附力越弱；分子芳香化程度越高，共轭双键越多，吸附力越强。不同洗脱剂洗脱能力由弱到强依次为：水、甲醇、丙酮、稀氢氧化钠、甲酰胺、二甲基甲酰胺、尿素。值得注意的是聚酰胺对酚类、黄酮类化合物的吸附是可逆的（鞣质除外），故特别适合于该类化合物的分离和脱鞣质处理。三是大孔吸附树脂法，其吸附原理是通过物理吸附（范德华力、氢键吸附）和分子筛性能。

根据物质分子大小差别进行分离：凝胶色谱法，其原理是利用分子筛原理分离物质，小分子进入凝胶颗粒内部，大分子化合物被排阻在外边难以进入，因此大分子物质首先被洗脱出柱。

根据物质解离程度不同进行分离：离子交换树脂色谱法，其原理是依据各成分解离度不同而分离，离子交换树脂外观为球形颗粒，不溶于水，但可在水中膨胀。

根据物质沸点不同进行分离：分馏法，其原理是混合组分中各成分的沸点不同而分离的一种方法。

中药化学成分结构研究的方法：在结构研究之前，需要对被测定结构的化合物进行纯度测定，然后采用分子式确定，如高分辨率质谱法（HR-MS）；质谱（MS）用于测定有机分子的分子量、求算分子式、推断结构信息；红外光谱（IR），在 4000~1500cm^{-1} 的区域为特征频率区，许多特征官能团，如羟基、氨基等，可据此进行鉴别；1500~600cm^{-1} 的区域为指纹区，可用于真伪鉴别；紫外光谱（UV）用于测定分子结构中具有共轭体系的化合物，推断化合物的骨架类型；核磁共振（NMR），^1H-NMR 可提供不同氢原子周围环境，主要为化学位移（δ），偶合常数（J）及质子数（积分面积）；$^{13}C-NMR$ 可提供不同碳原子周围环境，主要为化学位移和偶合常数等。

　　糖和苷类化合物是中药执业药师掌握的重点之一。包括糖及其分类、苷及其分类、糖和苷化学性质、多糖概念、含氰苷类化合物的常用中药，如苦杏仁（化学鉴别方法）、桃仁、郁李仁中《中国药典》的指标成分。

　　醌类化合物重点掌握结构与分类、理化性质、含醌类化合物的常用中药，如大黄、虎杖、何首乌、芦荟、决明子、丹参、紫草中主要有效成分的结构类型、《中国药典》的指标成分、生物活性。

　　香豆素和木脂素重点掌握结构与分类、理化性质、含香豆素类化合物的常用中药，如秦皮、前胡、肿节风、五味子、厚朴、连翘、细辛的主要化学成分及其结构类型、《中国药典》的指标成分、生物活性及临床应用中注意的问题。

　　黄酮类化合物重点掌握结构与分类、理化性质、含黄酮类化合物的常用中药，如黄芩、葛根、银杏叶、槐花、陈皮、满山红的主要有效成分及其结构类型、《中国药典》的指标成分、生物活性及临床应用中注意的问题。

　　鞣质重点掌握概念、结构与分类、理化性质、含可水解鞣质的中药，如五倍子的主要有效成分。

　　生物碱类是中药执业药师掌握的重点之一。包括概念、分布、结构和分类、理化性质、常见含生物碱中药，如苦参（理化性质）、山豆根（理化性质）、麻黄（理化性质）、黄连（理化性质）、延胡索、防己、川乌（毒性变化）、洋金花（理化性质）、天仙子、马钱子（结构与毒性、鉴别方法）、千里光、雷公藤的《中国药典》的指标成分、生理活性、临床应用中应注意的问题。

　　甾类化合物重点掌握强心苷的概念、苷元部分的结构与分类、糖部分的结构特征及其与苷元的连接方式、强心苷理化性质、含强心苷类化合物的常用中药，如香加皮、罗布麻叶的化学结构类型、毒性表现及临床应用中注意的问题；含强心苷元的常用中药，如蟾酥的化学成分结构及其化学性质；蜕皮激素的概念及其活性；胆汁酸结构特征及其鉴别、含胆汁酸成分的重要中药，如牛黄、熊胆的主要化学成分结构、《中国药典》的指标成分。

　　萜类和挥发油重点掌握萜类的含义、结构分类及其结构特征、环烯醚萜的理化性质、挥发油的概念及其化学组成、挥发油的通性和化学常数。含萜类化合物的常用中药，如穿心莲、青蒿、龙胆、薄荷、莪术、艾叶、肉桂的化学成分及其结构、《中国药典》的指标成分、临床应用中注意的问题。

　　皂苷类化合物重点掌握结构分类、理化性质、含三萜皂苷类化合物的常用中药，如人参、三七、甘草、黄芪、合欢皮、商陆、柴胡的化学成分及其结构、《中国药典》的指标成分；含甾体皂苷类化合物的常用中药，如麦冬、知母的主要化学成分。

　　其他成分重点掌握芳香族有机酸、含有机酸的常用中药，如金银花、当归、丹参、马兜铃的主要有机酸类成分，马兜铃的毒性，例如马兜铃酸具有较强的肾脏毒性；含其他成分的常用中药，如麝香、斑蝥、水蛭的主要化学成分及生物活性。

　　中药化学中生物碱类和苷类是学习的重点，糖和苷是学习其他苷类的重点，抓好糖和苷类，就是抓住了醌类、香豆素、木脂素、黄酮、皂苷和强心苷。含不同类型化学成分的常用中药是学习的重点，特别是这些中药中所含有的有效成分（《中国药典》中规定的指标成分）及其药理作用。中药化学各个章节学习有其自身规律，在内容上是：结构类型、理化性质、检识、提取分离、光谱特征和具体中药实例。在各章的结构分类和理化性质中，生物碱类结构复杂，是学习的难点，也是学习的重点。

目标检测答案

Chapter 1

一、单选题
1. A　2. B　3. C　4. E　5. E　6. A　7. E　8. C
二、多选题
1. ABCDE　2. ABCDE　3. ABCE　4. AE　5. CDE　6. AB　7. AE　8. ABDE

Chapter 2

一、单选题
1. E　2. A　3. C　4. E　5. E　6. A　7. E　8. A　9. C　10. B
二、多选题
1. ABCDE　2. CD　3. DE　4. BDE　5. ABCDE　6. ABE　7. ABE　8. ACD　9. ABD
10. ABCDE

Chapter 3

一、单选题
1. D　2. B　3. C　4. A　5. A　6. E　7. D　8. B　9. A　10. C
二、多选题
1. ABCDE　2. ABD　3. ABD　4. AD　5. BCE　6. CE　7. ABCE　8. ABCD
9. DE　10. AB

Chapter 4

一、单选题
1. C　2. C　3. A　4. B　5. C　6. A　7. D　8. E　9. B　10. D
二、多选题
1. BD　2. AB　3. AC　4. AB　5. AC　6. AE　7. CDE　8. ABCE　9. ABCDE
10. ABCE

Chapter 5

一、单选题
1. B　2. D　3. C　4. D　5. A　6. B　7. C　8. E　9. B　10. A

二、多选题

1. ADE 2. BD 3. ABCDE 4. BCE 5. BE 6. ACDE 7. ABDE 8. BDE 9. AC
10. ABDE

Chapter 6

一、单选题

1. C 2. D 3. C 4. E 5. A 6. C 7. D 8. B 9. A 10. A

二、多选题

1. BCE 2. ACD 3. ABCD 4. ACE 5. BDE 6. AB 7. ABD 8. ACE 9. BD
10. AC

Chapter 7

一、单选题

1. D 2. E 3. E 4. B 5. E

二、多选题

1. ABC 2. ABE 3. ABCD 4. BC 5. ACE

Chapter 8

一、单选题

1. C 2. D 3. B 4. C 5. A 6. C 7. A 8. E 9. A 10. E 11. C 12. D 13. E
14. B 15. D

二、多选题

1. DE 2. ABCE 3. ACD 4. ABCE 5. ACE 6. BCDE 7. ACD 8. ABCE 9. ACE
10. ACDE 11. BCD 12. CD 13. BD 14. ABCD 15. ABC

Chapter 9

一、单选题

1. A 2. C 3. C 4. C 5. B 6. D 7. A 8. B 9. A 10. C

二、多选题

1. AC 2. AB 3. BCDE 4. AC 5. ABCD 6. ABCE 7. ACDE 8. ABD 9. ABE
10. ACD

Chapter 10

一、单选题

1. B 2. D 3. B 4. A 5. A 6. D 7. A 8. C 9. D 10. B

二、多选题

1. AB 2. ABC 3. BCDE 4. ABC 5. ACD 6. BCDE 7. ACD 8. ADE 9. ABCD

10. ABDE

Chapter 11

一、单选题
1. C   2. C   3. B   4. C   5. A   6. B   7. D   8. C   9. C   10. B   11. B   12. D
二、多选题
1. ABC   2. ABDE   3. BC   4. ABDE   5. ABCDE   6. ADE   7. AB   8. ABD   9. CD
10. AD   11. ABCDE   12. ABE

Chapter 12

一、单选题
1. D   2. B   3. D   4. E   5. C   6. B   7. A   8. E   9. A   10. C
二、多选题
1. ABCD   2. ABCD   3. ABCDE   4. ABD   5. ACE   6. ABE   7. ABCD   8. BCE
9. BCE   10. ABCE

参考文献

[1] Kokate CK, Purohit AP, Gokhale SB. Pharmacognosy [M]. 39th ed. Abhyudaya Pragati, India: Nirali Prakashan, 2007.

[2] 高增平 . 中药化学 [M]. 英文版 . 北京：中国中医药出版社，2014.

[3] 冯卫生 . 波谱解析 [M]. 2 版 . 北京：人民卫生出版社，2019.

[4] 刘斌，倪健 . 中药有效部位及成分提取工艺和检测方法 [M]. 北京：中国中医药出版社，2007.

[5] 宋小妹，唐志书 . 中药化学成分提取分离与制备 [M]. 北京：人民卫生出版社，2004.

[6] Bensky D, Clavey S, Stoger E. Chinese Herbal Medicine: Materia Medica [M]. 3rd ed. Inc. Seattle, USA: Eastland Press, 2004.

[7] Hildebert Wagner, Rudolf Bauer, Dieter Melchart, et al. Chromatographic Fingerprint Analysis of Herbal Medicines: Thin-layer and High Performance Liquid Chromatography of Chinese Drugs[M]. 2nd ed. Vol.1. New York, USA: Springer Wien, 2011.

[8] John K Chen, Tina T Chen. Chinese Medical Herbology and Pharmacology [M]. Inc. City of Industry, USA: Art of Medicine Press, 2004.

[9] Dewick PM. Medicinal Natural Products, A Biosythetic Approach [M]. 3rd ed. The Atrium, England: John Wiley & Sons Lid, 2009.

[10] Ludwiczuk A, Skalicka-Woźniak K, Georgiev M I. Terpenoids/Pharmacognosy [M]. Pittsburgh, Pennsylvania.USA: Academic Press, 2017.

[11] Satyajit D. Sarker, Zahid Latif, Alexander I. Gray. Natural Products Isolation [M]. 2nd ed. Totowa, New Jersey. USA: Humana Press, 2006.

[12] 石任兵，邱峰 . 中药化学 [M]. 2 版 . 北京：人民卫生出版社，2016.

[13] 匡海学 . 中药化学 [M]. 北京：中国中医药出版社，2011.